MW00666838

Clinical Toxicology Testing

A Guide for Laboratory Professionals
Second Edition

Barbarajean Magnani, PhD, MD
Tai C. Kwong, PhD
Gwendolyn A. McMillin, PhD
Alan H.B. Wu, PhD
Editors

COLLEGE of AMERICAN
PATHOLOGISTS

Library of Congress Control Number: 2019950701
ISBN: 978-194109650-5

Printed in the USA

College of American Pathologists
325 Waukegan Road
Northfield, Illinois 60093
800-323-4040
cap.org

Contents

Contributors vi

Preface vii

Section I: Toxicology Testing in the Clinical Setting
Barbarajean Magnani, PhD, MD, Editor

Chapter 1
Introduction and Organizational Aspects of a Hospital Toxicology Laboratory 3
Tai C. Kwong, PhD, and Barbarajean Magnani, PhD, MD

Chapter 2
Supporting the Emergency Department 7
Barbarajean Magnani, PhD, MD, and Tai C. Kwong, PhD

Chapter 3
Laboratory Support of Chronic Opioid Therapy 17
Tai C. Kwong, PhD, and Barbarajean Magnani, PhD, MD

Chapter 4
Clinical Pathology Consultation for Pain Management Services 27
Barbarajean Magnani, PhD, MD, Nicholas Heger, PhD, and Tai C. Kwong, PhD

Chapter 5
Special Considerations in Pediatric Toxicology: Practical and Testing Perspectives 49
Robert A. Middleberg, PhD

Chapter 6
Workplace Drug Testing 66
Jennifer A. Collins, PhD, and Arthur M. Zebelman, PhD

Chapter 7
Regulatory Issues of Toxicology Laboratory Operations 76
Arthur M. Zebelman, PhD, and Jennifer A. Collins, PhD

Chapter 8
The Hospital Autopsy and Toxicology Testing 90
D. Kimberley Molina, MD, and Barbarajean Magnani, PhD, MD

Section II: Toxicokinetics and Methodologies for the Toxicology Laboratory
Alan H.B. Wu, PhD, Editor

Chapter 9
Pharmacokinetic Concepts for Toxicology and Therapeutic Drug Monitoring 101
Yashpal Agrawal, MD, PhD

Chapter 10
Pharmacogenomic Testing 112
Alan H.B. Wu, PhD, and Gwendolyn A. McMillin, PhD

Chapter 11
Laboratory-Based Screening Assays in Support of Pain Management 122
Tai C. Kwong, PhD, and Alan H.B. Wu, PhD

Chapter 12
Approaches to Broad-Spectrum Drug Testing in the Clinical Laboratory 129
Kara L. Lynch, PhD

Chapter 13
Method Validation in Toxicology Testing 140
Wieslaw Furmaga, MD, MS, and Yashpal Agrawal, MD, PhD

Chapter 14
Alternate Specimens for Drugs-of-Abuse Testing: Oral Fluid 157
Jennifer A. Collins, PhD

Chapter 15
Drug Testing in Hair, Sweat, Meconium, Cord Tissue and Breast Milk 170
Uttam Garg, PhD, and Gwendolyn A. McMillin, PhD

Section III: Specific Analytes
Tai C. Kwong, PhD, and Gwendolyn A. McMillin, PhD, Editors

Chapter 16
Ethanol 189
Graham R. Jones, PhD

Chapter 17
Non-Ethanol Volatiles and Ethylene Glycol 197
Graham R. Jones, PhD

Chapter 18
Cannabis 205
Paul J. Jannetto, PhD

Chapter 19
Club Drugs 214
Matthew D. Krasowski, MD, PhD, and Christine L.H. Snozek, PhD

Chapter 20
Cocaine 228
Daniel S. Isenschmid, PhD

Chapter 21
Amphetamines 239
Matthew D. Krasowski, MD, PhD, Christine L.H. Snozek, PhD,
and Stacy E.F. Melanson, MD, PhD

Chapter 22
Barbiturates 246
Matthew D. Krasowski, MD, PhD, Christine L.H. Snozek, PhD,
and Stacy E.F. Melanson, MD, PhD

Chapter 23
Benzodiazepines 253
Christine L.H. Snozek, PhD, Matthew D. Krasowski, MD, PhD,
and Stacy E.F. Melanson, MD, PhD

Chapter 24
Opioids I: Opiates and Semisynthetic Opioids 261
Matthew D. Krasowski, MD, PhD, and Gwendolyn A. McMillin, PhD

Chapter 25
Opioids II: Synthetic Opioids 270
Hoi-Ying Elsie Yu, PhD, and Nicholas Heger, PhD

Chapter 26
Novel Psychoactive Substances 282
Donna Papsun, MS

Chapter 27
Over-the-Counter Analgesics 300
Hoi-Ying Elsie Yu, PhD, and Gary L. Horowitz, MD

Chapter 28
Lead and Other Toxic Metals 309
Robert A. Middleberg, PhD

Chapter 29
Common Household and Environmental Toxicants 321
Christine L.H. Snozek, PhD, and Leland B. Baskin, MD

Section IV: Appendices and Index
Barbarajean Magnani, PhD, MD, Editor

Appendix A
Urine Toxic Screen Template 331
Nicholas Heger, PhD, and Barbarajean Magnani, PhD, MD

Appendix B
Serum Toxic Screen Template 337
Nicholas Heger, PhD, and Barbarajean Magnani, PhD, MD

Appendix C
Therapeutic Drug Monitoring Template 343
Nicholas Heger, PhD, and Barbarajean Magnani, PhD, MD

Appendix D
Frequently Asked Questions on Clinical Urine Drugs-of-Abuse Tests 355
Tai C. Kwong, PhD

Appendix E
CAP Proficiency Testing Surveys for Toxicology 361
Annabel Dizon, MT(ASCP)

Index 362

Contributors

Editors

Barbarajean Magnani, PhD, MD
Tufts University School of Medicine
Tufts Medical Center
Boston, Massachusetts

Tai C. Kwong, PhD
University of Rochester Medical Center
Rochester, New York

Gwendolyn A. McMillin, PhD
University of Utah
ARUP Laboratories
Salt Lake City, Utah

Alan H.B. Wu, PhD
University of California San Francisco
Zuckerberg San Francisco General Hospital
San Francisco, California

Contributing Authors

Yashpal Agrawal, MD, PhD
Rocky Mountain Regional VA Medical Center
University of Colorado, Denver
Aurora, Colorado

Leland B. Baskin, MD
Alberta Precision Laboratories
University of Calgary Faculty of Medicine
Calgary, Alberta

Jennifer A. Collins, PhD
MedTox Laboratories
Saint Paul, Minnesota

Annabel Dizon, MT(ASCP)
College of American Pathologists
Northfield, Illinois

Wieslaw Furmaga, MD, MS
UT Health San Antonio
San Antonio, Texas

Uttam Garg, PhD
Children's Mercy Hospital
University of Missouri, Kansas City School of Medicine
Kansas City, Missouri

Nicholas Heger, PhD
Tufts University School of Medicine
Tufts Medical Center
Boston, Massachusetts

Gary L. Horowitz, MD
Tufts University School of Medicine
Tufts Medical Center
Boston, Massachusetts

Daniel S. Isenschmid, PhD
NMS Labs
Horsham, Pennsylvania

Paul J. Jannetto, PhD
Mayo Clinic
Rochester, Minnesota

Graham R. Jones, PhD
Faculty of Medicine and Dentistry
University of Alberta
Edmonton, Alberta

Matthew D. Krasowski, MD, PhD
University of Iowa Hospital and Clinics
Iowa City, Iowa

Kara L. Lynch, PhD
University of California San Francisco
San Francisco, California

Stacy E.F. Melanson, MD, PhD
Brigham and Womens Hospital
Boston, Massachusetts

Robert Middleberg, PhD
NMS Labs
Horsham, Pennsylvania

D. Kimberley Molina, MD
Bexar County Medical Examiner's Office
San Antonio, Texas

Donna Papsun, MS
NMS Labs
Horsham, Pennsylvania

Christine L.H. Snozek, PhD
Mayo Clinic
Phoenix, Arizona

Hoi-Ying Elsie Yu, PhD
Geisinger Commonwealth School of Medicine
Geisinger Health
Danville, Pennsylvania

Arthur M. Zebelman, PhD
Laboratory Corporation of America
Seattle, Washington

Preface

This exciting new edition of *Clinical Toxicology Testing* brings updated and expanded chapters as well as new chapters to reflect the ever-growing field of toxicology in a clinical laboratory setting. The science of toxicology, in all its many basic and applied aspects, is a vast subject, and as Paracelsus put it: "What is not a poison? Only the dose makes a poison." Given the complexities of directing a toxicology laboratory, this book focuses on the issues facing the clinical laboratory director or pathologist in this role, as well as those in training in the field of laboratory medicine. The director of a clinical toxicology laboratory, either hospital/clinic based or free standing, typically has direct responsibility for a highly regulated and standardized drug testing menu.

The book is organized into three sections. Section one concentrates on toxicology testing in the clinical setting. Here we provide guidance and interpretation for specialized areas such as the emergency department, services treating chronic pain with opioid medications (with an additional chapter devoted to clinical pathology consultations for these services), and the hospital autopsy. This section also provides an introduction to such topics as workplace drug testing and relevant regulatory issues. Toxicology testing in children presents a variety of challenges, and a new chapter on special considerations in the pediatric population is included.

Section two addresses foundation topics such as toxicokinetic principles, pharmacogenomics, testing menus, methodologies, oral fluid testing, and other alternative matrices. A new chapter on validation procedures for laboratory-developed tests will guide the laboratory staff when bringing in a new assay.

Section three covers drugs and drug classes commonly encountered in toxicology testing, with a new chapter on novel psychoactive substances. Toxic metals as well as common household and environmental toxicants also are covered.

Finally, the appendices included at the end of the book provide templates for both urine and serum drug testing, therapeutic drug monitoring, frequently asked questions regarding urine toxicology testing, and information on the College of American Pathologists (CAP) proficiency testing surveys for toxicology.

The CAP Toxicology Committee (TxC), like other CAP scientific committees, is truly a vital international resource to the clinical laboratory industry, providing, as it does, proficiency testing, continuing education, and input on laboratory accreditation standards. The TxC has been fortunate to have as its members eminent scientific experts, many of whom have contributed to the writing of this book along with the many, equally renowned, invited contributors. Special thanks to Annabel Dizon, Senior Technical Specialist, Laboratory Improvement Programs, CAP, whose unwavering commitment to the TxC is greatly appreciated, and to Caryn Tursky, Editorial and Production Manager, for her diligent review of both the first and second editions of this work.

The reader will enjoy a comprehensive view of what is needed—and expected—when offering a clinical toxicology service. It is our hope that this second edition will serve as a useful complement to the first edition as well as a supplement to the specialized reference books utilized in the field today.

BJ Magnani, PhD, MD, FCAP
Boston, Massachusetts

Section I

Toxicology Testing in the Clinical Setting

Barbarajean Magnani, PhD, MD, Editor

Chapter 1. Introduction and Organizational Aspects of a Hospital Toxicology Laboratory
Tai C. Kwong, PhD, and Barbarajean Magnani, PhD, MD

Chapter 2. Supporting the Emergency Department
Barbarajean Magnani, PhD, MD, and Tai C. Kwong, PhD

Chapter 3. Laboratory Support of Chronic Opioid Therapy
Tai C. Kwong, PhD, and Barbarajean Magnani, PhD, MD

Chapter 4. Clinical Pathology Consultation for Pain Management Services
Barbarajean Magnani, PhD, MD, Nicholas Heger, PhD, and Tai C. Kwong, PhD

Chapter 5. Special Considerations in Pediatric Toxicology: Practical and Testing Perspectives
Robert A. Middleberg, PhD

Chapter 6. Workplace Drug Testing
Jennifer A. Collins, PhD, and Arthur M. Zebelman, PhD

Chapter 7. Regulatory Issues of Toxicology Laboratory Operations
Arthur M. Zebelman, PhD, and Jennifer A. Collins, PhD

Chapter 8. The Hospital Autopsy and Toxicology Testing
D. Kimberley Molina, MD, and Barbarajean Magnani, PhD, MD

Chapter 1

Introduction and Organizational Aspects of a Hospital Toxicology Laboratory

Tai C. Kwong, PhD
Barbarajean Magnani, PhD, MD

Introduction

Clinical toxicology can be defined as the analysis of drugs and toxins in body fluids for the purpose of patient care. The mission of the clinical toxicology laboratory is to effectively utilize available laboratory resources and expertise to provide clinically useful toxicology tests to support the needs of the patients. The two traditional clinical toxicology services are therapeutic drug monitoring (TDM) and emergency toxicology. TDM, the measurement of serum drug concentrations to aid in optimizing drug therapy, is beyond the scope of this book and will not be discussed except for those TDM tests that are also used in the assessment of suspected toxicity. (However, the reader is directed to chapter 9 for more general information on toxicokinetic concepts for toxicology and TDM, as well as the reference table found in appendix C). Emergency toxicology, on the other hand, is the accumulation of laboratory data to assist in the diagnosis and treatment of poisonings or drug overdoses. In recent years, the widespread abuse of prescription medications has placed additional demands on clinical toxicology laboratories. Consequently, clinical toxicology laboratories are now routinely performing urine testing of drugs of abuse for other clinical services—such as primary care practices, pain clinics, or rehabilitation medicine—that require compliance monitoring of their chronic pain patients on prescription opioids. These practitioners manage patients for compliance rather than for drug intoxication.

Different clinical services seek different answers from toxicology test results: for example, toxicity for a suspected drug overdose or exposure, abstinence in substance use disorder treatment, and compliance in pain management with chronic opioid therapy. Therefore, the scope of a clinical toxicology laboratory service should be designed to meet different clinical needs, each of which will depend on the clinical relevance of the tests and the impact of test results on the management of the patient (what to test for), and the availability of suitable analytical methods and technical resources (how to test for). This introductory chapter will discuss the organizational aspects of the hospital toxicology laboratory for dealing with different service-related challenges.

Emergency Toxicology

The goal of emergency toxicology is to provide *clinically useful* toxicology test results to support the needs of the poisoned or intoxicated patients in the emergency department. The clinical value of the results refers not only to the clinical utility of the test, but also to the timeliness of reporting toxicology results. It is impractical for any clinical laboratory to provide a full range of toxicological analyses in real time, mostly because of cost constraints and staffing problems; however, there are basic tests (Tier 1 tests) that should be offered in every hospital clinical laboratory because of their clinical relevance and the technical feasibility of rapid turnaround time, and hospitals with more resources and ability can offer more complex testing. Intoxicated patients, whose clinical presentation cannot be explained by the Tier 1 agents, may require additional tests (Tier 2 tests) that can be useful in identifying other agents that have clinical consequences.[1] Details can be found in chapter 2, *Supporting the Emergency Department.*

Toxicology Testing Supporting Other Clinical Services

In recent years, many toxicology laboratories have seen a significant increase in the utilization of the urine drug screens by other clinical services. For example, drug screens are ordered by obstetricians for pregnant patients with substance use disorders who are at risk for drug-related complications and by pediatricians for newborns suspected of drug exposure in utero. Drug screens are also central to drug dependency treatment programs, psychiatry, and addiction medicine for drug treatment/rehabilitation outcome. With the advent of the opioid epidemic, such screens are also used in pain management for monitoring patients on narcotic medications for compliance and for deterrence against diversion of drugs for street sale. Although these drug screens usually consist of a small panel of the most frequently abused drugs (much like the drug test list performed in emergency toxicology), there are service-specific needs (specimen types and drug list) that the clinical toxicology laboratory will have to address.

Most clinical drug testing activities are still based on urine, although other specimen types (eg, meconium and hair [newborns], and oral fluid [drug treatment/rehabilitation programs]) are beginning to gain in popularity in specific testing situations. Serum or plasma is useful in clinical toxicology, particularly in the emergency department setting, where more sophisticated methodologies for identifying specific analytes may be warranted (the reader is referred to chapter 2, *Supporting the Emergency Department*). However, urine as a drug testing specimen has many distinct advantages: the ease of urine collection and the relatively high drug concentrations make detection and quantitation possible with relatively inexpensive instrumentation. Moreover, there is vast field experience from many years of urine drug testing to draw on for analytical methodologies and the interpretation of results. Urine drug testing, however, also has the following distinct disadvantages: (1) urine drug concentrations are not related to drug effects, (2) the window of detection of 1 to 7 days only reflects recent use, and (3) urine specimens can be easily adulterated or tampered with. This last disadvantage is regarded as a particularly serious concern to many service providers, and the vigorous collection protocols designed to deter adulteration and tampering are intrusive and raise the issue of invasion of privacy. As a result of these disadvantages, the use of other specimen types is preferred when possible. The reader is referred to chapter 14, *Alternate Specimens for Drugs-of-Abuse Testing: Oral Fluid;* and chapter 15, *Drug Testing in Hair, Sweat, Meconium, Cord Tissue, and Breast Milk,* for details on the challenges posed by these alternate specimen types for the clinical toxicology laboratory.

Laboratories that want to support their pain management services will have to expand their test menu to include the frequently used opioids. The immunoassays that test for the typical opiates (designed with morphine and codeine as target analytes) do not detect the commonly used nonopiate opioid medications (such as fentanyl, methadone, and buprenorphine) and, depending on the assay used, may not have sufficient reactivity to detect low or even therapeutic doses of hydromorphone and hydrocodone (derivatives of morphine and codeine, respectively) or oxycodone. Laboratories can use commercially available, individual immunoassays that are specific for some of these drugs (oxycodone, methadone, buprenorphine, fentanyl) or resort to the use of chromatography–mass spectrometry assays. Readers should consult chapter 3, *Laboratory Support of Chronic Opioid Therapy;* chapter 4, *The Clinical Pathology Consultation for Pain Management Services;* and chapters 24 through 26 (opioids and emerging novel psychoactive substances) for details on this increasingly important toxicology laboratory service.

On-Site Testing

On-site testing is also referred to as *point-of-care testing* or *point-of-collection testing (POCT).* There has been much recent interest in the utility of rapid, easy-to-use, urine drug testing devices in a variety of settings: emergency departments, drug treatment programs, and pain service clinics. POCT devices require no sophisticated instrumentation or permanent laboratory, and they are generally easy to use and rapid, with results usually available within a few minutes. Many of these testing devices are "waived" tests and can be performed by personnel who are not trained clinical laboratory technologists. Although waived tests do not require proficiency testing (PT), performing PT can improve the quality of the drug testing program by helping to determine accuracy and reliability. Non–laboratory-trained individuals who perform POCT should also be screened for colorblindness because many of these devices have visual endpoints to determine positivity or negativity. The major advantage of POCT is the reduction in turnaround time; transporting of specimens to centralized laboratories for testing is time consuming and costly. Performing analysis at the site of collection and having results available without delay greatly increase the impact of test results. In the emergency department, it allows rapid implementation of therapeutic intervention (for a discussion of the pros and cons of on-site testing, see chapter 2, *Supporting the Emergency Department*). In drug treatment or pain management, particularly if done in the presence of patients whose test results were clinically unexpected, it is a powerful tool in deterring denial of drug use or noncompliance. Recent interest in oral fluid testing has resulted in the commercialization of devices for oral fluid collection and testing (for a discussion of oral fluid testing, see chapter 14).

The accuracy of testing by these devices is dependent on the experience and training of the operators. Laboratories considering the use of these devices should pay special attention to validation, quality control, and training protocols.

Definitive or Confirmation Testing and Adulterant Testing

Definitive Testing

Although the availability and rapidity with which toxicological analysis can be performed and reported is the focus of discussion, the importance of accuracy needs to be addressed. The analytical methods used in performing a drug screen—in particular, the immunoassays—lack the specificity for unequivocal identification of a drug. Hence, an immunoassay-positive result is only a presumptive positive result, requiring confirmation testing for definitive identification. Repeat analysis of the presumptive positive specimen using the same screening test method does not constitute confirmation, although it does serve to reduce random error. Definitive testing requires testing a new aliquot of the original specimen using a different analytical technique, one that is based on a different analytical principle and has greater specificity and at least equal sensitivity to that of the initial test. For example, a presumptive positive result obtained by an immunoassay for opiates cannot be confirmed by a second opiate immunoassay; a mass spectrometric assay, which can specifically identify the opiate involved, can provide confirmation. The reader is referred to chapter 12, *Approaches to Broad-Spectrum Drug Testing in the Clinical Laboratory,* for more information on definitive testing.

Although definitive testing is mandatory in forensic toxicology, the clinical toxicology laboratory routinely reports (unconfirmed) presumptive positive results, particularly when a rapid diagnosis of a suspected drug overdose is required. It is understood that interpretation of unconfirmed results by the physician is done within the context of both clinical and other laboratory findings. The laboratory report, however, must state accurately whether the positive result is a confirmed positive or an unconfirmed (presumptive) positive so that the treating physician can properly evaluate the toxicology result. For a template on specific language that can be used in the report or testing manual, refer to appendix A, *Urine Toxic Screen Template.* The template provides an example of wording that describes the limitations of testing, the analytes included in the urine screen, and one example of how several urine drug testing panels may be arranged.

Urine Adulterant Testing

The quality of testing, be it for clinical or forensic purposes, can only be as good as the quality of the specimen submitted for analysis. Individuals who want to escape detection of their drug use might attempt to tamper with the testing process to produce negative test results. Various methods of tampering include substitution with negative urine, dilution of the urine so that drug concentrations fall below the assay cutoffs for positivity and negativity, and addition of various chemicals to either inactivate the assays or chemically modify the analytes so that they become "invisible" to the initial and confirmation tests. Urine specimens can be easily tampered with, and thus the collection protocol must be designed to deter and detect attempts at tampering. An observed collection is the most effective way to guard against attempts at tampering, but it is invasive and is objectionable to both the donor and the collector. Simple procedures, such as visual inspection for unusual appearance and taking specimen temperature can be used in all collection protocols to assess the validity of a urine specimen, and these can be supplemented with urine creatinine and specific gravity measurements. Federal drug testing programs have published urine specimen collection guidance documents, a set of definitions for specimen validity, and a list of appropriate laboratory tests to assess specimen validity.[2-4] Although these requirements are specific for the federal drug testing programs, many of the procedures can be adapted for use in nonregulated workplace or clinical testing programs. The reader is referred to chapter 6, *Workplace Drug Testing;* chapter 14, *Alternate Specimens for Drugs-of-Abuse Testing: Oral Fluid;* chapter 15, *Drug Testing in Hair, Sweat, Meconium, Cord Tissue, and Breast Milk;* and chapters 3 and 4, relating to supporting chronic opioid therapy, for additional discussion.

Medical-Legal Testing

Medical-legal testing refers to activities that are medical in nature but with high potential of legal involvement or to legal (forensic) testing not related to patient care.

Clinical Testing With Legal Implications

Certain clinical tests have a higher potential for being involved in legal proceedings, for example, blood alcohol tests for motor vehicle accident patients, drugs-of-abuse tests for patients undergoing treatment for substance use disorders, or neonates suspected of drug exposure in utero. Therefore, a laboratory may choose to conduct these clinical tests using procedures and policies that meet both clinical and forensic laboratory standards. It should be borne in mind that these are medical tests, ordered by physicians for the diagnosis and care of patients, not for legal purposes. In most hospital settings, chain-of-custody is not performed. The testing needs to be implemented to meet the clinical laboratory standard of practice only, and the imposition of additional protocols in order to meet forensic standards is an administrative decision. Additional discussion can be found in chapter 7, *Regulatory Issues of Toxicology Laboratory Operations.*

Legal Testing

Some clinical toxicology laboratories have extended their expertise in alcohol testing and drugs-of-abuse testing into the arena of forensic testing (eg, traffic law enforcement, criminal justice and medical examiner systems, workplace urine drug testing programs). In doing so, the performance of legal testing must meet forensic, not clinical, laboratory standards. These forensic laboratory standards include the requirements for chain-of-custody protocols for specimens and aliquots, specimen seals, increased specimen and record security, appropriate confirmation testing, and a certifying review process. This is nonmedical testing and is a departure from the traditional mission of clinical toxicology. The forensic nature and specific requirements of workplace drug testing will be covered in chapter 6, *Workplace Drug Testing,* with additional discussion on forensic toxicology testing in chapter 8, *The Hospital Autopsy and Toxicology Testing.*

The clinical laboratory should be aware that a Supreme Court decision (Melendez-Diaz v Massachusetts[5]) now makes it more likely that laboratorians, technicians, and technologists will be called to court to testify if they have been involved in the analysis or acquisition of samples related to criminal (or civil litigation) cases (eg, homicides or driving under the influence [DUI] cases). Therefore, it is recommended that laboratory personnel become familiar with protocols for testifying in court. The laboratory should be aware that medical examiners and coroners have a specific exclusion within the Health Insurance Portability and Accountability Act of 1996 (HIPAA) that any and all information requested in a death investigation must be released to these offices as requested[6] (the reader is referred to chapter 8, *The Hospital Autopsy and Toxicology Testing,* for further discussion).

Summary

The clinical laboratory may be asked to provide toxicology testing that supports several sections of the hospital or patient care facility, each with its own objectives and needs. It is therefore incumbent upon the pathologist or clinical laboratory director to partner with various "end users" or customers to ensure that the laboratory can meet these needs and convey the limitations of the testing being offered.

Section I of this book specifically covers toxicology testing in the hospital or workplace setting, while Section II addresses specimen types and analytical methodologies that are commonly used in the clinical laboratory, as well as those used in more specialized toxicology laboratories. As pharmacogenomics becomes more mainstream, clinical laboratories may be asked to offer such testing, thus working in partnership with their clinical colleagues to ensure that the prescribed therapeutic drugs are efficacious while minimizing any harmful or adverse effects. Section III provides a review of the most frequently encountered analytes, including abused substances and toxic substances. The appendices present some reference templates or tables that can be adapted to any clinical toxicology laboratory, along with a series of frequently asked questions that pathologists face each day in their role as laboratory directors and information on the College of American Pathologists toxicology proficiency surveys.

References

1. Wu AH, McKay C, Broussard LA, et al; for the National Academy of Clinical Biochemistry Laboratory Medicine. National Academy of Clinical Biochemistry Laboratory Medicine practice guidelines: recommendations for the use of laboratory tests to support poisoned patients who present to the emergency department. *Clin Chem.* 2003;49:357-379.
2. Mandatory guidelines for federal workplace drug testing programs. 82 *Federal Register* 7920 (2017).
3. Urine Specimen Collection Handbook for Federal Agency Workplace Drug Testing Programs. Effective October 1, 2017. Substance Abuse and Mental Health Services Administration. https://www.samhsa.gov/sites/default/files/workplace/urine-specimen-collection-handbook-oct2017_2.pdf. Accessed May 29, 2019.
4. Urine Specimen Collection Guidelines. United States Department of Transportation. https://www.transportation.gov/sites/dot.gov/files/docs/resources/partners/drug-and-alcohol-testing/2567/urine-specimen-collection-guidelines-january-2018.pdf. Revised January 2018. Accessed May 29, 2019.
5. Melendez-Diaz v Massachusetts, 557 US 07-591 (2008).
6. Standards for Privacy of Individually Identifiable Health Information. Regulation Text.. § 164.512 Uses and Disclosures for Which Consent, an Authorization, or Opportunity to Agree or Object is Not Required. US Department of Health and Human Services. Office of the Assistant Secretary for Planning and Evaluation. https://aspe.hhs.gov/report/standards-privacy-individually-identifiable-health-information-regulation-text/%C2%A7-164512-uses-and-disclosures-which-consent-authorization-or-opportunity-agree-or-object-not-required. Accessed May 9, 2019.

Chapter 2

Supporting the Emergency Department

Barbarajean Magnani, PhD, MD
Tai C. Kwong, PhD

Introduction

The goal of emergency toxicology is to provide *clinically useful* toxicology test results to support the needs of the poisoned patients in the emergency department (ED). The clinical usefulness of the results refers not only to the clinical utility of testing, but also to the timeliness of reporting toxicology results. In a 2011 report from the Drug Abuse Warning Network (DAWN),[1] the number of drug-related ED visits was 790 per 100,000 people, with 402 and 458 visits per 100,000 people related to illicit drugs and pharmaceuticals, respectively. An increase in ED visits due to nonmedical use of pharmaceuticals from 2004 to 2011 represented a 132% change. In addition, the Centers for Disease Control and Prevention reported a 30% increase in ED visits related to opioid overdoses from July 2016 to September 2017.[2] The increase of patients presenting to the ED for complications due to prescribed, nonprescribed, and illicit drug use/misuse illustrates the need for the laboratory to have a robust toxicology service.

Because of the complexity of the diagnosis and treatment of poisoning, toxicology results, if available at the appropriate time, can influence the diagnosis and subsequent treatment of the poisoned patient. Emergency toxicology tests can validate drug history or identify drugs and toxins that were not previously suspected. Rapid laboratory identification or confirmation of the toxic agents is invaluable for those cases in which specific treatment is available and its prompt institution is critical: for example, *N*-acetylcysteine therapy for acetaminophen overdose, and ethanol or fomepizole infusion for methanol and ethylene glycol poisoning. Serum drug concentrations, in some instances, can be helpful in gauging the severity of intoxication and the need to initiate specific interventions, and ensuing determinations can be useful in monitoring and evaluating the effectiveness of the treatment procedure.

It is unrealistic to expect any clinical laboratory to provide a full spectrum of toxicological analyses in real time, mostly because of cost constraints and staffing problems. The laboratory and the ED should jointly decide on a toxicology service that is feasible within the financial and technical capability of the laboratory—a service that can still meet the basic needs of the treating physicians. The essential features that need to be considered include the following: (1) which drug assays should be available, (2) whether the assays should be qualitative or quantitative, (3) which specimen types (serum, urine, etc) should be used, (4) when the specimen should be obtained, and (5) what turnaround time (TAT) is acceptable.

There are published guidelines that address these issues and make recommendations regarding which serum/plasma and urine tests have the greatest impact on patient management and can be realistically delivered. However, as the illicit drug use landscape changes, additional analytes will need to be incorporated into the routine testing. In 2003, the National Academy of Clinical Biochemistry (NACB) and others recommended that the hospital clinical laboratory provide two tiers of toxicology testing.[3] Tier 1 tests include select serum or plasma quantitative tests and urine qualitative tests. These tests should be available at all times, on a stat basis, in any clinical laboratory that supports an active ED, regardless of the size or setting (rural or urban) of the institution. Tier 2 tests detect drugs or toxins not identified by Tier 1 tests, are more complicated and time consuming to perform, and may be referred to a reference laboratory.

Tier 1 Tests

The Tier 1 tests should be considered as the toxicology service essential to the support of an ED. Any clinical laboratory, including those that do not have advanced instrumentation, can provide these tests. Selection of the serum quantitative and urine qualitative tests should be based on the prevalence of the relevant drugs and toxins in the population served by the ED, the clinical usefulness of their early identification or quantitation, and the ability of the laboratory to perform the analyses with an acceptable TAT. The ED and the laboratory should jointly determine the list of Tier 1 tests. For example, some EDs may choose not to include cannabinoids (tetrahydrocannabinol [THC]) as part of their routine urine drug panel if it provides difficulties for follow-up and if it does not contribute significantly to the clinical picture; thus, its absence could provide a cost savings to the laboratory. However, other hospitals, such as a dedicated children's hospital, may want this analyte included on an initial screening panel because many consider it a "gateway" drug, and most pediatricians are willing to follow up with parents. In any case, THC should be available on the requisition list as a separate test for any practitioners who require it.

Another consideration is the impact of legalization of medical marijuana and recreational marijuana on the frequency of cannabinoids found in the urine. The state of Colorado legalized medical marijuana in 2000 and recreational marijuana in 2014. As a result, there has been an increase in ED visits associated with acute marijuana intoxication.[4] After legalization of medical marijuana, the prevalence of hospitalizations for marijuana exposure doubled in patients 9 years and older, and ED visits nearly doubled after legalization of recreational marijuana. Management of acute intoxication involves mostly supportive care of primarily neuropsychiatric and gastrointestinal symptoms. Cannabinoid hyperemesis syndrome has been identified in chronic marijuana users and has also contributed to increased ED visits.

Another consideration in determining a laboratory-specific test menu is the geographic utilization of certain drugs; for example, phencyclidine (PCP) use may not be geographically uniform throughout the United States[5] and therefore might not be included on the test menu if both the ED and the toxicology laboratory agree. It is most important is that there be a discussion between the laboratory and the ED to identify which tests are needed. Other considerations include the changing landscape of available drugs in the US, including prescribed and nonprescribed opioids. In November 2010, the Food and Drug Administration (FDA) notified health care professionals that propoxyphene was to be withdrawn from the market. This decision was based on evidence that the drug, even at therapeutic doses, can produce significant cardiac toxicity. Initial NACB guidelines included propoxyphene, but given that the number of patients receiving this drug will be reduced drastically with time, the need for testing for propoxyphene will have to be reassessed. The opioid crisis has increased the awareness of the misuse of medications prescribed for chronic noncancer pain, and, at a minimum, laboratories should include buprenorphine, oxycodone, and fentanyl in their toxicology screen. These drugs are available as FDA-cleared immunoassays and should be within the reach of all hospital laboratories.

It is also important for the ED and the toxicology laboratory to have the same definition of an acceptable TAT and to agree on a target TAT within which the laboratory can receive specimens and reasonably complete the analysis and report the results that are still clinically relevant to the acute care of an ED patient. Many consider 1 hour or less as the recommended TAT for Tier 1 tests, but this may be difficult to meet for some laboratories.[3] TAT is usually measured from the time the specimen reaches the laboratory until the time the result is reported. Specimens that are collected in the ED and then "sit" for a period of time are a potential source of frustration for both ED and laboratory staff. Every attempt should be made to send specimens as quickly as possible to the laboratory after they are collected. In an effort to reduce TAT, some laboratories may choose to use point-of-care testing (POCT) in order to accommodate a TAT of 1 hour or less. EDs may be reluctant to use centralized laboratory toxicology testing and choose POCT to improve TAT and clinical value.[6] One study demonstrated a reduction in TAT from 108 to 33 minutes when testing was switched from the core laboratory to POCT[7]; however, this testing was at least twice as expensive as that in the core laboratory (unit-cost basis) and increased the use of drugs-of-abuse testing, thereby increasing the cost of testing overall. Nevertheless, the increased cost of the POCT could be offset by the reduction in the length of stay in the ED. It is incumbent upon each laboratory to determine if the benefits of saving a small amount of time will actually translate into an overall savings for the hospital. Additional considerations when using POCT in the ED revolve around which department performs and has responsibility for these laboratory tests. Options include having the ED laboratory as a satellite of the core laboratory (ie, the ED laboratory is staffed and operated by the core laboratory personnel) or having the ED laboratory operated by ED staff, with the core clinical laboratory providing oversight. It is important in this regard to make sure the ED staff have demonstrated training and annual competency, and follow all the regulatory components necessary for laboratory accreditation.

With regard to analysis of other matrices, first gastric aspirate, vomitus, or stomach washings are useful specimens if they are obtained soon after ingestion and if pill fragments are noted; however, the analysis of gastric contents offers no advantage over urine, and drugs that are rapidly absorbed or not taken orally will not be detected. Oral fluid has been used successfully for alcohol testing and is gaining acceptance for drugs-of-abuse testing in the US (the reader is referred to chapter 14, *Alternate*

Table 2-1. Stat Quantitative Serum Toxicology Assays Required to Support an Emergency Department
Acetaminophen (paracetamol)
Lithium
Salicylate
Co-oximetry for oxygen saturation, carboxyhemoglobin, and methemoglobin
Theophylline
Valproic acid
Carbamazepine
Digoxin
Phenobarbital (if urine barbiturates are positive)
Iron
Transferrin (total iron-binding capacity [TIBC] or unsaturated iron-binding capacity [UIBC] assay if transferrin is not available)
Ethyl alcohol
Methyl alcohol
Ethylene glycol

From Wu A et al.[3] © 2003. Modified with permission of the American Association for Clinical Chemistry (AACC).

Specimens for Drugs-of-Abuse Testing: Oral Fluid, for further information on oral fluid testing).

Quantitative Serum Tests

Quantitative measurement of serum drug concentration is meaningful if drug concentration is correlated to toxicity or if knowledge of a specific drug concentration influences patient management. Serum tests for the following substances are suggested by the NACB guidelines and meet the above criteria: acetaminophen, salicylate, carbamazepine, valproate, phenobarbital, theophylline, digoxin, lithium, iron, transferrin (or total iron-binding capacity [TIBC]), ethanol; co-oximetry for carboxyhemoglobin and methemoglobin is also suggested (Table 2-1). Implementation of these quantitative serum tests in any laboratory supporting emergency medical care is feasible because these tests are usually available either as therapeutic drug monitoring assays (eg, digoxin, lithium) or clinical chemistry tests (eg, iron) in most, if not all, clinical chemistry laboratories.

Given the effectiveness of fomepizole as an antidote for methanol and ethylene glycol (EG) poisoning and the importance of early identification of methanol and EG, the quantitative assays for methanol and EG should be Tier 1 tests. Unfortunately, on-site availability of these tests is severely limited by the technical difficulties of the chromatographic methodologies, making them unavailable as Tier 1 tests in most hospital-based laboratories. Therefore, each hospital laboratory should have a reference laboratory or regional center where these tests can be referred if needed. An enzymatic assay is commercially available for EG, providing a useful screening to rule out the presence of EG, and modification of the assay allows quantification of serum concentrations.[8] Given that the test may be positive in the presence of increased lactic acid or lactate dehydrogenase activity,[9] positive screening tests should be confirmed by an alternate, more specific method, such as gas chromatography. An additional test that may provide useful information in overdoses of volatile substances (including EG) is the osmolal gap, which requires both the measured osmolality in mOsm/kg of solvent and calculated serum osmolarity in mOsm/L[10,11] (Figure 2-1).

Osmolal Gap =
Measured Osmolality – Calculated Osmolarity

The Reference Interval = 0 ± 5-10

Calculated Osmolarity = 2[sodium] + [glucose]/18 + [BUN]/2.8 = ~290 mOsm/L

Figure 2-1. How to calculate the osmolal gap. Serum sodium is measured in mEq/L, and glucose and blood urea nitrogen (BUN) are measured in mg/L. Both the measured osmolality and calculated serum osmolarity should be obtained from the same serum sample. See chapter 17, *Non-Ethanol Volatiles and Ethylene Glycol,* for more details.

Qualitative Urine Tests

The urine immunoassays for drugs of abuse are available as reagent kits for automated chemistry instruments or as POCT devices. These assays are used extensively because they can be performed at any time of the day and require low-to-moderate technical expertise.

There is a lack of consensus among clinical toxicology experts on the usefulness of a qualitative urine drug screen and, in particular, one that is composed of immunoassays for the common drugs of abuse (Table 2-2). Relevant issues include the poor specificity (inaccuracy) of the immunoassays,[12,13] the lack of correlation between the presence of drug or metabolite in urine and the toxic effects or clinical impairment, and the extended window of detection of drugs or metabolites after

Table 2-2. Stat Qualitative Urine Toxicology Assays Required to Support the Emergency Department
Amphetamines
Barbiturates
Benzodiazepines
Buprenorphine
Cocaine
Fentanyl
Opiates
Oxycodone
Phencyclidine
[Propoxyphene]
Tricyclic antidepressants

From Wu A et al.[3] © 2003. Modified with permission of the American Association for Clinical Chemistry (AACC).

the most recent use. Therefore, there is the perception that a urine drug screen has little impact on the acute care of a poisoned patient and that the screen serves more of a confirmatory or documentation purpose. Nevertheless, the use of a urine drug screen performed stat in emergency toxicology is widespread in the United States, and laboratory professionals are advised to consult the chapters on specific drug groups for the pharmacokinetic and toxicokinetic properties of these drugs, and chapter 11, *Laboratory-Based Screening Assays,* for detailed discussions on the limitations of immunoassay-based drug screens.

Tier 2 Tests

For intoxicated patients whose clinical signs cannot be explained by the Tier 1 agents, Tier 2 tests can be useful in identifying other agents that have clinical significance, for example, a more broad-spectrum drug screen or a trace metal analysis. These tests require complex analytical techniques (chromatography, atomic absorption spectrophotometry, mass spectrometry, etc), sophisticated expertise, and highly trained staff. Many of these tests are done infrequently, even in the largest hospitals, making it difficult to maintain competency and justify the costs of doing these tests. Tier 2 tests can be done on site, in a nearby laboratory, at a regional center, or in a reference laboratory. A cooperative effort undertaken to develop a regional toxicology center can provide a full spectrum of advanced toxicology service to support regional hospitals. The regional laboratory system has the advantages of avoiding duplication of laboratory facilities and of pooling regional workload to sustain proficiency in difficult, low-volume tests.

Unique Challenges Associated With Testing in the Emergency Department

Many victims of trauma—including those resulting from gun shots, stabbings, or motor vehicle accidents—or persons suspected of driving under the influence (DUI) will have some form of drug testing while in the ED. These cases, in addition to patients who may succumb to drug overdose or accidental poisoning, will necessitate the involvement of other outside agencies, including law enforcement or the medical examiner/coroner. Although drug testing in the ED is obtained to support and validate clinical findings, sometimes these results will be used in court in criminal or civil cases, or will help to determine the cause of death; the reader is referred to chapter 8, *The Hospital Autopsy and Toxicology Testing*. In these circumstances, it will be necessary for the laboratory to provide documentation of testing, results obtained, methodology used, and quality control results, if requested by law. In addition, the laboratory may be asked to provide any residual serum or urine specimens to the medical examiner/coroner, state police, or some other governmental agency. In consideration of the possible need for further testing in these types of cases, the ED and the laboratory may want to discuss an arrangement whereby an additional "gray top" or sodium fluoride/potassium oxalate tube is collected from the patient during the ED visit. Furthermore, clinical laboratories should keep a record of what specimens were released, as well as to whom they were released. Each laboratory should check for compliance with both the Health Insurance Portability and Accountability Act of 1996 (HIPAA) and the hospital legal or risk division regarding how this information should be documented. It is important to note, however, that medical examiners/coroners have a specific exclusion within the HIPAA law, in that any and all information requested in a death investigation must be released to these offices as requested.[14] An example of a policy for the release of specimens and the accompanying form can be found in Figures 2-2 and 2-3.

The clinical laboratory should be aware that a Supreme Court decision, Melendez-Diaz v Massachusetts,[15] now makes it more likely that laboratorians, technicians, and technologists will be called to testify in court if they have been involved in the analysis or acquisition of specimens related

Hospital Name

Hospital Name **Department of Pathology and Laboratory Medicine Policy**	**Subject:** Release of Laboratory Specimens	
Issuing Area: Laboratory Administration		
Original Procedure Date:		**Approved By:** Chief of Pathology Director of Laboratory Services

I. **Purpose**
The purpose of this policy is to define the process of releasing laboratory specimens to outside agencies.

II. **Eligibility**
All Staff of the [Department of Pathology and Laboratory Medicine].

III. **Forms**
Release of Laboratory Specimen Form (#).

IV. **Policy**
The laboratory is frequently asked to release patient-related specimens to other agencies for the purposes of further or confirmatory testing. It is the policy of the [Hospital Name and Department] that specimens can be released to the following entities:

ME/Coroner's Office | Organ Bank/ Donor Services | Local/State Police Officer/Trooper	
Authorized agent must provide:	• Documentation requesting specimens to be released • Proper identification (agency badge or state ID)
Lab technologist must complete:	• Release of Laboratory Specimen Form (#)
Other Individuals Not Listed Above: Contact Director of Operations or Medical Director [Department of Pathology and Laboratory Medicine] for advice.	

V. **Procedure for Release of Specimens**

1. If a request from a state Medical Examiner (ME)/Coroner's office is received, proceed with the procedure below. If a subpoena or search warrant is received, contact the Risk Management Department to review the documentation provided. Once approved by Risk Management, follow the below procedure.
2. Verify that we have requested specimens in the laboratory information system [LIS].
3. Pull all specimens that are requested.
4. Place the specimens in their original tubes and/or containers in a plastic specimen transport bag. Be sure that all specimens are capped with tightly fitting caps so that the content does not leak.
5. Complete the "Release of Laboratory Specimen Form" (refer to #).
6. Place the specimens and the form in the Send Out refrigerator in the bin labeled "ME/Coroner SPECIMENS."
7. Write the last name of the patient on the "ME/Coroner SPECIMENS" [dry erase board] in Send Outs.
8. When a representative from the requesting agency arrives in the laboratory to pick up the requested specimens:
   a. Verify their identification and make a copy of the agent's ID badge or license.
   b. Have them provide the copy of the search warrant, subpoena, or document requesting specific specimens (if not already obtained).
   c. Have them sign the "Release of Laboratory Specimen Form."
9. Place the completed form in the Release of Laboratory Specimens binder in Send Outs.
10. Direct all questions to the Director of Operations.

Author: **Dated:**

Figure 2-2. Example of a policy for release of specimens.

Hospital Name
Department of Pathology and Laboratory Medicine
Release of Specimen Form

Date of Request	
Patient Name	
Medical Record Number	
Date(s) Specimen Collected	
Specimen Types Requested	
Agency Requesting Sample	
Agency Representative (printed name)	
Hospital Tech Processing Request	

BELOW FOR LABORATORY USE ONLY

Released Specimens	
Order or Specimen Number	Specimen Type

Date and Time	
Supervisor or Senior Tech ID	
Agency Representative (printed name)	
Agency Representative (signed name)	

Attach any supporting documentation (subpoena, search warrant, etc).

Figure 2-3. Example of a form for release of laboratory specimens.

Table 2-3. Common Toxidromes, Toxic Symptoms, Toxidrome Agents, and Antidotes

Toxidrome	Signs and Symptoms	Common Toxidrome Agents	Antidotes
Anticholinergic	Red as a beet (erythema) Dry skin Delirium Mydriasis Hyperthermia Bowel and bladder (urgency and retention) Tachycardia	Jimson weed Antihistamines Phenothiazines Tricyclic antidepressants Over-the-counter sleep aids (antihistamines)	—
Cholinergic, muscarinic	D- Diarrhea U- Urination M- Miosis B- Bradycardia/bronchorrhea E- Emesis L- Lacrimation S- Salivation	Organophosphates Some mushrooms (*Amanita muscaria)*	—
Cholinergic, nicotinic	Nausea Vomiting Tachycardia Hypertension Muscle fasciculations Weakness or paralysis	Nicotine insecticides Tobacco Black widow spider venom Carbamates	—
Opioid (narcotic)	Central nervous system depression Miosis Hypotension Hypoventilation	Codeine Morphine Heroin Oxycodone Hydrocodone Meperidine Fentanyl	Naloxone

to criminal (or civil litigation) cases (ie, homicides, DUI cases). Therefore, it is recommended that laboratory personnel gain knowledge about testimony procedure if required to go to court. In these cases, the laboratory personnel can testify to obtaining a tube of blood or a container of urine labeled with the patient's name (eg, Jane Doe, MR #123456). Unless the laboratory technologist personally collected the specimen from Jane Doe, he or she cannot testify in court that the specimen is actually from "Jane Doe," but rather that the tube is labeled with Jane Doe's name. Although most clinical laboratories do not require chain of custody, they do follow good laboratory practice, which requires the labeling of specimens at the patient's bedside and using two forms of identification (eg, name, medical record number, and/or date of birth). All laboratories engaged in forensic toxicology testing should practice strict chain-of-custody procedures that clearly identify who collected the specimen and each person who has handled it subsequently.

Toxidromes

Historically, physicians and laboratory personnel were taught toxidromes, that is, signs and symptoms associated with a specific poison or drug. When considering a specific toxidrome, not only are the heart rate, respiratory rate, temperature, skin color, and pupil size of significance, but it is also important to take into consideration any odors associated with the patient (on clothes, breath, or body). Certain drugs or their metabolites may produce a specific odor that may point to the culprit drug (eg, the odor of garlic is associated with arsenic or organophosphate poisoning, and the odor of acetone is associated with isopropanol intoxication.)

However, toxidromes have become more difficult to identify in the acutely intoxicated patient, and this is primarily due to *polypharmacy*. Patients may ingest multiple drugs from different classes and present with seemingly mixed toxidromes—for example, drugs from the sedative-hypnotics class (benzodiazepines) or opioid toxidrome mixed with those of the sympathetic toxidrome (cocaine

Table 2-4. Commonly Encountered Toxic Agents

Toxic Agent(s)	Signs and Symptoms	Supportive Laboratory Tests	Antidotes
Acetaminophen (Tylenol compounds)	Phase 1: vomiting, nausea, gastrointestinal irritability, diaphoresis, and pallor; may last 12-24 hours Phase 2: latent period; slight improvement, but right upper quadrant pain, rise in LFTs Phase 3: hepatic necrosis; increased LFTs, increased PT, encephalopathy, death	Serum acetaminophen concentration 4 or more hours after a single ingestion, AST, ALT, glucose, PT, INR, lactate, serum creatinine, electrolytes, phosphate, hCG where appropriate as acetaminophen crosses the placenta, arterial blood gas	*N*-acetylcysteine (FDA-approved for PO or IV administration) as appropriate
Salicylates (Aspirin compounds)	Acute overdose: nausea, vomiting, abdominal pain, tinnitus at concentrations >20 mg/dL, coma, seizures	Serum salicylate concentration obtained 2 hours after ingestion, electrolytes, glucose, blood urea nitrogen (BUN), creatinine, baseline LFTs	—
Iron	Stage 1 (gastrointestinal) Stage 2 (latent) Stage 3 (metabolic/ cardiovascular) Stage 4 (hepatic) Stage 5 (delayed)	Serum iron concentration 4 hours after ingestion, glucose, CBC count, lactate, arterial blood gas, coagulation studies (PT), LFTs, electrolytes, hCG where appropriate	Deferoxamine
Cyanide	Moderate exposure: palpitations, dizziness, gastrointestinal symptoms, headache, hyperventilation High exposure: syncope, coma, seizures, cardiovascular collapse	Cyanide concentration	Cyanide antidote kit (amyl nitrite, sodium nitrite, and sodium thiosulfate)
Methanol (windshield washer fluid)	Ethanol-like intoxication, gastritis, visual disturbances, seizures, acute renal failure	Methanol concentration, osmolal gap, electrolytes (look for severe anion gap metabolic acidosis)	Ethanol, fomepizole (methylpyrazole or 4-methylpyrazole)
Ethylene glycol (antifreeze)	Ethanol-like intoxication, gastritis, seizures, dysrhythmias	Ethylene glycol concentration, osmolal gap, electrolytes (anion gap metabolic acidosis), calcium	Ethanol, fomepizole (methylpyrazole or 4-methylpyrazole)

LFT, liver function test; AST, aspartate aminotransferase; ALT, alanine aminotransferase; PT, prothrombin time; INR, international normalized ratio; hCG, human chorionic gonadotropin; FDA, Food and Drug Administration; PO, per os (orally); IV, intravenous; CBC, complete blood cell.

or amphetamines). The DAWN Report from 2011 revealed that there were approximately 2.5 million drug-related ED visits, of which about one-half were attributed to adverse reactions to pharmaceuticals and one-half to drug misuse or abuse, and about 25% involved drugs plus alcohol.[1] It is not surprising that ED visits involving misuse or abuse of pharmaceuticals rose approximately 52% from 2004 until 2011. Of the estimated 1.2 million ED visits involving the nonmedical use of pharmaceuticals, 29% were attributed to narcotic pain relievers. Of these, 44% were narcotic pain relievers only, while 56% of these visits included additional drugs.[16] In addition, when considering the application of toxidromes in the unconscious patient, the background prevalence of a specific agent should be considered. Specific geographic locations (even within a city) may mean that the availability of certain drugs would more likely produce the clinical presentation of the toxidrome than would another drug.[17]

Sympathetic, parasympathetic (cholinergic; muscarinic and nicotinic), anticholinergic, and opioid (narcotic) toxidromes are the most common. Thumbnail outlines of the classic toxidromes are found in Table 2-3; additional toxic agents commonly encountered in the ED are found in Table 2-4.[18-24] For detailed information about various drug classes or toxic agents, the reader is referred to the individual chapters within this book.

References

1. *Substance Abuse and Mental Health Services Administration, Drug Abuse Warning Network, 2011: National Estimates of Drug-Related Emergency Department Visits.* HHS Publication No (SMA) 13-4760, DAWN Series D-39. Rockville, MD: Substance Abuse and Mental Health Services Administration; 2013.
2. Opioid Overdoses Treated in Emergency Departments. Centers for Disease Control and Prevention. https://www.cdc.gov/vitalsigns/opioid-overdoses/. Updated March 16, 2018. Accessed June 19, 2019.
3. Wu A, McKay C, Broussard LA, et al. National Academy of Clinical Biochemistry Laboratory Medicine Practice Guidelines: recommendations for the use of laboratory tests to support poisoned patients who present to the emergency department. *Clin Chem.* 2003;49(3):357-379.
4. Kim HS, Monte AA. Colorado cannabis legalization and its effects on emergency care. *Ann Emerg Med.* 2016;68(1):71-75.
5. Bush DM. *Emergency Department Visits Involving Phencyclidine (PCP).* Rockville, MD: Center for Behavioral Health Statistics and Quality, Substance Abuse and Mental Health Services Administration; The CBHSQ Report: November 12, 2013.
6. Lager PS, Attema-de Jonge ME, Gorzeman MP, Kerkvliet LE, Franssen EJF. Clinical value of drugs of abuse point of care testing in an emergency department setting. *Toxicol Rep.* 2018;5:12-17.
7. Lewandrowski K, Flood J, Finn C, et al. Implementation of point-of-care rapid urine testing for drugs of abuse in the emergency department of an academic medical center: impact on test utilization and ED length of stay. *Am J Clin Pathol.* 2008;129(5):796-801.
8. Juenke JM, Hardy L, McMillin GA, Horowitz G. Rapid and specific quantification of ethylene glycol levels. *Am J Clin Pathol.* 2011;136:318-324.
9. Eder AF, Dowdy YG, Gardiner JA, Wolf BA, Shaw LM. Serum lactate and lactate dehydrogenase in high concentrations interfere in enzymatic assay of ethylene glycol. *Clin Chem.* 1996;42:1489-1491.
10. Jacobsen D, Bredesen JE, Eide I, Ostborg J. Anion and osmolal gaps in the diagnosis of methanol and ethylene glycol poisoning. *Acta Med Scand.* 1982;212(1-2):17-20.
11. Glaser DS. Utility of the serum osmol gap in the diagnosis of methanol or ethylene glycol ingestion. *Ann Emerg Med.* 1996;27:343-346.
12. Smith ML, Hughes RO, Levine B, Dickerson S, Darwin WD, Cone EJ. Forensic drug testing for opiates, VI: urine testing for hydromorphone, hydrocodone, oxymorphone, and oxycodone with commercial opiate immunoassays and gas chromatography–mass spectrometry. *J Anal Toxicol.* 1995;19:18-26.
13. Krasowski MD, Pizon AF, Siam MG, Giannoutsos S, Iyer M, Ekins S. Using molecular similarity to highlight the challenges of routine immunoassay-based drug of abuse/toxicology screening in emergency medicine. *BMC Emerg Med.* 2009;9:1-18.
14. Standards for Privacy of Individually Identifiable Health Information. Regulation Test..§ 164.512 Uses and Disclosures for Which Consent, an Authorization, or Opportunity to Agree or Object is not Required. US Department of Health and Human Services. https://aspe.hhs.gov/report/standards-privacy-individually-identifiable-health-information-regulation-text/%C2%A7-164512-uses-and-disclosures-which-consent-authorization-or-opportunity-agree-or-object-not-required. Published January 5, 2001. Accessed June 19, 2019.
15. Melendez-Diaz v Massachusetts, 557 US 07-591 (2008).
16. Crane, EH. *Emergency Department Visits Involving Narcotic Pain Relievers.* Rockville, MD: Center for Behavioral Health Statistics and Quality, Substance Abuse and Mental Health Services Administration; The CBHSQ Report: November 5, 2015.
17. Buckley NA, Whyte IM, Dawson AH. Diagnostic data in clinical toxicology—should we use a Bayesian approach? *J Toxicol Clin Toxicol.* 2002; 40(3):213-222.
18. McGregor T, Parkar M, Rao S. Evaluation and management of common childhood poisonings. *Am Fam Physician.* 2009;79(5):397-403.
19. Koren G. A primer of paediatric toxic syndromes or 'toxidromes.' *Paediatr Child Health.* 2007;12(6)457-459.

20. Farrell SE, Defendi GL. Acetaminophen Toxicity. Medscape. http://emedicine.medscape.com/article/820200-overview. Updated January 22, 2018. Accessed June 19, 2019.
21. Spanierman CS. Iron Toxicity. Medscape. http://emedicine.medscape.com/article/815213-overview. Updated February 4, 2019. Accessed June 19, 2019.
22. Mehta N, Ozick LA, Gbadehan E. Drug-Induced Hepatotoxicity. Medscape. http://emedicine.medscape.com/article/169814-overview. Updated December 8, 2016. Accessed June 19, 2019.
23. Camidge R, Bateman DN. Self-poisoning in the UK: epidemiology and toxidromes. *Clin Med.* 2003;3(2):111-114.
24. Farrell SE, Defendi GL. Acetaminophen Toxicity Treatment & Management. Medscape. https://emedicine.medscape.com/article/820200-treatment#d16. Updated January 22, 2018. Accessed June 19, 2019.

Chapter 3

Laboratory Support of Chronic Opioid Therapy

Tai C. Kwong, PhD
Barbarajean Magnani, PhD, MD

Introduction

The International Association for the Study of Pain defines chronic pain as pain lasting more than 3 months.[1] Drugs typically employed in the treatment of chronic pain are shown in Table 3-1 and include opioids as well as anti-inflammatory drugs and drugs used in the treatment of neuropathic pain. Opioid therapy for pain management has increased dramatically in recent years; opioid prescriptions per capita increased 7.3% from 2007 to 2012,[2] and the number of opioid prescriptions in 2012 amounted to 259 million—enough for every adult in the United States to have a bottle of pills.[3] Opioid-based pain therapy poses serious risks, including addiction and accidental overdose. In one report, more than 420,000 emergency department visits were related to misuse or abuse of opioid pain medications,[4] and, in another report, opioid overdose fatalities increased by 200% from the year 2000 to 2014.[5] In more recent years (2015-2016), opioid-related deaths associated with synthetic opioids have surpassed those with prescription opioids.[6] In 2016, fentanyl was associated with 45.6% of opioid-related overdose deaths (that figure was

Table 3-1. Drugs Used in the Treatment of Pain

Opioid agonists	Codeine (Tylenol #3) Fentanyl (Duragesic) Hydrocodone (Lorcet, Lortab, Vicodin) Hydromorphone (Dilaudid) Meperidine (Demerol) Methadone (Dolophine) Morphine (MS Contin) Sufentanil (Dsuvia) Oxycodone (OxyContin, Percocet) Oxymorphone (Numorphan) Buprenorphine (Buprenex, Subutex) Tramadol (Ultram) Propoxyphene (Darvon, Darvocet)	**Benzodiazepines and antianxiety agents**	Alprazolam (Xanax) Chlordiazepoxide (Librium) Clonazepam (Klonopin) Clorazepate (Tranxene) Diazepam (Valium) Lorazepam (Ativan) Oxazepam (Serax) Buspirone (Buspar)
Mixed agonists-antagonists	Buprenorphine with naloxone (Suboxone) Pentazocine with naloxone (Talwin Nx)	**Anti-inflammatories***	Ibuprofen Naproxen Acetaminophen Salicylates Cyclooxygenase-2 inhibitors
Antidepressants	Tricyclic antidepressants (amitriptyline, doxepin, imipramine, desipramine, nortriptyline) Selective serotonin reuptake inhibitors (citalopram [Celexa], fluoxetine [Prozac], fluvoxamine [Luvox], paroxetine [Paxil], sertraline [Zoloft]) Venlafaxine (Effexor) Bupropion (Wellbutrin) Duloxetine (Cymbalta)	**Drugs used to treat neuropathic pain (antiepileptics)**	Gabapentin (Neurontin) Pregabalin Carbamazepine Phenytoin

* Varied preparations available. Note: These agents may also be found as part of the above opiate preparations.

14.3% in 2010).[7] In 2017, the US Department of Health and Human Services declared a nationwide public health emergency regarding the opioid crisis.[8]

In response to the abuse of prescription opioids for chronic pain treatment, practice guidelines have been published to aid clinicians treating chronic pain patients with opioids.[9-15] In 2016, the Centers for Disease Control and Prevention (CDC) published a guideline for opioid prescriptions: "CDC Guideline for Prescribing Opioids for Chronic Pain—United States."[16] The guideline is aimed at primary care physicians, who are responsible for the majority of opioid prescriptions. The American Society of Addiction Medicine published a document detailing the technologies used in urine drug testing and the clinical utility of urine drug testing in the management of opioid therapy for chronic pain.[17] The American Association for Clinical Chemistry (AACC) published evidence-based recommendations for drug testing in support of opioid therapy in its *Laboratory Medicine Practice Guidelines*.[18] These guidelines share common elements in their recommended standards of practice in assessing the risk of opioid therapy and monitoring of therapy. For example, all of these guidelines recommended a comprehensive initial evaluation of the patient, an assessment of the risk and benefit of opioid therapy, and the use of a urine drug test before prescribing opioids (and periodically thereafter) to assess for prescribed medications as well as other controlled prescription drugs and illicit drugs.

In the context of these and other emerging guidelines, this chapter will focus on the role the clinical laboratory can expect to play in supporting the care of patients with chronic pain who are on opioid therapy. It will also address laboratory-related elements of urine drug testing that can best meet the specific needs of the patients.

Role of the Clinical Laboratory in Pain Management

Management of the patient with chronic pain on opioid therapy is challenging to medical providers. Routine urine drug screening can be used to identify use of nonprescribed medications, failure to use a prescribed medication (or use it regularly), and use of (undisclosed) alcohol and other illicit drugs.[19,20] Although urine drug testing cannot be used to determine how frequently a patient takes a medication or when it was last taken, the urine drug test remains an effective tool in supplementing behavioral monitoring of patients for their compliance with opioid therapy.[21] Therefore, practice guidelines have recommended the urine drug test as a laboratory tool that clinicians can rely on for ensuring safe and effective opioid therapy for their patients. Thus, clinical laboratories play an important role in supporting this clinical service (see also chapter 4, *Clinical Pathology Consultation for Pain Management Services*). The following sections will discuss the responsibilities and the roles of clinical laboratories in supporting safe and effective opioid therapy with positive clinical outcomes, which include designing the testing program, providing information on testing methodologies and their limitations, and offering assistance in results interpretation.

Design of Urine Drug Test Program

The clinical laboratory needs to partner with clinical disciplines that provide pain management services to design a drug testing program that best meets the clinical needs. This partnership will make decisions about all the elements of a testing program, many of which are not familiar to the providers: specimen matrix, specimen collection protocols, analytes to be included in the test menu, location of test performance, analytical methodologies, and testing strategies.

Specimen Matrix

Urine is currently the most commonly used matrix for pain management drug testing. Use of oral fluid has gained acceptance in recent years and is valued as an alternative to urine for its ease of collection and lower susceptibility to tampering. Oral fluid is also valued in situations where obtaining urine is difficult (an anuric patient) or awkward (witnessed collections). For compliance testing in pain management, urine testing is recommended over blood. Drugs in blood have short windows of detection, and urine provides information regarding drugs taken over a longer period of time. Use of urine also allows for detection of metabolites of drugs that may have already cleared the bloodstream. The use of oral fluid, blood, and other specimen matrices are discussed in detail in chapter 14, *Alternate Specimens for Drugs-of-Abuse Testing: Oral Fluid*; and chapter 15, *Drug Testing in Hair, Sweat, Meconium, Cord Tissue, and Breast Milk.* This chapter will focus on urine drug testing because current opioid prescription guideline recommendations on drug testing are based on urine.

The advantages of using urine specimens for drug testing include ease of collection, generally adequate sample volume for both initial and confirmation tests, and minimal preanalytical preparation for testing. In addition, concentrations of common analytes are sufficiently high for detection by currently available analytical methodologies. Moreover, the long history of drug testing on urine has given laboratorians and clinicians a vast body of knowledge to meet the analytical and interpretive challenges. Unfortunately, the use of a urine specimen does have the disadvantage of the relative ease of adulteration of the sample. Therefore, some urine drug testing programs may implement collection practices to deter attempts at adulteration, which may include the restriction of water access, use of colored agents in the toilet, and even the invasive collection protocol that requires observed collection using gender-specific collectors. In some cases, specimen validity testing may be warranted, which, at a minimum, should include taking urine temperature at time of collection and testing for specific gravity, creatinine, and pH.[18]

Test Menu and Testing Location

No single testing menu meets the needs of all pain clinics, and few laboratories can perform all drug assays in house. Table 3-2 shows a typical menu covering the frequently prescribed medications for pain management and commonly abused illicit drugs.[18,22] When selecting the menu, it is useful to work directly with the pain clinic, rehabilitation department, or primary care physicians to optimize the menu to reflect the prescription practice of medications and the prevalence and pattern of illicit drug use in the local area. In most instances, initial test menus by immunoassays are also limited by commercial availability of Food and Drug Administration (FDA)–cleared immunoassay test kits.

Most of these tests are also available in point-of-care testing (POCT) devices, some of which are "waived" tests that can be performed by personnel who are not clinical laboratory technologists. Thus, initial testing using POCT devices can be performed in a doctor's office or clinic, thereby offering the advantage of rapid turnaround time such that a provider can discuss test results with the patient during the patient's clinic visit. This real-time provider-patient interaction regarding test results can enhance the effectiveness of the drug test in the management of those patients who might be exhibiting aberrant drug behaviors. If the urine specimens are sent to a laboratory for testing, the turnaround time compared with POCT is generally longer and may not allow for real-time feedback to the patient. Laboratory testing, however, can be performed efficiently and cost effectively as a result of installation of high-throughput automation equipment for high-volume testing. The recent offering of direct, definitive testing by mass spectrometry (see below, under "Definitive First-Line Testing by Mass Spectrometry") is entirely laboratory based and, because of the technology involved, might even be restricted to regional or reference laboratories, thus further extending the turnaround time.

A laboratory can review its test result databases for test positivity and negativity rates to identify whether changes to the test menu should be made.[23,24] Drugs having low positive rates (eg, phencyclidine or methaqualone) could be eliminated from the test menu. However, clinicians may regard having a positive result for certain drugs, such as cocaine or amphetamines, as leading to serious consequences for the patient (dismissal from treatment program, discontinuation of opioid therapy, etc) and may opt to keep these drugs in the menu even if the positivity rates are low.

Testing Methodology: Initial Testing by Immunoassays

Initial testing ("screening") by immunoassays is still the most commonly used testing methodology because of lower cost, ease of use, adaptation to automated instrumentation, and rapid turnaround time. Nevertheless, immunoassays, whether they are used in POCT devices or laboratory chemistry analyzers, have limitations—namely, lower sensitivity and specificity compared with definitive testing methodologies based on mass spectrometry.

The assay immunospecificity and the cutoff used to designate a result as negative or positive determine the specificity and sensitivity of the immunoassay and therefore the clinical utility of immunoassay-based drug testing in pain management. Taking these limitations into consideration when interpreting test results will optimize the clinical utility of urine drug testing and assist clinicians in their clinical decision making in opioid pain management.[25,26] Immunoassay limitations include the qualitative nature of immunoassays, lack of specificity, inability to identify the reactive substances, and inadequate analytical sensitivity. The laboratory needs to communicate these limitations to pain treatment providers so they can utilize the urine drug test appropriately.

Immunoassays Are Qualitative Assays

The laboratory needs to ensure that providers understand the definition of a positive or negative result by immunoassay. Immunoassays are qualitative assays, and results are reported as positive or negative relative to the signal generated by the calibrator drug at the specified cutoff concentration. Thus, neither a positive nor negative result indicates the concentration(s) of the drug(s) present.[26]

Table 3-2. Testing Menu for Pain Management (Licit and Illicit Drugs)

Screening Assays (typical target analyte and cutoff options)	**Confirmation Assays** (drugs currently considered clinically relevant in each drug class)
Amphetamines/methamphetamines (*d*-amphetamine or *d*-methamphetamine) at 500 (1000) ng/mL	Amphetamine Methamphetamine Methylenedioxymethamphetamine (MDMA, ecstasy) Methylenedioxyamphetamine (MDA) Methylenedioxyethylamphetamine (MDEA) Phentermine
MDMA (ecstasy) at 500 ng/mL	MDMA (ecstasy) MDA
Barbiturates (secobarbital) at 200 [300] ng/mL	Amobarbital Butalbital Pentobarbital Phenobarbital Secobarbital
Benzodiazepines (nordiazepam) at 150 [200] ng/mL	Diazepam Nordiazepam Oxazepam Lorazepam Temazepam Hydroxyethylflurazepam (flurazepam metabolite) 7-Aminoclonazepam (clonazepam metabolite) α-Hydroxyalprazolam (alprazolam metabolite) 7-Aminoflunitrazepam (flunitrazepam metabolite) α-Hydroxytriazolam (triazolam metabolite)
Buprenorphine at 5 ng/mL	Buprenorphine Norbuprenorphine
Norbuprenorphine at 10 ng/mL	Norbuprenorphine
Cocaine (benzoylecgonine) at 150 [300] ng/mL	Benzoylecgonine Cocaine Cocaethylene (possibly)
Fentanyl at 1 ng/mL	Fentanyl Norfentanyl
Heroin (morphine) at 300 ng/mL; (6-acetylmorphine) at 10 ng/mL	Morphine 6-Acetylmorphine
Hydrocodone/hydromorphone at 300 ng/mL	Hydrocodone Hydromorphone
Methadone at 300 ng/mL Methadone metabolite (2-ethylidene-1,5-dimethyl-3,3-diphenylpyrrolidine [EDDP]) at 1000 ng/mL	Methadone EDDP
Opiates (morphine) at 300 ng/mL	Morphine Codeine Oxycodone Oxymorphone Hydrocodone Hydromorphone

Table 3-2. Testing Menu for Pain Management (Licit and Illicit Drugs) (continued)

Screening Assays (typical target analyte and cutoff options)	**Confirmation Assays** (drugs currently considered clinically relevant in each drug class)
Oxycodone at 100 ng/mL	Oxycodone Noroxycodone Oxymorphone
Propoxyphene at 300 ng/mL	Propoxyphene Norpropoxyphene
Tetrahydrocannabinol (THC) (Δ^9-THC- carboxylic acid) at 20 (50) (100) ng/mL	Δ^9-THC- carboxylic acid
Tramadol at 200 ng/mL	Tramadol
Others: phencyclidine (PCP), lysergic acid diethylamide (LSD) Serum: salicylate, acetaminophen	—

For example, an opiates assay gives a positive result (using 300 ng/mL cutoff) whether the morphine concentration is 300 ng/mL or 30,000 ng/mL. On the other hand, any drug concentration from 0 to 299 ng/mL will, theoretically, give a negative result. Therefore, it is important to emphasize that a negative result means that the drug, if present at all, is below the concentration at the assay cutoff and does not necessarily mean that the urine is devoid of drug.[22] This limitation of not knowing the concentration of the drug present can lead to inappropriate interpretation of the drug test result, which can have serious clinical implications.

Many immunoassays have been cleared by the FDA to run in a "semiquantitative" mode using assay parameters described in assay package inserts. The laboratory should remind providers that immunoassays detect not only the target analyte (calibrator drug), but also other immunoreactive drugs/metabolites present. Thus, the displayed semiquantitative result in nanograms per milliliter is not the concentration of the calibrator drug, but that of "calibrator equivalents."

Immunoassays Lack Immunospecificity and Specific Identification of Drug(s) Present

An immunoassay will detect all substances that have cross-reactivity with the assay antibody. Thus a positive immunoassay result can be a true positive or a false positive. Therefore, due to this lack of specificity, any positive immunoassay result must be considered a *presumptive* positive. Definitive testing by a more sensitive and specific method is required to determine whether the positive immunoassay result is a true positive or a false positive.

Among the most commonly used immunoassays are those for amphetamines, benzodiazepines, and opiates. These immunoassays detect not only the target analyte drug (calibrator), but also related drugs of that "class." A true-positive result of a class assay, however, does not identify the drug or drugs present. For example, a positive opiates assay result can be due to any of these combinations of opiates: morphine, morphine plus hydromorphone, or morphine plus hydrocodone plus hydromorphone. Consequently, the immunoassay cannot be used to monitor a patient on an opiate prescription for possible abuse of another (nonprescribed) opiate. Detection of such aberrant drug behavior will require ordering the definitive test that is capable of identifying the opiates present.

Immunoassays Lack Analytical Sensitivity

The assay immunoreactivity for a drug determines the analytical sensitivity (detection limit) for that drug. Class immunoassays, such as those for amphetamines, benzodiazepines, and opiates, can detect a large number of drugs or metabolites of that class, but with varying reactivities. For example, the opiates immunoassays will detect, with varying effectiveness, morphine (the target opiate) and other opiates and semisynthetic opiates such codeine, hydromorphone, hydrocodone, oxycodone, oxymorphone, and their metabolites.[26] Consequently, a low-reacting opiate, such as hydromorphone, may give a negative result because its concentration is below its threshold detection limit. One study reported immunoassay-based screens failed to detect 70% of urine samples that were positive for hydromorphone by mass spectrometry when present at low concentrations.[27] Likewise, benzodiazepines immunoassays have varying reactivities for commonly prescribed benzodiazepines.[28-30] Thus, a patient compliant with the dosage regimen can have a negative urine benzodiazepines result that is due to the immunoassay's poor sensitivity for the prescribed drug. This negative result is a clinical false negative in the context of monitoring compliance.[31]

Providers should be informed that drug detection limits do vary among assay manufacturers.[26] Thus, the same urine can test positive or negative depending on where the testing is performed because different laboratories may be using test reagents from different manufacturers. The laboratory should refer to the assay package insert for information on cross-reactivities of related drugs to assess the assay's ability to detect those drugs with low cross-reactivity. The package insert also lists substances that have been tested for possible interference with the assay to cause false-positive results. This information about the assay's specificity is required for proper interpretation of immunoassay test results and should be shared with providers.

Some immunoassays are FDA cleared for more than one cutoff: 1000 and 500 ng/mL cutoffs for the amphetamines assay, 2000 and 300 ng/mL for the opiates assay, and 300 and 150 ng/mL for the cocaine metabolite assay. The higher cutoffs may be too high for use in pain management drug testing. Choosing to use the lower cutoff will increase the detection rate. An FDA-cleared immunoassay can be modified for use with a cutoff below that of established thresholds.[32,33] Any test that is a modification of an FDA-cleared test becomes a laboratory-developed test and will require the laboratory to conduct extensive validation.

The higher opiates assay cutoff of 2000 ng/mL is used in workplace drug testing to minimize opiates positive results due to consumption of poppy seeds contaminated with morphine. Using this higher cutoff, however, is problematic for pain management drug testing because it will miss the detection of those opiate drugs, such as hydromorphone and hydrocodone, that have lower assay immunoreactivity and thus higher detection limits.[27]

Testing Methodology: Definitive Testing by Mass Spectrometry

Definitive assays based on mass spectrometry have the sensitivity and specificity to overcome the limitations of immunoassays described above. Pain management drug testing is clinical testing where confirmation of a positive result in an initial immunoassay is neither mandatory nor always necessary, as is the case with workplace or forensic testing. Ordering definitive testing is at the discretion of the physician (and can be in consultation with the pathologist or laboratory scientist), who may forgo definitive testing if the positive result is clinically expected or when there is no suspicion of aberrant drug behaviors.

Clinically, definitive testing is ordered typically because of one or more of the following clinical scenarios:

- When specific identification of the drug(s) present is necessary
- When a patient's immunoassay test result is negative for the prescribed drug (an unexpected negative; ie, the assay is thought to be able to detect a specific benzodiazepine or opiate that is prescribed to the patient)
- When a patient's immunoassay result is positive for a medication that is not prescribed (an unexpected positive)
- When a patient's immunoassay result is positive for an undisclosed illicit drug such as cocaine
- When the clinician suspects the patient is exhibiting aberrant drug behavior

Definitive testing by mass spectrometry has the following advantages:

- Specific identification of drugs and metabolites present
- Lower drug detection limits
- Quantitative measurement of drug concentrations
- Bypassing immunoassay for first-line testing

Specific Identification of Drug(s)

Definitive tests give specific identification of the drug or drugs present and therefore can confirm immunoassay positives as true positives and eliminate those that are false positives. Moreover, definitive tests will identify all drugs and metabolites of the same class that have contributed to an immunoassay true-positive result. For example, a patient on prescription morphine who is also using nonprescribed hydrocodone will test positive for both morphine and hydrocodone (and hydromorphone) by a definitive test, whereas the opiates immunoassay test will only be reported as positive.[25] In addition, the analytical sensitivity of definitive tests is capable of detecting drugs that are present in the urine of a compliant patient who tests negative with the immunoassays because of the low cross-reactivities of these drugs in immunoassays.[34]

Table 3-3. Opiate and Opioid Metabolites

Opiate/Opioid	Active Metabolites	Nonactive Metabolites
Buprenorphine	Norbuprenorphine	—
Codeine	Morphine Norcodeine Hydrocodone	—
Fentanyl	—	Norfentanyl
Heroin (diacetylmorphine)	6-Monoacetylmorphine Morphine	—
Hydrocodone	Hydromorphone Norhydrocodone Dihydrocodeine	—
Hydromorphone	6β-Hydromorphol	Hydromorphone-3-glucuronide
Levorphanol	Norlevorphanol	Conjugated levorphanol
Meperidine	Normeperidine	—
Morphine	Normorphine Hydromorphone Morphine-6-glucuronide	Morphine-3-glucuronid
Oxycodone	Oxymorphone	Noroxycodone
Pentazocine	*cis*-Hydroxypentazocine *trans*-Carboxypentazocine	—
Propoxyphene	Norpropoxyphene	—
Tramadol	*O*-Desmethyltramadol	Nortramadol

Quantitative Measurement of Drug Concentration

Definitive tests can be developed as quantitative assays to measure drug concentrations. Drug concentration in urine, however, cannot be used to verify compliance with a particular dosing regimen because of interindividual variations in drug absorption, metabolism, excretion, and volume of distribution.[35] Knowing drug concentrations, however, can be useful in determining if the second, unexpected opiate in the urine of a patient on an opiate prescription is due to nonprescription use of the opiate or to it being the minor metabolite of the prescribed opiate. For example, the presence of hydromorphone in the urine of a patient on prescribed morphine can be due to use of nonprescribed hydromorphone or to the hydromorphone being a minor metabolite of morphine.[36-38] Therefore, knowing the relative concentrations of morphine and hydromorphone can be helpful in determining the source of the unexpected hydromorphone. Likewise, for a patient on hydrocodone, a quantitative opiates assay can be helpful in determining the source of the detected hydromorphone, which is a metabolite of hydrocodone. The metabolites of the more common opioids can be seen in Table 3-3.

Pharmaceutical opiates contain low levels (<1.5%) of opiate contaminants that are produced during the manufacturing processes.[25,39] For example, oxycodone can be contaminated with hydrocodone,[40] and morphine can be contaminated with codeine.[41] These contaminants can be detected as unexpected positive results. Thus, hydrocodone, the contaminant of oxycodone, can be detected in a patient on high-dose oxycodone. Again, quantitative measurements of both the prescribed opiate and the unexpected opiate to determine their relative concentrations can differentiate between the two possible sources of hydrocodone.

Definitive First-Line Testing by Mass Spectrometry

The most common approach to performing a urine drug test is initial testing by immunoassays, with the positive results reflexed to definitive testing to eliminate the false positives resulting from the immunospecificity shortcoming of the immunoassays. With pain management drug testing, however, the positivity rate is high, making the screen-then-confirm paradigm inefficient and costly (excessive testing and increased turnaround time). Therefore, for those drugs with high immunoassay positive rates and high confirmation rates (the clinically expected positives that are prescription drugs and their metabolites), bypassing the initial immunoassay screens and going directly to confirmation testing for these drugs is one way to improve efficiency. Moreover, this reasoning is also applicable to those drugs with high clinical false-negative rates by immunoassay because of the low reactivities of the immunoassays for these drugs (eg, the opiates assay and hydrocodone and the benzodiazepines assay and clonazepam).[23,24] Bypassing immunoassays for first-line definitive testing has been shown to significantly improve turnaround time over the traditional screening-then-confirmation approach.[24] In recent years, some laboratories have explored bypassing immunoassays to perform first-line qualitative and quantitative testing by high-resolution mass spectrometry (HRMS) assays.[42-44]

Although modern mass spectrometry instrumentation has greatly improved its user-friendliness, this technology still has significant disadvantages that pose a challenge for its routine use in most clinical laboratories. Additional information on definitive testing by mass spectrometry and the use of HRMS in first-line or targeted testing can be found in chapter 12, *Approaches to Broad-Spectrum Drug Testing in the Clinical Laboratory.*

Interpretation and Consultation

Interpretation of drug test results can be challenging.[45-47] Poor understanding of the metabolism and urinary excretion patterns of the drugs being tested, as well as of the limitations of the analytical methods, may play a role. An incorrect interpretation of drug test results can lead to inappropriate medical decisions, such as discontinuation of opioid therapy or dismissal from a treatment program. The laboratory can play an important role in supporting clinicians to better understand the scientific and technical principles of drug testing and offering assistance regarding optimal test utilization and result interpretation.[48-49] The role of pathologists and laboratory scientists as clinical consultants in laboratory support of pain management is presented in detail in chapter 4, *Clinical Pathology Consultation for Pain Management Services.*

Summary and Conclusions

The expansion of opioid therapy in pain management has increased the demand for urine drug testing and opened new opportunities for the clinical laboratories performing the testing. The laboratory has an important role in the support of chronic opioid therapy. The laboratory must develop a drug testing program that meets the clinical needs of the treatment programs and provide educational and interpretation support to providers so that the appropriate tests are ordered and test results are interpreted correctly.

References

1. Classification of chronic pain: descriptions of chronic pain syndromes and definitions of pain terms. Prepared by the International Association for the Study of Pain, Subcommittee on Taxonomy. *Pain Suppl.* 1986;3:S1-226.
2. Institute of Medicine (US) Committee on Advancing Pain Research, Care and Education. *Relieving Pain in America: A Blueprint for Transforming Prevention, Care, Education, and Research.* Washington, DC: The National Academies Press; 2011.
3. Paulozzi LJ, Mack KA, Hockenberry JM. Vital signs: variation among states in prescribing of opioid pain relievers and benzodiazepines—United States, 2012. *MMWR Morb Mortal Wkly Rep.* 2014;63:563-568.
4. The DAWN Report: Highlights of the 2011 Drug Abuse Warning Network (DAWN) Findings on Drug-Related Emergency Department Visits. Rockville, MD: US Department of Health and Human Services, Substance Abuse and Mental Health Services Administration, Center for Behavioral Health Statistics and Quality. https://www.samhsa.gov/data/sites/default/files/DAWN127/DAWN127/sr127-DAWN-highlights.htm. February 23, 2013. Accessed June 12, 2019.
5. Rudd RA, Aleshire N, Zibbell JE, Gladden RM. Increases in drug and opioid overdose deaths—United States, 2000–2014. *MMWR Morb Mortal Wkly Rep.* 2016;64(50-51);1378-1382.
6. Rudd RA, Seth P, David F, Scholl L. Increases in drug and opioid-involved overdose deaths—United States, 2010–2015. *MMWR Morb Mortal Wkly Rep.* 2016;65(50-51):1445-1452.
7. Jones CM, Einstein EB, Compton WM. Changes in synthetic opioid involvement in drug overdose deaths in the United States, 2010-2016. *JAMA.* 2018;319:1819-1821.

8. HHS acting secretary declares public health emergency to address national opioid crisis. US Department of Health and Human Services. https://www.hhs.gov/about/news/2017/10/26/hhs-acting-secretary-declares-public-health-emergency-address-national-opioid-crisis.html. October 26, 2017. Accessed August 26, 2018.
9. VA/DoD Clinical Practice Guideline for Opioid Therapy for Chronic Pain. Department of Veterans Affairs. Department of Defense. https://www.healthquality.va.gov/guidelines/Pain/cot/VADoDOTCPG022717.pdf. V 3.0 2017. Accessed June 19, 2019.
10. Busse J, ed. The 2017 Canadian Guideline for Opioids for Chronic Non-Cancer Pain. National Pain Center. http://nationalpaincentre.mcmaster.ca/documents/Opioid%20GL%20for%20CMAJ_01may2017.pdf. Accessed June 19, 2019.
11. Wisconsin Medical Examining Board Opioid Prescribing Guideline—April 19, 2018. State of Wisconsin Department of Safety and Professional Services. https://dsps.wi.gov/Documents/BoardCouncils/MED/20180321MEBGuidelinesv8.pdf. April 19, 2018. Accessed June 19, 2019.
12. Interagency Guideline on Prescribing Opioids for Pain. 3rd ed. Washington State Agency Medical Directors' Group. http://www.agencymeddirectors.wa.gov/Files/2015AMDGOpioidGuideline.pdf. June 2015. Accessed June 19, 2019.
13. Manchikanti L, Abdi S, Atluri S, et al. American Society of Interventional Pain Physicians (ASIPP) guidelines for responsible opioid prescribing in chronic non-cancer pain, part 2: guidance. *Pain Physician.* 2012;15(Suppl 3):S67-S116.
14. Utah Clinical Guidelines on Prescribing Opioids for Treatment of Pain. Utah Department of Health. 2009. http://www.health.utah.gov/prescription/pdf/guidelines/final.04.09opioidGuidlines.pdf. Accessed June 19, 2019.
15. Chou R, Fanciullo GJ, Fine PG, Adler JA, Ballentyne JC, et al. Clinical guidelines for the use of chronic opioid therapy in chronic noncancer pain. *J Pain.* 2009;10:113-130.
16. Dowell D, Haegerich TM, Chou R. CDC guideline for prescribing opioids for chronic pain—United States, 2016. *MMWR Morb Mortal Wkly Rep.* 2016;65:1-49.
17. Jarvis M, Williams J, Hurford M, et al. Appropriate use of drug testing in clinical addiction medicine. *J Addiction Med.* 2017;11:163-173.
18. Langman LJ, Jannetto PH, eds. AACC Academy. Laboratory Medicine Practice Guidelines: Using Clinical Laboratory Tests To Monitor Drug Therapy In Pain Management Patients. https://www.aacc.org/-/media/Files/Science-and-Practice/Practice-Guidelines/Pain-Management/LMPGPain-Management20171220.pdf?la=en&hash=19670524407619F78999AB60731A24CB4901939D. Accessed June 19, 2019.
19. Michna E, Jamison R, Pham L, et al. Urine toxicology screening among chronic pain patients on opioid therapy: frequency and predictability of abnormal findings. *Clin J Pain.* 2007:23:173-179.
20. Couto J, Romney M, Leider H, et al. High rates of inappropriate drug use in the chronic pain population. *Popul Health Manag.* 2009;12:185-190.
21. Turner JA, Saunders K, Shortreed SM, et al. Chronic opioid therapy urine drug testing in primary care: prevalence and predictors of aberrant results. *J Gen Int Med.* 2014;29:1663-1671.
22. Kwong TC, Magnani BJ. Urine drug testing in opioid therapy for chronic pain management. In: Kwong TC, Magnani BJ, Rosano TG, Shaw LM, eds. *The Clinical Toxicology Laboratory.* 2nd ed. Washington, DC: AACC Press. 2013:447-458.
23. Melanson SEF, Ptolemy AS, Wason AD. Optimizing urine drug testing for monitoring medication compliance in pain management. *Pain Med.* 2013;14:1813-1820.
24. McMillin GA, Marin SJ, Johnson-Davis, Lawlor BG, Strathmann FG. A hybrid approach to urine drug testing using high-resolution mass spectrometry and select immunoassays. *Am J Clin Pathol.* 2015;143:234-240.
25. Pesce A, West C, Egan City K, Strickland J. Interpretation of urine drug testing in pain patients. *Pain Med.* 2012;13:868-885.
26. Kwong TC, Dasgupta A, Magnani BJ. Drug screening by immunoassays. In: Kwong TC, Magnani BJ, Rosano TG, Shaw LM, eds. *The Clinical Toxicology Laboratory.* 2nd ed. Washington, DC: AACC Press. 2013:411-422.
27. Mikel C, Almazan P, West R, et al. LC-MS/MS extends the range of drug analysis in pain patients. *Ther Drug Monit.* 2009;31:746-748.
28. Mikel C, Pesce AJ, Rosenthal M, West C. Therapeutic monitoring of benzodiazepines in the management of pain: current limitations of point of care immunoassays suggest testing by mass spectrometry to assure accuracy and improve patient safety. *Clin Chim Acta.* 2012;413:1199-1202.
29. Darragh A, Snyder ML, Ptolemy AS, Melanson S. KIMS, CEDIA, and HS-CEDIA immunoassays are inadequately sensitive for detection of benzodiazepines in urine from patients treated for chronic pain. *Pain Physician.* 2014;17:359-366.
30. West R, Pesce A, West C, et al. Comparison of clonazepam compliance by measurement of urinary concentration by immunoassay and LC-MS/MS in pain management population. *Pain Physician.* 2010;13:71-78.
31. Pyle-Eilola AL, Thornton DJ, Hays HL, Casavant MJ. Is this drug screen really negative?: special investigation of drug screening in pediatrics. *J Appl Lab Med.* 2017;1:437-440.

32. Wingert WE. Lowering cutoffs for initial and confirmation testing for cocaine and marijuana: large-scale study of effects on the rates of drug-positive results. *Clin Chem.* 1997;43:100-103.
33. Luzzi VI, Saunders AN, Koenig JW, et al. Analytic performance of immunoassays for drugs of abuse below established cutoff values. *Clin Chem.* 2004;50:717-722.
34. Pesce A, Rosenthal M, West R, et al. An evaluation of the diagnostic accuracy of liquid chromatography-tandem mass spectrometry versus immunoassay drug testing in pain patients. *Pain Physician.* 2010;13:273-281.
35. Nafziger AN, Bertino JS. Utility and application of urine drug testing in chronic pain management with opioids. *Clin J Pain.* 2009;25:73-79.
36. Cone EJ, Caplan YH, Moser F, Robert T, Black D. Evidence that morphine is metabolized to hydromorphone but not to oxycodone. *J Anal Toxicol.* 2008;32:319-323.
37. Wasan AD, Michna E, Janfaza D, Greenfield S, Teter CJ, Jamison RN. Interpreting urine drug tests: prevalence of morphine metabolism to hydromorphone in chronic pain patients treated with morphine. *Pain Med.* 2008;9:918-923.
38. Reisfield GM, Chronister CW, Goldberger BA, Bertholg R. Unexpected urine drug testing results in a hospice patient on high-dose morphine therapy. *Clin Chem.* 2009;55:1765-1769.
39. Haddox JD, Kupper RJ, Cone EJ. Clinical considerations for interpretation of unexpected results from urine drug testing. Poster presented at: 27th Annual Meeting of the American Academy of Pain Medicine; March 24-27, 2011; Washington, DC.
40. West R, West C, Crews B, et al. Anomalous observations of hydrocodone in patients on oxycodone. *Clin Chim Acta.* 2011;412(1-2):29-32.
41. West R, Crews B, Mikel C, et al. Anomalous observations of codeine in patients on morphine. *Ther Drug Monit.* 2009;31(6):776-778.
42. Rasmussen NN, Barker A, Strathmann FG. Lowering the bar for mass spectrometry: a comparison between immunoassay and rapid time-of-flight for presumptive screening of drugs in urine. *J Clin Lab Med.* 2018;2:535-542.
43. Thoren KL, Colby JM, Shugarts SB, Wu AH, Lynch KL. Comparison of information-dependent acquisition on a tandem quadrupole TOF vs a triple quadrupole linear ion trap mass spectrometer for broad-spectrum drug screening. *Clin Chem.* 2016;62:170-178.
44. Colby JM, Thoren KL, Lynch KL. Suspect screening using LC-QqTOF is a useful tool for detecting drugs in biological samples. *J Anal Toxicol.* 2018;42:207-213.
45. Reisfield G, Berthof R, Barkin R, et al. Urine drug test interpretation: what do physicians know? *J Opioid Manag.* 2007;3:80-86.
46. Reisfield G, Webb F, Bertholf R, et al. Family physicians' proficiency in urine drug testing interpretation. *J Opioid Manag.* 2007;6:333-337.
47. Starrels J, Fox A, Kunins H. They don't know what they don't know: internal medicine residents' knowledge and confidence in urine drug test interpretation for patients with chronic pain. *J Gen Intern Med.* 2012; 27:1521-1527.
48. Melanson S, Baskin L, Magnani BJ, et al. Interpretation and utility of drug abuse immunoassays: lessons from laboratory drug testing surveys. *Arch Pathol Lab Med.* 2010;134:735-739.
49. Moeller KE, Kissack JC, Atayee RS, Leey KC. Clinical interpretation of urine drug tests: what clinicians need to know about urine drug screens. *Mayo Clin Proc.* 2017;92:774-796.

Chapter 4

Clinical Pathology Consultation for Pain Management Services

Barbarajean Magnani, PhD, MD
Nicholas Heger, PhD
Tai C. Kwong, PhD

Clinical Pathology Consultations

Drug testing directly falls within the clinical laboratory, and therefore laboratory medicine physicians and scientists have become increasingly involved in growing their role as consultants to clinicians and other providers who manage patients with chronic noncancer pain using opioid medications. The premise behind urine drug testing to monitor patients on chronic opioid therapy is highlighted by several studies (previously discussed in chapter 3, *Laboratory Support of Chronic Opioid Therapy*) that assessed urine specimens collected from pain clinics. These studies have reviewed results from urine drug testing in patients prescribed opioids for their chronic pain with enlightening results.

One retrospective study included 470 pain clinic patients who provided a urine specimen, their current medication list, and the date and time the last medications had been taken.[1] Gas chromatography-mass spectrometry (GC-MS) was utilized for the analysis of the urine specimens, and two clinicians reviewed the results of the testing to determine if there was a correlation between the clinical data and the drug testing results. Of the patients, 55% had "clinically expected results" based on their prescriptions, while 12% of the patient urines did not have the prescribed opioid, 14.4% had an additional prescription drug, and 10.2% did not have the prescribed medication in their urine at all. Twenty-two percent of the urines contained an illicit substance, either cannabis (14.6%), cocaine (6.8%), or heroin (2%), and younger patients were more likely to have illicit substances as well as additional drugs in their urine. Adulteration of the urine (either an abnormal urine creatinine concentration or pH) was identified in 2.3% of patients.

One further study by Couto and colleagues[2] screened more than 900,000 urines from patients on opioid therapy to determine compliance/noncompliance as requested by their treating physician. Immunoassays were used for screening urines, and, if positive, the results were confirmed by either GC-MS or liquid chromatography-tandem mass spectrometry (LC-MS/MS). The results demonstrated that 38% of the urines did not contain the prescribed medication, while 29% had nonprescribed medications, and approximately 11% of the screens detected an illicit drug. However, since confirmatory testing was only performed on positive immunoassay results, it's uncertain as to the extent of their clinical false-negative rate. Even so, taken together these studies support the use of urine drug testing as an objective means of monitoring adherence to opioid therapy for patients with chronic noncancer pain.

Proper interpretation of drug testing results can be challenging to providers.[3] The limitations of the drug testing process (from specimen collection to analysis to reporting) are not fully appreciated by many ordering clinicians. In addition, many practitioners do not have the necessary training to understand specific drug metabolic pathways and pharmacokinetics, much less the limitations of the assays used to obtain the result. This deficit in knowledge may lead to an incorrect interpretation of the results, producing unanticipated consequences for the patient, such as termination of opioid therapy or even dismissal from the treatment program.[4] Several studies have looked at the aptitude of physicians to accurately interpret urine drug screening results and have uncovered a variety of problems with the interpretation.[5,6] Unfortunately, many clinicians fail to seek guidance from laboratory personnel such as pathologists or clinical scientists who are familiar with interpretations. In one study by Reisfield and colleagues,[5] participants at a family medicine course were quizzed on urine drug testing interpretation. None of the physicians were able to answer more than five of the seven questions correctly, and only 20% answered more than half the questions correctly. Further, only 23% of physicians specified that they would consult the laboratory if they received unexpected or abnormal findings on their patient. This statistic underscores the need for pathologists and laboratory scientists to promote themselves as a valuable resource for interpretation of urine drug testing results.

In a related study, the knowledge and confidence of urine drug test interpretation was assessed in internal medicine residents in training at an academic medical center using a similar tool.[6] The residents were tested with seven knowledge questions used in a previously published study by Reisfield and colleagues.[3,5] These questions presented a short scenario of a patient using various medications for pain management, or other substances, and then queried the reader to identify the expected compounds in the urine. For example:

- A patient taking an acetaminophen/codeine medication might have which of the following substances in their urine: codeine, morphine, oxycodone?
- In a patient using heroin, what substances would be expected in the urine: heroin, hydromorphone, morphine?

The internal medicine residents were also evaluated for their confidence in their ability to correctly interpret urine drug testing results. This survey revealed that the knowledge score mean was only three out of seven. While 55% of the residents felt confident in their ability to correctly interpret test results, 73% of the confident residents had a knowledge score of three or lower.[6] Although these surveys were several years ago, the gap in urine drug testing interpretation may still exist.

The pathologist or laboratory scientist, as the one who is conducting the testing, is obligated to work with clinicians ordering the drug tests to provide guidance on test utilization as well as result interpretation. The College of American Pathologists (CAP) offers interpretive challenges in their DMPM (Drug Monitoring for Pain Management) proficiency testing survey (see appendix E, *CAP Proficiency Testing Surveys for Toxicology*) by presenting clinical cases with drug testing results. Laboratory scientists and pathologists are asked to interpret the findings and determine if they are consistent with the patient's current medication and clinical scenario. These surveys provide educational challenges to help laboratory testing personnel learn how to render consultations for patients on chronic opioid therapy.

Establishing an open dialogue between treating clinicians and laboratory physicians/scientists is essential for understanding urine drug testing results that do not appear to support the patient's clinical state. Clinicians challenged with drug test interpretation should be able to turn to laboratory professionals for guidance and clarification.[4,7]

In some cases, a clinical pathology consultation may be warranted. When providing this service, the most appropriate CPT code is CPT 80500 or 80502.[8] Only a physician can provide a billable consultation and must fulfill the criteria as outlined: "A clinical pathology consultation is a service including a written report, rendered by the pathologist in response to a request from a physician or qualified health care professional in relation to a test result(s) requiring additional medical interpretive judgment. Report of a test result(s) without interpretive judgment is not considered a clinical pathology consultation." An 80500 consultation is limited, without review of the patient's history and medical records, while an 80502 consultation is comprehensive, for a complex diagnostic problem, with review of the patient's history and medical records. These consultations are also applicable for pharmacokinetic issues. An 80502 consultation should state the patient's problem, list of medications, results of drug testing, and an assessment of what the results mean (eg, consistent, not consistent with current medications) and/or recommendations for further monitoring or testing. Information derived from software programs about drug interactions may also be included and may be helpful to the ordering practitioner. For cases of clinical pathology (CP) consultations, see examples at the end of this chapter.

There are occasions where the treating physician can be helped with test result interpretation by a simple email or phone conversation, rather than a complex CP consultation. For example, the metabolism of certain benzodiazepines often produces confusing reports since many metabolites are themselves prescription medications (see Figure 4-1). Treating physicians may obtain results that appear inconsistent with the prescribed medication but are in fact consistent because the reported drug may be a metabolite of the prescribed medication. For example, a response to the statement from the practitioner, "My patient's report showed he took Serax (oxazepam) and I did not prescribe that," might be as follows:

> Dr. Jones,
>
> Regarding your patient's results: The definitive assay for benzodiazepines identified the presence of the benzodiazepine oxazepam (Serax). Please note that oxazepam is also a metabolite of temazepam (Restoril), clorazepate (Tranxene), and can sometimes be a minor metabolite of diazepam (Valium).
>
> Please call me if you have any further questions.

This same scenario is very common with prescribed opiates and opioids, and their metabolites. Definitive testing demonstrating the presence of hydrocodone and hydromorphone will be confusing if one is unaware that hydrocodone is metabolized to hydromorphone. Recently, studies have demonstrated that patients on high-dose morphine therapy for cancer pain have had small quantities of hydromorphone detected in their urine.[9-11] The patient may be suspected of obtaining unauthorized hydromorphone if the treating physician is unaware of the metabolic conversions (Figure 4-2). Investigations to date have shown hydromorphone to be less than 6% of the urinary morphine concentration in these cases, whereas higher

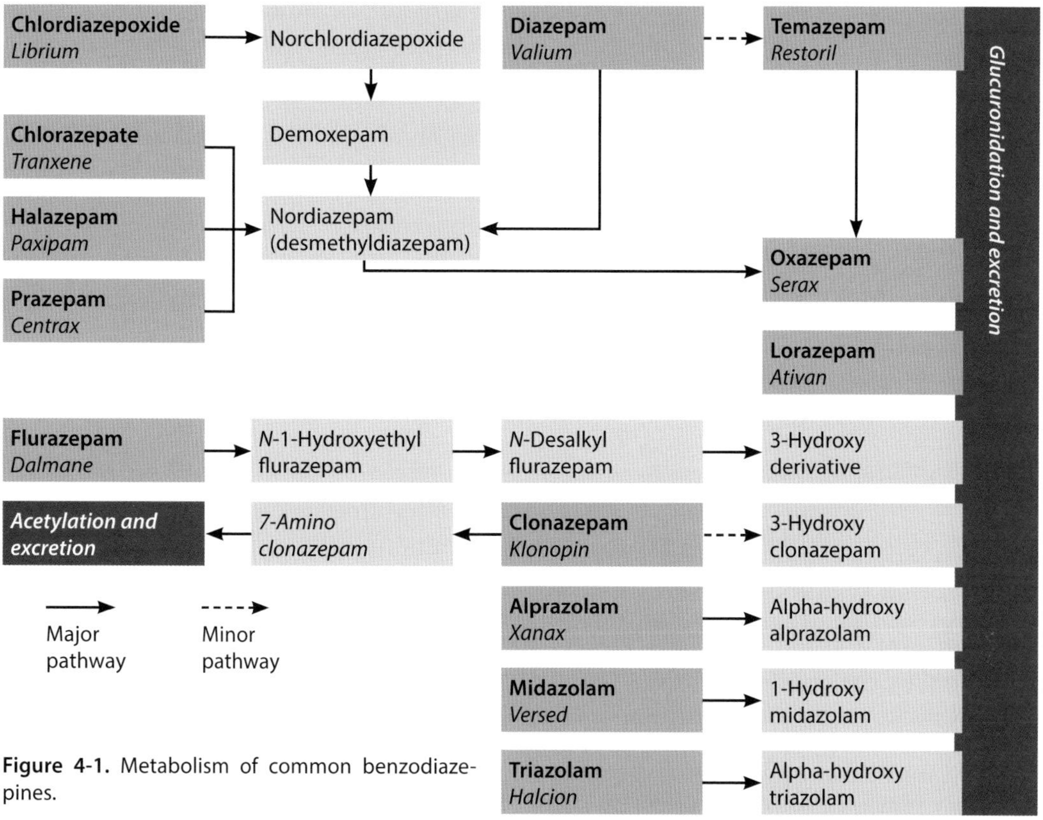

Figure 4-1. Metabolism of common benzodiazepines.

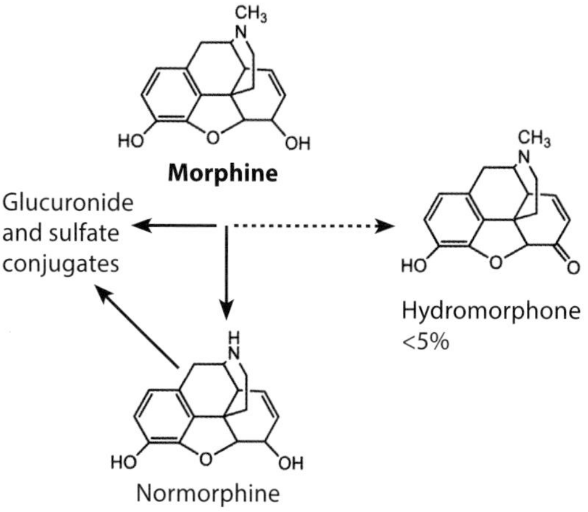

Figure 4-2. Metabolic pathways of morphine. Morphine is primarily excreted in the urine as glucuronide and sulfate conjugates. Small amounts of hydromorphone (<5% of the total morphine concentration) have been observed after administration of morphine in high doses (typically >150 mg/day for females and >200 mg/day for males).[9]

Table 4-1. Urinary Excretion Kinetics of Oxycodone (20-mg Dose)[16]

Time (hours)	Oxymorphone (ng/mL)	Oxycodone (ng/mL)
0	0	0
2.8	4714	9958
6.6	4393	5925
8.8	2457	2447
12/24	1006	679
24/36	524	283
36/48	425	21
48/60	132	0
60/72	60	0
72/84	38	0
84/96	34	0
96/108	0	0

percentages suggest administration of hydromorphone. Similarly, one may question whether oxycodone was spiked into the urine at collection or is being ingested by the patient as prescribed; the presence of the metabolite oxymorphone and or noroxycodone, particularly in conjunction with the parent compound oxycodone, is evidence that the patient is taking the drug (see Table 4-1).

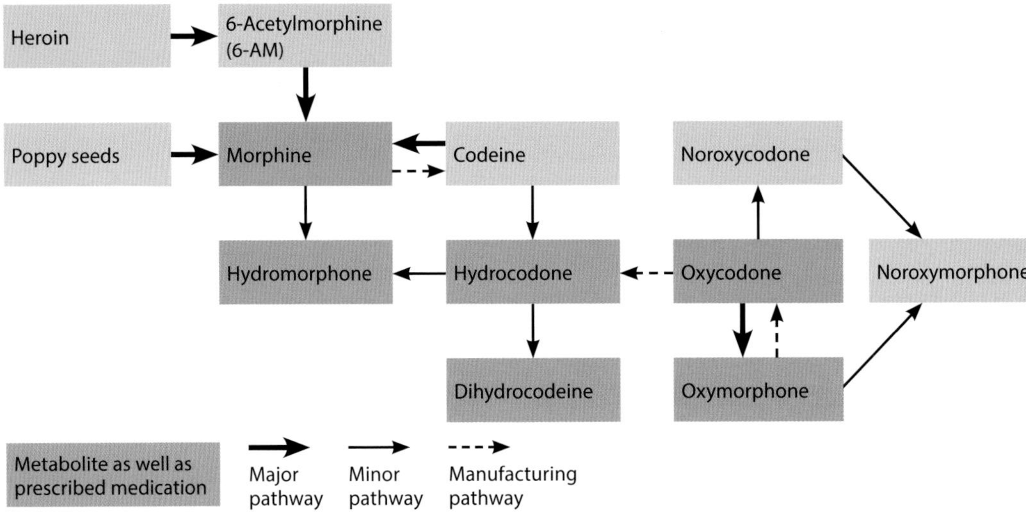

Figure 4-3. Metabolism of opiates/opioids.

For patients given morphine or codeine who may have previously abused heroin, confusion may occur if the definitive toxicology report states that both morphine and 6-acetylmorphine (6-AM) are found in the urine. The treating physician expects morphine as a metabolite but is unsure of the metabolite 6-AM, thinking it may be an expected metabolite of either morphine or codeine; it is not and in fact is only seen in patients abusing heroin, because heroin (diacetylmorphine) is first metabolized to 6-AM, with subsequent conversion to morphine (Figure 4-3). The window for detecting 6-AM is short: the average plasma half-life for heroin is 1 to 4 minutes and approximately 3 to 52 minutes for 6-AM.[12] Given the short half-life, it is possible for heroin abusers to have morphine present in the urine, but not 6-AM. Conversely, there are some patients who may have 6-AM in the urine with morphine concentrations less than 300 ng/mL, the opiates immunoassay cutoff used in most clinical laboratories.[13] Thus, testing for 6-AM can improve the detection of heroin use. Some immunoassays detect 6-AM in addition to morphine and codeine, and specific immunoassays for just 6-AM are available. The more common metabolites of the opiates/opioids can be seen in Table 4-2. When providing consultations, it is imperative to be able to explain the metabolic pathways and metabolites.

The urine opiates immunoassay is primarily designed to detect morphine and codeine, and to a lesser extent the semisynthetic opioids (depending on the assay used), while the synthetic opioids are not detected at all (see chapter 11, *Laboratory-Based Screening Assays in Support of Pain Management*). For example, the opiates immunoassay screen is negative for patients taking fentanyl. Thus, the laboratory may need to establish additional specific immunoassay screens or perform definitive testing. Examples of specific immunoassays include oxycodone (which is variably detected by the opiates assay), methadone, tramadol, buprenorphine, and fentanyl because these analytes are not detected with the traditional opiates immunoassay. However, in some cases the opiates immunoassay screen may be positive, but definitive testing is negative. Definitive testing may not include all well-characterized opioids. For example, opioid/opiates drugs included in a definitive testing panel may be laboratory specific and targeted to only certain drugs. Newly emerging designer opioids, which may cross-react with the opiates class immunoassay to produce a positive result, would not likely be included in definitive testing. For example, the typical definitive assay for fentanyl specifically identifies fentanyl and its metabolite norfentanyl. It does not identify acetylfentanyl, acrylfentanyl, butyrfentanyl, or other analogues of fentanyl that may cross-react with the fentanyl immunoassay screen.[14] Therefore, although the definitive testing was negative for fentanyl, other fentanyl derivatives may not be ruled out if the immunoassay screen was positive. These considerations may need to be addressed on a case-by-case basis and upon the knowledge that certain drugs/analogues may be prevalent in a particular geographical area.

Occasionally a request may be received to use a biological specimen other than urine for testing. The drugs discussed in this book are measured in other specimens, such as blood, oral fluid, sweat, hair, and nails, but these should be used with an understanding of their limitations (see specific chapters). The shortest windows of detection are seen

Table 4-2. Opiate and Opioid Metabolites

Opiate/Opioid	Active Metabolites	Nonactive Metabolites
Buprenorphine	Norbuprenorphine	—
Codeine	Morphine Norcodeine Hydrocodone	—
Fentanyl	—	Norfentanyl
Heroin (diacetylmorphine)	6-Monoacetylmorphine Morphine	—
Hydrocodone	Hydromorphone Norhydrocodone Dihydrocodeine	—
Hydromorphone	6β-Hydromorphol	Hydromorphone-3-glucuronide
Levorphanol	Norlevorphanol	Conjugated levorphanol
Meperidine	Normeperidine	—
Morphine	Normorphine Hydromorphone Morphine-6-glucuronide	Morphine-3-glucuronid
Oxycodone	Oxymorphone	Noroxycodone
Pentazocine	*cis*-Hydroxypentazocine *trans*-Carboxypentazocine	—
Propoxyphene	Norpropoxyphene	—
Tramadol	*O*-Desmethyltramadol	Nortramadol

with blood and oral fluid. As discussed in chapter 3, *Laboratory Support of Chronic Opioid Therapy,* blood is not an optimal specimen because many of the drugs for which testing is performed in the pain management setting have short half-lives and may be difficult to detect. Although the use of oral fluid as a specimen has gained favor recently, the pharmacokinetic profiles for many of the drugs in this matrix parallel that of the drugs in blood. Sweat has been used primarily for monitoring abstinence, not compliance. The longest windows of detection can be seen using hair and nails, and although these have been used to detect use of a drug, neither are good matrices for monitoring issues of compliance.

One of the few scenarios in which blood or oral fluid may be useful is in the testing of the patient with poor renal function. Another type of case in which serum measurements have been useful is that of the patient receiving fentanyl via a patch who has unexpectedly low fentanyl concentrations upon confirmation and who states that a new patch is needed more frequently than expected. A serum measurement at the end of the dosing cycle just before application of a new patch could confirm the patient's report.

Summary and Conclusions

The expansion of pain management in the United States has increased the demand for urine drug testing and opened new opportunities for the clinical laboratories performing the testing, as well as for the pathologist and laboratory scientist who may be called upon to provide expertise in the utilization of the tests and in interpretation of the results. To most effectively provide these services, pathologists and laboratory scientists must couple a solid knowledge of the drugs' pharmacokinetic and metabolic pathways with an understanding of the analytical methods.

■ ■ ■

Clinical Pathology Consultations

These consultations have been modified in order to protect patients' health information.

Case 1

Clinical Pathology Consultation

Comprehensive Review of patient's history and medical records 80502; complex diagnostic problem

Patient: NAME and MRN

Diagnosis: Chronic pain: opioid-requiring (ICD10-F11.20)

The patient is a 70-year-old female with a history of hypertension, migraines, depression, degenerative joint disease, and chronic pancreatitis. The patient also complains of chronic pain and stiffness in her joints. In June she fractured her right foot and is currently wearing a boot. She currently takes Dilaudid (hydromorphone) and MS Contin (morphine) for pain. During a recent visit with her primary care doctor, a urine drug screen was performed and found to be presumptively positive for buprenorphine, methadone, THC-cannabinoids, and opiates. The patient's physician has requested a formal toxicology consultation in light of the unexpected positive buprenorphine and methadone results.

Past Medical History (per EMR)

Pain, hand
Wrist drop
Headache
Chronic pain: opioid-requiring
Chronic pain opioid: 2 week refill
Hypertension
Pancreatitis, chronic
Dependence, continuous; MS Contin for chronic pancreatitis
Degenerative joint disease, hands
Pelvic pain
Peripheral neuropathy
Tobacco abuse
Migraine, classical
Depression

Social History (per EMR)

Tobacco: Current smoker, less than 1 pack per day.
Alcohol: Rarely.
Illicit drugs: Marijuana.

Medication List

Dilaudid 8 mg tabs (hydromorphone HCL) 1-4 tabs every 4 hours as needed for pain (max 8 day)
MS Contin 60 mg tb12 (morphine sulfate) 1 tablet 3 times a day
Atenolol 50 mg tabs (atenolol) take 1 tablet by mouth daily
Norvasc 10 mg tabs (amlodipine besylate) take 1 tablet by mouth daily
Lyrica 150 mg caps (pregabalin) 1 tab twice a day
Evista 60 mg tabs (raloxifene HCL) take 1 tablet by mouth once daily
Cyclobenzaprine hcl 10 mg tabs (cyclobenzaprine HCL) once a day as needed for muscle spasms
Omeprazole 20 mg cpdr (omeprazole) take 1 capsule by mouth twice daily
Ranitidine hcl 150 mg tabs (ranitidine HCL) take 1 tablet at bedtime

LABORATORY DATA:

Urine Toxicology Screen (immunoassay)

Urine collected (DATE)	
Amphetamines	Not Detected
Barbiturates	Not Detected
Benzodiazepines	Not Detected
THC-Cannabinoids	DETECTED
Cocaine	Not Detected
Ethanol	Not Detected
Methadone	DETECTED
Opiates	DETECTED
Oxycodone	Not Detected
Buprenorphine	DETECTED

Definitive Urine Toxicology Lab Results

Methadone quantitative, urine (LC-MS/MS) (Laboratory where testing was performed)

Urine collected (DATE)	Limit of Detection: 100 ng/mL
Methadone	2500 ng/mL
EDDP (methadone metabolite)	12000 ng/mL

Definitive Urine Toxicology Lab Results

Opiates expanded, urine (LC-MS/MS) (Laboratory where testing was performed)

Urine collected (DATE)	Limit of Detection: 50 ng/mL
Codeine	Negative
Hydrocodone	Negative
Hydromorphone	1700 ng/mL
Morphine	>15000 ng/mL
Norhydrocodone	Negative
Noroxycodone	Negative
Oxycodone	Negative
Oxymorphone	Negative

Definitive Urine Toxicology Lab Results

Heroin metabolite, urine (LC-MS/MS)
(Laboratory where testing was performed)

Urine collected (DATE)	Limit of Detection: 10 ng/mL
6-Acetylmorphine (heroin metabolite)	Negative

Definitive Toxicology Lab Results

Buprenorphine quantitative, urine (LC-MS/MS)
(Laboratory where testing was performed)

Urine collected (DATE)	Limit of Detection: 2 ng/mL
Buprenorphine	Negative
Norbuprenorphine	Negative

ASSESSMENT:

Methadone

The urine immunoassay drug screen performed on the specimen collected on (DATE) tested presumptively positive for methadone. Definitive testing by LC-MS/MS (liquid chromatography-tandem mass spectrometry) identified both methadone (2500 ng/mL) and the primary metabolite EDDP (12000 ng/mL), confirming in vivo metabolism of methadone. Methadone is a synthetic opioid used to treat opioid abuse and withdrawal symptoms as well as for chronic pain. Methadone has a long half-life (15-55 hours) and is detectable in urine for several days after the final dose.

Opiates

The in-house urine immunoassay drug screen performed on the specimen collected on (DATE) tested presumptively positive for opiates. This immunoassay is designed to cross-react with the naturally occurring opiates codeine and morphine, producing a positive result at concentrations of ≥150 ng/mL and ≥300 ng/mL, respectively. Definitive testing by LC-MS/MS identified morphine (>15000 ng/mL) and hydromorphone (1700 ng/mL) only. No other common opiates/opioids were detected (ie, codeine, hydrocodone, norhydrocodone, oxycodone, oxymorphone, noroxycodone).

Morphine can be found in urine following administration of morphine itself (eg, MS Contin) or as the metabolite of either codeine or heroin. The concentration of morphine found in the urine (>15000 ng/mL) is consistent with administration of morphine prior to the urine collection. Morphine has a half-life of 2 to 7 hours, and can be detected in the urine up to 2 to 3 days after the last dose. In light of the unexpected methadone immunoassay result and elevated morphine concentration, the urine sample collected on (DATE) was sent for definitive testing for heroin metabolites. The result of this analysis did not detect the heroin metabolite 6-acetylmorphine (6-AM). However, the absence of 6-AM does not rule out heroin use. Heroin, or diacetylmorphine, has an extremely short half-life (1-4 minutes) and is rapidly metabolized to 6-AM. 6-AM is also metabolized relatively quickly (3-52 minutes) to morphine.

Hydromorphone is a semisynthetic opioid (sold as Dilaudid) and is a major metabolite of hydrocodone (Vicodin) and a minor metabolite of morphine. Hydromorphone in the urine is consistent with administration of Dilaudid prior to the urine collection. However, given the concentration of hydromorphone was 1700 ng/mL, it is not possible to exclude that the hydromorphone is a metabolite of morphine. Hydromorphone has a plasma half-life of up to 9 hours and can be detected in urine 2 to 3 days after the last dose. Detection in the urine is dependent on both elimination patterns and the hydration status of the patient.

Note: Definitive testing did not include all well-characterized opiates/opioids (and as yet any newly emerging designer opioids) that may cross-react with the in-house opiates class immunoassay to produce a positive result. As such, it not possible to exclude administration of other opiates/opioids not specifically tested for here.

Buprenorphine

The in-house urine immunoassay drug screen performed on the specimen collected on (DATE) tested presumptively positive for buprenorphine. Definitive testing LC-MS/MS did not detect either buprenorphine or the primary metabolite norbuprenorphine. The buprenorphine immunoassay is not expected to cross-react with other individual opiates/opioids taken by this patient at low concentrations (ie, hydromorphone, methadone, morphine). However, when taken in combination, or at high concentrations (such as morphine or codeine), these opiates may be sufficient to produce a positive buprenorphine result. These findings suggest that the positive buprenorphine immunoassay result is a false positive. Buprenorphine is a semisynthetic opioid sold under the trade names Subutex (buprenorphine), Suboxone (buprenorphine and naloxone combination) and Butrans (transdermal patch), marketed for the treatment of opioid addiction. Due to its powerful analgesic and euphoric effects, buprenorphine may be abused or substituted for heroin or other opioids.

THC-Cannabinoids

The in-house urine immunoassay drug screen performed on the specimen collected on (DATE) tested presumptively positive for THC-cannabinoids.

Definitive testing was not performed. The in-house immunoassay detects metabolites of delta-9-tetrahydrocannabinol (THC), the primary psychoactive component of marijuana. The patient's urine may be positive for 2 to 7 days after use or for up to 1 month in chronic smokers.

CONCLUSION:

In conclusion, the patient's toxicology results are not consistent with the prescribed medications. The positive immunoassay methadone result, as confirmed by LC-MS/MS, indicates administration of methadone prior to the urine collection. Definitive testing for opiates identified morphine and hydromorphone, consistent with the patient's prescriptions for MS Contin and Dilaudid, respectively, although one cannot exclude the possibility of hydromorphone as a morphine metabolite.

Definitive testing for buprenorphine was negative, indicating that the urine immunoassay buprenorphine result was a false positive, most likely attributable to cross-reactivity of the combined effect of the other opioids present in the urine. Definitive testing for THC-cannabinoids was not performed. Further investigation into the patient's possible use of unprescribed drugs should be explored.

Pathologist's Name: ____________________, MD
Department of Pathology and Laboratory Medicine
DATE and TIME STAMP

Pearls

- With urine drug immunoassays, it is important to be familiar with cross-reactivity of both related and unrelated drugs, keeping in mind that a positive result may be attributable to the presence of one (or more than one) drug in the sample. An up-to-date and complete medication list of both prescribed and unprescribed drugs is essential.
- The absence of 6-AM in definitive testing does not exclude the possibility of heroin use. As heroin is metabolized rapidly to 6-AM and then relatively quickly to morphine, the absence of 6-AM may be a consequence of the time interval between last heroin use and urine collection. Similarly, the presence of morphine is not indicative of heroin use, as it may be the result of use of morphine-containing drugs, or as the metabolite of codeine, or consumption of contaminated poppy seeds. Avoid insinuation and overinterpretation regarding possible heroin use whenever 6-AM is not detected with definitive testing. Specific immunoassays for 6-AM are available.
- High concentrations of morphine (and codeine) can cross-react with buprenorphine immunoassays and produce a positive result.[15]

Case 2

Clinical Pathology Consultation

Comprehensive Review of patient's history and medical records 80502; complex diagnostic problem

Patient: NAME and MRN

Diagnosis: Opioid dependence with withdrawal (ICD10-F11.23)

The patient is a 30-year-old male with a past medical history of IV drug use, cardiomyopathy, recurrent pleural and pericardial effusion, and end-stage renal disease on dialysis. Outpatient hemodialysis in September with weekly drug screens were conducted to assess compliance with buprenorphine therapy. This continued until June of the following year when the hemodialysis catheter was replaced with a peritoneal dialysis catheter. At that time, outpatient dialysis was transferred to (HOSPITAL A), and weekly serum drug screening was not continued. The patient notes that he started using heroin in late August and denies use of other drugs, including cocaine, alcohol, and marijuana. He now presents to (HOSPITAL B) with symptoms of acute opioid withdrawal and the intention to enter an inpatient treatment program that will allow him to continue with peritoneal dialysis. The toxicology service was contacted to help determine what drugs the patient may have been taking in the time leading up to his current admission.

Past Medical History (per EMR)
IV drug use (heroin), on Suboxone
Cardiomyopathy
Pleural effusion
Pericardial effusion
End-stage renal disease (anuria)

Social History (per EMR)
The patient lives at home with his parents.
Denies using alcohol, marijuana, or cocaine.

Medication List (per email from CARE GIVER on DATE)
Acetaminophen
Amiodarone
Amlodipine
Gentamicin
Losartan
Metoprolol succinate
Buprenorphine-naloxone (Suboxone)

LABORATORY DATA:

Definitive Serum Toxicology Lab Results

General Toxicology Screen by LC-MS Q-Trap
(Laboratory where testing was performed)

Serum collected DATE	Result	Limit of Detection (ng/mL)
Cotinine (nicotine metabolite)	DETECTED	50
Acetaminophen	DETECTED	250
Gabapentin (Neurontin)	DETECTED	250
Fentanyl	DETECTED	10
Norfentanyl (fentanyl metabolite)	DETECTED	50
Lorazepam (Ativan)	DETECTED	100

Pertinent negative results include: 6-AM, morphine, buprenorphine, norbuprenorphine, methadone, EDDP, MDMA, amphetamine, methamphetamine, cocaine, benzoylecgonine, THC, metoprolol. For all drugs tested, see our online test directory.

Note: Drugs that fall below a cut-off concentration are reported as not detected; however, this does not necessarily mean the specimen is devoid of the specific drug.

ASSESSMENT:

Comprehensive toxicology testing was performed for this patient to identify the presence of a wide variety of prescribed and nonprescribed medications. Urine is the preferred matrix for detection of drugs as detection times are longer. Given that this patient is anuric, blood was collected shortly after admission and the serum was analyzed. Patients with altered renal function can exhibit altered drug disposition compared with patients with normal renal function. Length of time for detection can be affected by dosing interval, time since last dialysis, and other factors.

Cotinine

The broad-spectrum serum toxicology screen detected the presence of cotinine. Cotinine is the metabolite of nicotine and its presence is consistent with the use of tobacco products.

Acetaminophen

The broad-spectrum serum toxicology screen detected the presence of acetaminophen. The presence of acetaminophen may be attributed to administration of acetaminophen itself or an acetaminophen-containing drug at some point prior to the blood draw.

Gabapentin

The broad-spectrum serum toxicology screen detected the presence of gabapentin. Gabapentin, sold as Neurontin, is an analog of gamma-aminobutyric acid (GABA) and is prescribed for neuropathic pain and as an anticonvulsant. In patients with normal renal function, gabapentin is known to have a long half-life of up to 40 hours. The presence of gabapentin in the serum is consistent with administration of this drug at some point prior to the blood draw. Gabapentin is also known to be a widely abused drug.

Opioids (fentanyl and buprenorphine)

The broad-spectrum serum toxicology screen detected the presence of fentanyl and its metabolite norfentanyl. Fentanyl is a powerful synthetic opioid analgesic. According to the CDC, fentanyl is estimated to be 80 times more potent than morphine and more potent than heroin. Fentanyl may be administered in a variety of forms, including as a transdermal patch, nasal spray, sublingual spray, lozenges, or an injectable solution. Substitution of fentanyl for heroin in street preparations of this drug may lead to overdose due to the difference in potency. In patients with normal renal function, fentanyl has a half-life of up to 12 hours. The presence of fentanyl and norfentanyl is consistent with use of this drug prior to the blood draw. According to the medical record, the patient states that he last used "heroin" at 11 PM on (DATE). Following heroin use, the expected finding is the presence of the heroin-specific metabolite 6-acetylmorphine and its downstream metabolite morphine. Neither of these drugs was detected in the broad-spectrum analysis (limit of detection for both 6-acetylmorphine and morphine is 50 ng/mL). Therefore, it is most likely that the patient used fentanyl only prior to the blood draw.

The broad-spectrum serum toxicology screen DID NOT detect the presence of buprenorphine (limit of detection 500 ng/mL) or its metabolite norbuprenorphine (limit of detection 100 ng/mL). The absence of these drugs suggests that the patient has not recently taken buprenorphine. Buprenorphine is a semisynthetic opioid sold under the trade names Subutex (buprenorphine) and Suboxone (buprenorphine and naloxone combination), and is marketed for the treatment of opioid addiction. It is also used to treat moderately severe pain. Due to its powerful analgesic and euphoric effects, buprenorphine may be abused or substituted for heroin or other opioids. The serum half-life of buprenorphine in patients with normal renal function is approximately 37 hours. According to the Prescription Drug Monitoring Program, the patient has regularly picked up his prescription for Suboxone.

Benzodiazepines

The broad-spectrum serum toxicology screen detected the presence of lorazepam. Lorazepam (Ativan) is an intermediate-acting benzodiazepine with a serum half-life of 9 to 16 hours in patients with normal renal function. Detection of this drug is consistent with administration of lorazepam at some point prior to the blood draw. According to the Prescription Drug Monitoring Program, the patient has an active prescription for lorazepam.

CONCLUSION:

In conclusion, broad-spectrum serum toxicology testing was performed to identify prescribed and nonprescribed medications present upon the patient's arrival at (HOSPITAL B). The presence of fentanyl and its metabolite norfentanyl is consistent with the use of fentanyl prior to the blood (serum) collection. The absence of metabolites of heroin suggests that the patient most recently used fentanyl rather than heroin prior to admission. The presence of lorazepam is consistent with the patient's prescription. The presence of gabapentin (Neurontin) indicates that the patient used this drug prior to the blood collection. Further investigation into the patient's possible use of unprescribed drugs should be explored.

The absence of buprenorphine, despite an active prescription per the Prescription Drug Monitoring Program, suggests that the patient has not taken his prescription for Suboxone recently. Alternative scenarios should be considered, such as intermittent dosing, noncompliance, or prescription diversion.

Pathologist's Name: ____________________, MD
Department of Pathology and Laboratory Medicine
DATE and TIME STAMP

Pearls

- In anuric patients, alternate forms of assessment can be used, including testing of blood (serum), oral fluid, fingernails, or hair. Pathologists and laboratory scientists should be familiar with the limitations of each matrix and interpret the findings within the clinical context. Also, patients with altered renal function may exhibit differences in drug metabolism or pharmacokinetics, which adds an additional layer of complexity in the interpretation of results.
- When the patient's medication list or history of drug use is unclear (patient unable to communicate, medical record unavailable, etc), direct to definitive testing for a broad panel of various drug classes and compounds may be helpful.

Case 3

Clinical Pathology Consultation

Comprehensive Review of patient's history and medical records 80502; complex diagnostic problem

Patient: NAME and MRN

Diagnosis: Opioid use disorder, severe (ICD10-F11.20)

The patient is a 40-year-old man with a history of newly diagnosed heart failure. He presented to the hospital after experiencing dyspnea upon exertion and swelling in his legs. During his admission, he was found to have a 20% ejection fraction and diagnosed with heart failure. He is currently being evaluated for a heart transplant. The patient also has a previous history of hepatitis C and intravenous drug abuse, and states he has been clean for 10 years. During the patient's stay, a urine drug screen was performed and found to be presumptively positive for benzodiazepines, THC-cannabinoids, opiates, and oxycodone. The patient's physician has requested a formal toxicology consultation in light of the multiple positive urine drug screen results.

Past Medical History (per EMR)

Acute systolic (congestive) heart failure
Pneumonia, unspecified organism
Nicotine dependence, cigarettes, uncomplicated
Adjustment disorder with mixed anxiety and depressed mood
Opioid use disorder, severe

Social History (per EMR)

Family: Lived with girlfriend.
Tobacco: Prior smoker, quit "a few weeks ago."
Alcohol: Denies.
Illicit drugs: Former heroin user, but states he has been clean for 10 years. States he has been taking nonprescribed Percocet (acetaminophen-oxycodone combination; dosage unknown) for recent flank pain.

Medication List (per email from CARE GIVER)

Aspirin 81 mg by mouth daily
Carvedilol 6.25 mg by mouth, twice a day BID
Furosemide 80 mg by mouth, twice a day BID
Metolazone 5 mg by mouth as needed for shortness of breath
Nicotine 21 mg/24 hour patch, 1 patch daily

LABORATORY DATA:

Urine Toxicology Screen (immunoassay)

Urine collected DATE	
Amphetamines	Not Detected
Barbiturates	Not Detected
Benzodiazepines	DETECTED
THC-Cannabinoids	DETECTED
Cocaine	Not Detected
Ethanol	Not Detected
Methadone	Not Detected
Opiates	DETECTED
Oxycodone	DETECTED
Buprenorphine	Not Detected

Definitive Urine Toxicology Lab Results

Opiates expanded, urine (LC-MS/MS)
(Laboratory where testing was performed))

Urine collected DATE	Limit of Detection: 50 ng/mL
Codeine	Negative
Hydrocodone	Negative
Hydromorphone	1000 ng/mL
Morphine	4600 ng/mL
Norhydrocodone	Negative
Noroxycodone	920 ng/mL
Oxycodone	600 ng/mL
Oxymorphone	10000 ng/mL

Send-Out Urine Toxicology Lab Results

Benzodiazepines, urine (LC-MS/MS)
(Laboratory where testing was performed)

Urine collected DATE	Result	Limit of Detection (ng/mL)
Alphahydroxyalprazolam	Negative	25
Alphahydroxymidazolam	580 ng/mL	50
Alphahydroxytriazolam	Negative	50
Aminoclonazepam	Negative	25
Hydroxyethylflurazepam	Negative	50
Lorazepam	Negative	50
Nordiazepam	Negative	50
Oxazepam	Negative	50
Temazepam	Negative	50

ASSESSMENT:

Opiates and oxycodone

The in-house urine immunoassay drug screen performed on the specimen collected on (DATE) tested presumptively positive for opiates and oxycodone. Definitive testing by LC-MS/MS (liquid chromatography-tandem mass spectrometry) identified morphine (4600 ng/mL), hydromorphone (1000 ng/mL), oxycodone (600 ng/mL), oxymorphone (10000 ng/mL), and noroxycodone (920 ng/mL).

Morphine can be found in urine following administration of morphine itself (eg, MS Contin) or as the metabolite of heroin or codeine or after consumption of contaminated poppy seeds. Supplementary testing for the heroin-specific metabolite 6-acetylmorphine (6-AM) was not performed. Morphine has a serum half-life of approximately 2 to 7 hours and may be detected in the urine up to 2 to 3 days after the last dose

Hydromorphone is a semisynthetic opioid (sold as Dilaudid) and is a metabolite of hydrocodone (Vicodin). The presence of a small concentration of hydromorphone in the absence of hydrocodone and norhydrocodone may be the result of administration of hydromorphone itself or a waning dose of hydrocodone from several days prior. Of note, hydromorphone is also a very minor metabolite of morphine. The concentration of hydromorphone found in the urine specimen is not likely attributable to administration of morphine. Hydromorphone has a plasma half-life of up to 9 hours and can be detected in urine 2 to 3 days after the last dose.

Oxycodone in the urine, along with the active metabolite oxymorphone and inactive metabolite noroxycodone, is the expected finding in a patient taking oxycodone (Percocet) prior to the urine collection. Oxycodone is a semisynthetic opioid and is sold as both a stand-alone drug (OxyContin, Roxicodone) or in combination with acetaminophen (Percocet), aspirin (Percodan), or ibuprofen (Combunox). Oxycodone has a serum half-life of 3 to 6 hours and may be detected in the urine up to 2 to 3 days after the last dose. As with all opiates, detection in the urine is dependent on both elimination patterns and the hydration status of the patient.

The presence of oxycodone and its metabolites is due to administration of oxycodone prior to the urine collection. However, the source of the remaining opiates and opioids (ie, morphine and hydromorphone) in the urine is unclear. The concentrations of these drugs alone cannot determine which specific drugs were taken and when. Accordingly, the detection of multiple opiates and opioids in the urine may be the result of several scenarios such as administration of both prescribed and unprescribed medications, use of illicit substances, and/or detection of expected in vivo metabolites as part of definitive testing.

Note: Definitive testing did not include all well-characterized opiates/opioids (and as yet any newly emerging designer opioids) that may cross-react with the in-house opiates class immunoassay to produce a positive result. As such, it not possible to exclude administration of other opiates/opioids not specifically tested for here.

Benzodiazepines
The in-house immunoassay drug screen performed on the specimen collected on (DATE) tested presumptively positive for benzodiazepines. Definitive testing by LC-MS/MS identified the presence of alpha-hydroxymidazolam (580 ng/mL) only. Alpha-hydroxymidazolam is the metabolite of midazolam. Midazolam is a short-acting (half-life 1-4 hours) benzodiazepine prescribed as Versed and is used as a preoperative medication, sedative-hypnotic, and anesthetic induction agent. This definitive testing did not include all benzodiazepine family members that may produce a positive in-house benzodiazepines immunoassay result. As such, it not possible to exclude administration of other benzodiazepines not specifically tested for here. Benzodiazepines are a broad group of psychoactive drugs prescribed for the treatment of anxiety, insomnia, agitation, and seizure. Detection in the urine is dependent upon dose, metabolism, and hydration status of the patient.

THC-Cannabinoids
The in-house urine immunoassay drug screen performed on the specimen collected on (DATE) tested presumptively positive for THC-cannabinoids. Definitive testing was not performed. The in-house immunoassay detects metabolites of delta-9-tetrahydrocannabinol (THC), the primary psychoactive component of marijuana (and dronabinol), as well as its metabolites. The patient's urine may be positive for 2 to 7 days after use or for up to 1 month in chronic smokers.

CONCLUSION:
In conclusion, the patient's toxicology results are not consistent with the prescribed medications. The positive opiates result, as confirmed by LC-MS/MS, indicates administration of morphine (or a morphine prodrug such as heroin) and hydromorphone (or a hydromorphone prodrug such as hydrocodone) prior to the urine collection. Definitive testing for opiates also identified the presence of oxycodone and its metabolites oxymorphone and noroxycodone, which is the expected finding in a patient taking Percocet (oxycodone-acetaminophen combination). Definitive testing for benzodiazepines identified alpha-hydroxymidazolam, the primary metabolite of midazolam. Definitive testing for THC-cannabinoids was not performed. Further investigation into the patient's use of unprescribed drugs should be explored.

Note: A review of the Prescription Drug Monitoring Program (PDMP) database (accessed DATE) does not show any records of prescriptions for the drugs found during the toxicology testing on this patient (ie, morphine, hydromorphone, oxycodone, midazolam). In this state, prescriptions for medications dispensed to patients during inpatient or hospice stays are not recorded in the PDMP. The medical records from (HOSPITAL A) showing the medications administered and the date of discharge were not available at the time of this consultation. As such, it is not possible to rule out that the source of these medications may be the result of medications prescribed during an inpatient stay at another hospital within the last few days prior to admission to (HOSPITAL B).

Pathologist's Name: ____________________, MD
Department of Pathology and Laboratory Medicine
DATE and TIME STAMP

Pearls

- Prescription Drug Monitoring Program (PDMP) databases are used to track prescribing and dispensing data submitted by pharmacies and prescribers. Pathologists and laboratory scientists should be aware of the scope of information that is collected in the state in which they practice. Examples of this include which drugs/drug classes are monitored, how far back the database can track, whether drugs administered in inpatient or hospice settings are included, and whether the database can track prescriptions written by physicians in one state but are filled by a pharmacy in another state.
- Some drugs may be the metabolite of another drug but may also be a prescribed drug in their own right. It is important to understand both the major and minor metabolic pathways of drug classes before attempting to explain the source of a particular drug in the urine.

Case 4

Clinical Pathology Consultation

Comprehensive Review of patient's history and medical records 80502; complex diagnostic problem

Patient: NAME and MRN

Diagnosis: Chronic pain (ICD10-G89.29)

The patient is a 32-year-old woman with a history of right carpal tunnel syndrome. She reports that she previously had surgery to correct the carpal tunnel, but this exacerbated the associated pain. Her previous primary care physician prescribed Percocet (oxycodone-acetaminophen combination; 5-325mg tablets, 5 per day) and she also received a prescription for pain medication from her dentist (3 tablets of acetaminophen with codeine [Tylenol #3]) per the Prescription Drug Monitoring Program (PDMP). The patient also admits to getting pain medications from a relative (medication and dose unknown). A urine drug screen was performed at a recent visit and tested presumptively positive for opiates, oxycodone, and benzodiazepines. The patient's physician has requested a formal toxicology consultation in light of the unexpected positive benzodiazepine and opiates results.

Past Medical History (per EMR)

Carpal tunnel syndrome, right
Obesity

Social History (per EMR)

Family: Takes care of relatives.
Tobacco: No past use.
Alcohol: Unknown.
Illicit drugs: Unknown.

Medication List (per email from CARE GIVER on DATE)

Daily multivitamin caps (multiple vitamins-minerals) OTC
Percocet 5-325 mg tabs (oxycodone-acetaminophen) 1 tab by mouth every 4 hours as needed (average 5 pills/day)

LABORATORY DATA:

Urine Toxicology Screen (immunoassay)

Urine collected DATE	
Amphetamines	Not Detected
Barbiturates	Not Detected
Benzodiazepines	DETECTED
THC-Cannabinoids	Not Detected
Cocaine	Not Detected
Ethanol	Not Detected
Methadone	Not Detected
Opiates	DETECTED
Oxycodone	DETECTED
Buprenorphine	Not Detected

Definitive Urine Toxicology Lab Results

Opiates expanded, urine (LC-MS/MS)
(Laboratory where testing was performed)

Urine collected DATE	Limit of Detection: 50 ng/mL
Codeine	2400 ng/mL
Hydrocodone	370 ng/mL
Hydromorphone	320 ng/mL
Morphine	3100 ng/mL
Norhydrocodone	1100 ng/mL
Noroxycodone	790 ng/mL
Oxycodone	140 ng/mL
Oxymorphone	730 ng/mL

Send-Out Urine Toxicology Lab Results

Benzodiazepines quantitative, urine (LC-MS/MS)
(Laboratory where testing was performed)

Urine collected DATE	Result	Limit of Detection (ng/mL)
Alphahydroxyalprazolam	Negative	<25
Alphahydroxymidazolam	Negative	<50
Alphahydroxytriazolam	Negative	<50
Aminoclonazepam	Negative	<25
Hydroxyethylflurazepam	Negative	<50
Lorazepam	Negative	<50
Nordiazepam	200 ng/mL	<50
Oxazepam	1000 ng/mL	<50
Temazepam	320 ng/mL	<50

ASSESSMENT:

Opiates and Oxycodone

The in-house urine immunoassay drug screen performed on the specimen collected on (DATE) tested presumptively positive for opiates and oxycodone. Definitive testing by LC-MS/MS (liquid chromatography-tandem mass spectrometry) identified a number of opiates and opioids (and their metabolites) including morphine (3100 ng/mL), codeine (2400 ng/mL), hydrocodone (370 ng/mL), hydromorphone (320 ng/mL), norhydrocodone (1100 ng/mL), oxycodone (140 ng/mL), oxymorphone (730 ng/mL), and noroxycodone (790 ng/mL).

Oxycodone in the urine, along with the active metabolite oxymorphone and inactive metabolite noroxycodone, is the expected finding in a patient taking oxycodone prior to the urine collection. Oxycodone is a semisynthetic opioid and is sold as both a stand-alone drug (OxyContin, Roxicodone) or in combination with acetaminophen (Percocet), aspirin (Percodan), or ibuprofen (Combunox). The concentration in the urine cannot specifically determine how much and how often oxycodone was taken, but rather that it was taken prior to the urine collection. Oxycodone has a serum half-life of 3 to 6 hours and may be detected in the urine up to 2 to 3 days after the last dose. Detection in the urine is dependent on both elimination patterns and the hydration status of the patient.

Codeine in the urine can be the result of administration of some prescription antitussive cough medicines or analgesics such as Tylenol-Codeine tablets. Codeine is metabolized in vivo primarily into morphine, which can be further metabolized to hydromorphone (minor pathway). Through another minor metabolic pathway, codeine is metabolized to hydrocodone.

While hydrocodone is a minor metabolite of codeine, it is also sold as a stand-alone drug or in combination with acetaminophen (Vicodin, Lortab) or ibuprofen (Vicoprofen). Hydrocodone is metabolized into the active metabolite hydromorphone and inactive metabolite norhydrocodone. The presence of norhydrocodone in the patient's urine indicates that the patient most likely had taken hydrocodone prior to the urine collection. In addition to being an active metabolite of hydrocodone, hydromorphone is a semisynthetic opioid (sold as Dilaudid) and is also a minor metabolite of morphine. Hydrocodone and hydromorphone have a plasma half-life of up to 9 hours and can be detected in urine 2 to 3 days after the last dose.

Morphine can be found in urine following administration of morphine itself (eg, MS Contin) or as the metabolite of heroin and codeine. Supplementary definitive testing for the morphine-specific metabolite 6-acetylmorphine (6-AM) was not performed. Codeine and morphine have a serum half-life of approximately 1 to 4 and 2 to 7 hours, respectively, and may be detected in the urine up to 2 to 3 days after the last dose

The presence of oxycodone and its metabolites are due to administration of oxycodone prior to the urine collection. However, the source of the remaining opiates and opioids (ie, codeine, morphine, hydrocodone, hydromorphone, norhydrocodone) in the urine is most likely attributable to previously prescribed medications (Tylenol #3, ie, codeine) and nonprescribed medication (a relative's pain medication, possibly hydrocodone). However, the concentrations of these drugs and metabolites alone cannot determine which specific drugs were taken and when. Accordingly, the detection of multiple opiates and opioids in the urine may be the result of several scenarios such as administration of both prescribed and unprescribed medications, use of illicit substances, and/or detection of expected in vivo metabolites as part of confirmatory testing.

Note: Definitive testing did not include all well-characterized opiates/opioids (and as yet any newly emerging designer opioids) that may cross-react with the in-house opiates class immunoassay to produce a positive result. As such, it not possible to exclude administration of other opiates/opioids not specifically tested for here.

Benzodiazepines

The in-house urine immunoassay drug screen performed on the specimen collected on DATE tested presumptively positive for benzodiazepines. Definitive testing by LC-MS/MS identified oxazepam (1000 ng/mL), temazepam (320 ng/mL), and nordiazepam (200 ng/mL). Nordiazepam and temazepam are active metabolites of diazepam. Oxazepam is an active metabolite of both nordiazepam and tamazepam. Temazepam and oxazepam are also prescribed medications, Restoril and Serax, respectively, and have a plasma half-life from 3 to 13 hours depending upon dose and metabolism. Temazepam and oxazepam may be detected in the urine up to 5 to 7 days after the last dose. The presence of temazepam, nordiazepam, and oxazepam suggests the patient may have taken diazepam (Valium) prior to the urine collection. However, as nordiazepam is a common metabolite of multiple benzodiazepines, including chlordiazepoxide (Librium), diazepam, chlorazepate, prazepam, and others, it is not possible to exclude administration of other benzodiazepines not tested for here.

CONCLUSION:

In conclusion, the positive in-house urine oxycodone result, as confirmed by LC-MS/MS, is attributable to administration of oxycodone prior to the urine collection. Definitive testing also determined that the positive in-house opiates immunoassay result is due to the presence of multiple opiates and opioids (ie, morphine, codeine, hydrocodone, hydromorphone, norhydrocodone), which would be consistent with ingestion of Tylenol #3 (prescribed) and hydrocodone (not prescribed). Further investigation into the patient's use of unprescribed drugs should be explored.

Definitive testing for benzodiazepines identified oxazepam, temazepam, and nordiazepam. This finding is most consistent with administration of diazepam (Valium; not prescribed) prior to the urine collection. However, as nordiazepam is also an active metabolite of other benzodiazepines, it is not possible to exclude administration of other benzodiazepines not tested for here.

Pathologist's Name: ____________________, MD
Department of Pathology and Laboratory Medicine
DATE and TIME STAMP

Pearl

- Sometimes definitive testing will reveal a variety of compounds within the same drug class. It's important to examine the metabolic pathways involved. Concentrations alone cannot definitively determine which specific drugs were taken, how much, or when. The presence of these drugs in the urine may be the result of administration of both prescribed and unprescribed medications, the use of illicit drugs, detection of expected metabolites as part of definitive testing, or a combination of all these scenarios. When providing a possible explanation for the source of the drugs, avoid insinuation, accusation, or speculation. Stick with neutral/pragmatic phrases such as "alternative scenarios should be considered" and "use of other drugs cannot be ruled out."

Case 5

Clinical Pathology Consultation

Comprehensive Review of patient's history and medical records 80502; complex diagnostic problem

Patient: NAME and MRN

Diagnosis: Chronic pain: opioid-requiring (ICD10-F11.20)

The patient is a 50-year-old female with a history of chronic pain, rheumatoid arthritis, fibromyalgia, depression, anxiety, and migraine headache. Last year the patient was in a motor vehicle accident and suffered a fractured rib, which causes her pain. She currently takes Percocet (oxycodone-acetaminophen, 10-325 mg, 2 tabs every 6 hours as needed) and MS Contin (morphine, 15 mg tabs, 2 tabs per day) for pain. The patient also takes Ativan (lorazepam, 0.5 mg tabs, 1 tab per day), Fioricet (acetaminophen-caffeine-butalbital, 325-50-40 mg, 1-2 tabs every 4 hours as needed), isometheptene-acetaminophen-dichloral (2 pills at onset, may repeat at 1 hour), and trazodone (100 mg tabs, 1-2 tabs per day) for anxiety, migraine headache, and depression, respectively. A urine drug screen was performed and found to be presumptively positive for amphetamines, barbiturates, benzodiazepines, opiates, and oxycodone. The patient's physician has requested a formal toxicology consultation in light of the unexpected positive amphetamines results.

Past Medical History (per EMR)
History of motor vehicle accident
Rib pain, right sided
Chronic pain: opioid-requiring
Depression
Migraine, classical
Headache, tension
Stress
Insomnia
Fibromyalgia

Social History (per EMR)
Family: Married.
Tobacco: Never smoker.
Alcohol: Not disclosed.
Illicit drugs: Not disclosed.

Medication List (per email from CARE GIVER on DATE)
Percocet 10-325 mg tabs (oxycodone-acetaminophen) 2 every 6 hours as needed for pain
MS Contin 15 mg tb12 (morphine sulfate) 1 pill by mouth twice a day
Ativan 0.5 mg tabs (lorazepam) per psych
Tizanidine HCL 4 mg caps (tizanidine HCL) 2 tabs three times a day
Meloxicam 15 mg tabs (meloxicam) once a day as needed
Wellbutrin sr 150 mg tb12 (bupropion HCL) twice a day
Seroquel 100 mg tabs (quetiapine fumarate) per psych - once daily
Trazodone hcl 100 mg tabs (trazodone hcl) per psych - can take 1-2 pills daily
Aspirin ec 81 mg ec tab (aspirin) 1 once a day
Ranitidine hcl 150 mg tabs (ranitidine HCL) 1 pill twice daily - alternates with PPI
Plaquenil 200 mg tabs (hydroxychloroquine sulfate) once a day
Imitrex 50 mg tab (sumatriptan succinate) take 1 onset of headache as needed and may repeat in 2 hours up to 200 mg in 24 hours as needed
Fioricet 325-50-40 mg tab (acetaminophen-caff-butalbital) 1-2 tabs by mouth every 4 hours as needed for headaches, not to exceed 6 in a 24 hour period as needed
Isometheptene-apap-dichloral 65-325-100 mg caps (apap-isometheptene-dichloral) 2 pills at onset of headache and may repeat after 1 hour, as needed

LABORATORY DATA:

Urine Toxicology Screen (immunoassay)

Urine collected DATE	
Amphetamines	DETECTED
Barbiturates	DETECTED
Benzodiazepines	DETECTED
THC-Cannabinoids	Not Detected
Cocaine	Not Detected
Ethanol	Not Detected
Methadone	Not Detected
Opiates	DETECTED
Oxycodone	DETECTED
Buprenorphine	Not Detected

Definitive Urine Toxicology Lab Results

Amphetamines, urine (LC-MS/MS)
(Laboratory where testing was performed)

Urine collected DATE	Result	Limit of Detection (ng/mL)
Ephedrine	Not Detected	50
Pseudoephedrine	Not Detected	50
Phenylpropanolamine (PPA)	Not Detected	50
Norpseudoephedrine	Not Detected	50
Amphetamine	Not Detected	50
Phentermine	Not Detected	100
Methamphetamine	Not Detected	50
MDA	Not Detected	50
MDMA (Ecstasy)	Not Detected	50
MDEA	Not Detected	100

Definitive Urine Toxicology Lab Results

Meta-Chlorophenylpiperazine (m-CPP), urine (LC-MS/MS)
(Laboratory where testing was performed)

Urine collected DATE	Result	Limit of Detection (ng/mL)
m-CPP (Trazodone metabolite)	6700 ng/mL	1000

ASSESSMENT:

Amphetamines

The in-house urine immunoassay drug screen performed on the specimen collected on (DATE) tested presumptively positive for amphetamines. The in-house amphetamines class immunoassay is sensitive to amphetamine and methamphetamine, producing a positive result at a concentration of approximately 1000 ng/mL and higher. To a lesser degree, this assay will also pick up ecstasy (MDMA; 3,4-methylenedioxymethamphetamine) and its metabolites. Definitive testing by LC-MS/MS (liquid chromatography-tandem mass spectrometry) did not identify any amphetamines known to produce a positive result with this assay.

Definitive testing by LC-MS/MS was performed and identified the presence of meta-chlorophenylpiperazine (6700 ng/mL, limit of detection 1000 ng/mL). Meta-chlorophenylpiperazine (m-CPP) is the active metabolite of the antidepressants Trazodone and Nefazodone. m-CPP is known to cause false-positive results with some urine amphetamines immunoassays. The presence of m-CPP in the urine is consistent with administration of Trazodone at some point prior to the urine collection. Trazodone has a serum half-life of 3 to 7 hours and is metabolized extensively into the pharmacologically active compound m-CPP. m-CPP has also been identified in illicit tablets sold as ecstasy (MDMA).

In addition, isometheptene has been reported to produce false-positive urine amphetamine results with some immunoassays as well as Wellbutrin (bupropion). This was not explored with definitive testing.

Opiates

The in-house urine immunoassay drug screen performed on the specimen collected on (DATE) tested presumptively positive for opiates. This immunoassay is designed to cross-react with the naturally occurring opiates codeine and morphine, producing a positive result at concentrations of ≥50 ng/mL and ≥300 ng/mL, respectively. A positive urine opiates result is the expected finding in a patient taking MS Contin (morphine). Definitive testing to identify the specific opiate or opioid responsible for the positive urine opiates result was not performed. Morphine has a half-life of 2 to 7 hours and can be detected in the urine up to 2 to 3 days after the last dose.

Oxycodone

The in-house urine immunoassay drug screen performed on the specimen collected on (DATE) tested presumptively positive for oxycodone. A positive urine oxycodone result is the expected finding in a patient taking Percocet (acetaminophen-oxycodone combination). Definitive testing was not performed. Oxycodone is a semisynthetic opioid and is sold as both a stand-alone drug (OxyContin, Roxicodone) or in combination with acetaminophen (Percocet), aspirin (Percodan), or ibuprofen (Combunox). Oxycodone has a serum half-life of 3 to 6 hours and may be detected in the urine up to 2 to 3 days after the last dose. Detection in the urine is dependent on both elimination patterns and the hydration status of the patient.

Barbiturates

The in-house urine immunoassay drug screen performed on the specimen collected on (DATE) tested presumptively positive for barbiturates. A positive urine barbiturates result is the expected finding following administration of Fioricet prior to the urine collection. Definitive testing to identify the specific barbiturate responsible for the positive urine barbiturates result was not performed. Butalbital is an intermediate-acting barbiturate found in Fioricet (butalbital-acetaminophen-caffeine combination) and will produce a positive urine barbiturates result. Butalbital has a half-life of 61 hours and may be detected in urine for multiple days, depending upon the dose.

Benzodiazepines

The in-house urine immunoassay drug screen performed on the specimen collected on (DATE) tested presumptively positive for benzodiazepines. A positive urine benzodiazepines immunoassay result is the expected finding in a patient taking Ativan prior to the urine collection. Definitive testing to identify the specific benzodiazepine responsible for the positive urine benzodiazepine result was not performed. Lorazepam (sold as Ativan) is an intermediate-acting benzodiazepine with a serum half-life of 9 to 16 hours. In general, benzodiazepines can be detected in the urine up to several days after administration, depending upon the dose.

CONCLUSION:

The positive immunoassay amphetamines result, as confirmed by definitive testing for amphetamines and m-CPP, is most likely a false positive due to the presence of m-CPP (or possibility bupropion) from administration of trazodone (although isometheptene was not tested for). False-positive immunoassay drug screen results can also be due to nonspecific binding by prescription and nonprescription drugs or adulteration of the urine specimen. The positive opiates, oxycodone, barbiturates, and benzodiazepines results are consistent with the patient's prescriptions for MS Contin (morphine), Percocet (acetaminophen-oxycodone), Fioricet (acetaminophen-caffeine-butalbital), and Ativan (lorazepam), respectively. Definitive testing for these drugs was not performed.

One additional note is that the EMR states that the patient is prescribed Percocet, Fioricet, and isometheptene-acetaminophen-dichloral. If the patient were to ingest the maximum amount of tablets in 24 hours as written for, then the patient could potentially ingest 3900 mg of acetaminophen with just Percocet and Fioricet alone. However, with the isometheptene combination, an additional 1300 mg of acetaminophen could be taken. This would exceed the maximum recommended daily dose of acetaminophen. Studies have demonstrated that doses of acetaminophen greater than 4000 mg per day can result in liver damage.

Pathologist's Name: ____________________, MD
Department of Pathology and Laboratory Medicine
DATE and TIME STAMP

Pearls

- Pathologists and laboratory scientists should be knowledgeable about the sources of false positives with urine immunoassays. Bear in mind that while manufacturers perform interference studies to determine possible cross-reactivity by the most commonly encountered drugs and compounds, these efforts are not exhaustive. Sometimes it is only after an assay is brought to market that reports of false positives appear. Laboratorians should consult reputable medical literature for reports of false positives and integrate this knowledge into their consultations. Definitive testing for the compound assumed to be the cause of the false positive should be performed when appropriate and available.
- Some drugs are sold as combinations of both prescribed and/or over-the-counter drugs. Each drug's individual components and dose should be examined when reviewing the medication list. Pathologists and laboratory scientists should also be aware of the possible hidden additive effect of multiple medications which contain the same active ingredients and discuss it in the consultation when appropriate.
- Definitive testing was not performed because the immunoassay positive results were expected positive due to medication history. However, clinicians should understand that some immunoassays are class assays (eg, opiates or benzodiazepines), and specific identification of the drug(s) causing the positive result is not identified. Patients could take another drug in addition to, or instead of, the prescribed medication and obtain the desired class assay result (eg, prescribed codeine and instead using heroin will produce a positive opiates class result). Not ordering definitive testing to identify what drug or drugs are present is a clinical judgment and related to the degree of suspicion of aberrant drug behavior.

Case 6

Clinical Pathology Consultation

Comprehensive Review of patient's history and medical records 80502; complex diagnostic problem

Patient: NAME and MRN

Diagnosis: Opioid dependence, uncomplicated (ICD10-F11.20)

The patient is a 26-year-old female who presented to (HOSPITAL) for obstetric care at 36-2/7 weeks gestation. A urine drug screen performed on a specimen collected on (DATE 1) tested positive for fentanyl and cocaine. After further inquiry, the patient admitted to a history of IV drug use and alleges that although she was clean for the past 3 years, she relapsed approximately 3 weeks ago. She was admitted for observation due to concern for possible abruption during which time she developed withdrawal symptoms. The patient agreed to accept a referral to a methadone clinic and was started on 30 mg of methadone with a good response and was discharged on (DATE). The patient was readmitted to (HOSPITAL) on (DATE) for ruptured membranes, had an uneventful spontaneous vaginal delivery, and was discharged (DATE). At a follow-up postnatal visit on (DATE 2), a urine drug screen was performed and tested presumptively positive for fentanyl and methadone. The patient's OBGYN physician has requested a formal toxicology consultation regarding the positive drug screen results.

Past Medical History (per EMR)
None available.

Social History (per EMR)
Tobacco (1.5 packs per day at conception, now quit).
Heroin use with recent relapse.

Medication List (per email from CARE GIVER on DATE)
Iron supplementation
Methadone
Augmentin (amoxicillin/clavulanic acid); only prior to DATE 1 urine drug screen

LABORATORY DATA:

In-House Urine Toxicology Screen (immunoassay)

Urine collected DATE 1	
Amphetamines	Not Detected
Barbiturates	Not Detected
Benzodiazepines	Not Detected
THC-Cannabinoids	Not Detected
Cocaine	DETECTED
Ethanol	Not Detected
Methadone	Not Detected
Opiates	Not Detected
Fentanyl	DETECTED
Oxycodone	Not Detected
Buprenorphine	Not Detected

In-House Urine Toxicology Screen (immunoassay)

Urine collected DATE 2	
Amphetamines	Not Detected
Barbiturates	Not Detected
Benzodiazepines	Not Detected
THC-Cannabinoids	Not Detected
Cocaine	Not Detected
Ethanol	Not Detected
Opiates	Not Detected
Methadone	DETECTED
Fentanyl	DETECTED
Oxycodone	Not Detected
Buprenorphine	Not Detected

Send-Out Urine Toxicology Lab Results

Fentanyl, urine (LC-MS/MS)
(Laboratory where testing was performed)

Urine collected DATE 1	Limit of Detection: 0.50 ng/mL
Fentanyl	>100 ng/mL
Norfentanyl (fentanyl metabolite)	>100 ng/mL

Send-Out Urine Toxicology Lab Results

Cocaine Metabolite, urine (LC-MS/MS)
(Laboratory where testing was performed)

Urine collected DATE 1	Limit of Detection: 100 ng/mL
Benzoylecgonine	3600 ng/mL

Send-Out Urine Toxicology Lab Results

Fentanyl, urine (LC-MS/MS)
(Laboratory where testing was performed))

Urine collected DATE 2	Limit of Detection: 0.50 ng/mL
Fentanyl	Negative
Norfentanyl (fentanyl metabolite)	Interference

ASSESSMENT:

Fentanyl
The in-house urine immunoassay drug screen performed on the specimen collected on (DATE 1) tested presumptively positive for fentanyl. The specimen was sent to a reference lab for definitive testing by LC-MS/MS (liquid chromatography-tandem mass spectrometry) and identified fentanyl (>100 ng/mL; limit of detection 0.5 ng/mL) and the metabolite norfentanyl (>100 ng/mL; limit of detection 0.5 ng/mL). This finding is consistent with administration of fentanyl prior to the urine collection. The urine drug screen performed on the specimen collected on (DATE 2) also tested presumptively positive for fentanyl by immunoassay. Definitive testing by LC-MS/MS did not detect the parent drug fentanyl, and an assay interference was detected during definitive testing for the metabolite norfentanyl. As such, a result for norfentanyl cannot be reported.

Fentanyl is a powerful synthetic opioid analgesic. According to the CDC, fentanyl is estimated to be 80 times more potent than morphine and more potent than heroin. Fentanyl may be administered in a variety of forms, including as a transdermal patch, nasal spray, sublingual spray, lozenges, or an injectable solution. Substitution of fentanyl for heroin in street preparations of this drug may lead to overdose due to the difference in potency. Fentanyl has a half-life of up to 12 hours and may be detected in the urine for several days after administration, depending upon dose and hydration status of the patient.

Note: The definitive assay for fentanyl specifically identifies fentanyl and its metabolite norfentanyl. It does not identify acetyl-fentanyl, sufentanil, carfentanil, or other analogues of fentanyl that may cross-react with the in-house fentanyl immunoassay screen. Therefore, use of other fentanyl derivatives cannot be ruled out.

Cocaine

The in-house urine immunoassay drug screen performed on the specimen collected on (DATE 1) tested presumptively positive for cocaine. Definitive testing by LC-MS/MS identified the cocaine-specific metabolite, benzoylecgonine (3600 ng/mL; limit of detection 100 ng/mL). The presence of benzoylecgonine is consistent with use of cocaine prior to the urine collection.

Cocaine is used medically as a local anesthetic in ophthalmological and facial surgical procedures. It is also abused by injection, insufflation, or smoking due to its powerful stimulant effects. It has a short half-life of up to 1.5 hours. Adverse effects of cocaine use include anxiety, agitation, hyperactivity, hypertension, diaphoresis, mydriasis, and tachycardia.

Cocaine readily crosses the placenta and blood-brain barrier of the fetus. Fetal exposure to cocaine has been associated with growth retardation, shorter body length, smaller head circumference, and an increased incidence in premature birth. Possible longer term postnatal effects include deficits in higher executive functions including behavior, cognition, and memory.

Of note, some batches of fentanyl (sold as heroin) are cut with cocaine, unbeknownst to the user. Detection of benzoylecgonine in the urine of heroin or fentanyl users may be attributed to adulteration with cocaine.

Methadone

The in-house urine immunoassay drug screen performed on the specimen collected on (DATE 2) tested presumptively positive for methadone. This is the expected finding in patients prescribed methadone therapy. Definitive testing was not performed. Methadone is a synthetic opioid used to treat opioid abuse and withdrawal symptoms, and for chronic pain. Methadone has a long half-life (15-55 hours) and is detectable in urine for several days after the final dose.

CONCLUSION:

In conclusion, the positive in-house fentanyl and cocaine immunoassay results on urine specimen collected on (DATE 1), as confirmed with definitive testing by LC-MS/MS, are consistent with administration of fentanyl and cocaine prior to the urine collection. Further investigation into the patient's use of unprescribed drugs should be explored. Of note, fentanyl is sometimes substituted for heroin in street preparations of this drug and may also sometimes be adulterated with cocaine. The positive in-house fentanyl immunoassay result from the urine specimen collected on (DATE 2) appears to be a false positive. An unknown assay interference was observed during the LC-MS/MS analysis of the metabolite norfentanyl.

Unexpected false-positive immunoassay drug screen results can be due to nonspecific binding by prescription and nonprescription drugs or manipulation of the urine specimen. Definitive testing for methadone was not performed.

Pathologist's Name: __________________, MD
Department of Pathology and Laboratory Medicine
DATE and TIME STAMP

Pearls

- When a patient is pregnant and an unexplained urine drug test result is observed, definitive testing is a must. This is because some states mandate reporting of cases of suspected abuse or neglect as the result of drug use by the mother, and a false-positive result by urine immunoassay testing may have grave consequences. Drug metabolism and pharmacokinetics may be different in pregnant individuals, and some drugs may cross the placenta with potential impacts on the unborn.
- Street preparations of illicit drugs may be adulterated with other drugs in an attempt to make the end-product more desirable. Common combinations include cocaine with heroin or morphine ("speedball"), cocaine with levamisole (an anthelminthic drug used by veterinarians), and more recently fentanyl laced with cocaine. Some drugs may be substituted for other drugs (eg, fentanyl for heroin, or methamphetamine for cocaine), unbeknownst to the buyer. This can have serious consequences for the end-user, particularly in those who are opioid naïve and consume a powerful opioid such as heroin or fentanyl. Pathologists and laboratory scientists should be aware of these combinations when interpreting drug testing results and should stay up to date

with emerging patterns of combined drug use in their area.

- In some cases, the fentanyl immunoassay (eg, Immunalysis) is positive due to acetyl-fentanyl or other fentanyl analogs that are detectable by immunoassay but are not detectable by the LC-MS/MS assay that is set up for fentanyl and norfentanyl only.

Case 7

Clinical Pathology Consultation

Comprehensive Review of patient's history and medical records 80502; complex diagnostic problem

Patient: NAME and MRN

Diagnosis: Other psychoactive substance abuse with unspecified disorder (ICD10-F19.19)

The patient is a 40-year-old male with a past medical history of end-stage renal disease secondary to autosomal dominant polycystic kidney disease, hepatitis C, and heroin abuse (sober since 2011, currently on methadone). He had received a renal transplant in 2017 from a hepatitis C-positive donor and now presents to the nephrology clinic for a follow-up visit. A urine specimen was collected during the clinic visit, and urine drug screen was performed and tested presumptively positive for opiates, fentanyl, and methadone. The patient's physician has requested a formal toxicology consultation in light of the unexpected positive fentanyl and opiates results.

Past Medical History (per EMR)

Nephrolithiasis
Autosomal dominant polycystic kidney disease with stage V chronic kidney disease
Hypertension
Hyperkalemia
Rheumatic fever with heart murmur
Hepatitis C
Heroin abuse; sober since 2011
Depression
Deceased-donor kidney transplant

Social History (per EMR)

Family history: Both parents and 2 siblings alive.
Work/occupation: Currently not working.
Tobacco history: Former smoker, quit recently.
Alcohol: Denies.
Illicit drugs: Prior history of heroin use; sober for several years.

Medication List (per email from CARE GIVER on DATE)

Famotidine 20 mg tablet, 1 tablet orally once a day
Hydralazine HCl 50 mg tablet, 1 tablet with food orally twice a day
Labetalol HCl 200 mg tablet, 2 tablets orally twice a day
Methadone HCl 100 mg concentrate 10 mL (100 mg) orally once a day for a total of 100 mg
Mycophenolate Mofetil 500 mg tablet, 2 tablets orally twice a day
Sensipar 60 mg tablet, 1 tablet after a meal with food orally once a day
Tacrolimus 5 mg capsule, 1 capsule orally once a day
Testosterone cypionate 100 mg/mL solution, 1/2 mL intramuscular once a week
Valganciclovir HCl 450 mg tablet, 1 tablet orally once a day

LABORATORY DATA:

In-House Urine Toxicology Screen (immunoassay)

Urine collected DATE	
Amphetamines	Not Detected
Barbiturates	Not Detected
Benzodiazepines	Not Detected
THC-Cannabinoids	Not Detected
Cocaine	Not Detected
Ethanol	Not Detected
Methadone	DETECTED
Opiates	DETECTED
Oxycodone	Not Detected
Buprenorphine	Not Detected
Fentanyl	DETECTED

Send-Out Urine Toxicology Lab Results

Opiates expanded, urine (LC-MS/MS)
(Laboratory where testing was performed)

Urine collected DATE	Limit of Detection: 50 ng/mL
Codeine	Negative
Hydrocodone	Negative
Hydromorphone	Negative
Morphine	280 ng/mL
Norhydrocodone	Negative
Noroxycodone	Negative
Oxycodone	Negative
Oxymorphone	Negative

Fentanyl, urine (LC-MS/MS)
(Laboratory where testing was performed)

Urine collected DATE	Limit of Detection: 0.50 ng/mL
Fentanyl	>100 ng/mL
Norfentanyl	>100 ng/mL

ASSESSMENT:

Opiates

The in-house urine immunoassay drug screen performed on the specimen collected on (DATE) tested presumptively positive for opiates. This immunoassay is designed to cross-react with the naturally occurring opiates codeine and morphine, producing a positive result at concentrations of ≥150 ng/mL and ≥300 ng/mL, respectively. Definitive testing by LC-MS/MS (liquid chromatography-tandem mass spectrometry) identified morphine (280 ng/mL) only. No other common opiates/opioids were detected (ie, codeine, hydrocodone, hydromorphone, norhydrocodone, oxycodone, oxymorphone, noroxycodone).

Morphine can be found in urine following administration of morphine itself or as the metabolite of either codeine or heroin. Small amounts of morphine (and codeine) can be found in patients who ingest large quantities of poppy-seed–laden foods since some poppy seed batches are contaminated with naturally occurring morphine and codeine. To assess if the source of morphine is from contaminated poppy seeds, it is critical to know the time of urine collection in relation to the poppy seed consumption, since the higher morphine concentrations are found in urines collected within a few hours (eg, 6 hours) of consuming poppy-seed–laden foods. Morphine has a half-life of 2 to 7 hours, and can be detected in the urine up to 2 to 3 days after the last dose. Heroin, or diacetylmorphine, has an extremely short half-life (1-4 minutes) and is rapidly metabolized to 6-acetylmorphine (6-AM). 6-AM is also metabolized relatively quickly (3-52 minutes) to morphine. Definitive testing did not specifically assay for 6-AM in this urine specimen.

However, testing for 6-AM should not be overlooked because the morphine concentration is low, especially in a patient with history of heroin use. Some individuals who use heroin have low or little morphine in their urine but are 6-AM positive. Although the presence of 6-AM is a definitive marker of heroin use, the window of detection of 6-AM is narrow—6 to 12 hours after heroin use—and its detection can be missed if urine is not collected shortly after heroin use.

Note: Definitive testing did not include all well-characterized opiates/opioids (and as yet any newly emerging designer opioids), which may cross-react with the in-house opiates class immunoassay to produce a positive result. As such, it not possible to exclude administration of other opiates/opioids not specifically tested for here.

Fentanyl

The in-house urine immunoassay drug screen performed on the specimen collected on (DATE) tested presumptively positive for fentanyl. Definitive testing by LC-MS/MS identified both fentanyl (>100 ng/mL) and the metabolite norfentanyl (>100 ng/mL).

Fentanyl is a powerful synthetic opioid analgesic. According to the CDC, fentanyl is estimated to be 80 times more potent than morphine and more potent than heroin. Fentanyl may be administered in a variety of forms, including as a transdermal patch, nasal spray, sublingual spray, lozenges, or an injectable solution. Substitution of fentanyl for heroin in street preparations of this drug may lead to overdose due to the difference in potency. Fentanyl has a half-life of up to 12 hours and may be detected in the urine for several days after administration, depending upon dose and hydration status of the patient.

Note: The definitive assay for fentanyl specifically identifies fentanyl and its metabolite norfentanyl. It does not identify acetyl-fentanyl, sufentanil, carfentanil, or other analogues of fentanyl that may cross-react with our fentanyl immunoassay screen. Therefore, although the definitive testing identified fentanyl and norfentanyl, use other fentanyl derivatives cannot be ruled out.

Methadone

The in-house urine immunoassay drug screen performed on the specimen collected on (DATE) tested presumptively positive for methadone. This is the expected finding in patients prescribed methadone therapy. Definitive testing was not performed. Methadone is a synthetic opioid used to treat opioid abuse and withdrawal symptoms, and for chronic pain. Methadone has a long half-life (15-55 hours) and is detectable in urine for several days after the final dose.

CONCLUSION:

Definitive testing for opiates identified morphine only. Morphine in the urine can be the result of administration of morphine itself, codeine, or heroin. Low concentrations of morphine in the urine may be the result of consumption of poppy-seed–laden foods or ongoing metabolism from heroin use multiple days prior. Use of heroin cannot be excluded as definitive testing did not specifically assay for the heroin metabolite, 6-AM, given the low concentration of morphine. Definitive testing for fentanyl identified both fentanyl and the metabolite norfentanyl. Of note, fentanyl is sometimes substituted for, or combined with, heroin in street preparations of this drug. Further investigation into the patient's use of unprescribed drugs should be explored. The positive in-house methadone immunoassay results on the urine specimen collected on (DATE) are consistent with the patient's prescription of methadone. Definitive testing for methadone was not performed.

Pathologist's Name: __________________, MD
Department of Pathology and Laboratory Medicine
DATE and TIME STAMP

Pearls

- Definitive testing should be performed even when common causes of false positives are present. In the case above, the patient was prescribed a moderate dose of labetalol. Labetalol is known to cross-react with the urine fentanyl immunoassay and may therefore provide an easy and convenient explanation for the positive result. However, definitive testing was performed and identified both fentanyl and the metabolite norfentanyl as the source of the positive fentanyl immunoassay result. Failure to perform definitive testing even when common sources of false positives are possible can lead to an incorrect interpretation of results.
- When small concentrations of morphine (and sometimes codeine) are identified as part of definitive testing, pathologists and laboratory scientists may consider consumption of poppy seeds. Poppy seeds are known to be naturally contaminated with morphine and codeine, and ingestion of sufficient quantities can lead to a positive urine opiates immunoassay result. Linking poppy seed consumption to a positive opiates immunoassay result is challenging, as multiple factors including time, amount ingested, and concentration of morphine (and codeine) in the poppy seed batch can all influence whether a positive immunoassay result will be observed. A small concentration of morphine in the urine could also represent ongoing metabolism from administration of codeine or heroin at some point prior to the urine collection.[16]

References

1. Michna E, Jamison RN, Pham LD, et al. Urine toxicology screening among chronic pain patients on opioid therapy: frequency and predictability of abnormal findings. *Clin J Pain.* 2007;23(2):173-179.
2. Couto JE, Romney MC, Leider HL, Sharma S, Goldfarb NI. High rates of inappropriate drug use in the chronic pain population. *Popul Health Manag.* 2009;12(4):185-190.
3. Reisfield GM, Bertholf R, Barkin RL, Webb F, Wilson G. Urine drug test interpretation: what do physicians know? *J Opioid Manag.* 2007;3(2):80-86.
4. Moeller KE, Kissack JC, Atayee RS, Lee KC. Clinical interpretation of urine drug tests: what clinicians need to know about urine drug screens. *Mayo Clin Proc.* 2017;92(5):774-796.
5. Reisfield GM, Webb FJ, Bertholf RL, Sloan PA, Wilson GR. Family physicians' proficiency in urine drug testing interpretation. *J Opioid Manag.* 2007;3(6):333-337.
6. Starrels JL, Fox AD, Kunins HV, Cunningham CO. They don't know what they don't know: internal medicine residents' knowledge and confidence in urine drug test interpretation for patients with chronic pain. *J Gen Intern Med.* 2012;27(11):1521-1527.
7. Melanson SE, Baskin L, Magnani BJ, Kwong TC, Dizon A, Wu AH. Interpretation and utility of drug of abuse immunoassays: lessons from laboratory drug testing surveys. *Arch Pathol Lab Med.* 2010;134(5):735-739.
8. *CPT 2019: Professional Edition (CPT/Current Procedural Terminology).* Chicago, IL: American Medical Association; 2018.
9. Cone EJ, Caplan YH, Moser F, Robert T, Black D. Evidence that morphine is metabolized to hydromorphone but not to oxymorphone. *J Anal Toxicol.* 2008;32:319-323.
10. Reisfield GM, Chronister CW, Goldberger BA, Bertholf RL. Unexpected urine drug testing results in a hospice patient on high-dose morphine therapy. *Clin Chem.* 2009:55;1765-1768.
11. Wasan AD, Michna E, Janfaza D, et al. Interpreting urine drug tests: prevalence of morphine metabolism to hydromorphone in chronic pain patients treated with morphine. *Pain Med.* 2008;9:918-923.
12. Rook EJ, Huitema AD, van den Brink W, et al. Pharmacokinetics and pharmacokinetic variability of heroin and its metabolites: review of the literature. *Curr Clin Pharmacol.* 2006;1:109-118.
13. Crews B, Mikel C, Latyshev S, et al. 6-Acetylmorphine detected in the absence of morphine in pain management patients. *Ther Drug Monit.* 2009;31:749-752.
14. Helander A, Sztojanovic K, Villen T, Beck O. Detectability of fentanyl and designer fentanyls in urine by 3 commercial fentanyl immunoassays. *Drug Test Anal.* 2018;10:1297-1304.
15. Bottcher M, Beck O. Evaluation of buprenorphine CEDIA assay versus GC-MS and ELISA using urine samples from patients in substitution treatment. *J Anal Toxicol.* 2005;29:769-776.
16. Smith ML, Hughes RO, Levine B, et al. Forensic drug testing for opiates, VI: urine testing for hydromorphone, hydrocodone, oxycodone with commercial opiate immunoassays and gas chromatography-mass spectrometry. *J Anal Toxicol.* 1995;19:18-26.

Chapter 5

Special Considerations in Pediatric Toxicology: Practical and Testing Perspectives

Robert A. Middleberg, PhD

Introduction

The concept that children are not miniature adults in respect to pharmacotherapy was expressed in the early 1900s.[1] While distinctly different, pharmacology and toxicology share many of the same high-level basic concepts, eg, phamaco- and toxicokinetics, pharmaco- and toxicodynamics. It is by extension therefore that the basic premise whereby children are not small adults carries over into toxicology. Most differences between children and adults are noted at earlier ages of childhood, typically less than 5 years old, despite pediatrics normally defined to at least 21 years of age.[2] Nevertheless, responses to toxic substances in the developing child are influenced not only by physiological differences, but by epigenetic factors including routes of exposure and societal, psychosocial, behavioral, and other characteristics.[3]

For obvious reasons, much of what is known about toxic exposures in children is empirically based. Statistics gathered by various agencies and case reports of exposures often guide our current knowledge of toxicity in children. However, by gaining an understanding of developmental stages of factors influencing outcomes after exposure, predictive outcomes and preventive actions can be appreciated better. Specific examples of differences in toxic responses between children and adults also demonstrate the differential severity of toxic exposures in the pediatric population. Lastly, laboratories performing exposure testing in children must compensate for factors that differentiate this unique population.

Statistics

Each year, a multitude of statistics regarding pediatric exposures are made available in both the lay and scientific literature.[4] Unfortunately, often there is overlap and disparities between the same presented statistics based on the source of information. Notwithstanding these concerns, a number of solid, important data are available. Some limitations of the data include voluntary reporting versus mandatory reporting, thus resulting in an underreporting of exposures.[5]

Since 1995, there are roughly two million voluntary reports of exposure to chemicals, including drugs, to Poison Control Centers (PCCs) within the United States. More than half of those reports occur in children, mostly in children less than 3 years old.[6] Exposures in children generally can be further divided into two distinct groups, those 1 to 5 years old and 6 to 19 years old, with the former being relatively normally distributed, while the latter group is skewed toward the later ages. The younger group generally reflects either purposeful administration by parents or caregivers, or developmental inquisitiveness accompanied by ambulation; with older children, experimentation with drugs and other agents tends to predominate along with the maturing of suicidal intention.[7]

Fortunately, the majority of children exposed to drugs and other chemicals reported to PCCs recover without lasting effects, many of which never require hospitalization. Figure 5-1 shows the breakdown of substance types in children $\leq$5 years old as reported by PCCs in 2016; less than 1000 of these exposures resulted in major effects or death. Table 5-1 represents the percentage of all fatalities in 2016 for children according to age group as reported to PCCs. Since 1992, children comprise only 2% to 4% of all fatalities associated with drug or chemical exposures.[6] Until recently, deaths in younger

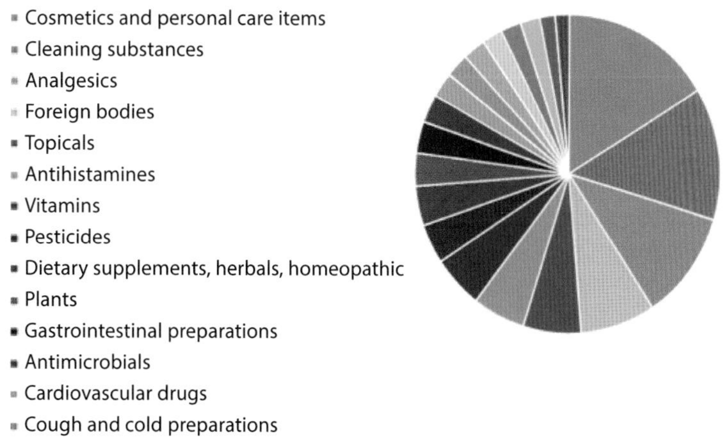

Figure 5-1. Top categories involved in pediatric exposures in 2016.[6]

Table 5-1. Percentage of All Poisoning Fatalities by Pediatric Age Group[6]

Age Group	Number of Fatalities	Percentage of All Fatalities*
≤5 years	24	1.7%
6-12 years	7	0.5%
13-19 years	42	3.0%

* Total fatalities at all ages due to poisoning = 1415.

children generally involved a preponderance of nonpharmaceutical agents; however, with the recent upswing in opioid-related deaths, analgesics now represent the number one cause of death in this population.[6,8] Medical examiner data related to young children reveals a much more diverse set of detected substances, in part due to the depth of toxicological analyses.[9] Data from individual centers as opposed to national databases is often more revealing in respect to pediatric poisoning. In one report, 8.4% of children brought to one hospital's emergency department with apparent life-threatening events were found to have significant positive toxicological screens; about half this number was positive for over-the-counter cold preparations, with no indication that the child was on such medication and no caregiver admitting administering a medication.[7]

In 1962, Kempe et al suggested that childhood poisoning can represent a form of child abuse.[10] The term *Munchausen by proxy*, a condition whereby individuals inflict suffering upon another to gain attention to themselves, was coined by Meadows in 1977.[11] Most often, this act involves a parent injuring a child to gather attention to themselves. While only scattered reports of this condition appeared prior to 1990, many reports of such poisonings have appeared in medical and legal literature.[7] In 1968, Weston described the need for toxicological evaluation if child abuse is suspected at autopsy.[12] Thus, the concept of nonaccidental poisoning of children is, remarkably, relatively new in respect to scientific literature. That such poisonings have occurred throughout history, however, is not new.[7]

Homicidal poisonings in the US are relatively rare. From 1999 to 2005, the overall reported estimated rate for homicidal poisonings was 0.26/million person years (total absolute number = 523). However, in infants, the rate was 2.05/million, approximately 8 to 9 times greater than the general population. Children age 1 to 4 years also had an elevated rate at 0.49/million. Children ≥5 years had homicidal poisoning rates comparable to the general population.[5] Historical and empirical evidence, including medicolegal and social issues as well as this author's experience, indicate that the rate of nonaccidental poisonings in the pediatric population, especially infants, is most likely underreported.[13]

General Toxicological Principles

The underlying reasons for differences in response to exposure to chemicals, including drugs, between children and adults are multivariate. In most cases, as children mature, the differences fade, but some remain into early adulthood as physical and mental functions progress. Physiologically, the majority of significant differences are noted in children less than 5 years old, beginning with the developing fetus. In utero exposure can result in four basic perturbations: embryolethality, developmental issues, growth retardation, and functional deficits, with the latter three potentially not fully realized until later in life.[7] The timing of in utero exposure often dictates the outcome, especially during organogenesis (4-8 months post gestation), but other times of exposures during development should not be considered free of potential adverse results.[14] The classic example of this phenomenon involved diethylstilbestrol (DES), a drug used by pregnant women from approximately 1940 to 1970. In all, approximately 10 million to 15 million women used the drug to, as advertised, prevent miscarriage. In the late 1960s, a few young women developed clear cell adenocarcinoma of the vagina, a disease that, up to that point, was observed in older women. Other vaginal abnormalities were also noted, eg, adenosis. Male offspring developed epididymal cysts, hypotrophic testes, and poor sperm quality. Epidemiological studies tracked these abnormalities to maternal use of DES, thus making DES one of the first compounds to be an endocrine disruptor. The effects of DES in affected families have expanded to over three generations of children.[15,16]

The root cause of differences between children and adults in response to chemical exposure in many situations are understood. These differences are often toxicokinetically and toxicodyanamically based. Other causes of such differences, eg, pathophysiology, are beyond discussion here but should be considered in assigning such differences.

Size

From birth to adulthood, the metamorphosis of man is remarkable. The changes are vast, but perhaps the most obvious is change in size. The term used to describe the nonlinear relationship

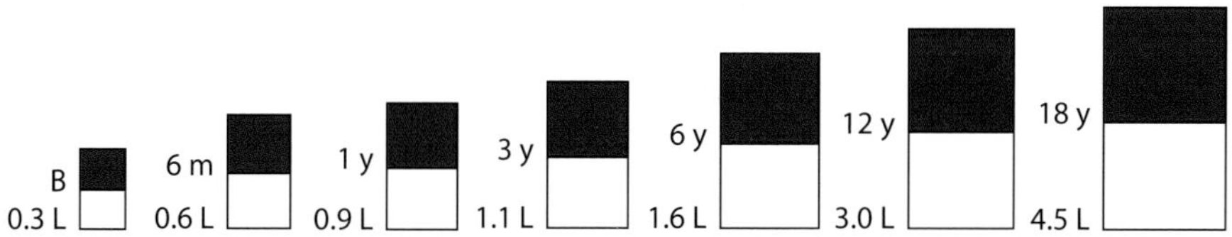

Figure 5-2. Approximate changes in blood volume with age. B, birth; m, months; y, year(s).

Modified from Collins KA, Byard RW, eds. *Forensic Pathology of Infancy and Childhood.* New York: NY; Springer Reference; 2014. Reproduced with permission.

between size and function is *allometry*. Allometric relationships can be described mathematically.[17] Some of the changes of significance as we grow include a 5.5-fold increase in weight and a 3-fold increase in surface area while we mature chronologically.[18] Blood volume increases approximately 16-fold between birth and adulthood (see Figure 5-2). Additionally, our percentage of total body water decreases over time, which affects volume of distribution (see Figure 5-3). Additionally, size is a major predictor of clearance, but such allometric parameters cannot be used to predict such things as drug metabolism due to rapid development of biotransformation capabilities. Drug dosing, on the other hand, may be influenced significantly by body size.[19-24]

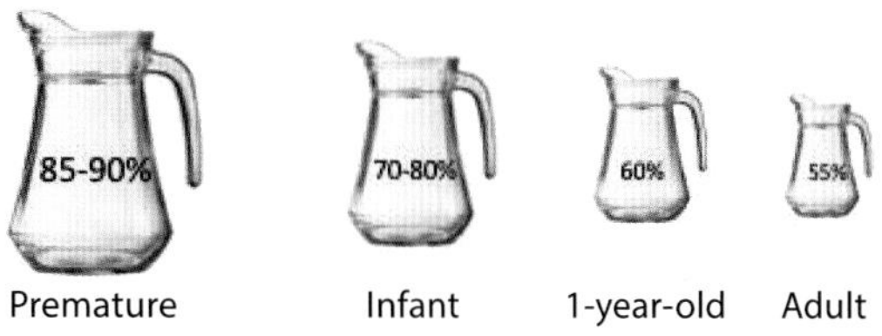

Figure 5-3. Approximate differences in total body water as a percentage of body weight during development.[22-23]

Toxicokinetics

Toxicokinetics (TK) is the mathematical description of the uptake and disposition of a chemical in the body. It is sometimes colloquially described as what the body does to a chemical. Classically, this encompasses absorption, distribution, metabolism, and excretion of a substance, with active transport considered another parameter in many circles.[25] A detailed explanation of each of these processes is not possible here; however, general highlights of factors affecting toxicokinetics in childhood that impact concentrations of chemicals in the body follows. In general, most, but not all, TK parameters mimic those of an adult by 10 years of age, with most differences appearing in children less than 6 years old.[7] The salient differences that impact exposure to toxicants in children are described below.

Absorption

For the young child, all routes of administration—oral, dermal, inhalation, rectal, etc—take on greater importance in respect to exposure to chemicals. Physiological differences generally lead to increased bioavailability for many substances. As a result, potential significant toxic outcomes might occur when compared to similar exposures in older children and adults. A number of factors affect absorption after oral exposure, including gastric and intestinal pHs, gastric emptying time and peristalsis, metabolic processes, whether the means of absorption is passive or active, bile acid and salt activity, digestive enzyme secretion, skin thickness, and lung development and maturation.[26]

A neonate is defined as a newborn up to 1 month old, whereas an infant is aged from 1 month to 1 year.[14] For the healthy neonate, exposure to substances generally occurs via ingestion of breast milk or formula and inhalation.[27] Most drugs and other chemicals are secreted into breast milk; however, it is estimated that less than 1% of a maternal dose is transferred to the child.[28] Even so, from a risk-benefit perspective, the recognized benefits appear to outweigh the risks in most cases.[29] In infancy, the gastric pH will be as high as it will ever be naturally (mean, 6.6; range, 1.4-7.8) The pH generally drops significantly within a day or two reaching adult values by 3 years old.[30] As gastric pH can be a determinant of bioavailability, its impact should not be overlooked, eg, orally administered penicillin G leads to greater bioavailability in neonates than older children as the compound is acid labile.[3]

Since absorption after oral exposure takes place mainly in the small intestine, gastric emptying is important. This parameter remains greater than adult values through the entirety of childhood. Even so, this does not correlate to increased absorption rates for most substances, and in fact most substances have a delayed rate of absorption in infants and young children, which often leads to lower achieved blood concentrations of absorbed substances.[13,24] This may be due, in part, to immature transport mechanisms in this younger cohort. On the other hand, it appears, at least based on L(+)-arabinose, that passive transport across the intestinal mucosa is mature in infants within approximately 4 months.[31]

In respect to skin, the stratum corneum becomes well developed at 34 weeks but still is not as mature as in older children and adults.[32] Neonates further develop the keratin exterior of skin over the first 3 to 5 days post birth. These initial days present significant exposure risk due to the absence of this critical barrier. Because of this, toxicities in infants due to percutaneous absorption of toxicants, eg, betadine (iodine), hexachlorophene, and phenol, have been observed. Additionally, the ratio of total body surface to body mass in neonates and infants is much greater than in older children and adults. Therefore, given the same amount of skin exposed to a given chemical, the younger child could absorb much more than the older group.[33,34] Subcutaneous and intramuscular administration of substances in the neonate and infant are influenced by factors such as decreased muscle mass, increased water content of muscle, and altered blood flow.[24,35]

While the liver represents the organ of greatest metabolic activity in respect to toxic exposures, the bioavailability of a substance can be influenced substantially by intestinal biotransforming enzymes, transporters, and gut microflora.[3] Based on ontogeny of biotransformation enzymes, eg, CYP450 isoforms, both decreased and increased activities are predictable. All of these factors are quantitatively different in young children and can therefore affect the amount of systemic chemical available to induce adverse effects. Absorption of rectally administered substances is highly variable from patient to patient and is influenced by the formulation, volume of diluent liquid, concentration of the substance, site of delivery (higher or lower rectum), presence of stool, pH of the rectal contents, rectal retention, and differences in venous drainage within the rectosigmoid region. Additionally, biotransformation capabilities are significant in respect to bioavailability via rectal administration. All of these factors often lead to mixed results in respect to toxicant absorption by this route.[36] Lastly, absorption of inhaled substances increases as lungs mature due to increases in the number of alveoli. Immature lung function also can have mixed effects on toxicant absorption by this route.[32]

Distribution

The process by which a xenobiotic moves from the site of absorption to other areas of the body is termed *distribution*. Qualitative and quantitative determinants of distribution include blood flow, total body water, body fat, storage of toxicants in tissues, protein binding, blood-brain barrier development, and tissue affinity.[37] Total body water can have wide extremes based on age and is greatest in premature babies (see Figure 5-3), reaching adult levels after about 1 year of age. Most of this water in neonates and infants is extracellular.[22-24] Body fat also follows an age-based pattern, with premature children and neonates having the lowest, reaching average adult levels by around 5 to 10 years of age.[38-40] In general, protein binding is lower in neonates. One consequence of this is a greater amount of drug in the free form, thus creating a greater dose-response effect. Additionally, endogenous substances, eg, bilirubin, that are present in neonates may compete for limited protein binding and can therefore preclude the binding of xenobiotics. Compounds known to be affected by decreased protein binding include phenytoin, salicylates, valproic acid, and ampicillin.[24] Due to the difficulty in performing experimental evaluations, there is controversy as to whether the blood-brain barrier is fully developed at birth. Evidence seems to indicate that at least at 4 months and older, there is little difference in this barrier compared to adults. In younger children, differences might exist, and given the fatty nature of the brain, this organ can serve as a depot for some substances. Further, an immature blood-brain barrier can expose this vital organ to toxic effects.[27,41]

Biotransformation (Metabolism)

The terms *biotransformation* and *metabolism* are not synonymous, even though they are used interchangeably by many individuals. While metabolism reflects the total fate of a substance following exposure, biotransformation is associated with the chemical changes to a substance that take place in an effort to hasten elimination or to detoxify a substance. For most substances, the liver is considered the organ where most biotransformation takes place. However, there are many sites within the body where such processes occur, including the kidney, gastrointestinal tract, lung, skin, testes, etc. Classically, biotransformation is broken down into phase I and phase II processes. Phase I involves an initial change to a substance, typically by oxidation, reduction, etc, and includes the cytochrome P450 isoforms. Phase II (conjugations) reactions further alter a molecule with the intent of hastening elimination, but this is not always the end result. Compounds do not have to undergo phase I or phase II processes to be eliminated from the body, and compounds can undergo only phase I metabolism, only phase II metabolism, or both. Biotransformation of a substance should not be confused with the term *detoxification*. Often,

Table 5-2. Differences in Elimination Half-Lives of Selected Compounds at Various Ages

Drug/Toxicant	Neonate	Infant	Children	Adult
Caffeine	103 h	—	—	6 h
Chloramphenicol	8-15 h	15-22 h	2.3-3.4 h	1.5-5 h
Diazepam	25-100 h	10 h	25 h	15-25 h
Mepiridine	22 h	—	—	3-4 h
Mepivicaine	8.7 h	—	—	3.2 h
Nortriptyline	56 h	—	—	18-22 h
2,3,7,8-Tetrachlorodienz-*p*-dioxin (TCDD)	1.6 y	—	—	3.2 y
Polychlorinated biphenyls (PCBs)	—	0.1-1.2 y	4.5-0.6 y	0.1-22 y

From Collins KA, Byard RW, eds. *Forensic Pathology of Infancy and Childhood.* New York: NY; Springer Reference; 2014. Reproduced with permission.

biotransformation leads to a more reactive species toxicologically or results in the formation of toxic by-products, eg, free radicals.[7,42,43]

The ontogeny of toxicant biotransformation is complex when considering both the nonenzymatic and enzymatic processes that facilitate such processes. Just considering the sheer number of enzymes involved, and related polymorphisms, can be overwhelming. Many enzymes of phase I and phase II biotransformation, including many cytochromes, are active in utero; however, most do not reach adult capabilities until after birth.[44] Shortly after birth, some enzyme activity exceeds that of adults, but biotransforming enzyme activity is generally less than that of adults. Due in part to biological variation, it is not possible to draw universal conclusions as to when each enzyme involved in biotransformation reaches adult levels. Excellent, detailed reviews of the subject are available.[45,46] It is known that some enzyme activity is not reached until adulthood. The differential development of these enzyme systems can lead to varied outcomes ranging from less toxicity to greater toxicity compared to an adult. For example, immature glucuronidation pathway in neonates produces the often fatal gray baby syndrome from chloramphenicol and codeine/morphine intoxication in infants,[47] while the toxicity of acetaminophen is reported to be mitigated in children due to an increased ability for sulfation.[48] Additionally, toxicogenetic influences, ie, enzyme polymorphisms that alter enzyme activity, such as ultra-rapid metabolism of codeine to morphine in breastfed infants, must be recognized.[49] Many of these factors result in differential bioavailability and residence times not only between children and adults, but between children of different age groups (see Table 5-2).

Table 5-3. Selected CYPs and Activity in the Developing Child[50]

CYP	Age Group	Comment
4A	Fetus	High concentrations
3A7	Fetus	High concentrations
2D6	Neonate	Active within a few hours of birth
2E1	Neonate	Active within a few hours of birth
3A4	Neonate	Activity begins to develop
2C8/9/18/19	Neonate	Activity begins to develop
1A2	Neonate	Activity begins to develop

In specific regard to the CYP series of enzymes, it is estimated that there is 20% to 70% of the activity of adults in neonates, infants, and children.[21] Table 5-3 provides developmental information on some specific CYP enzymes based on human liver microsomal studies.[50]

Non-CYP oxidation of many alcohols and aldehydes, including ethanol, are catalyzed by alcohol dehydrogenase (ADH).[42] While seven genes encode for ADH, class I ADH appears to play the most significant role in alcohol metabolism in humans. ADH is found in multiple locations within the body, with a preponderance, both in quantity and importance, in the liver.[50] ADH activity is not complete at birth, with fetuses having ADH activity approximately 10 to 100 times less than adults depending on the developmental stage. Children tend to reach adult levels of activity around 5 years of age.[51] Aldehyde dehydrogenase or aldehyde oxidase (AOX) biotransforms aldehydes, including acetaldehyde, the metabolite formed after alcohol dehydrogenase activity on ethanol. Neonates have 10% to 15% of the activity of AOX as adults, with a linear increase in activity to adult levels reached at 1 year of age.[45] Accumulation of acetaldehyde is responsible for many of the adverse effects of alcohol. As such, based on toxicological principles alone, the exposure of children, especially neonates and infants, to alcohol is contraindicated.

Specific examples of differences in phase II biotransformation exist, such as those mentioned above. Lastly, intestinal flora participate in both the degree of absorption as well as biotransformation of both endogenous compounds and xenobiotics. Such influences generally take place in the ileum and colon. Gastrointestinal flora colonization begins at birth with that obtained from the mother during birthing. Thereafter, a number of variables, including feeding and environmental factors, affect continued colonization, with bacterial flora reaching that of adults by 4 years of age. Additionally, whether a young child is breastfed or bottle fed will contribute to which bacteria predominate. Metabolic reactions by gut flora are generally reductive or hydrolytic in nature.[31,52,53]

As a general conclusion, and with some specific exceptions, based on the development of responsible physiological elements, children, especially young children, biotransform toxicants at slower rates than adults.

Excretion

Humans of all ages possess multiple means of excretion, eg, urine, feces, breath, sweat, and hair. The two most quantitatively important means of excretion are urine and bile (fecal). Renal elimination is often based on glomerular filtration and tubular secretion. Both processes reach adult capability at around 1 year of age. This developmental process is important to consider to mitigate toxicity with several compounds, eg, aminoglycosides, mainly due to decreased urinary excretion.[3] All of the processes involved in enterohepatic circulation are immature at birth, including bile synthesis, conjugation, transport, secretion, and reabsorption, reaching maturation at about 1 year of age.[26] As such, residence time for some substances may be either slowed or hastened compared to an adult.

In summary, toxicokinetics is a major determinant of toxicant concentrations in both children and adults. An appreciation of the toxicokinetic factors that define the differences between these two populations is necessary to understand, in part, potential effects following exposure to chemicals. This section has summarized many of the important differences, but it should be noted that many others exist. Figure 5-4 summarizes many of the most salient factors and the differences between children and adults.

Toxicodynamics

In contrast to toxicokinetics, toxicodynamics (TD) represents the effects of toxicant action. While the outward expression of toxic effects can be obvious, eg, seizures, it is the underlying cause or causes that define a particular outcome. These causes include binding and affinity to receptors, interactions with DNA, altered gene expression, modulation of mediator substances (eg, second messengers), interactions with or modulation of hormones, induced cell proliferation, cytotoxicity, and chronic changes in laboratory values, organ function, and histopathology.[7,54] Age-related maturation of biologic systems associated with toxic sequelae after exposure defines developmental TD.[55] The ability to properly assess TD in children is hampered by a number of factors including ethical factors, and studies are often performed in sick children. There has been substantial improvement for testing of drug or toxicant safety in children in the US and elsewhere, but certain limitations still do not equate to such studies in adults.[56-58]

It is well recognized that children and adults can have disparate responses to medications and toxic exposures. In children, it is often difficult to address TD differences without consideration of TK differences. In addition to previously noted causes, maturational differences in biochemical pathways can also put developing systems in jeopardy, eg, central nervous, endocrine, reproductive, and immune systems.[55] Because of this, many TD effects in young children may not be observed until later in life, eg, DES. A summary of observed TD differences compared to adults, potential consequences, and causes is found in Table 5-4.

Unlike TK, TD effects remain substantial in later childhood, especially in adolescents. Despite many developmental stages attaining biochemical and physiological maturation by this latter stage, some have not fully developed. A critical example is seen with the mesocorticolimbic circuitry, which continues to develop during this time period in

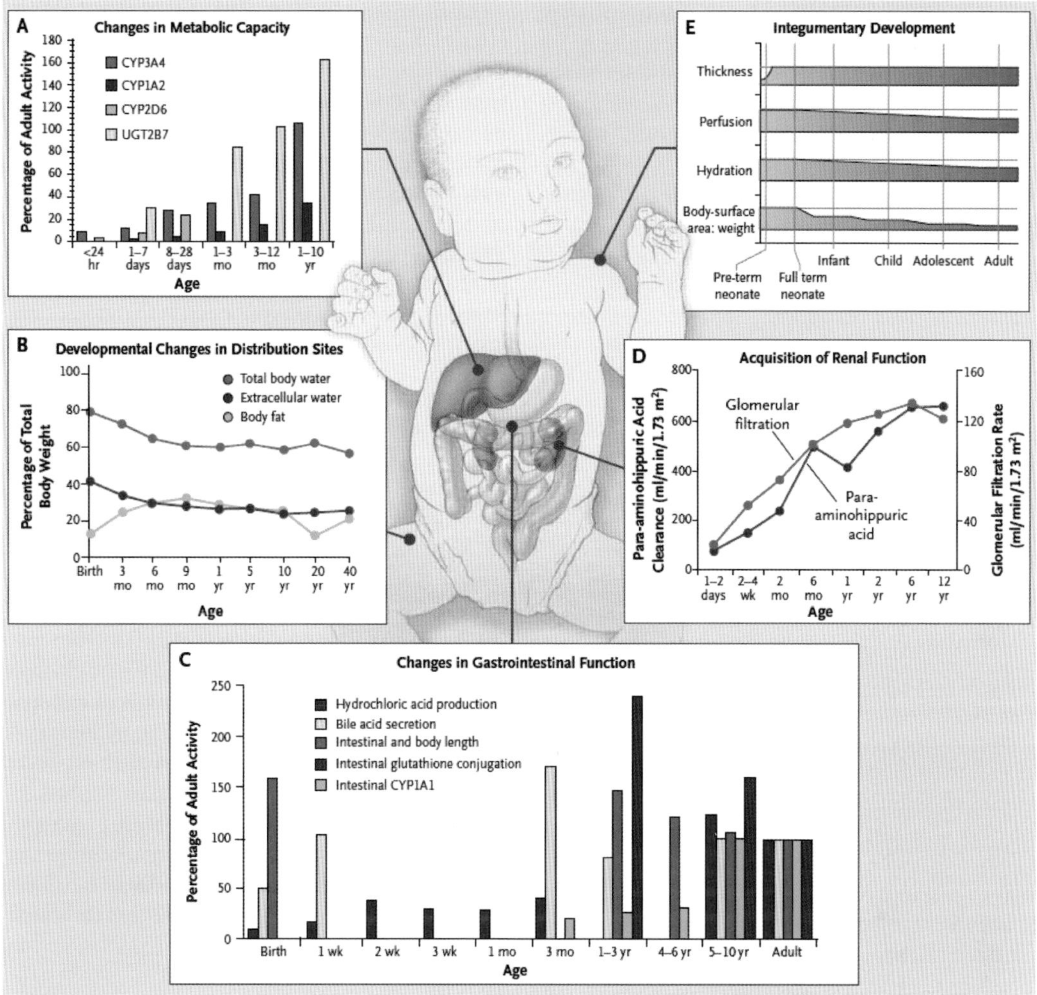

Figure 5-4. Toxicoketinetic developmental differences between children and adults that affect drug disposition. From Kearns GL et al.[3] Reproduced with permission of the Massachusetts Medical Society. © 2003.

Table 5-4. Some Common Toxicodynamic Outcomes in Children Compared to Adults[55,114]

Observed Effect Compared to Adults	Potential Consequence	Potential Cause
Increased/decreased potency	Unexpected effects at small or large doses or exposures	Receptor or target organ sensitivity; immature biochemical pathways
Increased/decreased efficacy	Under or exaggerated effects	Receptor or target organ sensitivity; immature biochemical pathways; toxicokinetic differences; not understood mechanisms
Target organ-specific toxicity or reduced toxicity at a given target organ	Damage to a specific target organ with related sequelae or lack of expected damage to a target organ	Susceptibility (eg, the brain) or lack of sensitivity to developing organs or organ systems
Paradoxical effects	Unexpected outcomes, eg, stimulation due to antihistamines	Underdeveloped target organs, cellular processes, receptors, modulators

Table 5-5. Substances That Can Be Fatal in Small Doses in Children[66,115]
Antimalarials
Antidysrhythmics
Benzocaine
Beta-blockers
Calcium channel blockers
Camphor
Clonidine (and other imidazolines)
Methyl salicylate (and other salicylates)
Opioids
Organophosphate pesticides
Sulfonylureas
Theophylline
Tricyclic antidepressants

Table 5-6. Esoteric Substances of Toxicological Concern Generally Unique to Children[6]
Automotive products
Building materials
Button batteries
Coins (other metal sources)
Cosmetics
Desiccants
Household products
Laundry detergent pods
Lead-containing objects
Nicotine (cigarette butts, vaping solutions, chewing tobacco)
Pica
Plants
Toothpaste

human development. In particular, processes utilizing neurotransmitters, eg, dopamine with the limbic system, play critical roles in attention, decision making, and motivational and emotional regulation. Interference with this critical developmental process has been associated with novelty-seeking and risk-taking behaviors, including substance abuse. Additionally, adolescence is heavily impacted by hormonal changes that, besides physiological effects, affect interactions with peers, which interplays with the previously mentioned behaviors.[59] Unfortunately, children will experiment with substances without concern for, or without careful consideration of, the consequences, with or without perceived peer influence.[60] Therefore, careful screening and education of children as young as 9 years of age for substance abuse is critical to help ward off possible long-term effects.[61] Lastly, the use of abused substances by this age group is associated with increased rates of attempted and death by suicide.[62-64] Impacts of exposure are not limited to drugs of abuse because other substances, including environmental agents, can also interfere with other critical developmental factors.[65]

Specific Examples of Toxicodynamic Impacts on Children

Many substances share similar toxicities in children and adults. However, there are also many substances that in small doses present significant toxic risks in children as opposed to adults (see Table 5-5). Additionally, some esoteric exposures generally unique in young children present challenges in both diagnosis and treatment (see Table 5-6). The following highlights some substances and their particular risks to children.

Salicylates

There are several aspects to salicylate exposure to young children that present significant risk. First, typical dosage units of salicylates (methysalicylate, bismuth subsalicylate) tend to be high. As a result, small exposures can have significant sequelae in children and include metabolic acidosis with resultant respiratory alkalosis, vomiting, and mental status changes.[66] Second, aspirin use in children with juvenile rheumatoid arthritis is associated with increased risk of hepatotoxicity due to effects on mitochondrial permeability transition leading to cell death.[67,68] Lastly, and of greater concern, is the connection between salicylate use in children and Reye syndrome. This syndrome, characterized by drowsiness, hypoglycemia, seizures, liver failure, coma, and death, can follow the use of aspirin in children with mild viral infection. After recognition of this link, the warning that salicylates should not be used in children with viral infection has led to a significant drop in the incidence of Reye syndrome.[69,70] (For additional information on salicylate poisoning, the reader is referred to chapter 27, *Over-the-Counter Analgesics.*)

Opioids

A complete discussion of the effects of opioids on children is not possible here; however, certain salient points should be noted. Children are typically exposed to opioids in three general ways: purposeful administration by a medical professional, parent, caregiver, or other individual; unintentional self-administration (eg, toddlers accessing parental medication); and intentional self-administration (eg, recreational use). From 2001 to 2008, the American Association of Poison Control Centers in the US reported about 29,000 visits to emergency departments due to opioid exposure in children ≤5 years of age, resulting in 20 deaths.[71] Between the years of 2004 to 2007 and 2012 to 2015, there was a doubling of childhood hospitalizations due to opioids. Most admissions were children between 12 and 17 years old, with one-third being <6 years old.[72] Since 2004, there have been 635 opioid-related deaths in children age 10 to 17 years old. Not surprisingly, 68% of such deaths occurred in children 16 years and older.[73]

Maternal exposure to opioids can have significant effects on the developing fetus. Neonatal abstinence syndrome (NAS), a withdrawal-type reaction, is not uncommon in neonates of opioid-using mothers, with signs and symptoms including central nervous system hypersensitivity, respiratory distress, autonomic dysfunction, and gastrointestinal disturbances. The severity of NAS is multifactorial, including which opioid was used, the dosage, the time since mother's last dose, the exposure duration, and the state of health of the neonate. NAS generally appears within 72 hours of birth but could be as long as 2 to 4 weeks, with effects lasting from 6 days to 8 weeks.[31,74]

It was once believed that children do not experience pain as significantly as adults. This premise is no longer accepted since it has been shown that the fetus attains peripheral, spinal, and supraspinal afferent pain transmission by 26 weeks post gestation, although descending inhibitory pathways develop later.[75] TK differences can influence TD outcomes of opioids up to and including death. For example, the elimination half-life of morphine is reported to be 7 to 10 hours in preterm neonates, 7 to 13 hours in term neonates, 1 to 4 hours in infants and other children, and 2 to 4 hours in adults.[76] These differences can be partially attributed to increased glucuronidation capabilities in the developing child.[77] Such differences must be taken into account when dosing morphine. Based on maturational processes associated with the lungs and respiratory-reflex responses, the use of opioids in neonates and infants may result in increased risk of opioid-related respiratory depression, with differences compared to adults eliminated after 3 to 6 months.

TK parameters of opioids in neonates tend to be different than those in adults, with elimination being slower but reaching or exceeding adult proportions in the first year of life. Metabolism in neonates may be slower than adults but may exceed that of adults in preschool and early school years. This may result in the need for higher dosages—a consideration in evaluating cases where children are prescribed opioids. There does not appear to be substantial differences in the TD of opioids in children compared to adults except in the neonatal period.[7,75,76]

As noted above, it is clear from hospitalizations that opioid abuse among adolescents has increased in recent years. In 2011, it was reported that less than 1% of adolescents in the US used heroin. However, 1.8%, 3.9%, and 4.9% of 8th, 10th, and 12th graders, respectively, used OxyContin (oxycodone). For hydrocodone, the corresponding statistics were 2.1%, 5.9%, and 8.1%, respectively.[78] As this author has seen many postmortem cases with unexpected opioid findings in children of various ages, it appears that other than infants, TD effects of these drugs leading to death are similar to those in adults. (For additional information on opiates, the reader is referred to chapters 24 and 25.)

Ethyl Alcohol

An estimated one in 10 pregnant women use alcohol at some point during pregnancy, with a small percentage (3.1%) being binge drinkers (≥4 drinks in one sitting).[79] Ethanol exposure to the developing child can have severe toxicological effects, including birth defects and developmental deficiencies. Fetal alcohol syndrome (FAS) is a condition that falls under the broader term of fetal alcohol spectrum disorder.[80] Characteristics of children born with FAS include facial dysmorphism, limb defects, cardiovascular defects, growth development issues, microcephaly, epicanthal folds, maxillary hypoplasia, short nose, thin upper lip, and mental retardation. Fetal alcohol effect (FAE), a lesser form of FAS, is associated with less alcohol use (eg, 1-2 oz/day). Manifestations of FAE include behavioral and learning difficulties that continue into adolescence.[14] No level of ethanol consumption is considered safe to the developing child in utero.[31] Estimates show that newborns metabolize alcohol at half the rate of adults.[81] As the use of alcohol by breastfeeding mothers as a means of increasing milk production, milk letdown, and relaxation of mother and infant is still prevalent, the decreased metabolic rate can be consequential to the child. One group of surveyed lactating women revealed that 25% were advised to drink alcohol by a physician. Unfortunately, it has been demonstrated that the use of alcohol in lactating women causes less milk production, infants to consume about 20% less milk, decreased sleep by the infant, and decreased motor skill maturation.[7,82]

A 2011 report revealed that 13%, 27%, and 40% of 8th, 10th, and 12th graders, respectively, consumed at least one alcoholic beverage within 30 days of being asked, reinforcing that alcohol remains a significant concern for teenagers.[78] As maturation of brain regions associated with drug reinforcement continue through adolescence, it can be expected that patterns of alcohol abuse would be different in adolescents compared to adults. Not surprisingly, long-term effects on neural and endocrine system maturation are also expected.[83] Neuropsychological effects, including short-term memory deficits, are associated with early to mid-adolescent heavy drinking.[7,84] Organic changes in adolescents with alcohol-related problems include smaller hippocampal volumes, with women more prone to brain shrinkage.[85,86] Hypoglycemia is a significant risk in children (ranging from infants to adolescents) that are exposed to alcohol.[87,88] The mortality rate in children with alcohol-induced hypoglycemia is reported to be as high as 25%.[7,89] (For more information on ethanol, the reader is referred to chapter 16.)

Carboxyhemoglobin (COHb) and Methemoglobin (MetHb)

Young children tend to be more susceptible to toxic sequelae of exposure to carbon monoxide (CO) and methemoglobin-inducing agents. There are a multitude of reasons for this sensitivity (see below), but in general, a young child has a higher basal metabolic rate with consequent higher tissue oxygen demand.[90] Significant amounts of fetal hemoglobin (Hbf) may still be present in children less than 6 months old. Hbf binds CO more avidly than adult hemoglobin, thus significantly increasing the half-life of the carboxyhemoglobin moiety as well as the concentration of COHb.[91,92] Therefore, given equal exposures, younger children may develop higher concentrations of COHb and/or be more susceptible to the effects of the toxin than adults. While a direct correlation between COHb levels and toxic sequelae across all age groups is not possible, COHb concentrations of >25% in children have a high degree of syncope associated with it and a higher degree of altered mental status, seizures, and death compared to adults.[93] It is important for the clinical laboratory scientist to understand that with some spectrophotometric-based measurement techniques, eg, some co-oximeters, interference of fetal hemoglobin may produce falsely elevated COHb.[94] (See also chapter 29, *Common Household and Environmental Toxicants.*)

Methemoglobin-inducing agents are plentiful, ranging from dietary and environmental substances (eg, meat preservatives and naphthalene) to industrial chemicals (eg, aromatic amines and nitrites) to drugs (eg, dapsone, rifampin).[95] Methemoglobin (where the iron in hemoglobin exists in the ferric [Fe^{+3}] state) is an oxidized form of hemoglobin. In this form, MetHb cannot transport oxygen.[96] Children less than 6 months of age are more susceptible to MetHb-inducing toxicities because[95]:

- Their Hb is more susceptible to oxidative stress.
- They are lacking significant enzyme necessary to reduce MetHb.
- Hbf may be more easily oxidized than normal hemoglobin.
- Hbf has a greater affinity for oxygen, thus it will not release oxygen to tissues as easily (left shift in the oxygen dissociation curve).
- MetHb causes an increase in oxygen affinity of the remaining normal hemoglobin—the "Bohr effect." (This same phenomenon holds for COHb as well.)[7]

Measurement of methemoglobin is challenging due to its rapid formation in some situations, eg, postmortem blood.[97] Thus, concentration of MetHb in infant deaths must be interpreted carefully, but this should not preclude the use of such testing when appropriate.

The few examples of specific substances above are meant to be a sampling of different substances and how responses in children differ from those in adults. Space limits a more expansive list, but it must be understood that such examples are plentiful. Even with education, children, even younger than 10 years old, are voluntarily exposed to substances. More modern examples include ingestion of laundry pods, cough syrup, synthethic cannabinoids, and diphenoxylate. As such, it is incumbent upon the practicing clinician and clinical laboratory scientist to be well versed in this ever-changing arena.

Other Issues

There are a host of other issues unique to the pediatric population in respect to toxicology. Space limits how many such topics can be covered. However, two areas of note include breastfeeding and analytical perspectives. Other areas that impact toxicological aspects of pediatric exposure that are not covered include epigenetics, disease states, detailed dosing requirements, homicidal administrations, and social aspects of pediatric poisoning.

Breastfeeding

Breastfeeding is recognized as the healthiest form of nourishment for the neonate, infant, and mother.[36,98] In respect to toxicology, breastfeeding presents a number of challenges (see also chapter 15, *Drug Testing in Hair, Sweat, Meconium, Cord Tissue, and Breast Milk*). It is often medically necessary for women to be on medications to maintain health before and after delivery. Additionally, there is no easy way to prevent environmental exposure to substances capable of being passed to the suckling child. Lastly, women who abuse substances while breastfeeding may put their child at risk for adverse effects. Nevertheless, when addressing these situations, there are three basis questions that should be addressed:

- Does the risk of drug use outweigh the benefits?
- Does a particular substance get into breast milk?
- Did the nursing child receive enough of a dose to cause illness or death?[7]

Whether the risk of exposure to a substance outweighs the benefit must not only be determined on a case by case basis between the patient and her physician, but must take into consideration TK and TD principles. A number of factors, including the need for a medication, effects of the substance on milk production, the amount of substance excreted into breast milk, extent of absorption of the substance by the infant, and ultimate effects on the child, must be considered. For many reasons short of potential harm to the infant, drugs of abuse are contraindicated during lactation. Similar blanket conclusions, short of radioactive substances, cannot be made for other substances.[99] In this respect, the LactMed searchable database (toxnet.nlm.nih.gov) is an extremely valuable tool for assessment of a particular compound and its toxicological relationship to breastfeeding.

Drugs and other toxicants enter breast milk through a series of complex processes. In brief, milk is produced in mammary tissue, and toxicants traverse alveolar mammary cells to get into breast milk. The processes involved in this transfer include transcellular diffusion, passive and ionophore-facilitated diffusion, intracellular diffusion (larger molecules), and other mechanisms.[7,100] While many substances make their way into breast milk, this does not correlate to any substantial risk to the child. The mere presence of a substance in breast milk does not portend any given adverse effect in the suckling child.[99,100] There are number of pharmacokinetic variables that are used to define the passage of drugs into breast milk; however, use of these variables to calculate the dose received by a child should not be performed in living or postmortem cases based on a measured blood concentration as the assumptions and variables are largely unfounded or not well grounded. Of particular concern is that toxicant accumulation in breast milk and the infant occur over time, thus making it virtually impossible to determine not only how much toxicant the mother was exposed to, but if the amount of substance in an infant came from a one-time or multiple exposures or from breast milk at all. Additionally, elimination kinetics and toxicogenomic factors in the nursing child, as well as how much milk was consumed in any given feeding, are typically unknown. Multiple other variables make such calculations tenuous at best.[7]

Whether adverse effects observed in a child are due to passage of toxicants in breast milk is not easily discerned, especially with drugs of abuse. Often, drug abusers predispose children to exposure possibilities via airborne concentrations, smoke, residue on parent's hands and face, etc. As such, accounting for the presence of a drug of abuse in a young child must preclude other means of exposure than just breast milk. Further, the presence of a drug of abuse in a child due to breast milk should not obviate other considerations for illness or death. Nevertheless, the prosecution of women accused of having passed drugs in breast milk resulting in the death of their child has occurred.[7,101-103] Based on current interest, one specific drug class is worth noting: opioids.

Opioids

The maternal use of oral narcotics during breastfeeding can cause infant drowsiness, central nervous system depression, and even death; thus, alternatives to opioids should be sought where possible.[104] Such potential safety issues are compound specific, and when used, the smallest dose and the shortest duration as possible should be considered.[105] Codeine has been reported to cause bradycardia and apnea as well as at least one reported death in breastfed infants. These effects have been partially attributed to maternal ultrarapid metabolism resulting in relatively high morphine concentrations in the infant.[106] Similar issues arise with hydrocodone. Morphine use in nursing mothers is

Table 5-7. Toxicological Analyses to Consider in Deaths Involving Children

Substance	Explanation
Carboxyhemoglobin, methemoglobin	Young children are particularly sensitive to exposure to carbon monoxide and methemoglobin-inducing agents. Concentrations not normally causing adverse effects in adults may be fatal in young children.
Drugs of abuse (comprehensive)	Children are often unknowingly exposed to such agents due to presence in the home or through second-hand smoke. Children in homes where drugs of abuse are synthesized may have in vivo only by-products or reagents associated with the synthesis of the intended agents. Adolescents may often experiment with such agents.
Therapeutic agents (comprehensive)	Given the multitude of therapeutic agents, both prescription and nonprescription, present in the home and available to children by other means, such agents should be included in all toxicological examinations of children. Younger children that die in the hands of caregivers should always be screened for therapeutic substances since such agents may be used to sedate a child.
Metals	Younger children may become toxic due to exposure to batteries, toys, etc that contain toxic metals. Signs and symptoms of toxic metal exposure may mimic other pathologies, precluding their diagnosis in the living patient.
Botanicals, fungi (eg, belladonna alkaloids; amatoxin)	Where and when appropriate, screening for toxicants found in plants, mushrooms, and other flora may be appropriate. Often, pathologic signs and symptoms precede death.
Alcohols and inhalants	Given the prevalence and widespread use of alcohols and inhalants in the pediatric population, such testing should be performed in all unexplained pediatric deaths.
Environmental agents (eg, pesticides, solvents)	Given the rapid toxicity of many such compounds, and the inability to detect most of these substances on routine toxicological screening, such agents must be considered in unexplained pediatric deaths.
Miscellaneous tests	Given specific histories and clinical pictures, consultation with a toxicologist to develop analyte-specific assays should be considered.

From Collins KA, Byard RW, eds. *Forensic Pathology of Infancy and Childhood.* New York: NY; Springer Reference; 2014. Reproduced with permission.

not necessarily contraindicated, while hydromorphone use should be limited. Oxycodone is contraindicated due to the high concentrations found in breast milk.[105] Methadone is a special case in that it is used not only for pain control, but in opioid dependence therapy. Numerous studies have evaluated the use of methadone in nursing mothers. While some discrete effects have been noted in infants born to mothers that used methadone during pregnancy, the use of methadone during and after pregnancy is not contraindicated, and its benefits far outweigh the concerns of heroin or other opioid abuse. Concentrations of methadone in breast milk in the first month of life and in infants have been demonstrated to be low. Methadone concentrations do accumulate in breast milk over time; however, this does not preclude the continued use of the substance by nursing mothers.[107-110]

While the community at large focuses on drug exposure in respect to breast milk, environmental agents present similar concerns. Data regarding such agents tends to be sparse, but that does not preclude adverse effects.[111,112] For example, many environmental agents are considered endocrine-disrupting substances, thus potentially adversely affecting maturational development of a child.[113]

Toxicological Analyses

Toxicological examination of specimens in pediatric patients should include testing that may not be routine in adults. Based on susceptibilities of children to various toxicants, especially younger children, the need for testing protocols that cover a broad range of possibilities should be utilized. In order to effectively assist in the clinical diagnosis of potential exposure to a toxicant, it is critical that the testing laboratory is provided as much history about the case as possible, including clinical signs and symptoms, as well as other laboratory test results. In addition to toxicological testing in children, inborn errors of metabolism should be excluded in unexplained illness or where toxicological agents were detected since mistaken identifications have been made.[7] For example, propionic acid was misidentified as ethylene glycol in a child with methylmalonic acidemia.[114] As toxicological findings are often unexpected in pediatric cases, and given the potential events that can follow, it is incumbent upon laboratories to utilize techniques that incontrovertibly identify toxicants. Table 5-7 outlines analyses that should be considered in cases involving children.

Techniques employed in toxicology laboratories should include methods that characterize substances based on their molecular structure. Today, the most common of such techniques employ mass spectrometry, including gas chromatography-mass spectrometry (GC-MS), liquid chromatography-mass spectrometry/mass spectrometry (LC-MS/MS), liquid chromatography-time of flight (LC-TOF), and inductively-coupled plasma-mass spectrometry (ICP-MS). It should be recognized, however, techniques based on mass spectrometry are not the only acceptable analytical tools.[7] Additionally, laboratories must be prepared to work with sample types and volumes substantially different than those obtained from adults. For example, blood spot and hair analyses may be suited to address limited collection volume and historical exposures, respectively.

Summary

Exposure of children, especially young children, to toxicologically active agents can have severe detrimental effects, up to and including death. Since toxic exposures to children have occurred throughout history, it is unlikely that such concerns will wane, and this is supported by statistics. It is clear that children often respond differently to exposure to toxic agents, and this, in part, is due to toxicokinetic and toxicodynamic differences. Clinicians and clinical laboratory scientists should understand these differences in order to put exposures in perspective for diagnostic, treatment, and medicolegal purposes. Lastly, it is incumbent upon laboratories performing analyses on specimens from pediatric patients to have techniques and procedures in place that capture the needs for this special population.

References

1. Jacobi A. General therapeutics of infancy and childhood. In: Robinson WJ, ed. *Contributions to Pediatrics*. New York, NY: The Critic and Guide Company; 1909.
2. Hardin AP, Hackell JM. Age limit of pediatrics. *Pediatrics*. 2017;140(3):2151.
3. Kearns GL, Abdel-Rahman SM, Alander SW, Blowey DL, Leeder JS, Kauffman RE. Developmental pharmacology: drug disposition, action and therapy in infants and children. *New Engl J Med*. 2003;349(12):1157-1167.
4. Qin A. Pediatric poisoning fatalities from 1972 through 2013. https://www.cpsc.gov/s3fs-public/PPPAMortality2013.pdf. Accessed January 10, 2019.
5. Shepherd G, Ferslew BC. Homicidal poisoning deaths in the United States 1999-2005. *Clin Toxicol (Phila)*. 2009;47:342-347.
6. Gummin DD, Mowry JB, Spyker DA, Brooks DE, Fraser MO, Banner W. 2016 Annual report of the American Association of Poison Control Centers' National Poison Data System (NPDS): 34th annual report. *Clin Toxicol (Phila)*. 2017;55(10):1072-1254.
7. Middleberg R. Pediatric toxicology. In: Collins KA, Byard RW, eds. *Forensic Pathology of Infancy and Childhood*. New York, NY: Springer Reference; 2014.
8. Liytovitz T, Manoguerra A. Comparison of pediatric poisoning hazards: an analysis of 3.8 million exposure incidents. *Pediatrics*. 1992;80(8):999-1006.
9. Campbell TA, Collins, KA. Pediatric toxicologic deaths: 10-year retrospective study. *Am J Forensic Med Pathol*. 2001;22(2):184-187.
10. Kempe CH, Silverman FN, Steele BF, Droegemueller W, Silver HK. The battered child syndrome. *JAMA*. 1962;181(1):17-24.
11. McClure, RJ, Davis PM, Meadow, SR, Sibert JR. Epidemiology of Munchausen syndrome by proxy, non-accidental poisoning, and non-accidental suffocation. *Arch Dis Child*. 1996;75:57-61.
12. Rogers D, Tripp J, Bentovim A, Robinson A, Berry D, Goulding R. Non-accidental poisoning: an extended syndrome of child abuse. *Br Med J*. 1976;1(6013):793-796.
13. Middleberg RA. The safety of commonly used therapeutic agents in the infant: a forensic toxicological perspective OTC preparations. Proceedings of the American Academy of Forensic Sciences Workshop, Postmortem Pediatric Forensic Toxicology. Issues in Childhood Poisoning. 1999.
14. Moore KL, Persaud TVN. *The Developing Human: Clinically Oriented Embryology*. Philadelphia, PA: Saunders; 2003.

15. Giusti R, Iwamoto K, Hatch E. Diethylstilbestrol revisited: a review of the long-term health effects. *Ann Intern Med.* 1995;122(10):778-788.
16. Newbold RR. Prenatal exposure to diethylstilbestrol (DES). *Fertil Steril.* 2008;89(S1):e55-e56.
17. Sumpter A, Anderson BJ. Pediatric pharmacology in the first year of life. *Curr Opin Anesthesiol.* 2009;22:469-475.
18. Rodman JH. Pharmacokinetic variability in the adolescent: implications of body size and organ function for dosage regimen design. *J Adolesc Health.* 1994;15:654-662.
19. Anderson B, Holford NHG. Tips and traps analyzing pediatric PK data. *Pediatr Anesth.* 2011;21:222-237.
20. Anderson BJ, Holford NHG. Understanding dosing: children are small adults, neonates are immature children. *Arch Dis Child.* 2013;98:737-744.
21. Mahmood I. Dosing in children: a critical review of the pharmacokinetic allometric scaling and modelling approaches in paediatric drug development and clinical studies. *Clin Pharmacokinet.* 2014;53:327-346.
22. International Life Sciences Institute. Total body water in infants. *Nutrition Rev.* 1963;21(4):113-115.
23. Raghaven, CV, Super DM, Chatburn RL, Savin SM, Fanaroff AA, Kalhan SC. Estimation of total body water in very-low-birth-weight infants by using anthropometry with and without bioelectrical impedance and H2[(18)O]. *Am J Clin Nutr.* 1998;68:668-674.
24. Koren G. Therapeutic drug monitoring principles in the neonate. *Clin Chem.* 1997;43(1):222-227.
25. Heringa MB, Brandon EFA, Bessems JG, Bos PMJ, eds. *RIVM Letter Report 055212001/2013.* The Netherlands: National Institute for Public Health and the Environment; 2013.
26. Scheuplein R, Charnley G, Dourson M. Differential sensitivity of children and adults to chemical toxicity. *Reg Toxicol Pharmacol.* 2002;35:429-447.
27. Makri A, Govela J, Balbus J, Parkin R. Children's susceptibility to chemicals: a review by developmental stage. *J Toxicol Environ Health B Crit Rev.* 2004;7:417-435.
28. Schreiber JS. Parents worried about breast milk contamination. *Pediatr Clin North Am.* 2001;49(5):1113-1127.
29. Bellows L, Moore R, Hunley J, Reeder A, Clark A. Benefits of Breastfeeding. Colorado State University Extension, Fact Sheet No. 9.385. 2013.
30. Miclat NN, Hodgkinson R, Marx GF. Neonatal gastric pH. *Anesth Analg.* 1978;57:98-101.
31. Heimann G. Enteral absorption and bioavailability in children in relation to age. *Eur J Clin Pharmacol.* 1980;18:43-50.
32. Blackburn-Tucker S. *Maternal, Fetal, and Neonatal Physiology: A Clinical Perspective.* 4th ed. Seattle, WA: Elsevier Saunders; 2013.
33. Bearer C. Environmental health hazards: how children are different from adults. *Future Child.* 1995;5(2):11-26.
34. Evans NJ, Rutter N. Development of the epidermis in the newborn. *Biol Neonate.* 1986;49:74-80.
35. Johnson PJ. Neonatal pharmacology-pharmacokinetics. *Neonatal Netw.* 2011;30(1):54-61.
36. Committee on Drugs. Alternative routes of drug administration: advantages and disadvantages. *Pediatrics.* 1997;100:143-152.
37. Lehman-McKeeman LD. Absorption, distribution and excretion of toxicants. In: Klassen CD, ed. *Casarett and Doull's Toxicology: The Basic Science of Poisoning.* 8th ed. New York, NY: McGraw-Hill Medical; 2013.
38. Gallagher D, Heymsfield SB, Heo M, Jebb SA, Murgatroyd P, Sakamoto Y. Healthy percentage body fat ranges: an approach for developing guidelines based on body mass index. *Am J Clin Nutr.* 2000;72:694-701.
39. Laurson KR, Eisenmann JC, Welk GJ. Body fat percentile curves for U.S. children and adolescents. *Am J Prevent Med.* 2011;41(4S2):S87-S92.
40. Schmelzle HR, Fusch C. Body fat in neonates and young infants: validation of skinfold thickness versus dual-energy x-ray absorptiometry. *Am J Clin Nutr.* 2002;76:1096-1100.
41. Webster R. Blood brain barrier maturation: implications for drug development. Pfizer Global Research and Development. Pharmacokinetics, Dynamics and Metabolism. http://www.ema.europa.eu/docs/en_GB/document_library/Presentation/2009/11/WC500009793.pdf. Accessed May 13, 2019.
42. Parkinson A, Ogilvie BW. Biotransformation of xenobiotics. In: Klaassen CD, ed. *Casarett and Doull's Toxicology: The Basic Science of Poisons.* 7th ed. New York, NY: The McGraw-Hill Companies; 2008.
43. Gregus Z. Mechanisms of toxicity. In: Klaassen CD, ed. *Casarett and Doull's Toxicology: The Basic Science of Poisons.* 7th ed. New York, NY: The McGraw-Hill Companies; 2008.
44. Blake JJ, Castro L, Leeder JS, Kearns G. Ontogeny of drug metabolizing enzymes in the neonate. *Semin Fetal Neonat Med.* 2005;10:123-138.
45. Hines R. The ontogeny of drug metabolism enzymes and implications for adverse drug events. *Pharmacol Ther.* 2008;118:250-267.
46. de Wildt SN. Profound changes in drug metabolism enzymes and possible effects on drug therapy in neonates and children. *Exp Opin Drug Metabol Toxicol.* 2011:7(8):935-948.

47. Choonara I, Rieder MJ. Drug toxicity and adverse drug reactions in children: a brief historical review. *Paediatr Perinat Drug Ther.* 2002; 5(1):12-18.
48. Penna A, Buchanan N. Paracetamol poisoning in children and hepatotoxicity. *Br J Clin Pharmacol.* 1991;32(2):143-149.
49. Neville KA, Becker ML, Goldman JL, Kearns GL. Developmental pharmacogenomics. *Pediatr Anesth.* 2001;21:255-265.
50. Jones AW. Biochemical and physiological research on the disposition and fate of ethanol in the body. In: Garriott, JC, ed. *Garriott's Medicolegal Aspects of Alcohol.* 5th ed. Tucson, AZ: Lawyers & Judges Publishing Company, Inc; 2008.
51. Pikkarainen PH, Raiha NCR. Development of alcohol dehydrogenase activity in the human liver. *Pediatr Res.* 1967;1:165-168.
52. Alcorn J, McNamara PJ. Pharmacokinetics in the newborn. *Adv Drug Deliv Rev.* 2003;55:667-686.
53. Strolin Benedetti M, Baltes EL. Drug metabolism and disposition in children. *Fundam Clin Pharmacol.* 2003;17(3):281-299.
54. Heinrich-Hirsch B, Madle S, Oberemm A, Gundert-Remy U. The use of toxicodynamics in risk assessment. *Toxicol Lett.* 2001;120:131-141.
55. Mulla H. Understanding developmental pharmacodynamics: importance for drug development and clinical practice. *Pediatr Drugs.* 2010;12(4):223-233.
56. Thaul S. FDA's authority to ensure that drugs prescribed to children are safe and effective. CSR Reports. Congressional Research Services. 2012.
57. Sinha G. EU law mandates drug testing in children. *J Nat Cancer Inst.* 2008;100(2):84-85.
58. Pasquali SK, Lam WK, Chiswell K, Kemper AR, Li JS. Status of the pediatric clinical trials enterprise: an analysis of the US Clinical Trials.gov registry. *Pediatrics.* 2012;130(5):e1269-e1277.
59. Stansfield KH, Kirstein CL. Neurochemical effects of cocaine in adolescence compared to adulthood. *Brain Res Dev Brain Res.* 2005; 159(2):119-125.
60. Bauman KE, Ennett ST. On the importance of peer influence for adolescent drug use: commonly neglected considerations. *Addiction.* 1996;91(2):185-198.
61. DuRant RH, Smith JA, Kreiter SR, Krowchuk DP. The relationship between early age of onset of initial substance use and engaging in multiple health risk behaviors among young adolescents. *Arch Pediatr Adolesc Med.* 1999;153:286-291.
62. Garlow SJ, Purselle DC, Heninger M. Cocaine and alcohol use preceding suicide in African American and white adolescents. *J Psych Res.* 2007;41(6):530-536.
63. Kelly TM, Cornelius JR, Clark DB. Psychiatric disorders and attempted suicide among adolescents with substance use disorders. *Drug Alcohol Depend.* 2004;73:87-97.
64. Kelly TM, Cornelius JR, Lynch KG. Psychiatric and substance use disorders as risk factors for attempted suicide among adolescents: a case control study. *Suicide Life Threat Behav.* 2002;32(3):301-312.
65. Gauderman WJ, Avol E, Gilliland F, et al. The effect of air pollution on lung development from 10 to 18 years of age. *New Engl J Med.* 2004;351(11):1057-1067.
66. Eldridge DL, Van Eyk J, Kornegay C. Pediatric toxicology. *Emerg Med Clin North Am.* 2007; 15:283-308.
67. Athreya BH, Moser G, Cecil HS, Myers AR. Aspirin-induced hepatotoxicity in juvenile rheumatoid arthritis. *Arthritis Rheum.* 1975;18(4): 347-352.
68. Trost LC, Lemasters JJ. Role of the mitochondrial permeability transition in salicylate toxicity to cultured rat hepatocytes: implications for the pathogenesis of Reye's syndrome. *Toxicol Appl Pharmacol.* 1997;147:431-441.
69. Choonara I, Gill A, Nunn A. Drug toxicity and surveillance in children. *Br J Clin Pharmacol.* 1996;42: 407-410.
70. Choonara I, Rieder MJ. Drug toxicity and adverse drug reactions in children: a brief historical review. *Paediatr Perinatal Drug Ther.* 2002;5(1):12-18.
71. Bond GR, Woodward RW, Ho M. The growing impact on pediatric pharmaceutical poisoning. *J Pediatr.* 2012;160(2):265-270.
72. Kane J, Colvin JD, Bartlett AH, Hall M. Opioid-related critical care resource use in US children's hospitals. *Pediatrics.* 2018;141(4).
73. Opioid-Related Deaths, Ages 10-17. The National Center for Fatality Review and Prevention. https://www.ncfrp.org/resources/quick-looks/opioid-related-deaths-ages-10-17/. Published November 2017. Accessed May 14, 2019.
74. Kaltenbach K, Berghella V, Finnegan L. Opioid dependence during pregnancy. *Obstet Gynecol Clin North Am.* 1988;25(1):139-151.
75. Berde CB, Sethna NF. Analgesics for the treatment of pain in children. *New Engl J Med.* 2002;347(14):1094-1103. Erratum in: *N Engl J Med.* 2011;364(18):1782.
76. Olkkola KT, Hamunen K, Maunuksela EL. Clinical pharmacokinetics and pharmacodynamics of opioid analgesics in infants and children. *Clin Pharmacokinet.* 1995;28(5):385-404.
77. McRorie TI, Lynn AM, Nespeca MK, Opheim KE, Slattery JT. The maturation of morphine clearance and metabolism. *Am J Dis Child.* 1992;146:972-976.

78. Johnston LD, O'Malley PM, Bachman JG, Schulenberg JE. Monitoring The Future. National Results On Adolescent Drug Use. Overview Of Key Findings 2011. The University of Michigan Institute for Social Research. 2012. http://monitoringthefuture.org/pubs/monographs/mtf-overview2011.pdf. Accessed May 14, 2019.
79. One in 10 pregnant women in the United States reports drinking alcohol. Centers for Disease Control and Prevention. https://www.cdc.gov/media/releases/2015/p0924-pregnant-alcohol.html. Press Release. Published September 24, 2015. Accessed November 25, 2018.
80. Frost EAM, Gist RS, Adriano E. Drugs, alcohol, pregnancy, and the fetal alcohol syndrome. *Int Anesth Clin.* 2011:49(1):119-133.
81. Idänpään-Heikkilä J, Jouppila P, Akerblom HK, Isoaho R, Kauppila E, Koivisto M. Elimination of metabolic effects of ethanol in mother, fetus and newborn infant. *Am J Obstet Gynecol.* 1972;112(3):387-393.
82. Mennella JA. Alcohol use during lactation: the folklore versus the science. In: Auerback KG, ed. *Current Issues in Clinical Lactation.* Burlington, MA: Jones & Bartlett Publishers; 2002.
83. Spear LP. Alcohol's effects on adolescents. *Alcohol Res Health.* 2002;26(4):287-291.
84. Brown SA, Tapert SF, Granholm E, Delis DC. Neurocognitive functioning of adolescents: effects of protracted alcohol use. *Alcohol Clin Exp Res.* 2002;24(2):164-171.
85. De Bellis MD, Clark DB, Beers SR, et al. Hippocampal volume in adolescent-onset alcohol use disorders. *Am J Psychiatry.* 2000; 157(5):737-744.
86. Hommer D, Momenan R, Ragan P, et al. Changes in CSF, ventricular, gray and white matter volumes in female alcoholics measured by automated segmentation of MRI images. Presented in the 1996 Joint Scientific Meeting of the Research Society on Alcoholism and the International Society for Biomedical Research on Alcoholism. Washington D.C. *Alcohol Clin Exper Res.* 1996;20(s2):1A-3A.
87. Lteif AN, Schwenk WF. Hypoglycemia in infants and children. *Endocrinol Metab Clin North Am.* 1999;28(3):619-646.
88. Ragan FA Jr, Samuels MS, Hite SA. Ethanol ingestion in children: a five year review. *JAMA.* 1979;242(25):2787-2788.
89. Ernst AA, Jones K, Nick TG, Sanchez J. Ethanol ingestion and related hypoglycemia in a pediatric and adolescent emergency department population. *Acad Emerg Med.* 1996;3(1):46-49.
90. Liebelt EL. Hyperbaric oxygen therapy in childhood carbon monoxide poisoning. *Curr Opin Pediatr.* 1999;11:259-264.
91. Snook CP. Carbon monoxide. In: Erickson TB, Ahrens WR, Aks SE, Baum CR, Ling LJ. *Pediatric Toxicology: Diagnosis and Management of the Poisoned Child.* New York, NY: The McGraw-Hill Companies, Inc; 2005.
92. Abelsohn A, Sanborn MD, Jessiman BJ, Weir E. Identifying and managing adverse environmental health effects, 6: carbon monoxide poisoning. *CMAJ.* 2002;166(13):1685-1690.
93. White S. Pediatric carbon monoxide poisoning. In: Penney D, ed. *Carbon Monoxide Toxicity.* Boca Raton, FL: CRC Press: 2000:463-491.
94. Vreman HJ, Ronquillo RB, Ariagno RL, Schwartz HC, Stevenson, DK. Interference of fetal hemoglobin with the spectrophotometric measurement of carboxyhemoglobin. *Clin Chem.* 1988;34(5):975-977.
95. Osterhoudt KC. Methemoglobinemia. In: Erickson TB, Ahrens WR, Aks SE, Baum CR, Ling LJ. *Pediatric Toxicology: Diagnosis and Management of the Poisoned Child.* New York, NY: The McGraw-Hill Companies, Inc; 2005.
96. Wright RO, Lewander WJ, Woolf AD. Methemoglobinemia: etiology, pharmacology and clinical management. *Ann Emerg Med.* 1999;34(5):646-656.
97. Reay DT, Insalaco SJ, Eisele JW. Postmortem methemoglobin concentrations and their significance. *J Forensic Sci.* 1984;29(4):1160-1163.
98. Howard CR, Lawrence RA. Breast-feeding and drug exposure. *Obstet Gynecol Clin North Am.* 1998;25(1):195-216.
99. Sachs HC. The transfer of drugs and therapeutics into human breast milk: an update on selected topics. *Pediatrics.* 2013;132:e796-e809.
100. Berlin CM, Briggs GG. Drugs and chemicals in human milk. *Semin Fetal Neonatal Med.* 2005;10(2):149-159.
101. Riparbelli L. Breastfeeding mother charged in infant's death. ABC News. http://abcnews.go.com/. Accessed December 6, 2012.
102. Hutchinson C. California woman claims meth-laced breast milk not cause of her baby's death. ABC News. http://abcnews.go.com. Accessed December 6, 2012.
103. Ariagno R, Karch SB, Middleberg R, Stephens BG, Valdes-Dapena M. Methamphetamine ingestion by a breast-feeding mother and her infant's death: people v Henderson. *JAMA.* 1995;274(3):215.
104. Morphine. LactMed: Drugs and Lactation Database. A TOXNET Database. https://toxnet.nlm.nih.gov/cgi-bin/sis/search2/f?./temp/~5S0Prq:1. Accessed May 14, 2019.

105. Boateng S, et al. Prescribing Guidelines for Pennsylvania. Safe Prescribing of Opioids in Pediatric and Adolescent Populations. Pennsylvania Department of Health, 2017. https://www.dos.pa.gov/ProfessionalLicensing/BoardsCommissions/Documents/PA%20Guidelines%20-Pediatric%20and%20Adolescent%20Populations.pdf. Updated September 19, 2017. Accessed May 13, 2019.
106. Madadi P, Shirazi F, Walter FG, Koren G. Establishing causality of CNS depression in breastfed infants following maternal codeine use. *Pediatr Drugs.* 2008;10(6):399-404.
107. Jansson LM, et al. Methadone maintenance and breastfeeding in the neonatal period. *Pediatrics.* 2008;121:106-114.
108. Glatstein MM, Garcia-Bournissen F, Finkelstein Y, Koren G. Methadone exposure during lactation. *Can Fam Physician.* 2008;54:1689-1670.
109. Farid WO, Dunlop SA, Tait RJ, Hulse GK. The effects of maternally administered methadone, buprenorphine and naltrexone on offspring: review of human and animal data. *Curr Neopharmacol.* 2008;6:125-150.
110. Jansson LM, Choo R, Velez ML, Lowe R, Huestis MA. Methadone maintenance and long-term lactation. *Breastfeed Med.* 2008;3(1): 34-37.
111. Leung HW, Kerger BD, Paustenbach DJ. Elimination half-lives of selected polychlorinated dibenzodioxins and dibenzofurans in breast-fed human infants. *J Toxicol Environ Health A.* 2006;69(6):437-443.
112. Landrigan PJ, Babasaheb S, Mattison D, McCally M, Garg A. Chemical contaminants in breast milk and their impacts on children's health: an overview. *Environ Health Perspect.* 2002;110(6):313-315.
113. Meeker JD. Exposure to environmental endocrine disruptors and child development. *Arch Pediatr Adolesc Med.* 2012;166(6):E1-E7.
114. Shoemaker JD, Lynch RE, Hoffman JW, Sly WS. Misidentification of propionic acid as ethylene glycol in a patient with methylmalonic acidemia. *J Pediatr.* 1992;120(3):417-421.
115. Calello DP, Henretig FM. Pediatric toxicology: specialized approach to the poisoned child. *Emerg Med Clin North Am.* 2014;32:29-52.

Chapter 6

Workplace Drug Testing

Jennifer A. Collins, PhD
Arthur M. Zebelman, PhD

Introduction

The United States' federal "War on Drugs," first declared by the Nixon administration in 1969, led to a wide variety of activities at both national and international levels, not least of which are continuing efforts at instituting and maintaining drug-free workplaces throughout the country. Drug use and abuse patterns have varied since the 1970s, and substance use issues continue to affect millions of adolescents and adults in the US.[1] The most recent Substance Abuse and Mental Health Services Administration (SAMHSA) data from the National Survey on Drug Use and Health provides insight into the magnitude of the problem and estimates of the association between employment status and rates of illicit drug use. For example, in 2016, of an estimated 26.6 million illicit drug users in the US aged 18 years or older, 18.0 million (67.8%) were employed either full or part time, representing 11.1% of the full-time and 14.4% of the part-time workforce. Likewise, most binge and heavy alcohol users were among the employed: of an estimated 64.1 million adult binge drinkers in 2016, 47.8 million (74.5%) were employed either full or part time, and 12.2 million (75.8%) of an estimated 16.1 million adult heavy drinkers were among the employed.[2] Although patterns of drug and alcohol use and misuse vary by industry, estimated costs to US companies are in the billions of dollars per year in lost productivity, workplace accidents and injuries, employee absenteeism, increased illness, and employee turnover.[3]

Workplace Drug Testing

Efforts to establish a drug-free federal workplace began in 1986 with a Reagan administration executive order, ultimately leading to the Department of Health and Human Services (HHS) Mandatory Guidelines for Federal Workplace Drug Testing Programs, published in 1988.[4] At that time, the National Institute of Drug Abuse (NIDA) was given the responsibility of administering the Federal Workplace Drug Testing Program. It was subsequently moved to SAMHSA, where it is administered today. When the Guidelines were first implemented on January 1, 1990, drug testing in both regulated and nonregulated workplaces increased dramatically.

Before 1990, most workplace drug testing was performed by clinical laboratories, and universally recognized standards for such testing did not exist. With publication of the Mandatory Guidelines, standards for testing personnel, methodologies, quality assurance, and cutoffs were established. Although the Guidelines specifically apply only to federal agencies and employers, they provide the basis for drug testing programs utilized by the Department of Transportation (DOT; 49 CFR Part 40), the Nuclear Regulatory Commission (NRC; 10 CFR Part 26), and many nonregulated employers across a wide variety of employment markets. The DOT represents the largest group of regulated entities, with more than 700,000 employers and approximately 12.1 million transportation employees performing safety-sensitive functions.[5] The Omnibus Transportation Employee Drug Testing Act of 1991,[6] passed by Congress after a high-profile subway accident in New York City, codified and expanded drug testing in the transportation industry. The requirements of the Act are incorporated into 49 CFR Part 40, and, within the DOT, the Office of Drug and Alcohol Policy and Compliance publishes, implements, and provides authoritative interpretations of these rules.[7] Drug testing program requirements detailed in Part 40 follow the scientific and technical aspects of the HHS Guidelines but have some provisions that differ. The NRC incorporates drug testing into a fitness-for-duty program in the nuclear power industry. Procedures used in the program are based on the HHS model, although components and cutoffs may differ.[8] Some states require that all workplace drug testing voluntarily conducted by employers follow either the HHS Guidelines or DOT regulations, including the use of a certified drug testing laboratory for specimen analysis. States that require the use of a certified laboratory may also recognize the College of American Pathologists (CAP) or the CAP Forensic Drug Testing (FDT) accreditations. The reader is advised to check the individual states' statutes to become familiar with requirements when providing drug testing services.

Since the original implementation in January of 1990, the HHS Guidelines have been revised five different times—in 1994, 1997, 2004, 2008, and 2017—to revise cutoffs, modify the test panel, and add specimen validity testing.[9] The most recent revision, effective October 1, 2017, incorporated the semisynthetic opioids hydrocodone, hydromorphone, oxycodone, and oxymorphone into the test panel and revised the interpretation of some specimen validity tests.[10] The current panel with included compounds and cutoffs is shown in Table 6-1. The DOT followed with a revision to 49 CFR Part 40, effective January 1, 2018, incorporating the same changes.[11] Use of alternate matrices (ie, oral fluid, hair, and sweat) has been proposed for inclusion in the Mandatory Guidelines; however, at the current time only urine is approved and fully implemented. Mandatory Guidelines for Federal Workplace Drug Testing Programs – Oral Fluid were published in a final version on October 25, 2019, with an effective date of January 1, 2020.[10] Full implementation is anticipated within 12 to 18 months when all stakeholders are prepared to meet the requirements of the Guidelines. Use of alternate matrices in toxicology testing is covered in detail in chapters 14 and 15.

Regulated Workplace Drug Testing

As indicated previously, the Mandatory Guidelines and derivatives thereof establish scientific and technical guidelines for workplace drug testing programs and establish a certification program for laboratories performing testing for regulated employees engaged in safety-sensitive environments (the National Laboratory Certification Program). The Guidelines include detailed standards for collection sites and individuals performing specimen collection, test panels and cutoffs, laboratory personnel, methodologies, quality assurance/quality control, certification and result reporting, and review/verification of laboratory results by a Medical Review Officer (MRO) before reporting a final result to an employer. For the specimen collection procedure, a split-specimen process is followed, whereby a specimen collected into a single collection cup is split into two separate bottles that are sealed and sent to the certified laboratory. The specimen must be accompanied by a federal custody and control form (CCF) that documents the donor ID, collection, and transport processes. The laboratory tests the "A" bottle and retains the "B" bottle for retesting at a second certified laboratory if requested by the donor through the MRO. Certified laboratories undergo periodic on-site inspections during which laboratory operations, standard operating procedures, personnel records, and reporting procedures are reviewed to ensure compliance with HHS requirements. Successful participation in a quarterly proficiency program provided by the HHS contractor administering the National Laboratory Certification Program is also required for continued certification. A list of certified laboratories is published monthly in the *Federal Register* and is also available online at http://www.samhsa.gov/workplace.

Testing must be performed under chain-of-custody protocols where all specimen and aliquot handling are documented. Test panels must comply with the analytes and cutoffs shown in Table 6-1. The testing process includes an initial test and, if positive, a second, confirmatory test performed on a separate aliquot of the original specimen. The initial test or screen is most often performed by immunoassay; however, alternate technologies are permitted by the Mandatory Guidelines. Confirmatory testing must be performed on an independent aliquot of the specimen using chromatographic methods with mass spectrometric detection. Only specimens with positive initial and confirmatory test results are reported as positive, and all analytical data and chain-of-custody documentation must be reviewed by a certifying scientist before reporting.

Another important feature of this program is the requirement to include specimen validity testing (SVT). Because results of workplace drug tests may have negative consequences for a donor, attempts to subvert the procedure by altering or tampering with the specimen may occur.[12] The three most common forms of alteration are urine dilution, substitution, and adulteration. The goal of dilution is to produce a specimen whose drug concentration is below the screening cutoff, which can be accomplished either by in vivo dilution through ingestion of large quantities of liquids or by in vitro dilution, whereby liquid is added to a previously voided sample. Substitution is the process whereby an external sample—from a different individual or purchased as a synthetic urine—is brought into the collection site and substituted for the donor's authentic specimen. Adulteration generally involves addition of a chemical or product that either interferes with the testing process or converts drugs or metabolites into by-products not measured in the analytical method. Laboratories are challenged with identifying such samples, but they also must be able to distinguish intentionally altered specimens from those resulting from normal physiological variability.

SVT consists of measurement of urine markers that can be interpreted to determine if a specimen is normal or abnormal on the basis of physiological characteristics.[13] Current HHS program requirements for urine include the following, at a minimum:

- Creatinine is measured on every specimen.

Table 6-1. Drug Test Cutoff Concentrations in Urine: Mandatory Guidelines for Federal Workplace Drug Testing Programs[10]

Initial Test Analyte	Initial Test Cutoff†	Confirmatory Test Analyte	Confirmatory Test Cutoff Concentration
Marijuana metabolites (THCA)‡	50 ng/mL§	THCA	15 ng/mL
Cocaine metabolite (benzoylecgonine)	150 ng/mL§	Benzoylecgonine	100 ng/mL
Codeine Morphine	2000 ng/mL	Codeine Morphine	2000 ng/mL 2000 ng/mL
Hydrocodone Hydromorphone	300 ng/mL	Hydrocodone Hydromorphone	100 ng/mL 100 ng/mL
Oxycodone Oxymorphone	100 ng/mL	Oxycodone Oxymorphone	100 ng/mL 100 ng/mL
6-Acetylmorphine	10 ng/mL	6-Acetylmorphine	10 ng/mL
Phencyclidine	25 ng/mL	Phencyclidine	25 ng/mL
Amphetamine Methamphetamine	500 ng/mL	Amphetamine Methamphetamine	250 ng/mL 250 ng/mL
MDMA MDA	500 ng/mL	MDMA MDA	250 ng/mL 250 ng/mL

THCA, Δ^9-tetrahydrocannabinol-9-carboxylic acid; MDMA, methylenedioxymethamphetamine; MDA, methylenedioxyamphetamine.

† For grouped analytes (ie, two or more analytes that are in the same drug class and have the same initial test cutoff):
Immunoassay: The test must be calibrated with one analyte from the group identified as the target analyte. The cross-reactivity of the immunoassay to the other analyte(s) within the group must be 80% or greater; if not, separate immunoassays must be used for the analytes within the group.
Alternate technology: Either one analyte or all analytes from the group must be used for calibration, depending on the technology. At least one analyte within the group must have a concentration equal to or greater than the initial test cutoff or, alternatively, the sum of the analytes present (ie, equal to or greater than the laboratory's validated limit of quantification) must be equal to or greater than the initial test cutoff.

‡ An immunoassay must be calibrated with the target analyte, THCA.

§ Alternate technology (THCA and benzoylecgonine): The confirmatory test cutoff must be used for an alternate technology initial test that is specific for the target analyte (ie, 15 ng/mL for THCA and 100 ng/mL for benzoylecgonine).

- Specific gravity is measured on any specimen with a creatinine concentration less than 20 mg/dL.
- pH is measured on every specimen.
- One or more tests for oxidizing adulterants (ie, nitrite, halogens, chromium VI) is performed on every specimen.

Additional testing may be performed for specimens exhibiting abnormal physical characteristics or abnormal responses in initial or confirmatory drug tests. The recently revised Guidelines provide an option to include additional validity biomarkers if such tests become available. If SVT results are outside the reference interval, specimens may be reported as *dilute, substituted, invalid,* or *adulterated.* The HHS definitions for those terms are as follows:

Dilute Specimen. A urine specimen with creatinine and specific gravity values that are lower than expected but are still within the physiologically producible ranges of human urine.

Substituted Specimen. A specimen that has been submitted in place of the donor's urine, as evidenced by creatinine and specific gravity values that are outside the physiologically producible ranges of human urine.

Invalid Result. The result reported by an HHS-certified laboratory when a positive, negative, adulterated, or substituted result cannot be established for a specific drug or specimen validity test.

Adulterated Specimen. A specimen that has been altered, as evidenced by test results showing either a substance that is not a normal constituent

Table 6-2. Specimen Validity Testing Reporting and Interpretation Criteria

Analyte	Interpretation	Criteria
Creatinine	Dilute	Creatinine ≥2.0 and <20.0 mg/dL SpGr >1.0010 and <1.0030
	Invalid	Creatinine <2.0 mg/dL SpGr acceptable (ie, SpGr >1.0010 and <1.0030) or SpGr ≤1.0010 Creatinine ≥2 mg/dL
	Substituted	Creatinine <2.0 mg/dL SpGr ≤1.0010 or ≥1.0200
pH	Invalid	pH ≥4.0 and <4.5 or pH ≥9.0 and <11.0
	Adulterated	pH <4.0 or ≥11.0
Oxidizing adulterants	Invalid	Oxidant present at or above specified level (eg, nitrite ≥200 and <500 mcg/mL); may include results from general oxidant reagents
	Adulterated	Specific adulterant is verified using a confirmatory test (eg, nitrite ≥500 mcg/mL, adulterant ≥ limit of quantitation)
Other		
Interference	Invalid	Assay interference in initial or confirmatory drug test
Biomarker	Invalid	Biomarker concentration not consistent with that established for human urine

From Department of Health and Human Services Mandatory Guidelines for Federal Workplace Drug Testing Programs.
SpGr, specific gravity.

for that type of specimen or showing an abnormal concentration of an endogenous substance.

Required actions by the employer when abnormal SVT results are reported are detailed in the Guidelines. A summary of SVT criteria and results interpretation is shown in Table 6-2. Clearly, current protocols for SVT in laboratories cannot detect all attempts at subversion, particularly with the plethora of products available for purchase on various internet sites.[14,15] The collection site environment and collection protocols can have a significant impact on the integrity of the collected specimen, and specific sections of the Guidelines address collection site security and integrity, as well as actions to take if the donor does not comply with the collection protocol. Both HHS and DOT publish handbooks that provide guidance for specimen collection personnel.[16,17]

Alcohol testing is also required for DOT-covered employees under the Omnibus Transportation Employee Drug Testing Act; however, it may be applied differently depending on the operating administration within the DOT. For example, pre-employment alcohol testing is not required by all agencies, and the US Coast Guard and Pipeline and Hazardous Materials Safety Administration (PHMSA) do not perform random alcohol tests.[18] Alcohol testing for DOT purposes does not involve a laboratory. It is performed at testing sites by personnel meeting the requirements of 49 CFR Part 40 Subparts J through O, using either breath or saliva for the initial test and breath for the confirmatory test, if necessary. Results below 0.020 g/dL are considered negative; results are reported directly to the Designated Employer Representative (DER); no additional review by an MRO is performed.

Nonregulated Workplace Drug Testing

Drug testing in the private sector in the US has largely followed the growth of drug testing in regulated industries. Recent estimates indicate that at least 66% of employers nationwide have some form of drug testing incorporated into hiring or

Table 6-3. Urine Drug Screening: Representative US Food and Drug Administration–Cleared Immunoassays

Test Analyte	Enzyme Immunoassay Cutoffs (ng/mL)
Amphetamines	1000, 500, 300
Methylenedioxymethamphetamine (MDMA, ecstasy)	500
Barbiturates	200, 300
Benzodiazepines	200, 300
Cocaine metabolite	300, 150
Opiates	300, 2000
Oxycodone	100, 300
Hydrocodone	300
Phencyclidine	25
Marijuana metabolites	20, 50, 100
Methadone	300
Methaqualone	300
Propoxyphene	300
Ethanol*	0.020 g/dL

* Ethanol assays are enzymatic rather than immunoassay

Table 6-4. Additional Immunoassays for Urine Specimens

Test Analyte	Enzyme Immunoassay Cutoffs (ng/mL)
Buprenorphine	5, 10
Tramadol	200
Meperidine	200
Methadone metabolite (2-ethylidene-1,5-dimethyl-3,3-diphenylpyrrolidine [EDDP])	300
Ethyl glucuronide*	250, 500, 1000
Fentanyl	1.0

* At this time, there is no Food and Drug Administration–cleared reagent kit for ethyl glucuronide. These tests may be validated and performed in laboratories as laboratory-developed tests.

employment policies.[19] Although no universal oversight or requirements exist for nonregulated testing programs, many are structured similarly to the federal program. In addition, the term *nonregulated* does not imply that these workplace drug testing programs are unregulated. Laboratories performing testing for nonregulated workplace drug testing programs must comply with a variety of federal and state laws that govern laboratory testing in general as well as laboratory testing for employment purposes. Although testing performed under the Mandatory Guidelines is exempt from state law, any other workplace drug testing program is subject to the laws of the state(s) in which the employer operates. Details of individual state laws and regulations may be obtained through state-specific websites as well as published resources that summarize requirements and related case law for workplace drug testing.[20-22] The regulatory environment for toxicology laboratories is covered in more detail in chapter 7, *Regulatory Issues of Toxicology Laboratory Operations*.

As in the regulated workplace, urine is the primary specimen type collected for nonregulated workplace drug testing programs, although alternate matrices are permitted in many states and are increasing in prevalence. Point-of-collection or point-of-care (POC) urine drug testing using "instant" or "on-site" test devices is also permitted for employment testing in many states; however, laboratory-based testing remains the prevalent model. Nonregulated drug testing programs for the workplace generally follow the SAMHSA model of laboratory-based testing, in other words, an initial screening test with confirmatory testing of initial test positive results. The primary difference between regulated and nonregulated workplace drug testing is that there are no single standard panel and cutoffs that must be adhered to. Although many employers adopt the panel required by SAMHSA, others utilize broader testing panels that may include 10 or more components. A sampling of initial immunoassay tests and cutoffs commonly available from multiple reagent vendors are shown in Table 6-3.

It should be noted that methaqualone and propoxyphene, included in Table 6-3, have very low prevalence because of limited availability in the US; however, they may be retained in testing panels on the basis of legacy program requirements or negotiated contracts. Some nonregulated testing programs incorporate more esoteric drugs when they apply to health care professionals or other unique employment environments. Examples of some additional tests that may be included are shown in Table 6-4.

Similar to regulated testing programs, nonregulated workplace drug testing programs generally require confirmatory testing for any initial test positive results. Methodologies used are consistent with regulated testing programs, namely, chromatography with mass spectrometry. Cutoffs are more variable, particularly for compounds that are not a part of regulated workplace testing, such as barbiturates and benzodiazepines. SVT is often not specifically addressed in state drug testing laws; however, many laboratories apply similar tests and reporting criteria to those required in the HHS Guidelines.

The Medical Review Officer

A major element common to all federal drug testing regulations, as well as to many state statutes, is the requirement that a qualified Medical Review Officer review and interpret laboratory-confirmed positive drug test results. The HHS Guidelines define an MRO as a licensed physician who reviews, verifies, and reports a specimen test result to the federal agency. MROs are expected to have knowledge of the pharmacology and toxicology of illicit drugs and prescription medications, and must have training and experience in relevant program components, such as (1) collection procedures, (2) chain of custody, (3) reporting and record-keeping requirements, (4) interpretation of results, and (5) procedures for review of results with donors, including assessment of legitimate medical explanations for abnormal results. Training on any revisions to the guidelines must be documented before reviewing any specimen results. Certification is achieved by passing an initial examination administered by a nationally recognized entity, followed by requalification training and re-examination at least every 5 years.[23] A list of HHS-approved boards for MRO certification is published annually in the *Federal Register*. The two primary resources for MRO training and certification are the American Association of Medical Review Officers and the Medical Review Officer Certification Council. SAMHSA provides a link to the current list of approved MRO certification entities and other MRO resources on their website at https://www.samhsa.gov/workplace/resources.

Pathologists may qualify and serve as MROs; however, they should be aware that federal regulations prohibit MRO–laboratory relationships in which an MRO is an employee of or has a financial interest in the laboratory. Nor can an MRO derive a financial benefit by directing a federal agency or employer to use a specific HHS-certified laboratory or have an agreement with a laboratory that may be viewed as a potential conflict of interest.[24] Most employers arrange for MRO services separately from their contract with a drug testing laboratory.

The review and interpretation of nonnegative laboratory test results is the central function of the MRO in workplace drug testing programs. Nonnegative results include those reported by the laboratory as positive for a drug or drug metabolite, substituted, adulterated, invalid, or rejected for testing. Staff under the direct supervision of the MRO may review and report negative and negative dilute results; however, the MRO must review a minimum of 5% of all negative results reported to ensure the accuracy of the review/reporting process. For all nonnegative results, the MRO must conduct an interview (telephone or in person) with the specimen donor to determine if there is a legitimate medical explanation for the laboratory findings. If, during the interview, the donor presents a legitimate medical explanation for the test result, the MRO must validate the medical record or medication information offered and maintain the documentation as part of the case record. If the donor does not provide acceptable documentation of a legitimate medical explanation for the laboratory result, the test is verified as positive, the adulterated or substituted specimen is verified as a refusal to test, and the invalid result is canceled, with a requirement for the donor to submit to another specimen collection under direct observation. MRO actions for reporting results to an employer are shown in Table 6-5.

Nonregulated drug testing programs may not be required to use an MRO. The use of an MRO is required by some states and not by others. Human Resources personnel may be chosen by employers to serve this function, particularly for preemployment testing.

Medical Review Officer's Interpretation of Results

The HHS guidelines and 49 CFR Part 40 both contain specific results interpretation and reporting criteria as well as required actions an MRO must take when reporting results. In addition, the *Medical Review Officer Guidance Manual for Federal Workplace Drug Testing Programs* provides detailed information related to the program requirements, testing methodologies, and drug and SVT results interpretation and scenarios.[25]

Interpretation of legitimate medical use of a substance has become more challenging with respect to marijuana and cannabinoids. Marijuana is the most prevalent drug found in both the federally mandated safety-sensitive workforce and in the general US workforce,[26] and the landscape with regard to marijuana legislation continues to change. At least

Table 6-5. Medical Review Officer Actions for Primary Specimen Reports[25]

Reported Primary Specimen Result	Medical Review Officer (MRO) Action
Negative	Report the negative result.
Negative and Dilute	Report the negative result and direct the federal agency to immediately collect another specimen from the donor.
Positive or Positive and Dilute	Contact the donor to determine if he/she has a valid medical explanation for the positive result. If the medical explanation for the positive result appears to be the following: a. Legitimate. Verify the result as negative and report a negative result to the federal agency. If the specimen was also reported as dilute, direct the federal agency to immediately collect another specimen from the donor. (It is recommended that the MRO contact the prescribing physician to discuss the possible impact that the medication may have on the safety aspects of the work performed by the donor. The MRO may inform the federal agency's designated representative that the donor is taking a medication that is restricted for an individual in that occupation or that the medication may affect the individual's ability to perform duties in a safety-sensitive occupation.) b. Not legitimate. Report the positive drug result to the federal agency. If the specimen was also reported as dilute, the MRO may choose not to report the dilute finding.
Substituted	Contact the donor to determine if he/she has a valid medical explanation for the substituted result. If the medical explanation for the substituted result appears to be the following: a. Legitimate. Report a negative result to the federal agency. b. Not legitimate. Report a "refusal to test" (substituted) to the federal agency.
Adulterated	Contact the donor to determine if he/she has a valid medical explanation for the adulterated result. *(Although the MRO is required to contact the donor and give the donor an opportunity to explain the adulterated result, the program criteria for adulteration definitively prove adulteration. There is no valid medical explanation.)* Report a "refusal to test" (adulterated) to the federal agency.
Invalid Result	Prior to reporting an invalid result to the MRO, the laboratory must contact the MRO to decide whether additional/different testing would be of use to obtain a definitive result EXCEPT when the invalid result is based on creatinine and specific gravity, pH, or a confirmatory nitrite test result ≥200 mcg/mL and <500 mcg/mL. For an invalid result based on pH in the 9.0 to 9.5 range: • Consider whether there is evidence of elapsed time and high temperature that could account for the result. Contact the collection site, Instrumented Initial Test Facility (IITF), and/or laboratory to discuss time and temperature issues. Contact the donor to determine if he/she has an explanation for the invalid result. If the medical explanation is legitimate or if pH is in the 9.0 to 9.5 range as a possible result of time and temperature for a first invalid result: • Report the test as canceled with the reason for the invalid result, and inform the federal agency that a recollection is not required because there is an acceptable explanation for the invalid result unless the federal agency plan requires a negative drug test result based on the reason for testing (eg, federal agency applicant/preemployment, return to duty, follow-up). • If the medical explanation is not legitimate and the pH is not in the 9.0 to 9.5 range due to time and temperature, report the test as canceled with the reason for the invalid result and direct the federal agency to immediately collect another specimen using a direct observed collection procedure. If a specimen is recollected using direct observation and that specimen is also reported as invalid: follow steps described in Chapter 5, Section 5.6.4 of the HHS *MRO Guidance Manual for Federal Workplace Drug Testing Programs.*

Table 6-5. Medical Review Officer Actions for Primary Specimen Reports (continued)

Reported Primary Specimen Result	Medical Review Officer (MRO) Action
Multiple Reported Results	Follow the review procedures above as appropriate for each reported result and report all verified positive and/or "refusal to test" results. Do not report invalid results for the primary specimen unless the split specimen is tested and reported as a failure to reconfirm.
Rejected for Testing	Report the test as canceled along with the reason for the cancellation and direct the federal agency to immediately collect another specimen from the donor.

33 states and the District of Columbia have laws legalizing marijuana for medical and/or recreational use.[27] Petitions to reschedule marijuana under the Controlled Substances Act (CSA) were denied by the US Drug Enforcement Administration in 2016, leaving marijuana as a Class I controlled substance, with no legitimate use under federal law.[28] The ruling of MROs on federally mandated drug testing must comply with federal law in this regard, as reiterated in the revised 49 CFR Part 40, which clarifies that the term *prescription* means "a legally valid prescription consistent with the Controlled Substances Act." This language reinforces the intent of the federally regulated workplace drug testing programs to follow the CSA regarding what an MRO may consider a legitimate medical explanation when reviewing positive results. It also clarifies that a prescription for medical marijuana, while legal in various states, cannot be considered legally valid because it is listed as a Schedule I substance under the CSA. This is consistent with the DOT's positions on medical[29] and recreational[30] marijuana posted on their website. On the other hand, this is not true for testing that is voluntarily conducted under the employer's own authority in those states that permit the medical use of marijuana. In those cases, the MRO must rely on the employer's policy with respect to determining positive results for marijuana and marijuana metabolites. The reader is referred to the individual analyte chapters in this book for further details on individual analytes and their interpretation.

Summary

Workplace testing for drugs of abuse is common in the United States. It is mandatory for many federal employees and individuals working in federally regulated industries and is also prevalent in nonregulated employment markets. Regulated testing is performed in accordance with specific rules and guidelines published in the *Federal Register* and with oversight by SAMHSA. Nonregulated testing programs have developed in concordance with federal programs and must comply with relevant federal and state laws governing diagnostic and workplace testing. MROs are important components of workplace drug testing and are responsible for interpreting and verifying test results in the context of relevant medical information. Testing programs have been revised over time to remain relevant to changing substance use demographics. Urine is currently the most commonly collected specimen for testing in these programs, but interest in use of alternate matrices, such as oral fluid and hair, continues to grow.

References

1. Ahrnsbrak R, Bose J, Hedden SL, Lipari RN, Park-Lee E. Key Substance Use and Mental Health Indicators in the United States: Results from the 2016 National Survey on Drug Use and Health. Substance Abuse and Mental Health Services Administration. https://www.samhsa.gov/data/sites/default/files/NSDUH-FFR1-2016/NSDUH-FFR1-2016.pdf. September 2017. Accessed June 7, 2019.
2. Results from the 2016 National Survey on Drug Use and Health: Detailed Tables. Substance Abuse and Mental Health Services Administration. Center for Behavioral Health Statistics and Quality. https://www.samhsa.gov/data/sites/default/files/NSDUH-DetTabs-2016/NSDUH-DetTabs-2016.pdf. September 7, 2017. Accessed June 7, 2019.
3. Bush DM, Lipari RN. *The CBHSQ Report: Substance Use and Substance Use Disorder by Industry.* Rockville, MD: Substance Abuse and Mental Health Services Administration, Center for Behavioral Health Statistics and Quality; April 16, 2015.
4. Mandatory guidelines for federal workplace drug testing programs; final guidelines; notice. 53 *Federal Register* 11970 (1988).

5. US Department of Transportation. Drug and Alcohol Testing. Resources for Key Persons. https://www.transportation.gov/odapc/employee. Updated April 29, 2019. Accessed June 7, 2019.
6. Omnibus Transportation Employee Testing Act of 1991. Public Law 102–143, Title V, 105 Stat. 917. https://www.transportation.gov/sites/dot.gov/files/docs/199111028_Omnibus_Act.pdf. October 28, 1991. Accessed June 7, 2019.
7. Office of Drug and Alcohol Policy and Compliance. US Department of Transportation. https://www.transportation.gov/odapc. Updated May 1, 2019. Accessed May 2, 2018.
8. Part 26—Fitness for Duty Programs. US Nuclear Regulatory Commission. http://www.nrc.gov/reading-rm/doc-collections/cfr/part026/. Updated May 16, 2019. Accessed May 2, 2018.
9. Revisions to the HHS Guidelines have been published in the following *Federal Register* volumes: 59 FR 29908 (June 9, 1994), 62 FR 51118 (September 30, 1997), 69 FR 19644 (April 13, 2004), 73 FR 71858 (November 25, 2008), and 82 FR 7920 (January 23, 2017).
10. Mandatory guidelines for federal workplace drug testing programs. Urine: 82 *Federal Register* 7920 (2017). Oral fluid: 84 *Federal Register* 57554 (2019).
11. Procedures for transportation workplace drug and alcohol testing programs: addition of certain schedule II drugs to the department of transportation's drug-testing panel and certain minor amendments. 82 *Federal Register* 52229.
12. Berge KH, Bush DM. The subversion of urine drug testing. *Minn Med.* 2010;93(8): 45-47.
13. Cook JD, Caplan YH, LoDico CP, Bush DM. The characterization of human urine for specimen validity determination in workplace drug testing: a review. *J Anal Toxicol.* 2000;24(7):579-588.
14. Dasgupta A. How people try to beat drug testing: issues with urinary adulterants and their detection. *Clinical Laboratory News.* https://www.aacc.org/publications/cln/articles/2015/february/drug-testing. February 1, 2015. Accessed June 7, 2019.
15. Kutz GD. Testimony before the Subcommittee on Highways and Transit, Committee on Transportation and Infrastructure, House of Representatives. Drug Testing: Undercover Tests Reveal Significant Vulnerabilities in DOT's Drug Testing Program. US Government Accountability Office. https://www.gao.gov/assets/120/118430.pdf. November 1, 2007. Accessed June 7, 2019.
16. Urine Specimen Collection Handbook for Federal Agency Workplace Drug Testing Programs: Effective October 1, 2017. Substance Abuse and Mental Health Services Administration. https://www.samhsa.gov/sites/default/files/workplace/urine-specimen-collection-handbook-oct2017_2.pdf. Accessed June 7, 2019.
17. Urine Specimen Collection Guidelines. US Department of Transportation. https://www.transportation.gov/sites/dot.gov/files/docs/resources/partners/drug-and-alcohol-testing/2567/urine-specimen-collection-guidelines-january-2018.pdf. Revised January, 2018. Accessed May 2, 2018.
18. What Employers Need to Know About DOT Drug and Alcohol Testing [Guidance and Best Practices]. Office of the Secretary, Office of Drug and Alcohol Policy and Compliance, US Department of Transportation. https://www.transportation.gov/sites/dot.gov/files/docs/ODAPC_Employer_Guidelines_%20June_1_2015_A.pdf. June 1, 2015. Accessed June 7, 2019.
19. HireRight Annual Employment Screening Benchmark Report. 2015 Edition. http://hosted-docs.ittoolbox.com/2015-employment-screening-benchmark-report_final.pdf. Accessed June 7, 2019.
20. Bernardo MA, Nieman MF. *Guide to State and Federal Drug-Testing Laws.* 16th ed. Reston, VA: Institute for a Drug-Free Workplace; 2013.
21. SAPAA Worldwide. Substance Abuse Program Administrators Association. http://www.sapaa.com/. Accessed June 7, 2019
22. DATIA. Drug and Alcohol Testing Industry Association. http://www.datia.org/. Accessed June 7, 2019.
23. Who may serve as an MRO? Mandatory guidelines for federal workplace drug testing programs. 82 *Federal Register* 7920 (2017). Subpart M, 13.1.
24. What types of relationships are prohibited between an MRO and an HHS-certified laboratory or an HHS-certified IITF? Mandatory guidelines for federal workplace drug testing programs. 82 *Federal Register* 7920 (2017). Subpart M, 13.10.
25. Medical Review Officer Guidance Manual for Federal Workplace Drug Testing Programs. Department of Health and Human Services, Substance Abuse and Mental Health Services Administration, Center for Substance Abuse Prevention, Division of Workplace Programs. https://www.samhsa.gov/sites/default/files/workplace/mro-guidance-manual-oct2017_2.pdf. Effective date October 1, 2017. Accessed June 7, 2019.
26. Drug testing index. Quest Diagnostics. https://www.questdiagnostics.com/home/physicians/health-trends/drug-testing/table1.html. Accessed May 6, 2018.
27. State Marijuana Laws in 2019 Map. https://www.governing.com/gov-data/safety-justice/state-marijuana-laws-map-medical-recreational.html. Current as of June 25, 2019. Accessed July 26, 2019.

28. DEA Announces Actions Related to Marijuana and Industrial Hemp. US Drug Enforcement Administration. https://www.dea.gov/divisions/hq/2016/hq081116.shtml. August 11, 2016. Accessed June 7, 2019.
29. DOT Office of Drug and Alcohol Policy and Compliance Notice (Medical Marijuana). US Department of Transportation. https://cms.dot.gov/sites/dot.gov/files/images/ODAPC%20Medical%20Marijuana%20Notice.pdf. October 22, 2009. Accessed June 7, 2019.
30. DOT Office of Drug and Alcohol Policy and Compliance Notice (Recreational Marijuana). US Department of Transportation. https://www.transportation.gov/sites/dot.gov/files/docs/odapc-notice-recreational-mj.pdf. December 3, 2012. Accessed June 7, 2019.

Acknowledgment

The authors would like to acknowledge Michael G. Bissell, MD, PhD, MPH, for his original version of this manuscript published in the first edition of this book.

Chapter 7

Regulatory Issues of Toxicology Laboratory Operations

Arthur M. Zebelman, PhD
Jennifer A. Collins, PhD

Introduction

This chapter discusses regulatory issues for laboratories in the United States, with emphasis on operating a clinical toxicology service within a hospital that provides general clinical laboratory support or a separate toxicology laboratory. Toxicology is a multifaceted science. The topics in this chapter are limited to drug testing for medical purposes and for forensic purposes, where drug testing, usually for drugs of abuse, is done for nonmedical purposes including employment-related screening and law enforcement. Specific state and local regulations and forensic regulations are not included in great detail. This is not a comprehensive compendium of the federal requirements or of the requirements for accreditation by the nonprofit programs with deemed status, the state programs, or of forensic accreditation. International Organization for Standardization or ISO 15189 certification of clinical laboratories is not common in the US, but a certification program is now available, and a brief description is included in this chapter. Last, there is a section on proficiency testing programs to help with selection of an appropriate program.

Clinical Laboratory Improvement Amendments of 1988 Certification

Clinical laboratories in the United States must be certified to perform clinical testing on human specimens. Laboratories are subject to the Department of Health and Human Services, Centers for Medicare and Medicaid Services (CMS), Part 493 Laboratory Requirements implementing the Clinical Laboratory Improvement Amendments of 1988 (CLIA). The authority for these laboratory requirements is Section 353 of the Public Health Service Act, sections 1102, 1861(e), the sentence following sections 1861(s)(11) through 1861(s)(16) of the Social Security Act 42 U.S.C. 263a, 1302, 1395x(e), and the sentence following 1395x(s)(11) through 1395x(s)(16). This part also applies to laboratories seeking payment under the Medicare and Medicaid programs. The requirements are the same for Medicare approval as for CLIA certification.[1]

A laboratory is defined under CLIA as "... a facility for the biological, microbiological, serological, chemical, immunohematological, hematological, biophysical, cytological, pathological, or other examination of materials derived from the human body for the purpose of providing information for the diagnosis, prevention, or treatment of any disease or impairment of, or the assessment of the health of, human beings. These examinations also include procedures to determine, measure, or otherwise describe the presence or absence of various substances or organisms in the body. Facilities only collecting or preparing specimens (or both) or only serving as a mailing service and not performing testing are not considered laboratories."[2]

CLIA requires clinical laboratories in the US to be either CLIA exempt or to possess one of the following CLIA certificates[3]:

Certificate of Registration. This certificate is required for a new laboratory to begin performing waived or nonwaived testing until they receive a Certificate of Waiver or Certificate of Accreditation. It is also required for a laboratory testing under a Certificate of Waiver that begins nonwaived testing.

Certificate of Waiver. This certificate allows a laboratory to perform waived testing only. There are no regularly scheduled inspections, but the laboratory is subject to announced or unannounced inspections. Laboratories are required to use only test systems that are classified as waived by the US Food and Drug Administration (FDA). The manufacturer's directions must be followed, and this requires documentation in records and worksheets. If it is not documented that the laboratory is following the manufacturer's directions, then the laboratory is not in compliance.

Certificate for Provider-Performed Microscopy (PPM) Procedures. This certificate is not applicable to the toxicology laboratory.

Certificate of Compliance. This certificate is issued after an inspection that finds the laboratory to be in compliance with all applicable condition level requirements.

Certificate of Accreditation. This certificate is issued on the basis of the laboratory's accreditation by a private nonprofit accreditation program approved by CMS (deemed status).

CLIA–Exempt Laboratories

The four categories of laboratories exempt from the CLIA regulations are as follows[4]:

(1) Any facility or component of a facility that only performs testing for forensic purposes;

(2) Research laboratories that test human specimens but do not report patient-specific results for the diagnosis, prevention or treatment of any disease or impairment of, or the assessment of the health of individual patients;

(3) Laboratories certified by the Substance Abuse and Mental Health Services Administration (SAMHSA), in which drug testing is performed which meets SAMHSA guidelines and regulations. However, all other testing conducted by a SAMHSA-certified laboratory is subject to this rule; and,

(4) Federal laboratories. Laboratories under the jurisdiction of an agency of the federal government are subject to the rules of this part, except that the Secretary [of HHS] may modify the application of such requirements as appropriate.

State Exemption From CLIA

A state may receive an exemption from CLIA if CMS determines that the state has a licensure program equal to or more stringent than the CLIA condition level requirements. New York and Washington have attained this exemption.

The New York Clinical Laboratory Evaluation Program issues annual permits to approximately 1000 laboratories and 900 patient service centers in New York State. In addition, the Clinical Laboratory Evaluation Program certifies approximately 3100 certificates of qualification to individuals to serve as directors or assistant directors. A New York clinical laboratory permit is required to perform laboratory tests on specimens obtained within the state. A permit is also required by clinical laboratories outside of New York that perform testing on specimens from New York. New York State had its own proficiency testing program up until January 2017.[5]

The Washington State Office of Laboratory Quality Assurance, Washington Medical Test Site Licensure Program provides Certificate of Waiver, Provider-Performed Microscopy Procedure, Categorized, and Accredited licenses. Inspections for the Categorized licenses are by Department of Health Laboratory Quality Assurance surveyors. Inspections for the Accredited licenses are by one of the approved private accreditation organizations: AABB (formerly American Association of Blood Banks), American Osteopathic Association (AOA), American Society for Histocompatibility and Immunogenetics (ASHI), the College of American Pathologists (CAP), the Commission on Laboratory Accreditation (COLA), and The Joint Commission.[6]

Forensic Testing Accreditation

A laboratory that performs forensic testing *only* is CLIA exempt and is not required to be CLIA licensed. Testing for preemployment, workplace, the criminal justice system, driving under the influence of drugs (DUID), blood and breath alcohol for traffic law enforcement, and medical examiner cases are in this category. Some states and other jurisdictions may have accreditation requirements for certain forensic testing. Accreditation programs for forensic testing include the CAP Forensic Drug Testing (FDT) Accreditation Program,[7] the American Board of Forensic Toxicology (ABFT) Laboratory Accreditation Program,[8] and the ANSI-ASQ National Accreditation Board (ANAB; formerly American Society of Crime Laboratory Directors Laboratory Accreditation Board [ASCLD/LAB])[9] programs. The reader is referred to chapter 8, *The Hospital Autopsy and Toxicology Testing*, for more information about postmortem toxicology.

Testing of certain federal employees under the SAMHSA regulations requires National Laboratory Certification Program (NLCP) certification. The requirements of an NLCP-certified laboratory are provided in the Mandatory Guidelines for Federal Workplace Drug Testing Programs. The most recent version was published on January 23, 2017, in the *Federal Register*.[10] If a forensic testing laboratory also performs clinical testing, it must be certified under the CLIA regulations for that testing.

The CAP Forensic Drug Testing Accreditation Program

The CAP FDT Accreditation Program is for laboratories performing workplace drug testing of urine, oral fluid, or hair. The program requires immunoassay screening and quantitative mass spectral confirmation of positive results performed either by the FDT-accredited laboratory or by referral to an FDT-accredited laboratory. The forensic requirements are comprehensive, supported by the CAP Accreditation Program Standards for FDT accreditation and enforced using four checklists: Forensic Drug Testing, Director Assessment, All Common, and Laboratory General. The laboratory inspections are by peers with forensic experience. For more information on workplace drug testing, the reader is referred to chapter 6, *Workplace Drug Testing*.

Forensic Testing in the Clinical Laboratory

Forensic drug testing may be performed in the clinical laboratory. If forensic specimens are co-mingled with clinical specimens with the same procedures, same instruments, and even the same batches, it may be difficult to isolate this forensic testing from the clinical testing. It is advisable to have policies and procedures that allow the clinical testing to be readily distinguished from the forensic testing.

Medical Testing With Legal Implications

All testing in the clinical laboratory may have legal implications under certain, often unpredictable, circumstances. Legal implications are more likely in drug testing of pregnant women, in labor and delivery, of newborns, of young children, of those involved in accidents, and in certain other circumstances. The laboratory may not be aware of a specimen that has legal implications. Unless ordered by law enforcement or the judicial system, specimens fall under clinical laboratory regulations. The laboratory may elect to follow chain-of-custody and other forensic procedures with these specimens, but there is no regulatory requirement that this be done. This decision may involve discussions with responsible persons in other departments and services, and the development of policies and procedures for documentation and specimen handling consistent with chain-of-custody testing.

CLIA does not include forensic requirements because forensic testing is exempt from those regulations.

Waived Tests

The FDA is responsible for approving commercial methods and their package inserts and for categorization as *waived, moderate,* or *high complexity.* A waived test must "employ methodologies that are so simple and accurate as to render the likelihood of erroneous results negligible" or "pose no reasonable risk of harm to the patient if the test is performed incorrectly."[11] However, one only needs to review proficiency testing results of waived point-of-care devices for drug screening to see that the likelihood of an erroneous result is not negligible. Under the current process, waiver may be granted to (1) any test listed in the regulation, (2) any test system for which the manufacturer or producer applies for waiver if that test meets the statutory criteria and the manufacturer provides scientifically valid data verifying that the waiver criteria have been met, and (3) test systems cleared by the FDA for home use.[11] A current list is maintained by the FDA and can be found at the FDA website.[12] Any modifications from the manufacturer's directions cause the test to no longer be waived. Waived testing does not require proficiency testing (although such testing is available), a concept that concerns many, and the laboratory director will need to decide whether to subscribe to proficiency testing. In addition, the accrediting programs may have their own requirements for proficiency testing.

There are a number of FDA-cleared, waived, immunochemical drug screening devices. A health care facility may elect to establish a "Waived Lab" with a Certificate of Waiver separate from the clinical laboratory, especially if the clinical laboratory director is not responsible for this testing.

Nonprofit Agencies with Deemed Status to Accredit Laboratories

CMS is authorized to grant private nonprofit accreditation agencies deemed status for accreditation of laboratories. The requirements of the accreditation organization must be equal to or more stringent than the CLIA requirements. There is an extensive review process, and CMS performs validation reinspections. At this time, programs with deemed status include the CAP, AABB, the AOA, The Joint Commission, COLA, and ASHI. The AABB and ASHI programs have focused accreditation programs. Effective June 30, 2010, COLA discontinued accreditation of the specialty of pathology—including histopathology, oral pathology, and cytology—but continues to accredit other specialties. The CAP Laboratory Accreditation Program (LAP) has the most comprehensive proficiency testing requirements and inspection checklists.

Five Condition Level Requirements for Accreditation

These five requirements consist of participation in proficiency testing, facility administration, quality systems, personnel, and inspection. They are described in detail in the CMS Part 493 Laboratory Requirements. More specifics are found in the CAP accreditation checklists and from the other nonprofit accrediting organizations.

First Condition Level Requirement: Proficiency Testing

CLIA regulations, Subpart H, include the requirements for proficiency testing.[13] Proficiency testing is not required by CLIA for laboratories with a Certificate of Waiver or for tests that are classified as waived by the FDA. This subpart lists by section of the laboratory the tests for which successful participation in proficiency testing is required ("regulated tests") and the specific requirements. Proficiency testing of the nonregulated analytes, including most analytes of interest in toxicology, is not required by CMS. The CAP accreditation program requires proficiency testing of most nonregulated analytes in accordance with good clinical and scientific laboratory practice.

The proficiency testing program must be approved by CMS. Three sets of five proficiency testing specimens per year are required. An 80% score is required for successful proficiency testing, except for certain tests, for example, some immunohematology tests, which require a 100% score. The laboratory must have a "successful" score on two of three consecutive proficiency testing events. CMS maintains a list of approved proficiency testing providers.[14] The CAP and other programs with deemed status may specify the proficiency testing programs approved for their accreditation programs. The "regulated analytes" with required participation in a CMS-approved proficiency testing program for toxicology are shown in Table 7-1, along with the CLIA-required criteria for acceptable performance.[15]

Most of the regulated analytes in toxicology are therapeutic drugs, and the required proficiency testing specimens are serum, plasma, or blood. Blood alcohol and blood lead are the only analytes that are not therapeutic drugs. Drugs of abuse and drugs in matrices other than serum, plasma, or blood are not included in the CMS-regulated analytes.

Serum, plasma, or blood alcohol (ethanol) is a regulated analyte, and the laboratory must subscribe to an approved proficiency testing program. It is important that the proficiency testing program be approved by the accreditation program used for the laboratory's accreditation. The providers of proficiency testing for alcohol and other volatiles are discussed in the section titled, "Proficiency Testing and Alternative Performance Assessment," below.

The evaluation of accuracy of the nonregulated analytes and the evaluation of proficiency testing results of the regulated and nonregulated analytes are covered under the "Quality Systems" condition level requirement, below.

Table 7-1. Regulated Analytes in Toxicology and Scoring on Proficiency Testing

Analyte	Target Value
Alcohol, blood	Target Value ± 25%
Blood lead	Target Value ± 10% or 4 mcg/dL (greater)
Carbamazepine	Target Value ± 25%
Digoxin	Target Value ± 20% or ± 0.2 ng/mL (greater)
Ethosuximide	Target Value ± 20%
Gentamicin	Target Value ± 25%
Lithium	Target Value ± 20% or ± 0.3 mmol/L (greater)
Phenobarbital	Target Value ± 20%
Phenytoin	Target Value ± 25%
Primidone	Target Value ± 25%
Procainamide (and metabolite)	Target Value ± 25%
Quinidine	Target Value ± 25%
Tobramycin	Target Value ± 25%
Theophylline	Target Value ± 25%
Valproic acid	Target Value ± 25%

Second Condition Level Requirement: Facility Administration

This requirement includes space, ventilation, utilities, and minimizing contamination. It also includes appropriate and sufficient equipment, instruments, reagents, materials, and supplies for the testing performed. Last, it includes safety and record retention.[16] Safety procedures must be established, accessible, and observed to ensure protection from physical, chemical, biochemical, and electrical hazards and from biohazardous materials.

It is a common misconception that safety is not included in the CLIA regulations. Even if safety were not included in CLIA regulations, there are several Occupational Safety and Health Administration (OSHA) and other federal, state, and local regulations and guidelines that require compliance, including the following:

- Air Contaminants—Permissible Exposure Limits, OSHA, 29 CFR 1910.1000
- General Housekeeping Requirements, OSHA, 29 CFR 1910.22
- Hazard Communication Standard, OSHA, 29 CFR 1910.1200
- Health Insurance Portability and Accountability Act of 1996[17] and subsequent regulations that include protected health information (confidentiality) and electronic medical records
- Medical Waste Tracking Act of 1988, Standards for the Tracking and Management of Medical Waste, Authority, 42 USC 69192,6992 et seq
- Occupational Exposure to Bloodborne Pathogens, Needlestick and Other Sharps Injuries, Final Rule, January 18, 2001, 29 CFR 1910

- Occupational Exposure to Bloodborne Pathogens, OSHA, 29 CFR 1910.1030
- Occupational Exposure to Hazardous Chemicals in Laboratories, OSHA, 29 CFR 1910.1450
- Occupational Injury and Illness Recording and Reporting Requirement, 29 CFR 1904 and 29 CFR 1952
- Personal Protective Equipment, OSHA, 29 CFR 1910.132
- Sanitation, Waste Disposal, OSHA, 29 CFR 1910.141
- Specifications for Accident Prevention Signs and Tags, OSHA, 29 CFR 1910.145
- Updated US Public Health Service Guidelines for the Management of Occupational Exposures to HBV, HCV, and HIV and Recommendations for Post Exposure Prophylaxis

The records retention requirements for toxicology are those of any CLIA-certified laboratory. The following are required to be retained for 2 years: (1) test requisitions and authorizations, (2) test procedures (standard operating procedures [SOPs]), (3) analytic systems records (including quality control, patient test records, and instrument printouts), (4) records of test system performance, (5) proficiency testing records, and (6) quality system assessment records and test reports.[18] It is acceptable for these records to be retained in electronic format providing they can be printed in their original format as appropriate. Although the record retention requirements are minimal for accreditation, there may be other factors to consider when determining how long to keep certain records. The potential for audits by the Office of Inspector General or Department of Health and Human Services may necessitate longer retention of certain records. The rule of thumb is to follow the most stringent of the applicable requirements, particularly if either the state or the accrediting agency has different retention requirements.

Third Condition Level Requirement: Quality Systems

The following is from the Part 493—Laboratory Requirements: Subpart K—Quality System for Nonwaived Testing: "Each laboratory that performs non-waived testing must establish and maintain written policies and procedures that implement and monitor a quality system for all phases of the total testing process (that is, preanalytic, analytic, and postanalytic) as well as general laboratory systems . . . . This must include a quality assessment component that ensures continuous improvement of the laboratory's performance and services through ongoing monitoring that identifies, evaluates and resolves problems."[19]

Quality Assurance (Assessment)/ Quality Management

The various "Q words" seem to be a difficult concept to understand and embrace. For this reason, the quality assurance (or assessment [QA])/quality management (QM) program in most clinical laboratories could stand improvement.

There must be documented policies and procedures for general laboratory systems QA, including preanalytic, analytic, and postanalytic phases of testing. There are specific requirements for the following aspects of testing:

- Test requisition
- Specimen submission, handling, and referral
- Procedure manual
- Test systems, equipment, instruments, reagents, materials, and supplies
- Method performance specifications and validation
- Maintenance and function checks
- Calibration and calibration verification
- Control procedures
- Comparison of same-test results when different methodologies, instruments, or sites are used
- Corrective actions
- Test records
- Analytic systems assessment
- Test report

The toxicology service must be included in the laboratory's QA/QM plan. Useful QAs for toxicology are not much different from those for other parts of the clinical laboratory. Assessments must include preanalytic, analytic, and postanalytic phases of testing. Items of special interest to the toxicology laboratory include (1) patient and specimen identification, (2) internal and external chain-of-custody documents (if created), (3) interpretation of analytic data, (4) scientific review of data, and (5) accurate reporting as appropriate to the specific laboratory. Chromatography and mass spectral methods require a significant amount of interpretation and attention to reporting, and are appropriate topics for assessment.

Proficiency Testing and Alternative Performance Assessment

Most of the analytes in clinical toxicology are not CLIA-regulated analytes. CLIA regulations require verification of their accuracy at least two times per year. The CAP LAP requires laboratories to participate in proficiency testing when available through the CAP or a CAP-approved alternate provider for most analytes. Alternative performance assessment is required for those tests for which there is no appropriate proficiency testing program or if the accrediting organization does not require proficiency testing for nonregulated analytes. The following is from the CAP *All Common Checklist*: "Appropriate alternative performance assessment procedures include participation in an external PT program not required by CAP; participation in an ungraded/educational PT program; split sample analysis with referral or other laboratories, split sample analysis with an established in-house method, use of assayed materials, clinical validation by chart review, or other suitable and documented means. It is the responsibility of the laboratory director to define such alternative assessment procedures and the criteria for successful performance in accordance with good clinical and scientific laboratory practice."[20]

Graded or ungraded proficiency testing programs are the methods most laboratories use to accomplish alternative performance assessment, when available. Proficiency testing programs are probably less expensive than the resources and time required to plan, develop, and implement an inhouse alternative performance assessment program that must be repeated at least every 6 months for each test and analyte. Proficiency testing programs generally provide more valid data than internal assessments and provide comparison data with other laboratories.

There are a number of programs for drug screening available from the American College of Physicians Medical Laboratory Evaluation (MLE) program,[21] the American Proficiency Institute (API),[22] the CAP (including programs cosponsored with the American Association for Clinical Chemistry [AACC]), and the Wisconsin State Laboratory of Hygiene (WSLH).[23] Pennsylvania provides proficiency testing material for use in their state programs. The websites of these organizations contain catalogs of the proficiency testing programs, which are updated annually. Many of these programs have applied for and attained approval for laboratories accredited by the CAP. The specific proficiency testing programs are addressed in more detail later in this chapter (the 2019 CAP proficiency survey offerings may be found in appendix E).

Evaluation of Proficiency Testing and Alternative Performance Assessment

Evaluation and corrective action of unsatisfactory proficiency testing and alternative performance assessments are required for both regulated and nonregulated analytes. The laboratory director is responsible for the method of assessment. There must be evidence of review of proficiency testing reports by the laboratory director or designee. Evaluations must include the cause of the unsatisfactory result, the corrective action taken, and an evaluation of whether patients' results could have been affected and, if so, the course of action taken. Results that are not graded for a variety of reasons or that the laboratory did not submit on time or at all also need evaluation. These evaluations and corrective actions must be documented and reviewed by the laboratory director or designee.

Method Validation

Many toxicology methods are laboratory-developed tests (LDTs), often referencing the scientific literature, and are essentially "home-brew" procedures without FDA clearance. Most gas chromatography, liquid chromatography, and mass spectral methods fall in this category. These require validation of the entire process, including applicability, accuracy, precision, interfering substances, cross-reactivity, reportable range of results, dilution protocol, reference intervals, calibration, and control procedures. The laboratory director is responsible for determining the method of validation. The FDA has taken recent interest in home-brew methods, so it behooves the laboratory to be aware of current regulatory requirements. Oversight of LDTs is within the authority granted to the FDA in 1976 to regulate all in vitro diagnostics as medical devices. The agency had exercised enforcement discretion for these tests until fairly recently, when the proliferation of more complex tests and diagnostic claims not fully supported with scientific evidence raised concerns. Because the FDA has indicated its intent to exercise greater oversight of LDTs, there has been significant dialogue between the laboratory community, the FDA, and other stakeholders to agree on a reasonable approach to this process. Final guidance has not been issued at this time.

A checklist is useful when developing a new test, whether FDA cleared or laboratory developed. An example of a checklist can be seen in Figure 7-1.

Fourth Condition Level Requirement: Personnel

CLIA regulations provide qualifications and responsibilities for the laboratory director, technical consultant, clinical consultant, technical supervisor, general supervisor, and testing personnel. The qualification requirements and responsibilities are quite detailed and specific.

The laboratory director's responsibilities are listed in CLIA, Subpart L, Sec. §493.1445(e)(1)

Name of Test:	Completed	Not Applicable	Comment
Calibration procedure			
Calculations			
Quality control (QC) procedure			
Specimen requirements			
Specimen storage and transport conditions			
Autoverification rules			
Interpretive comments			
Design specimen workflow to minimize ID errors			
Accuracy validation			
Imprecision validation			
Comparison with previous method			
Analytical measurement range (linearity)			
Limit of detection (LOD)			
Limit of quantitation (LOQ)			
Dilution protocol			
Sensitivity (non-FDA)			
Specificity (non-FDA)			
Interference/cross-reactivity testing			
Reference range			
Reporting protocol			
Critical values			
Harmonize systems measuring same analyte			
Standard operating procedure (SOP) written			
SOP approved			
New reagent lot validation procedure			
Activity menu for accrediting agency updated			
Proficiency testing enrolled			
Alternative test performance method developed			
Notify information technology			
Calculations in analyzer and LIS validated			
Interface and reporting validated			
Automated interpretations validated			
Preventive maintenance and function monitoring defined			
Safety considerations			
MSDS sheets obtained and filed			
Hazardous waste considerations			
Training and competency			
Ordering and suppliers specified			
Clinical indications defined			
Educate providers on indications and interpretation			
Backup plan for system failure			
Test directory updated			
Notify processing department			
Notify billing department			
Notify client services			
Notify marketing			
Cost accounting			

ID, identification; FDA, US Food and Drug Administration; LIS, laboratory information system; MSDS, material safety data sheet.

Figure 7-1. Example checklist for validation and institution of a new test.

through §493.1445(e15), Laboratory Director Responsibilities, 42CFR493.1455(e).[24] There are 15 responsibilities, some of which can be delegated to a designee and some cannot. This list is not as detailed as the CAP accreditation checklists but provides a useful overview of the requirements for the laboratory. These 15 responsibilities are as follows:

§493.1445(e)(1) Ensure that testing systems developed and used for each of the tests performed in the laboratory provide quality laboratory services for all aspects of test performance, which includes the preanalytic, analytic, and postanalytic phases of testing;

§493.1445(e)(2) Ensure that the physical plant and environmental conditions of the laboratory are appropriate for the testing performed and provide a safe environment in which employees are protected from physical, chemical, and biological hazards;

§493.1445(e)(3)(i) Ensure that the test methodologies selected have the capability of providing the quality of results required for patient care; (ii) Verification procedures used are adequate to determine the accuracy, precision, and other pertinent performance characteristics of the method; and (iii) Laboratory personnel are performing the test methods as required for accurate and reliable results;

§493.1445(e)(4)(i) The proficiency testing samples are tested as required under Subpart H of this part; (ii)The results are returned within the timeframes established by the proficiency testing program; (iii) All proficiency testing reports received are reviewed by the appropriate staff to evaluate the laboratory's performance and to identify any problems that require corrective action; and (iv) An approved corrective action plan is followed when any proficiency testing result is found to be unacceptable or unsatisfactory;

§493.1445(e)(5) Ensure that the quality control and quality assessment programs are established and maintained to assure the quality of laboratory services provided and to identify failures in quality as they occur;

§493.1445(e)(6) Ensure the establishment and maintenance of acceptable levels of analytical performance for each test system;

§493.1445(e)(7) Ensure that all necessary remedial actions are taken and documented whenever significant deviations from the laboratory's established performance characteristics are identified, and that patient test results are reported only when the system is functioning properly;

§493.1445(e)(8) Ensure that reports of test results include pertinent information required for interpretation;

§493.1445(e)(9) Ensure that consultation is available to the laboratory's clients on matters relating to the quality of the test results reported and their interpretation concerning specific patient conditions;

§493.1445(e)(10) Ensure that a general supervisor provides on-site supervision of high complexity test performance by testing personnel qualified under §493.1489(b)(4);

§493.1445(e)(11) Employ a sufficient number of laboratory personnel with the appropriate education and either experience or training to provide appropriate consultation, properly supervise and accurately perform tests and report test results in accordance with the personnel responsibilities described in this subpart;

§493.1445(e)(12) Ensure that prior to testing patients' specimens, all personnel have the appropriate education and experience, receive the appropriate training for the type and complexity of the services offered, and have demonstrated that they can perform all testing operations reliably to provide and report accurate results;

§493.1445(e)(13) Ensure that policies and procedures are established for monitoring individuals who conduct preanalytical, analytical, and postanalytical phases of testing to assure that they are competent and maintain their competency to process specimens, perform test procedures and report test results promptly and proficiently, and whenever necessary identify needs for remedial training or continuing education to improve skills;

§493.1445(e)(14) Ensure that an approved procedure manual is available to all personnel responsible for any aspect of the testing process; and

§493.1445(e)(15) Specify, in writing, the responsibilities and duties of each consultant and each supervisor, as well as each person engaged in the performance of the preanalytic, analytic, and postanalytic phases of testing, that identifies which examinations and procedures each individual is authorized to perform, whether supervision is required for specimen processing, test performance or result reporting and whether supervisory or directory review is required prior to reporting patient test results.

Responsibilities (e)(3), (4), (5), (6), (7), (12), (13), and (14) can be reapportioned to a technical supervisor in writing.

Responsibilities (e)(8) and (9) can be reapportioned to a clinical consultant in writing.

Responsibilities (e)(1), (2), (10), (11), and (15) cannot be reapportioned.

Competency Evaluation of Technical Staff

A competency evaluation of technical staff must be performed at 6 months, 12 months, and annually thereafter. Competency evaluation may be more involved with LDTs in toxicology if they involve extraction, operating and maintaining chromatography and mass spectrometry instruments, and interpreting results. The CLIA regulations include six required elements of these evaluations[25]:

- Direct observations of routine patient test performance, including patient preparation, if applicable, specimen handling, processing, and testing
- Monitoring the recording and reporting of test results
- Review of intermediate test results or worksheets, quality control records, proficiency testing results, and preventive maintenance records
- Direct observation of performance of instrument maintenance and function
- Assessment of test performance through testing previously analyzed specimens, internal blind testing samples, or external proficiency testing samples
- Assessment of problem-solving skills

Fifth Condition Level Requirement: Inspection

CLIA requires biennial inspections of all certified laboratories, except those with a Certificate of Waiver. The CAP requires an interim self-inspection on alternating years between on-site inspections. Inspections are performed by the accrediting organization, be it CMS, a CMS agent such as a state program inspector, the licensure department of a CLIA-exempt state (New York and Washington), or a nonprofit accreditation program granted deemed status by CMS (AABB, ASHI, CAP, COLA, or The Joint Commission). CMS provides a Certificate of Compliance or a Certificate of Accreditation after any deficiencies cited during the inspection are corrected.

After a complaint, or for other reasons, additional inspections may be performed by CMS, CAP, or the agency or program that accredits the laboratory. CMS or a CMS agent may inspect a laboratory with a Certificate of Waiver for complaints, to assure that laboratory testing does not constitute an imminent and serious risk to public health, to determine whether the laboratory is performing tests beyond the scope of their certificate, and to collect information regarding the appropriateness of tests specified as waived. CMS or a CMS agent will perform a certain percentage of reinspections after inspections by CMS agents, of CLIA-exempt programs, and of those performed by deemed-status programs for validation purposes.

ISO 15189

ISO 15189:2007 is an international standard that "specifies requirements for quality and competence particular to medical laboratories. It is for use by medical laboratories in developing their quality management systems and assessing their own competence, and for use by accreditation bodies in confirming or recognizing the competence of medical laboratories."[26] The CAP now offers CAP 15189—Accreditation to the ISO 15189:2007 Standard. ISO 15189:2007 does not replace the CAP LAP accreditation in the United States, but it is used for accreditation of laboratories in many countries.

Alcohol and Volatiles Proficiency Testing

Alcohol (ethanol) is a CLIA-regulated analyte with required proficiency testing in a CLIA-approved program and with CLIA-regulated grading criteria. This is addressed in the section titled, "First Condition Level Requirement: Proficiency Testing," above. There are four CLIA-approved proficiency testing programs for alcohol. API offers quantitative serum alcohol and qualitative acetone testing. The CAP/AACC Whole Blood Alcohol/Ethylene Glycol/Volatiles (AL1) and CAP/AACC Serum Alcohol/Ethylene Glycol/Volatiles (AL2) surveys both include acetone, ethanol, ethylene glycol, isopropyl alcohol, and methanol. MLE offers serum alcohol and acetone testing. WSLH offers testing for serum alcohol, qualitative acetone, and semiquantitative acetone.

Immunoassay Urine Drug Screen Proficiency Testing

Proficiency testing programs for laboratories performing immunoassay screens on urine and not chromatographic or mass spectral analyses are offered by API, CAP, MLE, and WSLH. The programs differ in the number of proficiency testing challenges per shipment, number of shipments per year, and the breakdown of peer groups. The test menus of the programs are similar, covering most of the commonly available instrument-based and point-of-care devices. To be more or less challenging to the participant and to determine how different methods compare at different concentrations of drug, the programs may differ in the amount of drug present. Catalogs from the sponsoring organizations are published each year, and the latest publication should be consulted for the most up-to-date information.

The API proficiency testing program in 2019 included 27 drugs or drug groups in urine, including:

- 6-Acetylmorphine
- Acetaminophen
- Alcohol
- Amphetamines
- Barbiturates
- Benzodiazepines
- Buprenorphine
- Cannabinoids
- Carisoprodol
- Cocaine metabolites
- Cotinine
- Fentanyl
- Hydrocodone
- Lysergic acid diethylamide (LSD)
- Meperidine
- Methadone
- Methadone metabolite (EDDP)
- Methamphetamines
- Methaqualone
- Methylenedioxymethamphetamine (MDMA)
- Opiates
- Oxycodone
- Phencyclidine
- Propoxyphene
- Tramadol
- Tricyclic antidepressants
- Zolpidem

The CAP/AACC Urine Drug Testing (Screening) (UDS) proficiency testing program in 2019 included 21 drugs or drug groups, including:

- Acetaminophen
- Amphetamine
- Amphetamine/methamphetamine group
- Barbiturate group
- Benzodiazepine group
- Benzoylecgonine/cocaine metabolites
- Buprenorphine and metabolites
- Delta-9-THC-COOH
- Ethanol
- Fentanyl
- Lysergic acid diethylamide (LSD)
- Methadone
- Methadone metabolite (EDDP)
- Methamphetamine
- Methaqualone
- Methylenedioxymethamphetamine (MDMA)
- Opiate group
- Oxycodone
- Phencyclidine
- Propoxyphene
- Tricyclic group

The concentrations of drugs are variable, designed to evaluate the sensitivity of the various kit methods and to challenge around those concentrations. Participants are graded against peers at their stated cutoff concentration. The group assays are challenged with different drugs within the group to allow participants to evaluate the specificity of their methods.

The MLE proficiency testing program in 2019 included 29 drugs and drug groups in urine, including:

- 6-Acetylmorphine
- Acetaminophen
- Amphetamines
- Barbiturates
- Benzodiazepines
- Buprenorphine
- Cannabinoids
- Carisoprodol
- Cocaine metabolites
- Cotinine
- Ethanol
- Fentanyl
- Hydrocodone
- LSD
- MDMA
- Meperidine
- Methadone
- Methadone metabolite (EDDP)
- Methamphetamines
- Methanol
- Methaqualone
- Opiates (morphine trihydrate)
- Oxycodone
- Oxymorphone
- Phencyclidine
- Propoxyphene
- Tramadol
- Tricyclic antidepressants
- Zolpidem

For laboratories holding New York State clinical laboratory permits, the New York State Department of Health Wadsworth Center used to provide a routine drug testing module, including amphetamines, barbiturates, benzodiazepines, benzoylecgonine, ethanol, fentanyl, methadone, opiates, phencyclidine, propoxyphene, tetrahydrocannabinol (THC)-cannabinoids, and tricyclic antidepressants.[27] As of January 1, 2017, the New York State Department of Health no longer provides proficiency testing samples itself.

The WSLH proficiency testing program in 2018 included 21 drugs or drug groups in urine, including acetaminophen, 6-acetylmorphine, amphetamines, barbiturates, benzodiazepines, buprenorphine, cannabinoids, cocaine metabolites, cotinine, methadone metabolite (EDDP), ethanol (alcohol), MDMA, methadone, methamphetamine, methaqualone, morphine, opiates, oxycodone, phencyclidine, propoxyphene, and tricyclic antidepressants.

Broad-Spectrum Urine Drug Screening Proficiency Testing

Laboratories utilizing chromatographic and mass spectral methods in addition to immunoassay require a more comprehensive proficiency testing program. There are programs for urine, serum, and whole blood. The providers are largely limited to the CAP and the proficiency testing program for SAMHSA National Laboratory Certification Program (NLCP)-accredited laboratories.

The CAP Urine Toxicology (UT) proficiency testing program is for laboratories that test urine with chromatographic and/or mass spectral methods to identify specific drugs. It is for qualitative results only. Chromatographic methods include thin-layer chromatography, gas chromatography, and liquid chromatography. This testing program is appropriate for the various types of mass spectrometry. It is appropriate for initial immunoassay screening, with follow-up of positive results with another, more definitive, method to confirm the immunoassay and to identify the specific drug or metabolite; it is not appropriate for immunoassay screening without confirmation. It is also appropriate for primary chromatographic or mass spectral screening. The UT menu includes more than 120 drugs, although not all drugs are challenged every year. A large number of the drugs are not detectable with the commonly used immunoassays.

The CAP/AACC Forensic Urine Drug Testing (Confirmatory) (UDC) proficiency testing program is designed for workplace urine drug screening; it consists of immunoassay screening of drugs of abuse followed by quantitative mass spectral quantitative confirmation. It is a collaborative effort of the CAP and the AACC. There are four shipments of 10 urine specimens per year. In 2019 it included:

- 6-Acetylmorphine
- Alpha-hydroxyalprazolam
- Amphetamines
- Benzoylecgonine
- Buprenorphine
- Butalbital
- Codeine
- Delta-9-THC-COOH
- Hydrocodone
- Hydromorphone
- Lorazepam
- Methadone
- Methadone metabolite (EDDP)
- Methamphetamine
- Methaqualone
- Methylenedioxyamphetamine (MDA)
- Methylenedioxyethylamphetamine (MDEA)
- Methylenedioxymethamphetamine (MDMA)
- Morphine
- Norbuprenorphine
- Nordiazepam
- Norpropoxyphene
- Oxazepam
- Oxycodone
- Oxymorphone
- Phencyclidine
- Phenobarbital
- Propoxyphene
- Secobarbital
- Temazepam
- Creatinine
- pH
- Specific gravity

The UDC survey was developed as a companion to the CAP FDT Accreditation Program. The urine drugs of abuse are not CLIA-regulated analytes, and there is no federal requirement to participate. There are requirements in some states for FDT and/or SAMHSA NLCP accreditation for workplace testing. The latest state regulation should be checked for guidance.

Drug Monitoring for Pain Management Proficiency Testing

The CAP offers the Drug Monitoring for Pain Management (DMPM) survey, developed for the rapidly expanding needs of this medical specialty. As of 2018, this program challenges from a list of 56 drugs and drug metabolites, with three specimens in each of two shipments per year. It also includes two "dry" challenges per year that require no testing but present a case study with toxicology results that require an interpretation.

Whole Blood, Serum, and Plasma Drug Screening Proficiency Testing

The CAP Serum Drug Screening (SDS) proficiency testing program includes tests for quantitative acetaminophen and salicylate, qualitative and semiquantitative acetone, qualitative barbiturate group, qualitative benzodiazepine group, and total tricyclic antidepressants. The barbiturate, benzodiazepine, and tricyclic groups are targeted at the serum immunoassays.

The CAP Toxicology (T) proficiency testing program is designed for laboratories testing both urine and serum with chromatographic and/or mass spectral methods to identify specific drugs. It includes paired urine and serum specimens as well as serum-only specimens. It includes serum quantitative testing. The test menu includes 137 drugs—the same drugs as for the UT survey, with the exception of any that are pharmacologically found only in serum. As with the UT survey, not all drugs are challenged every year. Several drugs were added to the survey in 2018, including aripiprazole, gabapentin, pregabalin, and topiramate.

The CAP Forensic Toxicology (Criminalistics) (FTC) proficiency testing program in 2019 included 74 drugs and drug metabolites of interest to the forensic community. Forensic testing is not CLIA regulated. It may be of interest to medical examiners, laboratories that perform tests for DUID, and clinical laboratories performing broad-spectrum drug screening on whole blood. The laboratory should determine whether the FTC or Toxicology survey (or both) is appropriate for the testing performed.

Vitreous Fluid, Postmortem Proficiency Testing

Laboratories performing postmortem toxicology may also use the CAP Vitreous Fluid, Postmortem (VF) survey that provides challenges for eight substances found in vitreous fluid.

Urine Adulteration Proficiency Testing

API offers a proficiency testing program Urine Adulteration Test, including creatinine, nitrite, pH, and specific gravity.

The CAP UDC survey offers creatinine, pH, and specific gravity. The CAP also offers a broader proficiency testing product for adulterant and specimen integrity assessment: the Urine Drug Adulterant/Integrity (DAI) proficiency survey, which provides samples containing normal and abnormal levels of creatinine and abnormal amounts of glutaraldehyde, nitrite, and oxidants, as well as specimens of normal and abnormal pH and specific gravity.

Oral Fluid Proficiency Testing

Oral fluid is now commonly used for drugs-of-abuse testing. As of August 2019, the specifics of testing oral fluid in the federally mandated drug testing programs have not been published in final form. It seems clear, however, that such standards will be published, and there is little doubt that this will increase the use of oral fluid testing for drugs of abuse. The CAP currently offers an oral fluid proficiency survey called Oral Fluid for Drugs of Abuse (OFD). For 2019 it contains 25 drugs and drug metabolites for use in laboratories performing screening, confirmation, and quantitation. Oral fluid testing is fully covered in chapter 14, *Alternate Specimens for Drugs-of-Abuse Testing: Oral Fluid.*

Summary

This chapter provides a review of the various options for certification of clinical and forensic toxicology laboratories. The toxicology laboratory is virtually always a federally regulated entity that does testing with potential legal implications and often performs medical testing as well. Although laboratories may accomplish toxicology testing through waived or nonwaived assays, the condition level requirements for accreditation must be fulfilled. As part of the CLIA requirements for proficiency testing, there are many options available to the laboratory director, and selection of an appropriate proficiency testing program involves detailed knowledge of the toxicology test menu and complexities of the testing methods.

References

1. US Department of Health and Human Services, Centers for Medicare and Medicaid Services. Laboratory Requirements. Title 42 CFR Part 493, Clinical Laboratory Improvement Amendments of 1988, Subpart A. General provisions. Sec. 493.1. Basis and scope. 42CFR493.1. https://www.ecfr.gov/cgi-bin/text-idx?SID=1248e3189da5e5f936e-55315402bc38b&node=pt42.5.493&rgn=div5#se42.5.493_11 Accessed August 15, 2019
2. US Department of Health and Human Services, Centers for Medicare and Medicaid Services. Laboratory requirements. Title 42 CFR Part 493, Clinical Laboratory Improvement Amendments of 1988, Subpart A. General provisions. Sec. 493.2. Definitions. 42CFR493.2. https://www.ecfr.gov/cgi-bin/text-idx?SID=1248e3189da5e5f936e-55315402bc38b&node=pt42.5.493&rgn=div5#se42.5.493_12. Accessed August 15, 2019.
3. US Department of Health and Human Services, Centers for Medicare and Medicaid Services. Laboratory requirements. Title 42 CFR Part 493, Clinical Laboratory Improvement Amendments of 1988, Subpart A. General provisions. Sec. 493.5. Categories of tests by complexity. 42CFR493.5. https://www.ecfr.gov/cgi-bin/text-idx?SID=1248e3189da5e5f936e55315402bc-38b&node=pt42.5.493&rgn=div5#se42.5.493_15. Accessed August 15, 2019.

4. US Department of Health and Human Services, Centers for Medicare and Medicaid Services. Laboratory requirements. Title 42 CFR Part 493, Clinical Laboratory Improvement Amendments of 1988, Subpart A. General provisions. Sec 493.3. Applicability. 42CFR493.3. https://www.ecfr.gov/cgi-bin/text-idx?SID=1248e3189da5e5f936e55315402bc38b&node=pt42.5.493&rgn=div5#se42.5.493_15. Accessed August 15, 2019.
5. Clinical Laboratory Evaluation Program. New York State Department of Health, Wadsworth Center. https://www.wadsworth.org/regulatory/clep. Accessed August 15, 2019.
6. Washington State Department of Health, Office of Laboratory Quality Assurance. License Types, Requirements, and Applications. https://www.doh.wa.gov/LicensesPermitsandCertificates/FacilitiesNewReneworUpdate/LaboratoryQualityAssurance/Licensing/Applications. Accessed August 15, 2019.
7. College of American Pathologists. www.cap.org. Accessed August 15, 2019.
8. American Board of Forensic Toxicology. www.abft.org. Accessed August 15, 2019.
9. ANSI National Accreditation Board (ANAB). https://www.anab.org/forensic-accreditation. Accessed August 15, 2019.
10. Department of Health and Human Services, Substance Abuse and Mental Health Services Administration. Mandatory guidelines for federal workplace drug testing programs. 82 Federal Register 7920 (2017).
11. US Department of Health and Human Services, Centers for Medicare and Medicaid Services. Laboratory requirements. Title 42 CFR Part 493. Clinical Laboratory Improvement Amendments of 1988, Subpart A. General provisions. Sec. 493.15. Laboratories performing waived tests. 42CFR493.15. https://www.ecfr.gov/cgi-bin/text-idx?SID=1248e3189da5e5f936e55315402bc38b&node=pt42.5.493&rgn=div5#se42.5.493_115. Accessed August 15, 2019.
12. CLIA—Clinical Laboratory Improvement Amendments—Currently Waived Analytes. US Food and Drug Administration. https://www.accessdata.fda.gov/scripts/cdrh/cfdocs/cfClia/analyteswaived.cfm. Accessed August 15, 2019.
13. US Department of Health and Human Services, Centers for Medicare and Medicaid Services. Laboratory requirements. Title 42 CFR Part 493. Clinical Laboratory Improvement Amendments of 1988, Subpart H. Participation in proficiency testing for laboratories performing nonwaived testing. Sec. 493.801 through 493.865. https://www.ecfr.gov/cgi-bin/text-idx?SID=1248e3189da5e5f936e55315402bc38b&node=pt42.5.493&rgn=div5#sp42.5.493.h. Accessed August 15, 2019.
14. CLIA Approved Proficiency Testing Programs—2019. Centers for Medicare and Medicaid Services. www.cms.hhs.gov/CLIA/downloads/ptlist.pdf. Accessed August 15, 2019.
15. US Department of Health and Human Services, Centers for Medicare and Medicaid Services. Laboratory requirements. Title 42 CFR Part 493. Clinical Laboratory Improvement Amendments of 1988, Subpart I. Sec. 493.937. Toxicology. https://www.ecfr.gov/cgi-bin/text-idx?SID=1248e3189da5e5f936e55315402bc38b&node=pt42.5.493&rgn=div5#se42.5.493_1937 Accessed August 15, 2019.
16. US Department of Health and Human Services, Centers for Medicare and Medicaid Services. Laboratory requirements. Title 42 CFR Part 493, Clinical Laboratory Improvement Amendments of 1988, Subpart J. Facility administration for nonwaived testing. Sec. 493.1100 through 493.1105. https://www.ecfr.gov/cgi-bin/text-idx?SID=1248e3189da5e5f936e55315402bc38b&node=pt42.5.493&rgn=div5#sp42.5.493.j. Accessed August 15, 2019.
17. US Public Law 104-191, Health Insurance Portability and Accountability Act of 1996. https://www.govinfo.gov/content/pkg/PLAW-104publ191/html/PLAW-104publ191.htm. Accessed August 15, 2019.
18. US Department of Health and Human Services, Centers for Medicare and Medicaid Services. Laboratory requirements. Title 42 CFR Part 493, Clinical Laboratory Improvement Amendments of 1988, Subpart J. Facility administration for nonwaived testing. Sec. 493.1105. Standard: retention requirements. 42CFR493.1105. https://www.ecfr.gov/cgi-bin/text-idx?SID=1248e3189da5e5f936e55315402bc38b&node=pt42.5.493&rgn=div5#se42.5.493_11105. Accessed August 15, 2019.
19. US Department of Health and Human Services, Centers for Medicare and Medicaid Services. Laboratory requirements. Title 42 CFR Part 493, Clinical Laboratory Improvement Amendments of 1988, Subpart K. Quality system for nonwaived testing. Sec. 493.1200. Introduction. 42CFR493.1200. https://www.ecfr.gov/cgi-bin/text-idx?SID=1248e3189da5e5f936e55315402bc38b&node=pt42.5.493&rgn=div5#se42.5.493_11200. Accessed August 15, 2019.
20. Laboratory Accreditation Program. *All Common Checklist.* Northfield, IL: College of American Pathologists; August 22, 2018:COM.01500.
21. Laboratory proficiency testing program. American College of Physicians. www.acponline.org/running_practice/mle/. Accessed August 26, 2019.
22. American Proficiency Institute. www.api-pt.com. Accessed August 15, 2019.

23. Wisconsin State Laboratory of Hygiene. www.slh.wisc.edu/. Accessed August 15, 2019.
24. US Department of Health and Human Services, Centers for Medicare and Medicaid Services. Laboratory requirements. Title 42 CFR Part 493, Clinical Laboratory Improvement Amendments of 1988, Subpart M. Personnel for nonwaived testing. Sec. 493.1445(e)(1) through 493.1445(e15). Standard; laboratory director responsibilities. 42CFR493.1455(e). http://edocket.access.gpo.gov/cfr_2004/octqtr/42cfr493.1445.htm. October 1, 2004. Accessed August 4, 2011.
25. US Department of Health and Human Services, Centers for Medicare and Medicaid Services. Laboratory requirements. Title 42 CFR Part 493. Clinical Laboratory Improvement Amendments of 1988, Subpart M. Personnel for nonwaived testing. Sec. 493.1451(b)(8) through (b)(9). Standard: technical supervisor responsibilities. 42CFR493.1451. http://edocket.access.gpo.gov/cfr_2004/octqtr/42cfr493.1451.htm. October 1, 2004. Accessed August 4, 2011.
26. International Organization for Standardization. www.iso.org. Accessed August 15, 2019.
27. New York State Department of Health, Wadsworth Center, Proficiency Testing. https://www.wadsworth.org/regulatory/clep/pt. Accessed August 15, 2019.

Acknowledgment

The authors would like to acknowledge Wayne R. Markus, MD, for his original version of this manuscript published in the first edition of this book.

Chapter 8

The Hospital Autopsy and Toxicology Testing

D. Kimberley Molina, MD
Barbarajean Magnani, PhD, MD

Introduction

Deaths that are due to drug toxicity most often fall under the jurisdiction of a medical examiner (ME; usually an appointed forensic pathologist) or coroner (usually an elected official), but the sheer magnitude of both prescription and illicit drug use and misuse makes it likely that hospital pathologists will come across such cases during their careers.

The Centers for Disease Control and Prevention reported more than 63,000 drug-induced deaths in the United States in 2016, most commonly caused by opiate and opioid drugs and cocaine.[1] In addition, in some jurisdictions, intoxication deaths may be deferred to hospital pathologists because of limited ME resources. Therefore, at least a rudimentary understanding of toxicology, specifically postmortem and forensic toxicology, is necessary for the hospital pathologist.

It has long been known that poisons can result in death; however, Dr Mathieu Joseph Bonaventure Orfila brought forensic toxicology to the forefront in the early 1800s with the publication of his treatise, *Traité des Poisons*. The scientific methods used by Dr Orfila to discover and delineate cases of poisoning formed the foundation for the field of forensic toxicology. The principles he presented led to an increased understanding of deaths due to intoxication, as well as to multiple criminal convictions, and form the basis of many of the testing methodologies and scientific practices used today.

Unfortunately, there are no pathognomonic signs of poisonings found either clinically or at autopsy, although there are features suggestive of such. In addition, because many intoxicants are not detected upon routine clinical drug screens (including the newer synthetic opiates, cannabinoids, and psychoactive substances), treating physicians and pathologists must maintain a high degree of suspicion and must understand the principles of postmortem toxicology in order to correctly assess and interpret results in a suspected drug toxicity death.

Per the National Association of Medical Examiners (NAME) autopsy performance standards, deaths due to apparent intoxication by alcohol, drugs, or poisons require autopsy examinations.[2] This necessity was further described in a recent NAME position paper published in response to the overwhelming opioid epidemic.[3] In this paper, the authors list indications for ordering toxicology testing in the investigation of a death (Table 8-1). Thus, if the clinical pathologist thinks that there is any indication that a drug toxicity may have played a role in a death, before performing the autopsy or ordering any testing, the pathologist should consult the appropriate medicolegal death authority, whether that be the local coroner or ME. Simply ordering toxicology testing on a deceased person may have serious medicolegal implications, and these should be thoroughly discussed and understood before commencing any examination (see "Medicolegal Issues," below).

Table 8-1. Indications for Toxicology Investigation After a Death
Known history of prescription opioid or illicit drug use, misuse, or abuse
Evidence of opioid or illicit drug abuse revealed by scene investigation
Autopsy findings suggesting a history of illicit drug abuse (including needle marks, hepatic cirrhosis, and cases in which birefringent crystalline material is within foreign body giant cells in the lungs)
Massive lung edema and froth in airways present with no grossly visible explanation (eg, heart disease) or other nontoxicological explanation (eg, seizure)
Potential or suspected smugglers of illicit drugs (mules)
No unequivocal cause for death identified at autopsy
Decedents with a potential natural cause of death visible at autopsy whenever a drug may have precipitated or contributed to death by an additive mechanism, such as opioid-induced respiratory depression
Traumatic deaths

From Davis et al.[3] Reproduced with permission from the National Association of Medical Examiners.

The Autopsy

Any autopsy examination must begin with a review of the circumstances of death. In the medicolegal setting, this may mean reviewing the scene and witness statements of what was occurring at or near the time of death. In the hospital setting, this means a thorough review of the decedent's medical chart, which includes (1) how the decedent presented to the hospital (signs, symptoms, and laboratory values); (2) the hospital course; (3) pertinent medical history, including medication history; and (4) the events that occurred at or near the time of death. The pathologist should discuss the case with the treating physicians to determine if there are any specific clinical concerns that an autopsy may be able to address. The medical record review will often ascertain whether a drug may have caused or contributed to death or if there is a clinical concern of that nature. Medical record review is also critical in assisting the pathologist in determining which type of toxicological analysis is necessary or if other additional testing may be helpful. For example, a patient with a chronic, unrelenting dermatitis may be suffering from thallium poisoning.[4] In such a case, a pathologist may obtain a sample of blood, kidney, hair, or nail tissue for heavy metal testing, as well as a skin biopsy to evaluate for necrosis of the sebaceous glands and hair follicles, commonly found in thallium poisoning.

Once the records have been reviewed and the pathologist is comfortable with the clinical scenario, the autopsy begins with an external examination. This examination focuses on documenting distinguishing characteristics (eg, scars, tattoos, eye color) as well as signs of trauma or natural disease. The following observations could provide clues that a drug(s) may have been a factor in the death:

- Decedents having expired as a result of opiate intoxication may exhibit a pink tinge or frothy "foam cap" around the mouth or nose (Figure 8-1).
- Needle track marks (linear scars within the antecubital fossae or overlying veins along the anterior forearms) may suggest chronic intravenous drug use (Figure 8-2).
- Small skin ulcerations or abscesses may result from skin popping of cocaine or heroin.
- Fenestration of the nasal septum can occur with chronic cocaine insufflation.
- Chronic dental grinding may lead to wear of the incisors in methamphetamine abusers.
- Lead poisoning may result in so-called lead lines, or Burton lines (blue lines along the gums).
- Carbon monoxide and cyanide poisoning may result in cherry-red lividity.
- Cyanide poisoning is often associated with a bitter almond smell (although the ability to detect this odor is genetically determined and is absent in 20-40% of the population);.

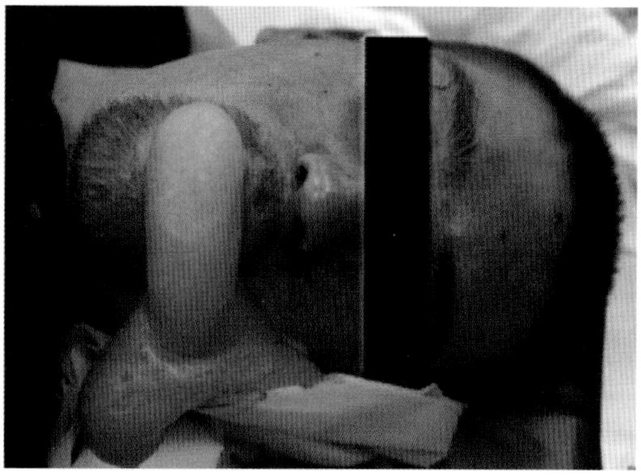

Figure 8-1. Example of a "foam cone" often seen in overdose deaths.

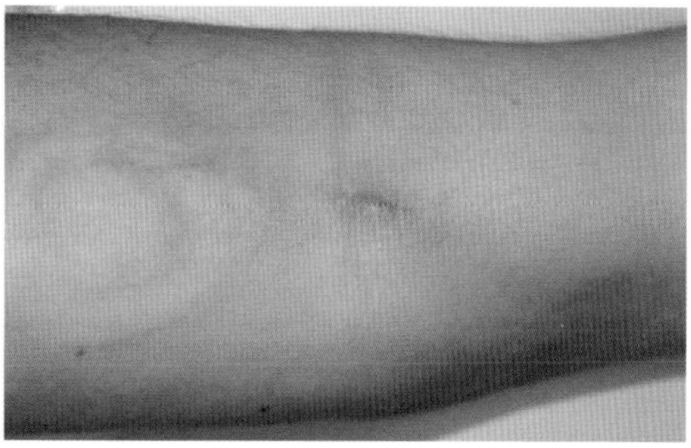

Figure 8-2. Needle track mark.

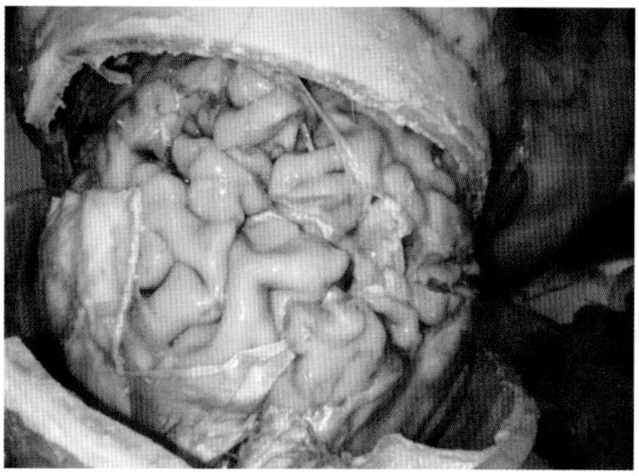

Figure 8-3. Bluish-green discoloration of brain tissue from methylene blue.

- Methylene blue, utilized in the treatment of methemoglobinemia and cardiovascular collapse, can produce a bluish-green discoloration of the brain (Figure 8-3).
- Mees' lines (white lines across the nails) may indicate heavy metal poisoning, such as from arsenic or thallium.

The external examination should also include assessment of the vaginal vault and intergluteal

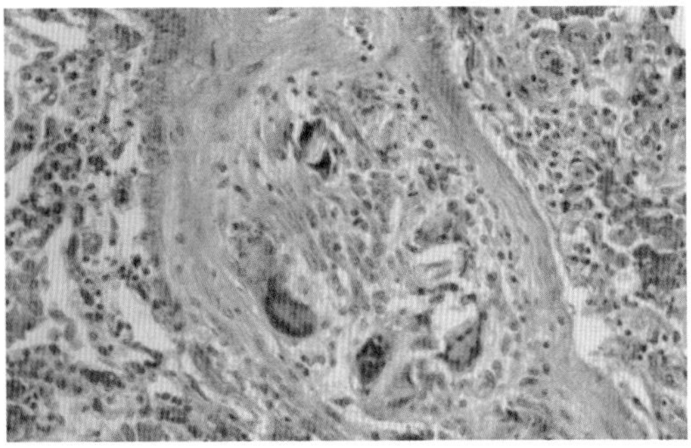

Figure 8-4. Talc granuloma within the lung of an intravenous drug user.

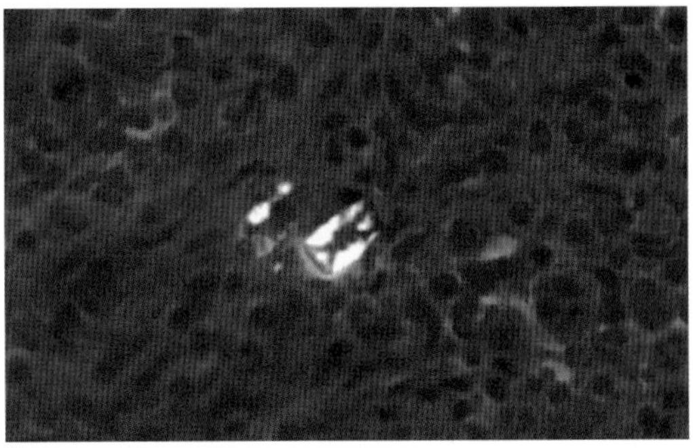

Figure 8-5. Starch granule (birefringent foreign material) in lung, exhibiting a Maltese cross pattern.

cleft for packets of drugs. Although not pathognomonic for drug toxicity, such findings may lead the pathologist to suspect intoxication and to suggest which toxicology tests should be ordered.

The results of the medical record review and external examination are then correlated with the internal examination. Intoxicating substances do not result in characteristic internal findings, although nonspecific findings may be present. For example, heavy edematous lungs, cerebral edema, and bladder distention are often present in deaths due to intoxication (particularly from central nervous system depressants), although these may also be seen in cases of cerebral hypoxia due to heart failure and in medical states of overhydration.[5]

Correlating autopsy findings with the medical history can also lead a pathologist to suspect the use of intoxicants. For example, the presence of a large heart in a young person without a significant medical or family history or the characteristic gross appearance of idiopathic, hypertrophic, subaortic stenosis may be a result of chronic stimulant use. Occasionally, internal examination can lead to unexpected findings, including the presence of baggies or balloons in the intestinal contents. Drug "mules" often swallow these items filled with illicit substances for transport.[6] If a baggie or balloon ruptures during transport, death can be caused by massive, rapid intoxication.[7] The presence of such material in the intestinal contents should lead the pathologist to order appropriate toxicological testing.

Most hospital autopsies also include microscopic examination of the major organs. Although there are no pathognomonic findings seen under the microscope of deaths due to poisonings, some findings can be suggestive. In individuals who inject medications intravenously, foreign-body giant cell granulomas containing polarizable material—such as talc, starch, or methylcellulose, which are often used as fillers to either cut illicit drugs or as part of the pill composition—may be present surrounding the pulmonary vessels (Figure 8-4). Birefringent material can also be seen within lung tissue without giant cell granulomas (Figure 8-5). Intranuclear inclusions in hepatocytes and renal epithelium (as well as basophilic stippling in red cells) can be seen in cases of lead poisoning. Ingestion of ethylene glycol can lead to polarizable crystals of calcium oxalate within the renal tubules. Focal dropout lesions in myocardium with small foci of lymphocytes or contraction band necrosis, as well as small vessel arteriosclerosis, may be seen in cocaine or sympathomimetic drug users. Each of these findings can lead the pathologist to become suspicious and to order the appropriate toxicological testing for the specific substance in question.

Natural disease processes can also be the result of medication use or misuse. Hepatic cirrhosis commonly occurs with chronic ethanol use. Intravenous drug use can lead to endocarditis and its consequences, often resulting in death. Amiodarone toxicity can cause significant pulmonary disease, which can lead to death. Numerous medications can cause Stevens-Johnson syndrome or, at the more severe end of the spectrum, toxic epidermal necrolysis, which may prove fatal.[8,9] Fatal anaphylactic reactions to medications can also occur. By convention, all of these types of deaths are classified as "natural" with respect to the manner of death, even though they can be traced back to substance use. An exception would occur if a superimposed acute intoxication also contributed to death. For example, in the case of a heroin addict who dies of a combination of endocarditis and acute heroin intoxication, the death would be considered an accident. If there is a question about the role a drug may or may not have played, the pathologist would be well served to consult their local ME before death certification.

Specimen Collection

For the most accurate toxicological examination, the best specimen is peripheral antemortem blood obtained just after an intoxicating event is suspected or upon hospital admission. For example, if a patient presents to the hospital after overdosing on heroin but survives in the hospital for 7 days, the best specimen on which to perform toxicology testing is the one from presentation, 7 days before death. If the intoxication is believed to be an interaction of medications given in the hospital, blood specimens obtained immediately before death may be the preferred specimen. For this reason, hospital laboratories that see a population prone to overdose and death may wish to retain admitting blood specimens longer than the College of American Pathologists or state guidelines dictate. However, given that many clinical laboratories are constrained for space with respect to storage of specimens, it may only be possible to retain specimens that come from selected patients, for example, those admitted from the emergency department.

The pathologist should collect and sequester all available blood and urine specimens from the hospitalization of the deceased patient. If it is later determined that there is no need for these specimens, they can be discarded. Because many specimens are discarded within a few days of collection as part of the routine laboratory work flow, it is best to sequester these specimens as soon as it is known that there will be an autopsy. Occasionally, a patient is seen in the emergency department who does not survive, and any specimens collected during the emergency department visit may be requested by the ME if the case is transferred to his or her jurisdiction.

If antemortem blood is not available, the best postmortem specimen is peripherally obtained blood, in order to minimize the effects of postmortem redistribution. Postmortem redistribution occurs after death, as drugs are released from protein-bound molecules and intracellular locations. Drugs diffuse down a concentration gradient, and a spuriously elevated concentration may result if blood is collected centrally (see "Interpretation of Toxicology Results," below). Research has shown that peripheral blood is less affected by postmortem redistribution than is central blood.[10] The preferential order for obtaining blood in a postmortem case would be femoral blood, followed by (in rank order) blood obtained from the (1) subclavian vessels, (2) iliac veins, (3) superior or inferior vena cava, (3) aorta or pulmonary artery, and (4) heart; ideally, blood should be collected from both the heart and a peripheral site.[11] At least 50 mL of blood should be obtained via a clean large-bore needle attached to a clean syringe and placed into a glass container preserved with a fluoride-oxalate additive (2% weight/volume fluoride and 5 mg/mL oxalate)—a grey top Vacutainer tube includes these additives if a larger container is not available. The fluoride preservative inhibits bacterial growth and certain metabolic processes (such as the action of peripheral esterases) to prevent in vitro metabolism of drugs, especially cocaine. Some drugs will bind to the polymers in plastic, so glass containers are preferable. Subdural and epidural clots should also be collected because these may be useful in accidents where drug ingestion may have played a role.

In addition to blood, the pathologist should obtain urine on all cases where available, along with bile, vitreous humor, and hair in those cases where such specimens may be useful. Urine and bile are collected by inserting a clean large-bore needle attached to a clean 10-cc syringe into the respective viscera and withdrawing the fluid. The specimens should then be placed into sterile, glass, red top tubes (no additives). If desired, a clean razor can be used to obtain 100 mg to 200 mg of hair from the body. Scalp hair is preferable because it is usually the longest. The hair should then be placed into a new, unused, dry-specimen container. The root and distal ends of the hair should be clearly marked with transparent tape because this may become important in cases of chronic poisoning. Hair grows at approximately 1 cm to 1.5 cm per month, and in cases of heavy metal poisoning, analysis of the hair can provide a time line for exposure. Vitreous humor is obtained by inserting a clean 16- or 18-gauge needle through the lateral sclera of the eye, being careful to avoid the cornea, and gently extracting the fluid. Vigorous suction on the syringe can lead to retinal detachment and aspiration of tissue into the fluid, contaminating the specimen. The fluid obtained from each eye may be combined into a single clean, glass, red top tube.

Tissue specimens may also be collected, including from spleen, skeletal muscle, liver, kidney, brain, and fat. Tissue is often helpful in specific situations, but its routine use, instead of blood, is not recommended. For example, in decomposed bodies, skeletal muscle and spleen are useful specimens. Approximately 50 g of tissue should be collected with a clean blade and placed into a clean, unused, dry-specimen container. If liver is collected, the sample should be taken from the deep right lobe to limit diffusion from the stomach and intestines. Muscle should be obtained from the quadriceps to limit diffusion but also because it is a large and easily accessible muscle.

Stomach contents are normally collected when an oral drug overdose is suspected. The entirety of the gastric contents should be measured—because the total volume is necessary to calculate the drug concentration—and collected into a clean dry-specimen container.

Where possible, all specimens should be transferred to the laboratory and tested under proper chain-of-custody procedures. Although hospital laboratories usually do not routinely collect specimens using chain-of-custody procedures, they do follow good laboratory practice of specimen identification and documentation of testing personnel. Analysts or laboratory technologists performing the testing should be aware that they may be called to testify in a court of law regarding chain of custody as well as the specific testing performed. Hospitals should also be aware of any specific requirements or local laws that may potentially affect the testing. For example, in Texas, anyone performing toxicological testing for potential criminal determination is required to have a license to do so.

Specimen Selection

The most crucial element of toxicological analysis is specimen selection. A living patient has limited specimens available for laboratory analysis, whereas postmortem specimens are usually available in plenty. Analysis can be performed on fluids or tissues, but simply being able to perform an analysis does not mean the data obtained will be useful. Blood is the best specimen for determining death resulting from drug overdose. Blood is easy to obtain and process, and most of the available data regarding therapeutic, toxic, and lethal drug concentrations come from blood. To limit the effects of postmortem redistribution, quantification should be performed on peripheral blood samples when available.

Urine can be a useful medium for drug screening and identification of drug metabolites, but the concentrations obtained are rarely helpful in interpretation. Urine drug concentrations commonly reflect that a drug was ingested hours, sometimes days, before death. In addition, urinary excretion (and concentration) of a drug can be dependent upon the urine environment (eg, pH) and not solely on the blood concentration.

Vitreous humor (fluid) is an excellent specimen that can be used as an alternative to blood. Vitreous fluid is relatively isolated and stable, which allows for less effect of postmortem redistribution and decomposition. Its isolation can also be of assistance when dealing with substances with short half-lives, because they or their metabolites can often be found in the vitreous fluid even after they have been cleared from the blood. For example, 6-monoacetylmorphine (6-MAM) can often be found in the vitreous fluid in heroin overdoses even when it can no longer be detected in the blood. Vitreous fluid is also an excellent specimen to use if the drugs of interest are highly water soluble, including ethanol, barbiturates, and carbamates. The average vitreous humor:blood ethanol concentration ratio is approximately 1.2 in the postabsorptive phase.[12] The small quantity of vitreous fluid available for analysis limits its routine use.

Bile is an easy specimen to obtain, although it is available in limited quantities. Certain drugs can be concentrated in the bile (eg, benzodiazepines and opioids), making interpretation of concentrations difficult.

Tissue specimens (eg, liver, kidney, skeletal muscle, brain) are often available in abundance in postmortem cases but are markedly susceptible to postmortem redistribution. Some drugs may accumulate in certain tissues, such as tricyclic antidepressants (TCAs) in the liver and heart. Sometimes this tendency to accumulate in tissues can be useful, as with pesticides in fat or heavy metals in the kidney, but it can make the interpretation of concentrations difficult. Published reports of tissue concentrations in therapeutic, toxic, or lethal cases are often not available.

Analysis of stomach contents can be helpful, especially when an oral drug overdose is suspected. The utility of gastric drug concentrations is, however, circumspect. If a drug is present in the stomach, even at high concentrations, it may simply reflect a recent ingestion and not necessarily reflect the blood concentration or pharmacologic effects. A massive amount of drug in the gastric contents, however, is more likely to indicate a suicidal overdose rather than an accident in the appropriate setting.

Hair is an excellent specimen to show chronicity of drug use but has little value in determining acute use or the relationship with death.

Ordering of Toxicology Testing

The decision to order toxicology testing should be based upon the case at hand and in consultation with the appropriate medicolegal death investigation authority. Comprehensive drug testing is often only available in the ME setting or at reference laboratories. Hospitals often do not possess the equipment, staffing, or materials necessary to perform such testing. The NAME position paper on the investigation of opioid-related deaths provides recommendations regarding when to perform toxicology testing for controlled substances (Table 8-1)[3]; however, caution should be used before ordering any testing, and the local medicolegal death-investigating authority should be consulted before undertaking any such testing.

In the medicolegal setting, a battery of screening tests is often utilized to look for as many intoxicating agents as possible, including drugs of abuse as well as commonly used prescription and over-the-counter medications, such as antipsychotic, antidepressant, anxiolytic, pain, cough, and cold medications. Screens for heavy metals, cannabinoids, and other additional drugs or drug classes are also available and can be ordered as needed; however, hospital toxicology testing is usually more directed in nature. After a review of the medical records and consultation with treating physicians, the hospital pathologist will generally know which medications and drugs are of interest.

Screening for drugs or medications will depend upon the laboratory methods available at a specific hospital and whether the testing is done on site or is ordered through a reference laboratory. Most hospitals use a urine immunoassay drugs-of-abuse screen for initial toxicology testing, although care must be used when determining that a death is not drug related on the basis of the results of such testing. As discussed previously, the presence of a drug in the urine often reflects that a drug was ingested hours, sometimes days, before death and may not indicate current toxicity. In addition, urine drug screens may miss commonly abused drugs, such as synthetic opiates and cannabinoids; for example, specific immunoassays are required for certain analytes such as fentanyl, buprenorphine, and oxycodone. Immunoassays are also unreliable because of cross-reactivity and inhibiting substances, leading to false-negative or false-positive results.

In addition to urine drugs-of-abuse screens, hospitals may also employ assays for serum barbiturates, benzodiazepines, salicylates, acetaminophen, TCAs, and ethanol, which are commonly used in compliance or overdose testing. There are also specific assays for therapeutic drug monitoring, which may be useful if the deceased person was taking anticonvulsants, lithium, or digoxin, for example; however, because these assays are for serum, not whole blood, they may be of limited utility in postmortem testing because of redistribution issues. If the drug of interest is one for which the hospital or reference laboratory is able to test, it is recommended that the laboratory be contacted directly to elucidate the type of specimen required before collection because some specimens require special handling. For example, specimens collected for testing of volatiles (eg, fluorocarbons, hydrocarbons) need to be collected in glass screw-top containers because the volatile gases can escape through rubber stoppers, and royal blue metal-free tubes are necessary for trace metal analysis. Of note, commercial immunoassays are not approved to assay postmortem blood specimens because of potential matrix effects that could affect accuracy.

Interpretation of Toxicology Results

Interpretation of toxicology results depends on many factors. Individual variations result in a marked difference in drug concentrations in normal healthy volunteers.[13] This variation is often magnified in hospitalized patients, who may not be able to metabolize drugs appropriately. Drug metabolism is dependent upon many variables, including organ function and volume of distribution. Hospitalized patients may have decreased organ function—especially with respect to the heart, liver, and kidneys—all of which can be critical in drug metabolism and excretion. In addition, hospitalized patients may have pathologic fluid accumulations (ascites, anasarca), which can dramatically affect drug distribution.

The principle of postmortem redistribution and how it can affect toxicology results must be understood by pathologists. After death, the heart stops and the blood ceases to flow. When this occurs, the blood begins to separate, resulting in changes in the hematocrit and in the distribution of drugs within the blood itself. Enzymes and microbes can alter drugs directly or the transport proteins to which they bind. All of these factors contribute to the changing environment of the blood and surrounding tissues, resulting in changes in pH, solubility, binding properties, and so forth. These environmental changes can result in the diffusion of drugs both into and out of the blood and to or from the surrounding tissues—a phenomenon known as *postmortem redistribution*. In his research, Pounder found that the volume of distribution (V_d) of a specific drug strongly affects this redistribution process, with drugs with higher V_d having a greater tendency toward redistribution.[10] Postmortem drug concentrations must be interpreted with this principle in mind. For example, digoxin has been shown to have such significant postmortem release into the blood that vitreous fluid is the specimen of choice when digoxin intoxication is suspected; TCAs are also well known to be subject to postmortem redistribution and should be interpreted with caution. In general, utilization of peripheral blood samples for quantification minimizes, but does not eliminate, the inaccuracies due to postmortem redistribution.

Pathologists must also understand how the method of testing and the specimen used can affect interpretation. In some cases, immunoassays lack specificity and may give erroneous results due to cross-reactivity or the presence of inhibiting substances, whereas chromatography (either gas or liquid) paired with mass spectrophotometry is considered the "gold standard" in forensic toxicology. Issues regarding methodology are discussed in more detail in subsequent chapters. The specimen used for testing is also critical because of the effects of postmortem redistribution, as well as when making comparisons to known values. Most therapeutic concentration data are obtained in living patients from tests performed on serum from peripheral blood specimens. Comparing these data with those of whole-blood specimens from central locations or tissues can lead to erroneous interpretation. It is best to compare data from the same source tissue performed by the same methodology, but data are often not available. Published compilations of drugs and their toxic concentrations in blood, urine, and tissues are available.[14-17]

Knowledge of the specific drugs in question, including the metabolism, mechanisms, side effects, and pharmacologic properties, is critical to analyzing the result. For example, gamma-hydroxybutyrate (GHB) and succinylmonocholine (a metabolite of succinylcholine) can be created in vivo, and thus their presence alone may not constitute intoxication. In contrast, strychnine is significant at any concentration. Chronic use of many medications, especially the opioids, can result in drug tolerance. The chronicity of use must be considered when interpreting the significance of a given concentration, particularly in those patients receiving high-dose opiates for end-of-life palliative care.

The majority of drugs are affected by a drug-metabolizing enzyme, most of which are a part of the CYP450 system. Although most drugs are the substrates of this system, some drugs may activate (upregulate) or inhibit the same enzyme system. Thus, the concurrent use of multiple medications metabolized by the CYP450 system may lead to accumulation (or depletion) of one or more drugs. Knowledge of metabolic pathways can also assist the pathologist in assessing the effects of postmortem redistribution. The concentration of the parent drug can be compared with that of its metabolite to determine acute versus chronic administration, even if both are found at elevated concentrations. For example, in deaths where TCAs are detected, the parent compound:desmethyl metabolite ratio is important in determining whether death was due to an overdose or to some other cause, such as heart disease. In a patient who is taking therapeutic doses of a TCA, the ratio would be less than 2 and usually less than 1, whereas in the overdose scenario, the ratio would be expected to be greater than 2.[18] This is particularly important in light of the fact that TCAs undergo significant postmortem redistribution and may exhibit high concentrations even when an overdose did not occur.[19,20]

In patients taking multiple prescribed and over-the-counter medications, additional consideration must be given to the possible overlapping, even synergistic, side effects of the drugs. Polypharmacy is extremely common and can lead to drug reactions and interactions that must be understood when interpreting toxicology results. The presence of multiple drugs, even at low or "therapeutic" concentrations, can cause serious morbidity and even death. Drugs with similar side effects, such as respiratory or cardiac depression, can be fatal when combined, even when not taken in elevated doses. Benzodiazepines are commonly considered to be "safe" medications (ie, they have a high therapeutic index) because they are relatively nontoxic, even at high doses and concentrations; however, when benzodiazepines are combined with ethanol, the effect is often lethal because of their additive, or synergistic, effects. In addition to respiratory or cardiac depression, medications can combine in other ways to produce toxicity. If two drugs that prolong the QT interval are taken together, the effect may be cumulative and lead to a fatal cardiac arrhythmia (eg, cocaine and antihistamines). Many medications have central nervous system effects, either directly or through neurotransmitters, and in combination they can lead to toxicity. For example, toxicity is increased when cocaine and heroin are combined (known as a speedball) or with the combined use of stimulants and antipsychotic medications.

In addition, pathologists must correlate the toxicology findings with the circumstances of death. The mere presence of a drug in either blood or urine does not mean that it contributed to death. For example, drugs likely did not play a role in a patient who presents to the hospital complaining of chest pain who recently used heroin and is subsequently diagnosed with a myocardial infarct and dies, but drugs may play a role if the history involves cocaine use rather than heroin.

Medicolegal Issues

The general pathologist must understand when the medical examiner/coroner (ME/C) needs to become involved in the investigation of a death. In some jurisdictions, the hospital pathologist and ME/C may have a long-standing relationship in which the ME/C defers nonviolent cases, such as intoxications, to the hospital pathologist. In these cases, the agreed-upon protocol should be followed. However, the pathologist should always consider the potential legal implications of any testing performed and its outcomes. It is best for the pathologist to consult the ME before requesting any sort of toxicological testing so as to discuss these issues and their potential implications.

If there is not an existing agreement between the ME/C and the hospital pathologist, the ME/C should be contacted regarding all suspected drug overdose deaths. The ME/C will probably take jurisdiction of the case and perform the examination of the body. The ME/C will probably also request that any hospital admission blood or urine samples be sent along with the body. As previously stated, if requested, the hospital pathologist should collect all available blood still retained within the clinical laboratory (the blood bank often keeps specimens the longest). The specimens should be clearly labeled with the name of the decedent and his or her medical record number, as well as the date and time the specimens were obtained. The blood specimens should be released to the ME/C along with the body and all available medical records. Clinical laboratories should keep a record of what specimens were released as well as to whom they were released. Please see Figures 2-2 and 2-3 in chapter 2, *Supporting the Emergency Department,* for examples of a policy and form for release of laboratory specimens.

Each laboratory should check for compliance with both the Health Insurance Portability and Accountability Act (HIPAA) and the hospital legal or risk department as to how this information should be documented. It is important to note, however, that MEs/Cs have a specific exclusion within the HIPAA law that any and all information requested in a death investigation must be released to these offices as requested.[21]

In cases where the ME/C has released jurisdiction, if, either before or after examining the body, the pathologist thinks that a drug intoxication probably caused or contributed to death, the ME/C should be contacted immediately. The ME/C may or may not take jurisdiction of the case at that point. If the ME/C office does take jurisdiction and the pathologist has already completed the examination, the report should be completed and sent to the ME/C for review, along with any other requested materials. The ME/C may request additional testing or ask for postmortem fluid or tissue specimens, so it is recommended that nothing be destroyed until after the review.

A Supreme Court decision now renders it more likely that laboratorians, technicians, and technologists will be called to court to testify if they have been involved in the analysis or acquisition of specimens related to criminal (or civil litigation) cases (eg, homicides, driving under the influence [DUI] cases).[22] Therefore, it is recommended that laboratory personnel become familiar with testimony protocol. Furthermore, all laboratories engaged in forensic toxicology testing should practice strict chain-of-custody procedures, if possible.

A report issued by the Research Council of the National Academies has noted significant variability in the quality of toxicological analysis across the country.[23] Strong quality assurance programs and implementation of proficiency testing is recommended, if not already in practice, because this is likely to be mandated in the future.

In light of the issues discussed above, it is imperative that pathologists have a good working relationship with their local ME/C office. Pathologists often identify cases, either before or after their examination, that should have been reported to the ME/C. They should feel comfortable contacting the ME/C to discuss these cases. The clinical pathologist can also use the local forensic pathologist as a resource when deliberating on difficult cases, whether toxicology related or not, as well as to obtain insight and assistance should courtroom testimony become necessary. In addition, many ME/C offices employ a forensic toxicologist who may aid in the interpretation of postmortem toxicology results.

Summary

A main clinical principle taught in medical schools is to treat the patient, not the laboratory results. This same principle applies to the autopsy and toxicology. Toxicology results must be interpreted in the context of the entire case, including the circumstances of death, the autopsy findings, medical history, and so forth. Toxicology is one element of the puzzle, and although it may play a key role, it is not the entire picture. The hospital pathologist should have a basic understanding of toxicology principles and how they apply to postmortem examinations. Laboratories and pathologists involved in sporadic forensic casework might find it useful to have a forensic laboratory, forensic pathologist, and/or toxicologist available for consultation.

References

1. Provisional Counts of Drug Overdose Deaths, as of 8/6/17. Centers for Disease Control and Prevention, National Center for Health Statistics. https://www.cdc.gov/nchs/data/health_policy/monthly-drug-overdose-death-estimates.pdf. Accessed June 7, 2019.
2. Standard B3, Selecting Deaths Requiring Forensic Autopsy, Forensic Autopsy Performance Standards, National Association of Medical Examiners. Approved Sept 2016.
3. Davis GG and the National Association of Medical Examiners and American College of Medical Toxicology Expert Panel on Evaluating and Reporting Opioid Deaths. Complete republication: National Association of Medical Examiners position paper: recommendations for the investigation, diagnosis, and certification of deaths related to opioid drugs. *J Med Toxicol.* 2014;10:100-106.
4. Cvjetko P, Cvjetko I, Pavlica M. Thallium toxicity in humans. *Arh Hig Rada Toksikol.* 2010; 61:111-119.
5. Delaveris GJM, Hoff-Olsen P, Rogde S. Nonnatural deaths among users of illicit drugs. *Am J Forensic Med Pathol.* 2015;36(1):44-48.
6. Sporer K, Firestone J. Clinical course of crack cocaine body stuffers. *Ann Emerg Med.* 1997;29:596-601.
7. Norfolk G. The fatal case of a cocaine body-stuffer and a literature review: towards evidence based management. *J Forensic Leg Med.* 2007;14(1):49-52.
8. Tartarone A, Lerose R. Stevens-Johnson syndrome and toxic epidermal necrolysis: what do we know? *Ther Drug Monit.* 2010;32(6):669-672.
9. Stern R, Divito S. Stevens-Johnson syndrome and toxic epidermal necrolysis: associations, outcomes, and pathobiology: thirty years of progress but still much to be done. *J Invest Dermatol.* 2017;137(5):1004-1008.
10. Pounder D. The nightmare of postmortem drug changes. *Leg Med.* 1993:163-191.
11. Randall BB, Fierro MF, Froede RC. Practice guideline for forensic pathology. Members of the Forensic Pathology Committee, College of American Pathologists. *Arch Pathol Lab Med.* 1998;122:1056-1064.
12. Levine B, Caplan YH. Alcohol. In: Levine B, ed. *Principles of Forensic Toxicology.* 3rd ed. Washington, DC: AACC Press; 2010:175-190.
13. Eichelbaum M, Ingelman-Sundberg M, Evans W. Pharmacogenomics and individual drug therapy. *Annu Rev Med.* 2006;57:119-137.
14. Schulz M, Schmoldt A. Therapeutic and toxic blood concentrations of more than 800 drugs and other xenobiotics. *Pharmazie.* 2003;58:447-474.
15. Molina D. *Handbook of Forensic Toxicology for Medical Examiners.* New York, NY: CRC Press; 2009.
16. Musshoff F, Padosch S, Steinborn S, Madea B. Fatal blood and tissue concentrations of more than 200 drugs. *Forensic Sci Int.* 2004;142(2-3):161-210.
17. Baselt RC. *Disposition of Toxic Drugs and Chemicals in Man.* 8th ed. Foster City, CA: Biomedical Publications; 2008.
18. Apple F. Postmortem tricyclic antidepressant concentrations: assessing cause of death using parent to metabolite ratio. *J Anal Toxicol.* 1989;13:197-198.
19. Apple F, Bandt C. Liver and blood postmortem tricyclic antidepressant concentrations. *Am J Clin Pathol.* 1988;89:794-796.
20. Rohrig T, Prouty R. A nortriptyline death with unusually high tissue concentrations. *J Anal Toxicol.* 1989;13:303-304.
21. Health Insurance Portability and Accountability Act of 1996. Uses and disclosures for which consent and authorization or opportunity to agree or object is not required, Part g) Standard: uses and disclosures about decedents.
22. Melendez-Diaz v Massachusetts, 557 US 07-591 (2008).
23. Committee on Identifying the Needs of the Forensic Sciences Community, National Research Council. *Strengthening Forensic Science in the United States: A Path Forward.* Washington, DC: The National Academies Press; 2009.

Section II

Toxicokinetics and Methodologies for the Toxicology Laboratory

Alan H.B. Wu, PhD, Editor

Chapter 9. Pharmacokinetic Concepts for Toxicology and Therapeutic Drug Monitoring
Yashpal Agrawal, MD, PhD

Chapter 10. Pharmacogenomic Testing
Alan H.B. Wu, PhD, and Gwendolyn A. McMillin, PhD

Chapter 11. Laboratory-Based Screening Assays in Support of Pain Management
Tai C. Kwong, PhD, and Alan H.B. Wu, PhD

Chapter 12. Approaches to Broad-Spectrum Drug Testing in the Clinical Laboratory
Kara L. Lynch, PhD

Chapter 13. Method Validation in Toxicology Testing
Wieslaw Furmaga, MD, MS, and Yashpal Agrawal, MD, PhD

Chapter 14. Alternate Specimens for Drugs-of-Abuse Testing: Oral Fluid
Jennifer A. Collins, PhD

Chapter 15. Drug Testing in Hair, Sweat, Meconium, Cord Tissue, and Breast Milk
Uttam Garg, PhD, and Gwendolyn A. McMillin, PhD

Chapter 9

Pharmacokinetic Concepts for Toxicology and Therapeutic Drug Monitoring

Yashpal Agrawal, MD, PhD

Introduction

Drug levels are measured to determine if the measured drug concentration is within the therapeutic range or when toxicity is suspected. Therapeutic drug monitoring (TDM) and the reporting of drug levels is a common practice in laboratories. However, interpretation of drug levels requires an understanding of some of the key pharmacokinetic parameters, as well as an understanding of the concept of drug steady-state levels. It is important to point out that not all drugs require TDM. Drugs that do not produce toxicity at therapeutic dosages do not generally require monitoring. The purpose of TDM is to optimize drug therapy for individual patients such that the efficacy of the drug is maximized and toxicity is minimized.

The *therapeutic range* for a drug reflects a range of drug concentrations for which the probability of a clinical response is high and the probability of unacceptable drug toxicity is low. When toxicity results, pharmacological principles can help in understanding the absorption and elimination kinetics of the drug in question. This information can be used to estimate when the serum concentration of the drug can be expected to drop back into the therapeutic range or to help decide between the choice of specific antidote therapy versus the use of physical methods (eg, charcoal adsorption) to reduce further drug absorption by the body. Indications for TDM are listed in Table 9-1. A list of the common drugs monitored by TDM is provided in Table 9-2. In this chapter, we will review the pharmacokinetic principles as they relate to TDM and toxicology.

Table 9-1. Indications for Therapeutic Drug Monitoring
Drugs with narrow therapeutic index
Drugs with predictable relationship between toxicity and drug concentration
Drugs showing variability in ADME due to age, sex, race, renal or hepatic disease, etc
Drugs with pharmacodynamic variability, eg, warfarin

ADME, absorption, distribution, metabolism, and excretion.

Pharmacokinetics and Pharmacodynamics

The traditional way to think about the concepts of pharmacokinetics and pharmacodynamics is that pharmacodynamics represents "the effects of the drug on the body," and pharmacokinetics is "the effects of the body on the drug." Thus, the pharmacodynamic response comprises the pharmacological effects of the drug binding to its receptors, whereas the Absorption, Distribution, Metabolism, and Excretion (ADME) of the drug are pharmacokinetic concepts.[1]

Drug Absorption

Absorption refers to the process of the transfer of drug from the site of administration to the systemic circulation. Drugs can be administered in multiple ways (eg, oral, intravenous, subcutaneous, intramuscular). The choice of the route of administration depends on the desired goal. For example, vancomycin, which is absorbed poorly, may be administered orally if the desired effect is local, as in *C difficile* gastroenteritis; or vancomycin may be administered intravenously when high serum levels are needed rapidly, as in severe infections. A drug with a high rate of absorption would be expected to have a rapid onset of action.

Bioavailability

Bioavailability is the percentage of drug that reaches the systemic circulation. For drugs that are absorbed orally, the fraction of the administered oral dose that is delivered to the systemic circulation is known as the bioavailability of the drug. Bioavailability is not usually calculated for drugs that are absorbed poorly, but it can be very useful in estimating the expected drug absorption for TDM and toxicological purposes. In the management of drug toxicity, bioavailability of the drug can be reduced by delaying gastric emptying using pharmacological agents or by using activated charcoal to reduce the extent of drug absorption. Bioavailability does not take into account the rate of absorption, only the extent of absorption.

The amount of drug reaching the systemic circulation = Bioavailability (F) × Dose (D).

Table 9-2. Common Therapeutically Monitored Drugs for Which Proficiency Testing Is Available From the College of American Pathologists*

Acetaminophen	Imipramine	**Primidone**
Amikacin	**Itraconazole**	**Procainamide**
Amitryptyline	Lacosamide	**Quinidine**
Caffeine	Lamotrigine	Rufinamide
Carbamazepine	Levetiracetam	Salicylate
Carbamazepine, free	Lidocaine	Sirolimus (rapamycin)
Clozapine	**Lithium**	Tacrolimus
Cyclosporine	Methotrexate	Teriflunomide
Desipramine	Mycophenolic acid	**Theophylline**
Digoxin	***N*-Acetylprocainamide (NAPA)**	**Tobramycin**
Digoxin, free	Nortriptyline	Topiramate
Disopyramide	Oxcarbazepine metabolite	Tricyclics, total
Ethosuximide	**Phenobarbital**	**Valproic acid**
Everolimus	**Phenytoin**	Valproic acid, free
Fluconazole	Phenytoin, free	Vancomycin
Gabapentin	**Posaconazole**	**Voriconazole**
Gentamicin	Pregabalin	Zonisamide

* Drugs in bold are regulated drugs for proficiency testing purposes and are reportable to the Centers for Medicare and Medicaid Services.

Example 1

Calculate the expected bioavailability in a patient known to have ingested 10 mg of digoxin. Because bioavailability is approximately 80%, $F \times D$ can be calculated as 0.80×10 mg = 8 mg. The clinical impact of bioavailability calculations should never be considered in isolation but together with other key pharmacokinetic parameters discussed in the text. In some cases, the above equation needs to be multiplied by a factor, S, which corrects for the fraction of drug that is active ($S \times F \times D$).

First-Pass Metabolism

Drugs can undergo a variety of processes before they reach the systemic circulation. They can pass through the gastrointestinal mucosa, where they have the potential to be metabolized or even be pumped back into the lumen by certain cytochrome P450 enzymes. After being absorbed from the intestinal mucosa, the drug molecules enter the portal vein into the liver. In the liver, the drugs can undergo extensive hepatic metabolism even before entering the systemic circulation. This *first-pass metabolism* can be significant for certain drugs (eg, lidocaine), and as a result, drugs such as lidocaine are not given orally. After passage through the liver, drugs reach the lungs via the inferior vena cava, enter the right side of the heart, to the lungs, to the left side of heart, and into the arterial circulation, from which they are eliminated via a variety of processes.

Peak absorption occurs when the rate of absorption equals the rate of elimination. Peak absorption should not be confused with completion of absorption.

Drug Distribution

When the drug reaches the systemic circulation, it is ready to be transported to the peripheral tissues. This process is dependent both on the blood flow to the tissues as well as on the affinity of the drug for the tissues. Thus, drugs that are highly bound to plasma proteins, such as albumin, will show higher concentrations in plasma than in tissues. It is common for laboratories to use serum as the specimen type for drug measurements, although measurement of drug concentrations from plasma should yield similar results. The differences between serum and plasma drug levels can be exaggerated for drugs and other substances that distribute inside of red blood cells (eg, heavy metals) rather than in the serum or plasma.

Key Pharmacokinetic Parameters and Concepts

The following topics are important for the understanding of pharmacokinetics and toxicokinetics:

- Volume of distribution (V_d)
- Clearance (Cl)
- Elimination rate constant (K_e) and the half-life ($t_{1/2}$)
- Steady-state levels
- Area under the curve (AUC) calculations

Volume of Distribution

The volume of distribution (V_d) is a hypothetical volume in liters or milliliters that relates serum drug concentrations to the amount of drug in the body. It is important because it determines the *loading dose* that is required to achieve a particular *steady-state* concentration immediately after the drug is administered. Once the drug is absorbed, it equilibrates between the serum and the tissues and organs of the body.

For some drugs that are distributed primarily in blood, the V_d is quite small (5-7 L); for others with wide tissue distribution, the V_d can be large (500 L). Thus, V_d is the volume of the compartment necessary to account for the drug if it were present throughout the body at the same concentration as in plasma. When the V_d is high (eg, >1 L/kg), it implies that the drug is bound to tissues or is mostly outside the plasma compartment. Therefore, in cases of drug toxicity, procedures that are effective for rapid reduction of toxic levels of drug in plasma, such as hemodialysis or exchange transfusions, are not likely to be very effective when the V_d is high. A related factor affecting V_d is the amount of drug that is bound or free in the serum and in tissues. Drugs that are tightly bound to proteins like albumin cannot be removed by hemodialysis because the albumin-drug complex will not cross the dialysis membranes. The albumin-drug binding is important clinically because when the patient is given another albumin-binding drug, it may displace the first drug from albumin, with resultant high levels of free drug in the plasma.

Example 2

Acetaminophen is about 10% to 20% bound to plasma proteins. For acetaminophen, the V_d is about 1.0 L/kg, and highest tissue concentrations are found in the periportal liver tissue and renal medulla. In contrast, aspirin is about 60% bound to plasma proteins, and the V_d is about 0.15 L/kg to 0.2 L/kg. Thus, hemodialysis and exchange transfusions are a treatment option in aspirin toxicity but not in acetaminophen toxicity.

Drug Elimination

The kidneys and the liver are the major organs for excretion of drugs. Excretion via skin, sweat, and gastrointestinal tract also occurs to some extent. Water-soluble drugs and metabolites are excreted by the kidneys using a combination of glomerular filtration, tubular reabsorption, and secretion. Hepatic metabolism or biotransformation of drugs is performed by the cytochrome P450 system of enzymes. These biotransformations can be grouped into phase I reactions (eg, oxidations, reductions, or hydrolytic changes) and phase II reactions, dealing with biochemical conjugation (eg, glucuronidation, methylation, or acetylation). Phase I reactions lead to *functionalization* of the drug by addition or uncovering of functional groups that may undergo subsequent metabolism by phase II enzymes. Phase II reactions are biosynthetic in nature, such as glucuronidation of drugs. Both phase I and phase II reactions allow the drug to become more polar and thus be excreted more easily. Induction or inhibition of the liver enzymes can increase or decrease drug metabolism, but sometimes biotransformation results in *metabolic activation* of the drug, which can happen when the drug metabolite is more toxic than the parent drug (eg, amitriptyline is demethylated to nortriptyline). The pharmacogenomic aspects of the cytochrome P450 system are discussed in chapter 10, *Pharmacogenomic Testing.* Biliary excretion via the liver is another route to remove drugs from the systemic circulation into the gastrointestinal tract.

Clearance

Clearance is defined as the volume of serum or plasma completely cleared of the drug per unit of time, typically in milliliters per minute. Clearance by the liver or kidney depends on two interrelated parameters: the *blood flow (BF)* to the kidney or liver and the ability of the tissue or organ to metabolize or eliminate the drug. The latter is measured by the *extraction ratio (ER),* which is calculated by measuring the concentration of drug entering the organ and leaving the organ, expressed as a percentage. Thus, Clearance = BF × ER.

Example 3

In a patient with liver blood flow of 1.5 L/min and drug extraction ratio of 0.8, the liver clearance is 1.5 L/min × 0.8 = 1.2 L/min. In other words, a drug with an ER of 0.8 indicates that 80% of the drug flowing through the liver will be cleared in the first pass. If the drug is also cleared by the kidney, then the kidney clearance should be added to the hepatic clearance.

Drug ERs are not measured in clinical laboratories, but this information can be used in toxicology to classify drugs into those having low and high hepatic ERs. When the liver ER is low, it implies that most of the drug is bound to serum protein. Therefore, drug interactions that displace the bound drug will lead to an increase in free drug levels, and the free drug hepatic clearance will increase or even decrease if hepatic cytochrome P450 enzymes are inhibited. Metabolism of drugs with low liver ERs (eg, diazepam, phenytoin, warfarin) is not very sensitive to a decrease in liver blood flow, as may occur in congestive heart disease or liver disease. In contrast, drugs with high liver ERs (eg, morphine, lidocaine) are quite sensitive to liver blood flow because drug metabolism depends on the amount of drug delivered to the liver. Clearance is affected by various factors: body weight, body surface area, blood flow, the function of organs (eg, liver and kidney), plasma protein binding, and genetic polymorphisms of the cytochrome P450 system.

For pharmacokinetic dosing calculations, in individuals older than 18 years, the creatinine clearance is usually calculated using the Cockcroft-Gault equation[2] (Equation 1).

Equation 1

Creatinine clearance in mL/min = [(140 – age in years) × (body weight in kg) × (0.85 if female)] / (72 × serum creatinine in mg/dL)

The creatinine clearance reflects the glomerular filtration rate (GFR). Because the Cockcroft-Gault equation was derived from only 249 patients, attempts have been made to determine more robust equations for determination of the GFR and, by proxy, creatinine clearance. The Cockcroft-Gault equation, however, continues to be used in hospital settings because many of the drug package inserts present drug data that are based on the Cockcroft-Gault equation. An alternative method to estimate the GFR utilizes the equation for modification of diet in renal disease (MDRD).[3] However, this equation has not been extensively validated for pharmacokinetic dosing nor has it been studied in all ethnic groups, in children, or in very old individuals. In the MDRD equation, values greater than 60 mL/min/kg are not reported as an exact value but are reported simply as, for example, ≥60 mL/min/1.73 m^2. A newer equation, the Chronic Kidney Disease Epidemiology Collaboration (CKD-EPI) equation, allows the reporting of estimated GFR (eGFR) as an exact value greater than 60 mL/min/1.73 m^2. Note the difference in units between the Cockcroft-Gault equation (mL/min) and the MDRD/CKD-EPI equations (mL/min/1.73 m^2). To convert mL/min/1.73 m^2 from the MDRD equation to mL/min from the Cockcroft-Gault equation, the results from the MDRD equation must be multiplied by $(\text{weight in kg}/70\text{ kg})^{0.7}$.

The National Kidney Disease Education Program performed a study[4] to compare the Cockcroft-Gault and MDRD equations, and it was found that, for the majority of patients and for most drugs tested that did not have narrow thresholds for toxicity, there was little difference in the drug dose that would be administered using either equation to estimate kidney function. However, for drugs with a narrow therapeutic index, the Cockcroft-Gault equation was less reliable in assessing the risk of kidney damage.

In the presence of a reduced creatinine clearance, drug dosage will usually need to be decreased or the drug dosage interval will need to be increased. Where systemic drug clearance is highly dependent on renal clearance, such as for vancomycin, one can estimate the patient's renal clearance of the drug distinct from nonrenal clearance (eg, hepatic). This can be done by reviewing the package insert (eg, renal vancomycin clearance is approximately 75% of creatinine clearance) or by use of nomograms.[5] If the drug is metabolized extensively in the liver, dose adjustments may also be needed in the presence of cirrhosis or other liver diseases. Although creatinine clearance can be used to monitor renal function, liver function is measured by monitoring the Child-Pugh score, which is then used to modify the dose or dosing interval.

Elimination Rate Constant. The elimination rate constant (K_e) is the fraction of the total amount of drug in the body removed per unit of time by first-order kinetics. It can be calculated from the clearance (Cl) and the volume of distribution (V_d).

Equation 2

$K_e = Cl/V_d$

Example 4

If clearance (Cl) is 79.9 mL/min and the average V_d for vancomycin is 0.7 L/kg or 49 L (49,000 mL) for a 70-kg person, the K_e can be calculated as follows:

$K_e = 79.9$ mL/min / 49,000 mL

$K_e = 0.0016306$/min, or 0.16 % of the V_d is cleared per minute.

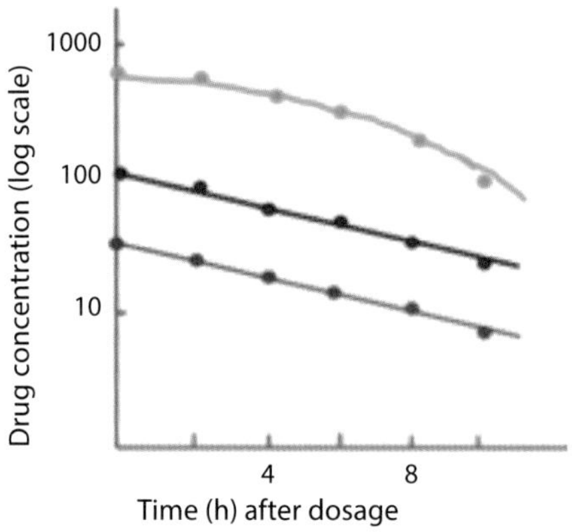

Figure 9-1. First-order kinetics (linear pharmacokinetics) of drug elimination. Note the log scale on the Y-axis and compare with Figure 9-2, which shows first-order kinetics using a linear Y-axis. The blue dots (sample times) and line show the linear elimination profile of a drug, and the red dots (sample times) and line show the drug elimination profile of that drug at twice the dose. As discussed in the text, the amount of drug eliminated is proportional to the concentration of the drug, but the kinetic parameters—such as clearance (Cl), volume of distribution (V_d), and half-life ($t_{½}$)—do not change; in other words, in linear kinetics, the pharmacokinetic parameters are dose independent. For comparison, the green dots (sample times) and line shows a typical elimination profile for saturable kinetics (zero-order kinetics, dose-dependent nonlinear kinetics); compare with Figure 9-2.

In first-order kinetics (nonsaturable enzyme kinetics, dose-independent linear pharmacokinetics), the amount of drug eliminated diminishes logarithmically over time and is proportional to the drug concentration; as a result, the *fraction* of drug eliminated remains constant and independent of the dose (Figure 9-1). In other words, the pharmacokinetic parameters such as Cl and V_d that are used to calculate the K_e, as well as the $t_{½}$, do not vary with drug dose because most drugs follow first-order kinetics.

For some drugs whose metabolism is saturable (eg, alcohol, phenytoin), a constant *amount* of drug is metabolized, which is characterized by zero-order kinetics (dose-dependent nonlinear pharmacokinetics; Figure 9-2). Thus, if at saturation the body metabolizes 10 mL of alcohol per hour and 40 mL was ingested, the $t_{½}$ will be 2 hours. If 80 mL of ethanol was ingested, the $t_{½}$ will be 4 hours; in other words, the half-life varies depending on the amount of ethanol ingested. The difference between first-order and zero-order kinetics thus has important implications in treatment decisions, as well as in time to achieve steady-state levels (see below). Nonlinear pharmacokinetics is discussed later in this chapter.

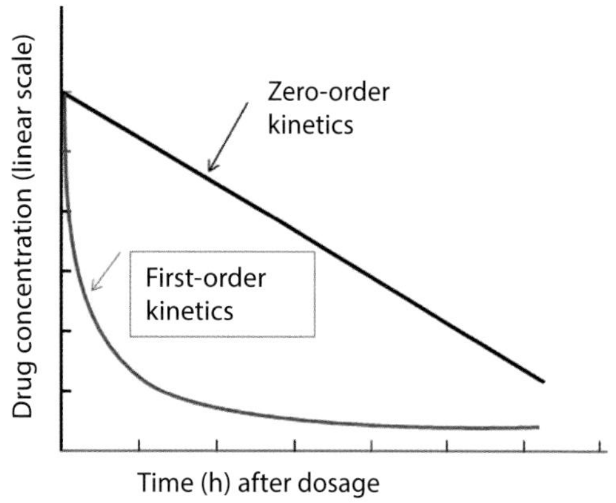

Figure 9-2. Plasma concentration–time curve. Drug elimination by zero-order kinetics (black line) and first-order kinetics (blue line) is shown after a loading dose. Note the linear scale on the Y-axis. If a logarithmic Y-axis scale were to be used to plot first-order kinetics, the plot would resemble a straight line similar to that for zero-order kinetics. A logarithmic Y-scale makes it easier to calculate the half-life estimates of drugs that follow first-order kinetics.

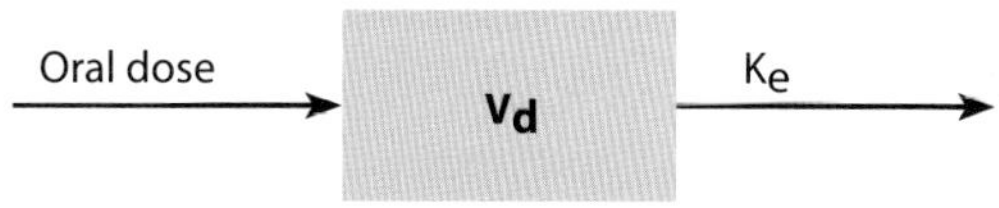

Figure 9-3. One-compartment model of pharmacokinetics for a drug given orally. When the drug is given intravenously, there is no absorption phase and the drug distributes in V_d instantaneously. K_e = elimination rate constant; V_d = volume of distribution. From Bauer LA.[13] Modified with permission of McGraw Hill.

Ethanol concentrations can be expressed in various ways: 0.01% w/v = 10 mg/dL = 10 mg%.

Compartmental Models of Pharmacokinetics

After the administration of a drug, its subsequent disposition inside the body can been described using one-, two-, or three-compartment models.

One-Compartment Model

In a one-compartment model, the body is considered as a single compartment (V_d), and the given drug (IV or orally) is assumed to distribute almost instantaneously between the blood and the tissues. Its elimination by metabolism can be characterized by its elimination rate constant, K_e. If the drug distribution in tissues is not rapid, one may still use the one-compartment model, providing that the duration of the distribution phase in tissues and the infusion times are small compared with the half-life of the drug and if little drug is eliminated during the distribution phase (Figure 9-3).

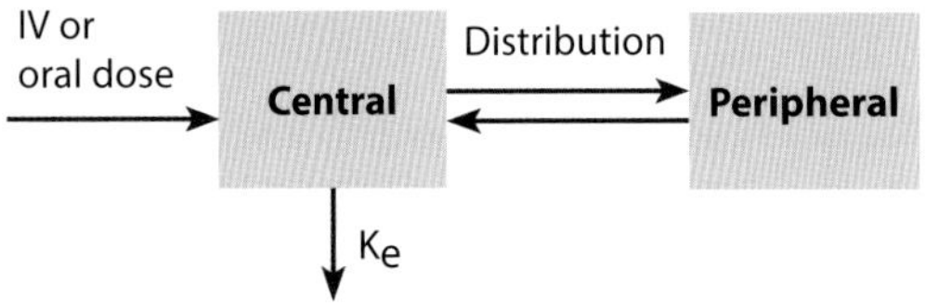

Figure 9-4. Two-compartment model of pharmacokinetics for an orally or intravenously administered drug that distributes in the tissue. K_e = elimination rate constant. From Bauer LA.[13] Modified with permission of McGraw Hill.

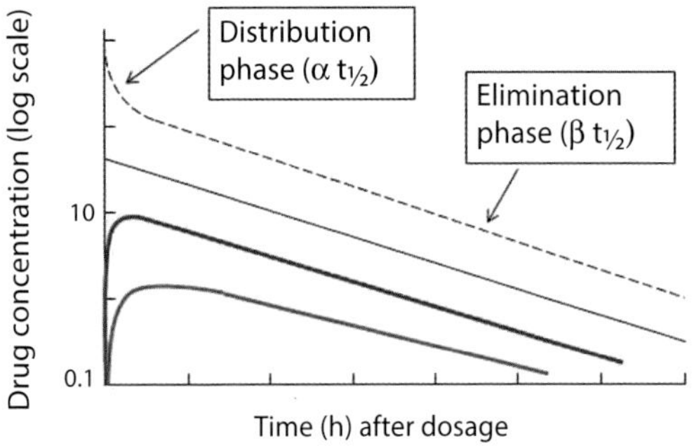

Figure 9-5. Plasma concentration–time curve for drugs that follow one- or two-compartment pharmacokinetics. The solid black line shows the serum concentration graph for a drug that follows one-compartment model pharmacokinetics after an intravenous bolus. Drug distribution occurs instantaneously, and serum concentration declines in a straight line (semi-log scale). Oral absorption of a rapidly absorbed drug (red line) and a slowly absorbed drug (blue line) is shown schematically. The dashed line represents the plasma concentration–time plot for a drug that follows a two-compartment pharmacokinetic model after an intravenous bolus. During the initial distribution phase, drug is distributing between blood and tissues, and, depending on the specific drug, elimination via kidneys and liver may or may not occur. During the elimination phase, drug is being eliminated from the body. The biphasic decay of drug levels during the distribution phase is called the *alpha half-life* ($\alpha\ t_{1/2}$) and during the elimination phase is known as the *beta half-life* ($\beta\ t_{1/2}$).

Two-Compartment Model

In the two-compartment model, the body is considered to be a central compartment where the drug is administered and equilibrates quickly (Figure 9-4). This central compartment, in practice, is composed of the vascular compartment and organs with high blood flow. This is similar to the one-compartment model described previously. From the central compartment, the drug then distributes to another peripheral compartment, which represents tissues that equilibrate slowly with blood. The elimination can be represented by a constant, K_e. Thus, a loading dose calculated on the basis of total V_d could cause serious toxicity if the drug resides and acts when in the central compartment and distributes slowly into the peripheral tissue compartment. A good example of this is the IV injection of potassium, which can cause serious toxicity, including death, by its actions in the central compartment before distributing to the peripheral compartment. In contrast, even high levels of plasma digoxin (central compartment) do not cause toxicity as long as digoxin levels at its site of action in the peripheral compartment (heart tissue) are low. Thus, a second important feature of multiple-compartment pharmacokinetics relates to the time at which drug plasma concentrations should be measured. In the example above, digoxin concentrations should be measured at a time when the drug has distributed in tissues. Thus, plasma digoxin levels measured less than 6 hours after an oral dose are not likely to be meaningful because the drug has not had time to distribute to heart tissues.

Half-Life

The half-life ($t_{1/2}$) of a drug is the time required for the total amount of drug in the body or the serum concentration to be reduced by 50%. It describes how quickly serum concentrations of the drug decrease after administration of the drug. When reviewing half-life data, one should note whether the distribution half-life ($\alpha\ t_{1/2}$) or the elimination half-life ($\beta\ t_{1/2}$; Figure 9-5) is being referred to. The terminal half-life and elimination half-life are synonyms, but by using the term "elimination" half-life, it indicates the mechanism of decay of the drug levels. These differences in terminology are usually insignificant for drugs that follow one-compartment kinetics, but they can be meaningful for those that have a distribution phase (Figure 9-5). For drugs that follow multiple-compartment kinetics, during the initial distribution phase the decrease in drug concentration is due to distribution of drug to the tissues, after which the drug enters the elimination phase, and the time taken to eliminate half the *remaining fraction* is the terminal half-life.[6]

Because half-life is a function of the elimination rate constant (K_e), the $t_{1/2}$ can be estimated in one of two ways:

Equation 3

$$t_{1/2} = 0.693/K_e$$

Equation 4

$$t_{1/2} = 0.693\,(V_d/Cl)$$

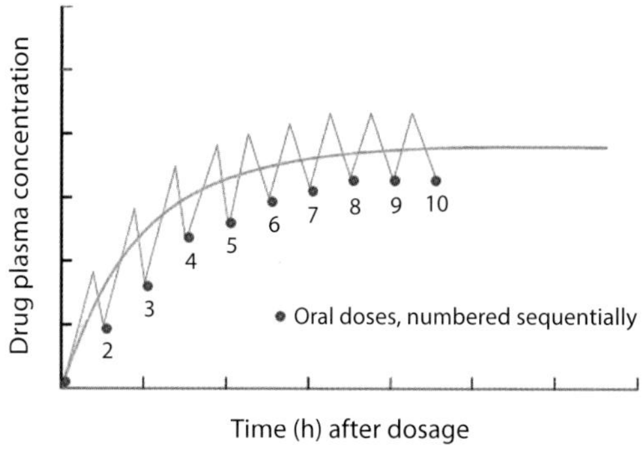

Figure 9-6. A hypothetical plot of drug plasma concentrations versus time after drug administration in a patient with normal hepatic and renal function. Oral doses were administered sequentially. Typically, it takes one half-life to reach 50%, two half-lives to reach 75%, three half-lives to reach 87.5%, four half-lives to reach 93.75%, and five half-lives to achieve 95% of steady-state concentrations. Drug elimination also follows the same kinetics, in other words, 50% of the drug is eliminated after one half-life, 75% after two half-lives, 87.5% after three half-lives, and approximately 93.75% after four half-lives are reached. In practice, steady state is assumed to have been achieved after four half-lives, or, alternatively, a drug is believed to be completely eliminated after four half-lives. When drugs are given by continuous intravenous administration, the blue line approximates the plasma concentrations.

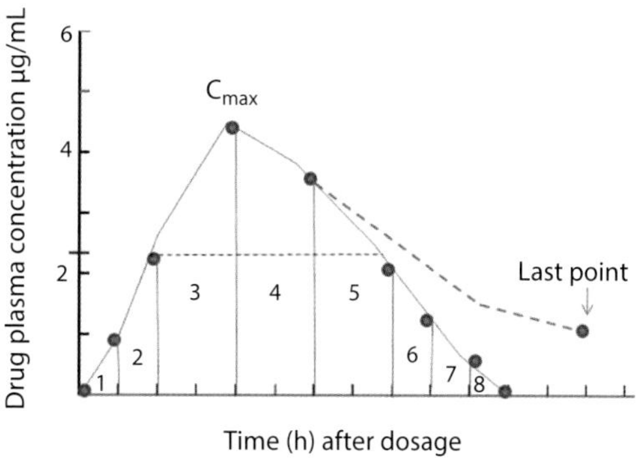

Figure 9-7. Area under the curve (AUC) calculation and related parameters. After a single oral dose, the C_{max} represents the peak concentration, which in this example is achieved at 4 hours (T_{max}). Every drug has a minimally effective concentration (in this example shown as a horizontal mark on the y-axis at 2.2 µg/mL). When that concentration is reached, it represents the onset of drug action (at 2 hours), which lasts until the plasma drug concentration falls below the minimally effective concentration up to approximately 8 hours (shown as the red dashed horizontal line between 2 and 8 hours). The AUC is calculated by constructing triangles or trapezoids, using vertical lines from the measured plasma levels, until the last measured level has been utilized. The calculation of the AUC beyond the last measured level requires more complex calculations when plasma levels do not return to zero but essentially tends to infinity (blue dash line). In the usual AUC curve, the first and the last segments are triangles, with trapezoids in between. The area of these triangles and trapezoids can be added up to provide the AUC (see Example 7). From Khan and Reddy.[8] Copyright 2000. Modified with permission of Taylor & Francis Group LLC.

Example 5

Using data from Example 4, the $t_{1/2}$ can be calculated by using Equation 3 as follows: 0.693/0.0016306 = 425 min; or by using Equation 4 as follows: 0.693 (49000 mL / 79.9 mL/min) = 425 min.

Concept of Steady State

At steady state (Figure 9-6), the rate of drug administration equals the rate of drug elimination, and, as a result, drug levels remain essentially constant. The best time to take serum samples for drug levels is after steady state has been achieved.

Time of Sampling

In the presence of drug toxicity, the sample may be collected at any time, but the general recommendation is to allow at least three to four half-lives to elapse before taking a sample. Samples should preferably be collected during the elimination phase (Figure 9-5). It is worth remembering that age, sex, body weight, diet, pharmacogenomics, and so forth can affect ADME parameters, and these may affect the interpretation of drug levels. Trough levels are preferred because they represent the lowest concentration of drug in the blood. Trough samples (as opposed to peak samples) are preferred because they are less sensitive to errors due to potential delays in absorption (C_{max}; Figure 9-7). Trough samples are best collected about 30 minutes before the next dose, and peak samples (usually after an IV infusion) are best collected usually about 30 minutes to 1 hour after the infusion. This allows some time for the drug to equilibrate (ie, distribution phase; Figure 9-5) before sample collection. Peak levels (before steady state) may be useful (eg, when giving antibiotics) to determine the maximum concentration achieved. Peak samples are useful when monitoring aminoglycosides because the ratio of the peak concentration to the minimal inhibitory concentration (MIC) is important for their bactericidal activity. A peak level represents the highest level of drug in the body; however, peak levels can be very misleading, especially if the drug undergoes tissue distribution and acts on tissues (eg, digoxin, lithium). The drug package insert should be consulted to determine the best time to take the peak and trough samples in relation to the dosing schedule. A third type of sample is the "random" level, which is collected at any time, for example if ongoing drug toxicity is suspected.

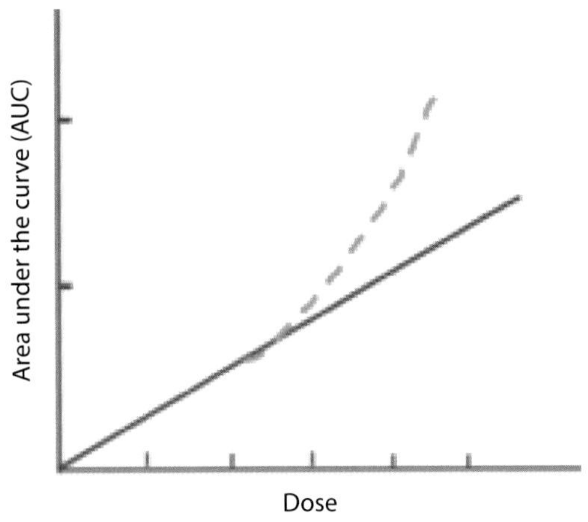

Figure 9-8. Drug dose plotted against drug area under the curve (AUC) or plasma concentrations. As the drug dose is increased, the plasma concentrations increase proportionally (blue line). However, certain drugs that undergo saturable kinetics (zero-order kinetics, nonlinear kinetics) can show a disproportionate increase in plasma concentrations as the drug dose is increased (green dashed line).

Area Under the Curve

The area under the curve[7] (AUC; Figure 9-7) is mostly a research tool but offers another way of looking at the curve of drug plasma level versus time (compare with Figure 9-5, log Y-axis). AUC calculations are performed to evaluate the extent of drug absorption after a single dose. AUCs can be used to compare absorption between two drugs, with the larger AUC signifying a better absorption. A variety of other pharmacokinetic parameters can be derived (Figure 9-7), including the peak concentration (C_{max}), the time of peak concentration (T_{max}), the onset of drug action, and the duration of drug action.

Example 7

The area of a triangle is calculated as (w × h)/2; the area of a trapezoid is calculated as 1/2 × w × sum of parallel sides, where *w* is the width and *h* is the height of the plasma drug concentration versus time curve.

Segment 1: (w × h)/2 = (1 hr × 1 μg/mL)/2 = 0.5 μg·hr/mL

Segment 2: ½ × w × sum of parallel sides = ½ × 1 hr × (1 + 2.2 μg/mL) = 1.6 μg·hr/mL

Segments 3, 4, 5, 6, 7, 8 …

Sum of segments 1 to 8 are added to obtain the AUC. In practice, AUC is frequently calculated using fewer data points and with software programs.

Nonlinear Pharmacokinetics

Up to this point, we have focused on linear (first-order) kinetics. The main cause of the nonlinear (zero-order) kinetics[8] is saturation of any of the ADME processes. Thus, as examples, saturation of the enzymes involved in first-pass metabolism, protein binding sites, metabolic reactions, tubular reabsorption, and secretion mechanisms can all contribute to nonlinear kinetics. The characteristic of nonlinear pharmacokinetics (Figure 9-8) is that at saturating or high drug doses, the plasma concentrations can change disproportionately (usually increase). Another term for saturation kinetics is *capacity-limited kinetics/metabolism*, which is defined by Michaelis-Menten kinetics. The two terms that are clinically relevant are the V_{max} and the K_m values (Figure 9-9). V_{max} represents the maximum velocity of the reaction rate, and K_m represents the drug concentration at half the V_{max}. An approximation of the V_{max} and K_m values can be made from a plot of the drug concentration versus the enzymatic reaction rate (Figure 9-9); however, for a more accurate estimation of the V_{max} and the K_m values, the Lineweaver-Burk plot[9] must be constructed. If enzyme induction occurs, that will raise the V_{max} without affecting the K_m, and, correspondingly, in the presence of competitive inhibitors, the K_m value of the drug increases without affecting the V_{max}. In the presence of noncompetitive inhibition, the V_{max} decreases, but the K_m remains unchanged.

Phenytoin is one of the drugs that undergoes capacity-limited pharmacokinetics, even at therapeutic concentrations. The liver enzymes that metabolize phenytoin become saturated (V_{max}), and, as a result, small changes in a maintenance dose can disproportionately increase plasma steady-state concentrations (Figure 9-8). This has significant implications for how drugs that undergo capacity-limited kinetics are eliminated (clearance) and the time taken to achieve steady-state. Under the usual first-order kinetics, the clearance of the drug and the $t_{1/2}$ are constants because the rate of drug administration correlates with the steady-state levels. This relationship changes under capacity-limited conditions. As the drug dose is increased (eg, above the K_m value), saturating concentrations (V_{max}) are reached (Figure 9-9), the clearance decreases, the plasma concentrations increase, and the $t_{1/2}$ increases and is no longer constant as it was under first-order kinetics. The increase in $t_{1/2}$ with a decrease in clearance is also predicted on the basis of Equation 4, which shows that $t_{1/2}$ and clearance are inversely related. This is important for the dosing of phenytoin because both the V_{max} (maximum rate of metabolism, expressed as the dose in mg/kg/day) and the K_m (plasma drug concentration at which the rate of metabolism is 50% of the

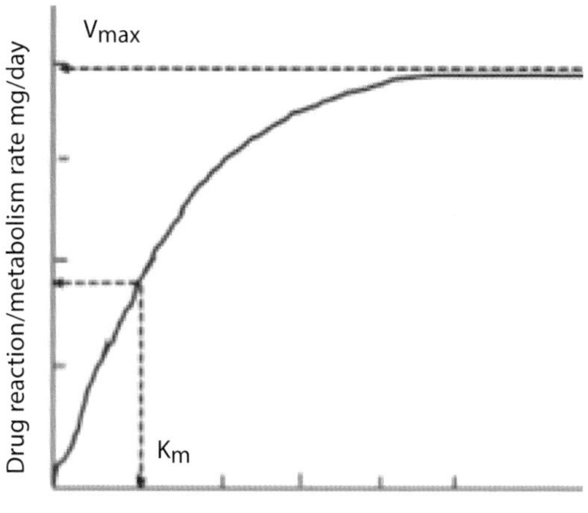

Figure 9-9. Effect of drug concentration on the enzymatic reaction rate. V_{max} represents the maximum velocity of the reaction rate, and K_m represents the drug concentration at half the V_{max}. It can be seen that at low drug concentrations (below the K_m value), the reaction rate is linear (ie, proportional to the drug concentration). As the drug concentration increases, the reaction rate starts to slow down, and at very high drug doses, the reaction rate/metabolic rate becomes saturated and there is no further increase in reaction velocity (V_{max}); in other words, the reaction rate becomes independent of the drug concentration (zero-order kinetics).

V_{max}, expressed as mg/L) vary in individual patient populations, perhaps depending on their CYP450 status.

Considerations in the Interpretation of Therapeutic Drug Monitoring Results

Assay Characteristics

It is useful to understand the assay characteristics, including (1) potential cross-reactivity (see chapter 11, *Laboratory-Based Screening Assays in Support of Pain Management*), (2) total drug level versus free drug levels, (3) whether the parent drug is being measured or also metabolites, and (4) whether the metabolites are pharmacologically active (eg, for parent drugs diazepam, lidocaine, amitriptyline, *N*-acetylprocainamide).

Free Drug Levels[10]

One must consider whether total drug (bound + free) or only free drug is being measured. When the free fraction of a drug that is highly bound to a plasma protein is constant, the free drug levels can be consistently estimated from the total drug levels, and the measurement of the free drug levels becomes unnecessary. It is when the drug exhibits variability in the free drug levels at therapeutic concentrations that the determination of the free drug levels becomes useful. Free drug levels are commonly used for drugs that are highly bound to proteins (usually >80%) or when the drug must traverse the blood-brain barrier for its site of action. It is worth noting that it is the free drug that interacts with its drug receptor and causes the physiological action. Free drug assays are technically more demanding than the total drug (bound + free) assays and may not always be available. A common technique to separate free from bound drug is by equilibrium dialysis or ultrafiltration using a membrane filter that will allow the free drug to pass, but not the protein bound drug. The College of American Pathologists provides proficiency testing for four free drug measurements (free digoxin, free phenytoin, free valproic acid, and free carbamazepine), discussed briefly below.

Free Digoxin Levels

Digoxin is only about 30% bound to proteins, and free digoxin levels are measured infrequently. Its site of action is the myocardial tissue. It is important to know the type of assay, free digoxin versus free-plus-bound digoxin, that is being used in the laboratory to monitor digoxin toxicity. If DigiFab (Digoxin Immune Fab ovine) therapy is planned to reverse the toxicity, it is crucial to obtain the digoxin level before initiation of therapy. When DigiFab is given, it binds to the free digoxin in plasma and renders the drug inactive. As digoxin is bound by DigiFab, the tissue-plasma equilibrium of digoxin is disturbed, and digoxin moves from the tissues back to the plasma, where it is captured by the DigiFab antibody. As a result, a total serum digoxin assay performed on a sample collected after the administration of DigiFab can give an erroneously high level because of the recognition of digoxin bound to the antibody in the assay. A free digoxin assay might have some value in this situation, but the levels of free digoxin are expected to be quite low.

Free Phenytoin Levels

Please also refer to the discussion on nonlinear pharmacokinetics. Phenytoin is a drug that is about 90% bound to plasma proteins and about 10% is free or unbound, with its site of action being the brain tissue. Phenytoin is bound mostly to albumin, and, as a result, binding is decreased in renal failure or conditions resulting in hypoalbuminemia. The phenytoin binding to plasma proteins is also susceptible to displacement by many other drugs, such as valproic acid. Free phenytoin measurements can be useful if protein binding is affected as the result of hypoalbuminemia, renal disease, liver disease (impact on CYP450 enzymes), or in the presence of multiple drug therapy, where displacement of phenytoin from plasma proteins might occur. In laboratories where free phenytoin levels are not available, the Sheiner-Tozer equation and its derivatives may be used to estimate the corrected total phenytoin levels, taking into account the possibility of reduced binding to albumin.[11]

Free Valproic Acid

Valproic acid is about 85% bound to plasma proteins, but the binding and clearance is concentration dependent[10] and is saturable with respect to albumin concentrations. Generally, the number of binding sites on a plasma protein such as albumin are finite, and the molar concentration of the binding protein (eg, albumin) far exceeds the molar concentration of the drug. As a result, the number of unbound binding sites on the plasma protein remain in excess and unchanged at therapeutic concentrations. Such a situation provides a predictable free drug fraction. Drugs such as valproic acid exhibit a concentration-dependent plasma protein binding within their therapeutic range because the molar concentration of valproic acid is higher than the molar concentration of the binding protein. As a result, the level of the free valproic acid can vary with the concentration and the level of the binding proteins. Thus, free valproic acid levels are generally higher and variable in the presence of hypoalbuminemia.

The binding of valproic acid is also affected by a variety of other factors, such as patient age, where younger patients may have lower albumin levels (ie, higher free valproic acid levels) and older patients have elevated free fatty acid levels (ie, higher free valproic acid levels). The unbound or free fraction of valproic acid is also known to be elevated in late pregnancy, renal disease, and hepatic disease because of the decrease in albumin levels in these conditions. The free valproic acid level is also susceptible to displacement interactions by other drugs and compounds, such as salicylates and nonsteroidal anti-inflammatory drugs (NSAIDs), and by uremia. Attempts have been made to calculate the free fraction of valproic acid using various equations derived from linear and nonlinear pharmacokinetics, but that has been difficult. Any clinical interpretation of a free valproic acid level needs to be interpreted in light of these clinical variables.

Free Carbamazepine Levels

The case for measurement of free carbamazepine levels is less clear, and, in most cases, knowledge of the total carbamazepine levels should suffice. Free carbamazepine levels could be considered in the presence of ongoing polytherapy with valproic acid when complex interactions can occur. In this situation, valproic acid can inhibit the metabolism of carbamazepine via CYP3A4 enzyme inhibition and also displace carbamazepine from albumin binding sites, thus increasing free carbamazepine levels. Carbamazepine is about 80% bound to plasma proteins such as albumin and α1-acid glycoprotein. The drug is metabolized by the cytochrome P450 system to the active metabolite carbamazepine 10,11-epoxide. Whereas the binding of carbamazepine to albumin is fairly consistent at about 80%, the active metabolite carbamazepine 10,11-epoxide is only bound to albumin at about 50%. During chronic carbamazepine therapy, the metabolite levels vary between 15% and 50% of total carbamazepine concentrations. During carbamazepine overdose, the albumin binding sites get saturated, and the metabolite concentrations may increase to even 80% of carbamazepine concentrations. Carbamazepine 10,11-epoxide is also known to increase in the presence of drug therapy with phenytoin and valproate sodium.

Interpretation of Drug Concentrations

The clinical history, including dosing information, must be utilized to determine whether the drug concentrations were collected at steady state. Assuming steady-state concentrations were collected and the drug concentrations are within the therapeutic range, the patient is expected to experience a therapeutic effect unless the drug-receptor interaction is hindered for any reason. If, on the other hand, the drug concentrations are higher than the expected therapeutic range, one must consider causes, such as increased bioavailability, the patient is taking more drug than prescribed, clearance (renal/hepatic) has decreased, or the patient's condition has led to an increase in plasma protein concentrations and drug binding. If the drug concentrations are less than the therapeutic range, the reverse applies, namely, reduced bioavailability, patient is taking less drug than prescribed, increased clearance, or decreased plasma protein binding.

It is best to avoid interpreting drug concentrations that were collected before achieving steady state, although similar considerations as above apply. In this instance, one must now also take into account the possibility of errors due to the incomplete distribution of drug between the plasma and tissue compartments.

References

1. Elbarbry F. *ABCs of Pharmacokinetics.* Fawzy Elbarbry (self published); 2017.
2. Beringer PM. *Winter's Basic Clinical Pharmacokinetics.* 6th ed. Philadelphia, PA: Wolters Kluwer Health; 2018.
3. Cockcroft DW, Gault MH. Prediction of creatinine clearance from serum creatinine. *Nephron.* 1976;16:31-41.
4. Glomerular Filtration Rate (GFR) Calculators. National Institute of Diabetes and Digestive and Kidney Diseases. https://www.niddk.nih.gov/health-information/communication-programs/nkdep/laboratory-evaluation/glomerular-filtration-rate-calculators. Accessed May 29, 2019.
5. Laboratory Evaluation. Frequently Asked Questions. National Institute of Diabetes and Digestive and Kidney Diseases. https://www.niddk.nih.gov/health-information/communication-programs/nkdep/laboratory-evaluation/frequently-asked-questions. Accessed May 29, 2019.
6. Vancomycin. Global RPh. http://www.globalrph.com/vancomycin_dilution_renal.htm. Updated September 6, 2017. Accessed May 13, 2019.
7. Toutain PL, Bousquet-Malou A. Plasma terminal half-life. *J Vet Pharmacol Ther.* 2004;27:427-439.
8. Khan MA, Reddy IK. *Pharmaceutical and Clinical Calculations.* 2nd ed. Boca Raton, FL: CRC Press; 2000.
9. Mehvar R. Principles of non-linear pharmacokinetics. *Am J Pharm Educ.* 2001;65:178-184.
10. Lineweaver H, Burk D. The determination of enzyme dissociation constants. *J Am Chem Soc.* 1934; 56(3):658-666.
11. Barre J, Didey F, Delion F, et al. Problems in therapeutic drug monitoring: free drug concentration monitoring. *Ther Drug Monit.* 1988;10:133-143.
12. Kiang TK, Ensom MH. A comprehensive review on the predictive performance of the Sheiner-Tozer and derivative equations for the correction of phenytoin concentrations. *Ann Pharmacother.* 2016;50:311-325.
13. Bauer LA. *Applied Clinical Pharmacokinetics.* 2nd ed. New York, NY: McGraw-Hill Medical; 2008.

Chapter 10

Pharmacogenomic Testing

Alan H.B. Wu, PhD
Gwendolyn A. McMillin, PhD

Introduction

Historically, clinical laboratory testing designed to guide pharmacotherapy decisions is based on characterization of a drug response phenotype, such as metabolic enzyme activity or concentrations of drugs or drug metabolites, and evaluating other biomarkers of drug response, such as cholesterol concentrations for patients treated with cholesterol-lowering drugs. Thus, the drug response phenotype may reflect pharmacokinetics, pharmacodynamics, or the combination of both. Pharmacogenomics (PGx) describes the correlation of genetic test results, for one or several genes, with a drug response phenotype. Unlike most testing designed to characterize a drug response phenotype, PGx testing can be performed before a drug is administered, and thus the results can be used to inform drug and dose selection decisions. PGx test results are often utilized to qualify or disqualify a person for a particular drug or drug dose, using predictive algorithms derived from a population with similar genetic, clinical, and demographic profiles. Professional consensus guidelines and drug labeling have been published for specific gene-drug pairs wherein well-characterized genotype-phenotype relationships are described. Together these tools contribute to achieving the vision of personalized medicine. Testing to support personalized medicine offers new opportunities for clinical laboratories to make significant contributions to health care.

The desire to improve the performance of therapeutic drugs stems from the knowledge that (1) the efficacy of the most widely used therapeutic drugs on the market today averages only around 50% (range of 25% for chemotherapeutics to 80% for analgesics)[1] and (2) the incidence of serious adverse drug reactions is estimated to be 2 million per year in the United States (resulting in about 100,000 deaths).[2] The Institute of Medicine was instructed by the US Congress to carry out a comprehensive study of drug safety and to find means to prevent or reduce medication errors, followed in 2015 by President Obama's "Precision Medicine Initiative."[3] The current opioid epidemic that has escalated rates of both drug addiction and accidental drug overdose has intensified demand to develop and implement PGx and other testing opportunities that can guide or mitigate risks of drug therapy decisions.

Many facilities have initiated preemptive PGx testing to improve future pharmacotherapy decisions.[4] Reduced costs of therapy and improved outcomes have been demonstrated for some applications. However, PGx cannot explain all of the drug response phenotypes, so the degree to which adverse drug events and medication errors can be reduced through PGx testing is unknown. Errors associated with incorrect writing or dispensing of prescriptions, patients not following physicians' dosing recommendations, or uninformed polypharmacy decisions will not be corrected by genetic testing. However, adverse events due to inherited sensitivity or resistance to a specific drug or drug dose may be identified by PGx testing and can be used to minimize the likelihood of an adverse drug reaction. For example, implementation of PGx testing for abacavir has reduced the incidence of hypersensitivity reaction and is now the standard of care for patients who are being considered for abacavir therapy.[5] The success of other PGx applications, such as for warfarin and tamoxifen, has been less fruitful (see discussion below for more details). The success of a PGx program requires a multidisciplinary effort. Stakeholders include medical professionals, payers, and regulators, as well as experts in clinical pharmacology, medical genetics, and diagnostics research. A major component of a successful PGx program is the education of physicians who use the medications for which PGx data are relevant.

There are significant ongoing research efforts conducted by academia and the pharmaceutics industry in discovering new gene associations that predict drug effects and adverse outcomes for existing and novel therapeutics. In some cases, the need for a companion laboratory test (ie, the need for a certain test result before a drug is given) will be a barrier to the adoption of that drug because the pharmaceutics industry may opt to develop safer and more efficacious alternatives that do not require companion testing. In other cases, PGx tests will help salvage drugs that might not normally receive clearance or perhaps even those that have been removed from the market if either (1) the toxicity profile can be significantly eliminated or reduced with clinical laboratory testing, such as a detection of a genetic biomarker of vulnerability to toxicity; or (2) if the probability of efficacy is well correlated with a genetic signature. As suggested earlier, there are many examples of successfully implemented clinical PGx applications, and there are also examples of applications that have not been adopted clinically. In the end, it is likely that a minority of current and future drugs will require PGx testing, just as today only a few drugs require routine therapeutic monitoring. Therefore, important studies and decisions lie ahead with regard to which drugs are most appropriate for testing, how testing is to be conducted and reimbursed, how tests results are reported and interpreted, and demonstrating the medical and economic benefits of testing.

Definitions and Terminology for Pharmacogenetics and Pharmacogenomics

The completion of the Human Genome Project in 2003 can be thought of as the birth of the field of pharmacogenetics and pharmacogenomics.[6] *Pharmacogenetics* can be is defined as the use of small numbers of polymorphisms in genes that are relevant to a drug's disposition or efficacy. *Pharmacogenomics* involves a larger collection of factors (eg, age, renal function, co-morbidities) that contribute to the variability of drug responses. This may include genes that regulate phase I oxidative drug metabolism (especially the cytochrome P450 family of enzymes [CYPs]), phase II drug conjugation (eg, glucuronosyltransferases and *N*-acetyltransferases), transport factors (eg, organic anion transporters), immune mediators, and proteins associated with drug response (eg, ion channels and ligand-gated receptors). Despite the different definitions, these terms have been used interchangeably, and here the abbreviation *PGx* is used to represent both pharmacogenetics and pharmacogenomics. Certainly, personalized medicine includes genetics, but there are also nongenetic factors (eg, overexpression or underexpression of proteins, co-medications, health, and lifestyle factors) as well as cultural and personal beliefs that determine the appropriateness of therapeutics. These factors are beyond the scope of this chapter; only germline PGx tests will be described.

Drivers of Clinical Pharmacogenomics

The US Food and Drug Administration's Center for Drug Evaluation and Research (CDER) has enacted new labeling requirements for selected drugs where polymorphisms have been linked to either a reduction in drug efficacy or an increased incidence of adverse events and has been a driver for implementation of clinical pharmacogenomics. The current drug listing for pharmacogenomics and companion testing is available on the CDER website.[7] There are now more than 500 drug labels that contain PGx information and more than 3000 clinical associations described between specific gene variants and drugs. This relabeling initiative now imposes a medico-legal implication in cases where an adverse event has occurred. For example, if a patient suffers an adverse event that is directly linked to the use of a drug, and the prescribing physician did not know that the individual was predisposed to that adverse event as the result of a genetic polymorphism, that physician may have difficulty defending a medical malpractice lawsuit, given that a warning for that event was present on the drug's label. These drug relabeling mandates will probably drive the need for PGx from medical efficacy to a "defense of medicine practice." Regardless of the driver, the implementation and proper utilization of PGx will incrementally improve medical care.

Although PGx is an attractive concept, the implementation into routine clinical practice has been slow. The barriers to implementation include regulations, technology access, costs and reimbursements, and demonstration of effectiveness. Many of the drugs listed by the CDER as recommending PGx testing have been in routine use for many years (eg, warfarin, codeine, and clopidogrel). As a result, most physicians have many years of experience using these drugs and believe that pharmacogenomics testing is unnecessary. The CDER has also indirectly affected the direction of the pharmacology industry. Because many of these drugs are off patent with generic formulations available, there is little incentive for the pharmacology industry to support pharmacogenomics trials or encourage laboratories to implement pharmacogenomics testing. Quite the contrary, it has stimulated this industry to create next-generation drugs where pharmacogenomics *does not* have influence on efficacy or toxicity. For example, a new drug might be metabolized by a series of CYP enzymes, and therefore the presence of a single pharmacogenomics variant will not reduce its rate of metabolism. Ads by the pharmaceutical industry to potential new users (doctors and their patients) state that there are cost savings by eliminating PGx testing. What is not stated in these ads is that the costs of these drugs are higher than the generic versions, even when considering the one-time cost of pharmacogenomics testing performed on the latter drugs. Where appropriate, this will be discussed in the subsequent sections.

Table 10-1. Example Consensus Nomenclature for Common Predicted Pharmacogenomic Phenotypes[8]

Gene Category	Predicted Phenotype	Genetic Definition(s)†	Example Diplotypes
Drug-metabolizing enzyme	Ultrarapid metabolizer	• More than two copies of normal function alleles • Two copies of increased function alleles	*CYP2D6*1/*2xN* *CYP2C19*17/*17*
	Rapid metabolizer	• Combination of normal function and increased function alleles	*CYP2C19*1/*17*
	Normal metabolizer	• Combination of normal function, decreased function, and/or loss-of-function alleles (gene specific) • Two copies of normal function alleles	*DPYD*1/*1* *CYP2D6*1/*4*
	Intermediate metabolizer	• Combination of normal function, decreased function, and/or loss-of-function alleles (gene specific)	*CYP2C9*1/*3* *DPYD*1/*2* *TPMT*1/*3A*
	Poor metabolizer	• Combination of loss-of-function alleles and decreased function alleles (gene specific) • Two copies of loss-of-function alleles	*CYP2C9*2/*3* *CYP2D6*4/*4* *UGT1A1*28/*28* *TPMT*2/*3A* *CYP3A5*3/*3*
Drug transporter	Increased function	• One or more increased function alleles	*SLCO1B1*1/*14*
	Normal function	• Two copies of normal function alleles	*SLCO1B1*1/*1*
	Decreased function	• Combination of normal and decreased or loss-of-function alleles	*SLCO1B1*1/*5*
	Poor function	• Combination of decreased function and loss-of-function alleles	*SLCO1B1*5/*5*
High-risk genotype	Positive	• One or two copies of the high-risk allele	*HLA-B:5701* *HLA-B:1502*
	Negative	• No copies of high-risk alleles	

† The definition depends on the specific gene.

Drug Examples

It would be impractical and beyond the scope of this chapter to describe all PGx associations. Examples of gene-drug pairs that are supported by published consensus guidelines are listed in Table 10-1. In addition, some representative examples of clinical PGx and the lessons learned thus far are described below.

Warfarin

Warfarin is an anticoagulant used widely to prevent and/or treat thrombotic disease for patients with atrial fibrillation, acute coronary syndromes, stroke, valve disease and replacement, deep venous thrombosis, and pulmonary emboli. It is supplied as a racemic mixture of *(R)*- and *(S)*-enantiomers, with the latter form having the most anticoagulant activity. The standard dose is 5 mg/day. The degree of anticoagulation due to warfarin is monitored by the prothrombin time and targeting an international normalized ratio (INR) value between 2.0 and 3.0. Patients who have INR values above this limit are at risk for bleeding complications, including subarachnoid hemorrhage, whereas those below this limit are subject to venous and arterial thrombosis.

Table 10-2. Pharmacogenomic Examples With the Highest Levels of Evidence From the PharmGKB, Including Published Guidelines from Either CPIC or DPWG, and FDA Label Comments

Gene or Allele	Generic Drug Name	Comment in FDA Labeling			
		Testing Required	Testing Advised	Actionable	Not Available
*HLA-B*57:01*	Abacavir		X		
CYP2D6 *CYP2C19*	Amitriptyline			X	
*HLA-B*15:02*	Carbamazepine	X†			
CYP2C19	Clopidogrel		X		
CYP2D6	Codeine			X	
UGT1A1	Irinotecan			X	
CFTR	Ivacaftor	X			
TPMT	Mercaptopurine		X		
G6PD	Rasburicase	X			
SLCO1B1	Simvastatin				X
CYP3A4	Tacrolimus				X
CYP2D6	Tamoxifen	X			
CYP2C9 *VKORC1*	Warfarin			X	

PharmGKB, Pharmacogenomics Knowledge Base; CPIC, Clinical Pharmacogenetics Implementation Consortium; DPWG, Dutch Pharmacogenetics Working Group; FDA, US Food and Drug Administration.
† In patients with ancestry in genetically at-risk populations, mainly Asians.

The optimum warfarin dose to achieve stable anticoagulation is dependent on a number of demographic, clinical, dietary, and PGx factors. For example, the rate of metabolism is reduced with increased age, resulting in lower dose requirements. In contrast, obese patients require higher warfarin dosing. Warfarin is converted to inactive metabolites by CYP2C9, which is coded from the gene of the same name. Variant alleles that affect expression and/or function of the protein are described as "star" alleles, designated with an asterisk.[8] Table 10-2 lists drugs where there is substantial evidence linking common PGx variants with a predicted drug response. Patients with one or two loss-of-function 2C9 alleles (common examples include **2* and **3*) have high drug levels, resulting in over-anticoagulation (INR >3.0) at the standard dose due to reduced rates of metabolic inactivation that lead to accumulation of the active parent drug.[9] The presence of co-medications that induce or inhibit CYP2C9 activity will also affect warfarin pharmacokinetics. Warfarin exerts its biological activity by blocking vitamin K epoxide reductase complex 1 (VKORC1), a key enzyme needed to recycle vitamin K from the oxidized to the reduced form. Reduced vitamin K is necessary for the activation of coagulation factors II, VII, VIII, and X. A common mutation in the promoter region *(c.-1639G>A)* of the associated gene *(VKORC1)* is associated with an extended elimination half-life for warfarin and a decreased warfarin dose requirement.[10] Variants in another gene that codes for an enzyme involved in recycling of vitamin K *(CYP4F2)* are associated with increased warfarin dose requirement during the first few weeks of therapy.

Given these variables that affect warfarin efficacy, only a minority of patients who are given the standard dose achieve the target INR. As a result, many patients suffer adverse events, particularly during the initial warfarin administration period. Dosing algorithms based on genetic and nongenetic factors have been established that improve the prediction of stable anticoagulation. For example, the International Warfarin Pharmacogenetics Consortium published a widely cited dosing algorithm, and the website WarfarinDosing.org provides online dosing calculators.[11] The implementation of a dosing algorithm is expected to reduce adverse-event rates of bleeding and thrombosis, and clinical guidelines for implementation have been published. That said, several randomized trials have published outcomes data, with mixed conclusions.[12,13] Although most of these trials have demonstrated better compliance with targeted INR goals, only one recent trial (Genetic Informatics Trial [GIFT]) has demonstrated improved efficacy.[14] In the meantime, direct oral anticoagulants are now available (eg, dabigatran, apixaban, edoxaban, and rivaroxaban), none of which have known PGx interactions.

One could argue that PGx testing could be cost effective if it were used to select optimum therapy instead of to optimize warfarin dosing. In the ENGAGE AF-TIMI 48 Trial, the medical efficacy of warfarin was equivalent to edoxaban for patients who did not carry loss-of-function variants in *VKORC1* and *CYP2C9*.[15] It may be cost effective to perform pharmacogenomics testing on all patients, and reserve use of the more expensive edoxaban drug for the minority of patients who have *VKORC1* and *CYP2C9* variants. Unfortunately, marketing pressures are such that the direct oral anticoagulants are rapidly becoming the oral anticoagulant of choice in the United States and western world, and pharmacogenomics testing for warfarin has not been used.

One lesson learned by the warfarin example is that PGx testing may not change physician or patient behavior. Adjustment of warfarin dose based on INR, as per historical clinical guidelines, does not directly take into consideration the impact of PGx variation, and current algorithms do not consider changes in diet that impact vitamin K concentrations. In addition, algorithms and dose calculators best reflect the population (age, sex, disease status, co-medications, etc) used to develop the dosing tool, in a well-controlled clinical trial, and may not be appropriate for other populations.

Tamoxifen

Tamoxifen is a selective estrogen receptor modulator used to treat women with breast cancer after mastectomy or chemotherapy to reduce recurrence. This adjuvant hormonal therapy is effective for women whose tumors were positive for estrogen and/or progesterone receptors. Tamoxifen is

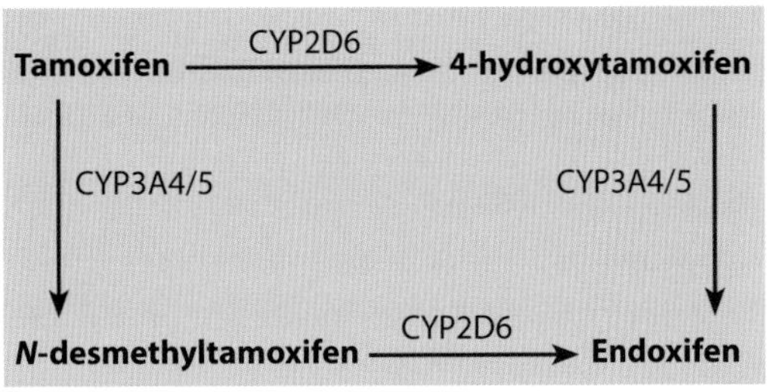

Figure 10-1. Metabolic pathway for tamoxifen (prodrug) to *N*-desmethyltamoxifen (major inactive metabolite), 4-hydroxytamoxifen (minor, <10% active metabolite), and endoxifen (minor, <10% active metabolite).

a prodrug that requires conversion to pharmacologically active metabolites, including 4-hydroxytamoxifen active metabolites through CYP2D6 and endoxifen through CYP3A4/5 enzymes (Figure 10-1). Patients who have loss-of-function alleles such as the **4, *5,* or **36* have no enzyme activity, whereas others may have decreased-function alleles such as **9, *10, *17,* and **41.* Clinical outcomes studies have shown that patients who are predicted to be poor metabolizers (eg, have two copies of loss-of-function *CYP2D6* alleles) have reduced relapse-free time, disease-free survival, and proportion free of progression.[16,17] Guidelines suggest that CYP2D6 poor metabolizers use an alternate antiestrogen therapy, such as aromatase inhibitors for postmenopausal women, or escalate the dose. For CYP2D6 intermediate metabolizers (eg, one loss-of-function allele and one decreased function allele), dose escalation or alternate therapy should be considered. However, some patients predicted to exhibit a normal *CYP2D6* phenotype experience significant dose-related adverse effects or disease progress and/or relapse, such that the value of PGx for all tamoxifen patients has been questioned. The *CYP2D6* gene is incredibly complex, and few laboratories look for all possible variants. As such, it is possible that variants could be missed and phenotype predictions could be inaccurate. Furthermore, it is not clear if dose adjustments can adequately overcome the impact of *CYP2D6* variation. Additional factors known to influence the success of tamoxifen include other drug-metabolizing enzymes, adherence, co-medications, estrogen receptor changes, and other potential changes to the disease pathophysiology. As a consequence, a therapeutic range for steady-state endoxifen concentrations has been proposed.

Although PGx may be useful for patients considering tamoxifen therapy, a lesson learned by the tamoxifen example is that therapeutic drug monitoring may be a more effective dose optimization strategy than PGx. Another lesson learned is that genetic testing may not be sensitive enough or specific enough to detect all phenotypically relevant variants.

Irinotecan

Irinotecan is a topoisomerase 1 inhibitor that acts as a chemotherapeutic agent by preventing DNA from unwinding. It is mainly used in conjunction with other agents, such as 5-fluorouracil and leucovorin, for the treatment of colon cancer. It has also been used to treat other malignancies such as brain cancer, leukemias, and lymphomas. Irinotecan is a prodrug that undergoes metabolism to the active metabolite SN-38, which is then inactivated to SG-38N by the uridine 5'-diphosphate (UDP)-glucuronosyltransferase 1A1 isoenzyme.[18] The *UGT1A1* gene is polymorphic, with variable numbers of TA dinucleotides in the promoter region (ranging from five to eight copies). The functional (normal) number of TA repeats is six, which is described as the *UGT1A1*1* allele. Patients with seven TA repeats (*UGT1A1*28*) have reduced expression of the UGT1A1 protein and a reduced ability to convert irinotecan to SN-38.[19] Other variant alleles have also been described that lead to reduced expression.

An accumulation of SN-38 produces significant diarrhea (grade III-IV), neutropenia (grade III-IV), and hematologic toxicity.[20] To minimize these problems, patients who have two copies of reduced function alleles, such as *UGT1A1 *28/*28,* should be given alternate chemotherapeutic drugs or lower irinotecan doses (100 mg/m^2).[21] In contrast, higher doses that will maximize therapeutic efficacy (eg, 300 mg/m^2) can be given to patients that do not carry deleterious *UGT1A1* variants, with considerably less risk of complications. In many practices, PGx testing is not performed; instead, irinotecan is routinely administered in lower doses, in combination with other chemotherapeutic agents. *UGT1A1* variants are also now associated with dosing guidelines for atazanavir, which has become the predominant application of *UGT1A1* testing. Of note, the *UGT1A1*28/*28* genotype is also associated with Gilbert syndrome. These individuals have a mild increase in total and indirect bilirubin due to the inability to conjugate bilirubin.[22]

Lessons learned with the irinotecan example include the fact that clinical practice may change to prevent the need for PGx testing, and also that applications for a PGx test may change from the original indication, including different drug-gene and disease associations.

Clopidogrel

Clopidogrel is an oral antiplatelet drug that binds to the P2Y12 receptor of platelets and is used to inhibit thrombosis and platelet aggregation, thereby reducing the incidence of cardiovascular disease. The standard daily dosage of clopidogrel is 75 mg. For a significant number of patients, this dosage is inadequate to prevent thrombosis. There are many causes of "clopidogrel resistance," including variable rates of metabolism and pharmacokinetic response, variable absorption, drug-drug interactions, noncompliance, and alternate pathways toward platelet activation.[23] Clopidogrel resistance can be determined by testing the ability of platelets to aggregate in blood after therapeutic doses. Clinical studies have shown that many patients who are clopidogrel resistant have reduced 6-month adverse medical outcomes of death, nonfatal myocardial infarction, or thrombosis.[24]

For many patients, genetic polymorphism in *CYP2C19* is the cause of clopidogrel resistance. Clopidogrel is a prodrug that is metabolized to an active metabolite by this enzyme. Patients who carry a loss-of-function allele, such as the **2* or **3,* are unable to produce this metabolite.[25]

Several clinical studies have shown that patients who carry one or more copies of the **2* or **3* genotype associated with poor metabolism suffer a higher incidence of adverse cardiac events than the wildtype.[26,27] In these cases, increasing the clopidogrel loading or maintenance dose, such as to 150 mg/day, may be sufficient to overcome resistance.[28] At this point, it is unknown whether or not the rate of bleeding will increase at the higher clopidogrel dose. It is also not well characterized how genetic variation leading to increased expression (eg, **17*) impacts dosing. One of the concerns about the clopidogrel association is that *CYP2C19* testing may not be available fast enough to impact dosing decisions. Newer antiplatelet drugs that do not require metabolic activation, such as prasugrel, may also be an alternative for those who are clopidogrel resistant.[29]

Lessons learned from the clopidogrel PGx example include the fact that the results of testing are most useful when available in a clinically relevant time frame to assure that the results can be used to guide therapy. In addition, the pharmaceutical industry may respond to PGx variability by offering drugs that do not have PGx implications.

Thiopurine Drugs

The thiopurine drugs include azathioprine, 6-mercaptopurine, and thioguanine (TG). They are used for a variety of diseases, including hematologic cancer and chronic inflammatory diseases, and to prevent solid organ transplant rejection.[30] The thiopurines are prodrugs and must be converted to 6-thioguanosine nucleotides (6-TNGs), the active metabolites by hypoxanthine-guanine phosphoribosyl transferase, in order to exert their cytotoxic effects. Within hematopoietic cells, dGS is principally deactivated through the thiopurine methyltransferase (TPMT) pathway. At therapeutic dosages, genetic impairment or deficiency of this enzyme leads to an accumulation of active TG nucleotides. Clinical complications of TG include myelosuppression, neutropenic sepsis, and hepatotoxicity.[31] The **2, *3A,* and **3C* alleles of *TPMT* account for the majority of patients who have intermediate or low TPMT enzyme activity.[32] Evaluating TPMT metabolic status is currently standard of care for naïve patient populations that are likely to receive high-dose thiopurine therapy (eg, acute lymphoblastic leukemia patients), but TPMT metabolic status is not necessarily evaluated in patient populations that will receive low-dose thiopurine therapy (eg, psoriasis patients).

As an alternative to genotyping, some investigators have advocated measurement of TPMT enzyme activity within erythrocytes, in part because genotyping does not account for all causes of TPMT deficiency. An advantage of phenotyping is that it can detect the influence of non-TPMT metabolism on thiopurine drugs. For example, variation in other genes, such as *NUDT15,* may also influence sensitivity to thiopurine drugs, and TPMT activities are lower in Africans and African Americans, requiring the use of ethnic-specific reference intervals.[33] These factors are more likely be detected through phenotype testing than by genotype testing. Disadvantages of phenotype testing include the fact that TPMT activity is affected by blood transfusions (sometimes necessary in treating these patients) and prior administration of thiopurine drugs, as well as co-medications. Phenotyping also requires fresh whole blood samples to assure that the integrity of the erythrocyte membranes is sufficient to withstand aggressive washing and packing of the cells before testing. False low enzyme activity is a likely consequence of specimen mishandling. An advantage of genotype testing is that it can be performed using buccal swab or saliva samples, which are not generally affected by transfusions or co-medications. Genotyping can also be performed with archived specimens or with specimens collected after the thiopurine drug has been administered.

Lessons learned through the thiopurine application include the sensitivity and specificity of genotyping versus phenotyping, as well as several logistical variables. In addition, because most adverse drug reactions to thiopurine drugs are dose related, the standard strategy is to start with a low amount. This allows time to identify and manage adverse drug reactions. This is in contrast to pretherapeutic screening, which is common for patients who are candidates for high-dose therapy.

Abacavir

Stevens-Johnson syndrome (SJS) and toxic epidermal necrolysis (TEN) are debilitating diseases characterized by severe systemic rash of the skin and mucous membranes due to a delayed hypersensitivity reaction. SJS involves skin detachment of less than 10% of the body surface area, SJS/TEN overlap has 10% to 30% of body surface detachment, and TEN has detachment of more than 30% of the surface area.[34] Many therapeutic drugs can cause SJS/TEN in a minority of patients after a few weeks of exposure. The severity of the hypersensitivity reaction is intensified if a drug is discontinued and then resumed. The antiretroviral drug abacavir is commonly associated with SJS/TEN.[35] Mechanistically, this drug-induced SJS/TEN is immune mediated and is not dose dependent. Caucasians have a high incidence of *HLA-B*5701.*[36] In a prospective study, Mallal et al found no cases of SJS/TEN among 666 subjects negative for this allele.[5] In contrast, of 47 white subjects with this allele, 22 (47%) developed immunologically confirmed hypersensitivity reaction. PGx testing for *HLA-B*5701* is standard of care and is incorporated into many dosing guidelines and drug-labeling documents. Although genotyping remains the method of choice, screening methods based on flow cytometry to detect HLA-B17 antigens (including B57 and B58) are also available.[37] The availability of flow cytometry enables this testing to be more widely applied.

Lessons learned with the abacavir example include the fact that some PGx-related adverse drug reactions are not dose dependent. As such, the appropriate response when an individual is a carrier of an *HLA-B*5701* allele is to avoid the drug. Another lesson is that this reaction is inherited in an autosomal dominant fashion, such that the presence of one allele is sufficient to illicit the phenotype.

Codeine

Codeine is a widely used pain management and antitussive medication. Like many other drugs discussed in this chapter, codeine must be activated by metabolism to produce its therapeutic effects. Codeine is converted to morphine through a demethylation reaction mediated primarily by CYP2D6. In a normal metabolizer, approximately 10% of a codeine dose is converted to morphine.

Conversion of codeine to morphine would be inadequate for CYP2D6 poor metabolizers and would be excessive for ultrarapid metabolizers. As such, both extremes of metabolizer phenotypes should avoid codeine because of the potential for toxicity. Administration of codeine to a person with the ultrarapid metabolizer phenotype is a significant safety concern because higher than expected concentrations of morphine can be produced, leading to risk of unintentional overdose and opioid toxicity. For example, nursing women with an ultrarapid metabolizer phenotype for CYP2D6 can deliver much higher than expected morphine concentrations to their babies in the breast milk. Children who receive codeine for pain control after tonsillectomy and adenoidectomy are also vulnerable to potentially deadly opioid-induced respiratory depression. A similar PGx vulnerability to opioid-induced toxicity exists for other opioids that utilize CYP2D6 for activation, such as tramadol. Other genes are also probably involved in the pharmacodynamics of opioids, such as *OPRM1* and *COMT.*

A recently published "shortlist" of 10 genes that are recommended for evaluation in pain management includes *CYP2D6,* as well as seven other genes related to pharmacokinetic processes that affect select opioids: *ABCB1, ABCC3, COMT, CYP3A4, CYP3A5, SLC22A1,* and *UGT2B7.*[38] A review by Nerenz and Tsongalis[39] presents overlapping genes *ABCB1, COMT, CYP2D6, CYP3A4* and an additional gene that codes for another drug-metabolizing enzyme, *CYP2B6.* This difference in selection of the most relevant genes by two well-respected groups of authors demonstrates that consensus for routine PGx in pain management is inconsistent and requires additional study.

Summary

The implementation and success of PGx in routine clinical practice require a collaborative effort of (1) physicians, clinical pathologists and laboratorians, pharmacists, and pharmacologists; (2) the in vitro diagnostics industry; and (3) regulatory agencies. Portability of results and standardization of clinical decision support are also necessary. Although PGx touches nearly all medical disciplines, the early adopters are oncologists, cardiologists, psychiatrists, and rheumatologists. With regard to the clinical expertise needed to run a clinical PGx service, pharmacologists are routinely engaged for questions on drug selection, dosing, and efficacy, while the clinical toxicologists provide the expertise on adverse reactions and the clinical scientists for testing issues.

Although genotype analysis requires testing of DNA, PGx does not generally have the ethical issues surrounding testing for genetic diseases. Individuals with unusual or rare genotypes will probably not be denied employment, advancement in the workplace, or access to life insurance policies. It is hoped that analysis for genes that affect drug metabolism, transport, and excretion is only used to make therapeutics safer and more effective.

Previously, molecular diagnostic testing was restricted to academic and reference laboratories because of the high degree of complexity required. However, the technology for testing nucleic acids is becoming more robust and automated. There are US Food and Drug Administration–cleared testing platforms and assays now available for targeting select genes and gene variants.[40] Most laboratories utilize assays that target only the most common clinically actionable PGx variants and often for very discrete applications. Some laboratories have utilized massively parallel sequencing methods and are exploring whole-exome or whole-genome testing with PGx interpretations. Using this approach, it may be possible in the foreseeable future for individuals to pretest their DNA for all of the relevant PGx genes during health, in advance of their need for therapeutics. In this way, the information will be immediately available for therapeutic selection and dose adjustments. Undoubtedly, new genomic associations will be uncovered for current and future medications, making PGx information even more valuable.

References

1. Spear BB, Heath-Chiozzi M, Huff J. Clinical application of pharmacogenetics. *Trends Mol Med.* 2001;7:201-204.
2. Lazarou J, Pomeranz BH, Corey PN. Incidence of adverse drug reactions in hospitalized patients: a meta-analysis of prospective studies. *JAMA.* 1998;279:1200-2005.
3. Committee on Identifying and Preventing Medication Errors, Board on Health Care Services; Aspden P, Wolcott JA, Bootman JL, Cronenwett LR, eds. *Preventing Medication Errors.* Washington, DC: The National Academies Press; 2007.
4. Pulley JM, Denny JC, Peterson JF, et al. Operational implementation of prospective genotyping for personalized medicine: the design of the Vanderbilt PREDICT project. *Clin Pharmacol Ther.* 2012;92(1):87-95.
5. Mallal S, Phillips E, Carosi G, et al. HLA-B*5701 screening for hypersensitivity to abacavir. *N Engl J Med.* 2008;358:568-579.

6. Collins FS, Morgan M, Patrinos A. The Human Genome Project: lessons from large-scale biology. *Science*. 2003;300:286-290.
7. Table of Pharmacogenomic Biomarkers in Drug Labeling. US Food and Drug Administration. https://www.fda.gov/drugs/science-research-drugs/table-pharmacogenomic-biomarkers-drug-labeling. Updated March 26, 2019. Accessed May 17, 2019.
8. Caudle KE, Dunnenberger HM, Freimuth RR, Peterson JF, Burlison JD, Whirl-Carrillo M. Standardizing terms for clinical pharmacogenetic test results: consensus terms for the Clinical Pharmacogenetics Implementation Consortium (CPIC). *Genet Med*. 2017;19:215-223.
9. Schwarz UI, Ritchie MD, Bradford Y, et al. Genetic determinants of response to warfarin during initial anticoagulation. *N Engl J Med*. 2008;358:999-1008.
10. Wadelius M, Pirmohamed M. Pharmacogenetics of warfarin: current status and future challenges. *Pharmacogenomics J*. 2007;7:99-111.
11. Johnson JA, Caudle KE, Gong L, et al. Clinical Pharmacogenetics Implementation Consortium (CPIC) Guideline for Pharmacogenetics-Guided Warfarin Dosing: 2017 Update. *Clin Pharmacol Ther*. 2017;102(3):397-404.
12. Caraco Y, Blotnick S, Muszkat M. CYP2C9 genotype-guided warfarin prescribing . enhances the efficacy and safety of anticoagulation: a prospective randomized control study. *Clin Pharmacol Ther*. 2008;83:460-470.
13. Anderson JL, Horne BD, Stevens SM, et al. Randomized trial of genotype-guided versus standard warfarin dosing in patients initiating oral anticoagulation. *Circulation*. 2007;116:2563-2570.
14. Gage BF, Bass AR, Lin H, et al. Effect of genotype-guided warfarin dosing on clinical events and anticoagulation control among patients undergoing hip or knee arthroplasty: the GIFT randomized clinical trial. *JAMA*. 2017;318(12):1115-1124.
15. Mega JL, Walker JR, Ruff CT, et al. Genetics and the clinical response to warfarin and edoxaban: findings from the randomised, double-blind ENGAGE AF-TIMI 48 trial. *Lancet*. 2015;385(9984):2280-2287.
16. Bradford LD. CYP2D6 allele frequency in European Caucasians, Asians, Africans and their descendants. *Pharmacogenomics*. 2002;3:229-243.
17. Goetz MP, Knox SK, Suman VJ, et al. The impact of cytochrome P450 2D6 metabolism in women receiving adjuvant tamoxifen. *Breast Cancer Res Treat*. 2007;101:113-121.
18. Innocenti F, Ratain MJ. Pharmacogenetics of irinotecan: clinical perspectives on the utility of genotyping. *Pharmacogenomics*. 2006;7:1211-1221.
19. Maitland ML, Vasisht K, Ratain MJ. TPMT, UGT1A1 and DPYD: genotyping to ensure safer cancer therapy? *Trends Pharmacol Sci*. 2006;27:432-437.
20. Cote JF, Kirzin S, Kramar A, et al. UGT1A1 polymorphism can predict hematologic toxicity in patients treated with irinotecan. *Clin Cancer Res*. 2007;13:3269-3275.
21. Hoskins JM, Goldberg RM, Qu P, Ibrahim JG, McLeod HL. UGT1A1*28 genotype and irinotecan-induced neutropenia: dose matters. *J Natl Cancer Inst*. 2007;99:1290-1295.
22. Bosma PJ, Chowdhury JR, Bakker C, et al. The genetic basis of the reduced expression of bilirubin UDP-glucuronosyltransferase 1 in Gilbert's syndrome. *N Engl J Med*. 1995;333:1171-1175.
23. Lau WC, Gurbel PA. Antiplatelet drug resistance and drug-drug interactions: role of cytochrome P450 3A4. *Pharm Res*. 2006;23:2691-2708.
24. Price, MJ, Endemann S, Gollapudi RR, et al. Prognostic significance of post-clopidogrel platelet reactivity assessed by a point-of-care assay on thrombotic events after drug-eluting stent implantation. *Eur Heart J*. 2008;29:992-1000.
25. Xie HG, Kim RB, Wood AJ, Stein CM. Molecular basis of ethnic differences in drug disposition and response. *Annu Rev Pharmacol Toxicol*. 2001; 41:815-850.
26. Mega JL, Close SL, Wiviott SD, et al. Cytochrome P450 polymorphism and response to clopidogrel. *N Engl J Med*. 2009;360:354-362.
27. Simon T, Verstuyft C, Mary-Krause M, et al; French Registry of Acute ST-Elevation and Non–ST-Elevation Myocardial Infarction (FAST-MI) Investigators. Genetic determinants of response to clopidogrel and cardiovascular events. *N Engl J Med*. 2009;360:363-375.
28. Bonello L, Camoin-Jau L, Arques S, et al. Adjusted clopidogrel loading doses according to vasodilator-stimulated phosphoprotein phosphorylation index decrease rate of major adverse cardiovascular events in patients with clopidogrel resistance: a multicenter randomized prospective study. *J Am Coll Cardiol*. 2008;51:1404-1411.
29. Wiviott SD, Braunwald E, McCabe CH, et al. Prasugrel versus clopidogrel in patients with acute coronary syndromes. *N Engl J Med*. 2007; 357:2001-2015.
30. Sahasranaman S, Howard D, Roy S. Clinical pharmacology and pharmacogenetics of thiopurines. *Eur J Clin Pharmacol*. 2008;64:735-767.
31. Connell WR, Kamm MA, Ritchie JK, Lennard-Jones JE. Bone marrow toxicity caused by azathioprine in inflammatory bowel disease: 27 years of experience. *Gut*. 1993;34:1081-1085.

32. Tai HL, Krynetski EY, Yates CR, et al. Thiopurine-S-methyltransferase deficiency: two nucleotide transitions define the most prevalent mutant allele associated with loss of catalytic activity in Caucasians. *Am J Hum Genet.* 1996;58:694-702.
33. Heckmann JM, Lambson EMT, Little F, Owen EP. Thiopurine methyltransferase (TPMT) heterozygosity and enzyme activity as predictive tests for the development of azathioprine-related adverse events. *J Neurol Sci.* 2005;231:71-81.
34. Bastuji-Garin S, Rzany B, Stern RS, Shear NH, Naldi L, Roujeau JC. Clinical classification of cases of toxic epidermal necrolysis, Stevens Johnson syndrome, and erythema multiforme. *Arch Dermatol.* 1993;129:92-96.
35. Lucas A, Nolan D, Mallal S. HLA-B*5701 screening for susceptibility to abacavir hypersensitivity. *J Antimicrob Chemother.* 2007;59:591-593.
36. HLA-B*57:01 for Abacavir Sensitivity. ARUP Laboratories. http://www.aruplab.com/guides/ug/tests/2002429.jsp. Accessed May 17, 2019.
37. Martin AM, Krueger R, Almeida CA, Nolan D, Phillips E, Mallal S. A sensitive and rapid alternative to HLA typing as a genetic screening test for abacavir hypersensitivity syndrome. *Pharmacogenet Genomics.* 2006;16:353-357.
38. Matic M, de Wildt SN, Tibboel D, van Schaik RHN. Analgesia and opioids: a pharmacogenetics shortlist for implementation in clinical practice. *Clin Chem.* 2017;63(7):1204-1212.
39. Nerenz RD, Tsongalis GJ. Pharmacogenetics of opioid use and implications for pain management. *J Appl Lab Med.* 2018;2(4):622-632.
40. Wu AH, Babic N, Yeo KJ. Implementation of pharmacogenomics into the clinical practice of therapeutics: issues for the clinician and the laboratorian. *Per Med.* 2009;6:315-327.

Chapter 11

Laboratory-Based Screening Assays in Support of Pain Management

Tai C. Kwong, PhD
Alan H.B. Wu, PhD

Introduction

Chronic pain affects a significant number of Americans. A National Institutes of Health study estimated that 25.3 million adults (11.2% of the population) experienced chronic pain, defined as pain every day for the last 3 months.[1] Chronic pain treatment based on opioid therapy has increased dramatically in recent years, as reflected in the quadrupling of the sales of opioid pain drugs from 1999 to 2010[2,3] and a 7.3% increase in opioid prescriptions per capita from 2007 to 2012.[4] Unfortunately, this extensive use of prescription opioids has been accompanied by a rise in opioid medication misuse and opioid-related overdoses. Deaths attributed to opioids, most of which were the natural and semisynthetic opioids, increased by 200% from year 2000 to 2014.[5] The epidemic has continued to worsen, such that in more recent years (2015-2016), deaths due to synthetic opioids (including fentanyl but not methadone) have increased by 100%.[6]

In response to the abuse of prescription opioids for chronic pain treatment, several state or specialty organizations published practice guidelines to aid clinicians in treating chronic pain patients with opioids.[7-15] In 2016, the Centers for Disease Control and Prevention (CDC) published a guideline for opioid prescription: CDC Guideline for Prescribing Opioids for Chronic Pain—United States, 2016. The guideline includes a comprehensive initial evaluation of the patient and an assessment of the risk/benefit of opioid therapy. When assessing risk and addressing harms of opioid use, the guidelines state that "clinicians should use urine drug testing before starting opioid therapy and consider urine drug testing at least annually to assess for prescribed medications as well as other controlled prescription drugs and illicit drugs."[16] Despite the various practice guidelines recommending the use of the urine drug test in chronic opioid therapy, reimbursement of this laboratory test continues to decline.

Some of the patients on opioid therapy exhibit aberrant drug behaviors such as the use of undisclosed medications, non-use of prescribed medication, or an undisclosed use of alcohol and illicit drugs. The urine drug test is an objective means of documenting some of the aberrant drug behaviors; it is more efficacious than self-reporting in revealing recent opioid use and can be used to supplement behavioral monitoring.[17]

Urine is currently the most commonly used matrix for pain management drug testing, but oral fluid testing is gaining acceptance because of the ease of oral fluid collection.[18-20] Drug testing typically involves an initial test *(screening)* by a panel of immunoassays. Immunoassay positive results are then subjected to secondary testing *(definitive testing)* using methods based on mass spectrometry. The use of immunoassays in urine and oral fluid drug testing is discussed in detail here.

Immunoassay-Based Urine Drug Test

Initial testing (screening) by immunoassays is still the most commonly used testing method because of lower cost, ease of use, adaptation on automated instrumentation, and rapid turnaround time.

Certain variables will determine the immunoassay test menu that best meets the clinical needs of a treatment program. The laboratory needs to establish a partnership with drug treatment providers in arriving at a drug testing program that best meets their clinical needs and expectations. The laboratory needs to learn the prescription practices of medications of various treatment programs and the prevalence and pattern of illicit drug use in the local area. A typical menu would include immunoassays to detect the commonly prescribed pain management medications (eg, morphine, codeine, tramadol, fentanyl, buprenorphine, oxycodone, hydrocodone, and oxycodone/oxymorphone) as well as frequently abused illicit drugs (eg, amphetamines, benzodiazepines, cannabinoids, and cocaine).[15,21] The laboratory has to inform the providers that laboratories employ commercially available, US Food and Drug Administration (FDA)-cleared immunoassay reagent kits and that it is not able to test for new "designer" drugs that have recently become popular. Testing for these new drugs may have to be referred to highly specialized reference laboratories that have the expertise and resources to undertake the challenges to develop and validate in-house assays (laboratory-developed tests) to detect these drugs.

Immunoassay testing can be carried out at a central laboratory or at the site of collection (ie, point of collection [POC]). If the urine specimens are sent to a laboratory for testing, analysis can be performed on chemistry analyzers. Automation and high-throughput instrumentation make it possible for laboratories to perform high-volume urine drug testing with improved efficiency and cost effectiveness. Laboratory-based testing, however, suffers from the disadvantage of longer turnaround time due to extra time incurred in courier pickup and transportation to the laboratory.

Many of these immunoassay-based tests are also available in POC testing devices. Moreover, some of the POC tests are "waived" tests that can be performed by personnel other than clinical laboratory technical staff. Thus, screening using POC devices can be performed in a doctor's office or clinic, making results available for a provider to discuss test results with the patient during the clinic visit. This provider-patient interaction on test results in real time can enhance the effectiveness of drug testing as a management tool for those patients who might be exhibiting aberrant drug-related behavior.

Limitations of Urine Drug Test Immunoassays

The clinical utility of immunoassay-based drug testing in pain management is dependent on two immunoassay parameters that determine the sensitivity and specificity of the immunoassay: the immunospecificity of the assay antibody and the assay cutoff. The immunospecificity determines the detection limit of the drug, and the cutoff defines a result as negative or positive. Having the knowledge of these immunoassay properties is essential in arriving at an accurate interpretation of test results that will assist clinicians in their clinical decision making and in optimizing the clinical utility of the urine drug test in opioid pain management.[22,23] Nevertheless, immunoassays have limitations, which can be addressed by definitive testing methods based on mass spectrometry. Discussed in detail below are the following limitations: immunoassays are qualitative; lack the ability to provide specific identification of the drug(s) present; have inadequate immunospecificity, which can result in false-positive results; and suffer from inadequate analytical sensitivity for some commonly prescribed pain management drugs.

Immunoassays Are Qualitative Assays

Most immunoassays are run in a qualitative mode; results are designated as positive or negative relative to the calibrator drug at assay cutoff concentration. Thus, neither a positive nor a negative result provides the concentration(s) of the drug(s) present.[23] For example, a urine specimen containing morphine at 300 ng/mL or 30,000 ng/mL will give a positive result by the opiates assay using the 300 ng/mL cutoff. On the other hand, morphine concentrations ranging from 0 ng/mL to 299 ng/mL will yield a negative opiates assay result. Therefore, a negative result should not be interpreted only as evidence that the urine is devoid of drug, but possibly that the drug, if present, is below the concentration (as calibrator drug equivalent concentration) of the assay cutoff. Therefore, a "negative" opiates assay result in a urine containing 299 ng/mL of morphine is negative because of assay cutoff, not necessarily because of patient noncompliance, ie, the patient is taking the drug but the laboratory test is indicating otherwise (see below). Such a negative result can be considered a "clinical false negative" in the context of patient noncompliance, with serious clinical consequence. Obviously, a clinician provided with a quantitative result would be able to interpret the drug test differently depending on concentrations of the drug.[21]

Many of the immunoassays cleared by the FDA can be run in a "semiquantitative" mode using instrument parameters listed in assay package inserts; results are presented in concentration units, for example, nanograms per milliliter (ng/mL). Because an immunoassay will detect all substances that have immunoreactivity with the assay antibody, it will detect not only the calibrator drug (target drug), but also related drugs/metabolites, but with varying reactivities. Thus, immunoassays are class assays, and one should note that a semiquantitative concentration result, displayed in ng/mL, is not the concentration of the calibrator drug but rather the sum of immunoreactivities of all reactive substances as calibrator-equivalents in nanograms per milliliter.

Immunoassays Do Not Give Specific Identification of Drug(s) Present

Immunoassays are class assays, able to detect not only the target analyte drug (calibrator), but also related drugs and metabolites of that "class" when they are present in concentrations sufficiently high for detection. Thus, most immunoassays, as class assays, are labeled as those for the amphetamine, benzodiazepine, and opiate families of drugs. It follows that an immunoassay's positive result does not identify the drug or drugs present. For example, the following three combinations of opiates will give the same positive result by an opiates assay: morphine, morphine plus hydromorphone, or morphine plus hydrocodone plus hydromorphone. Consequently, it is not possible to use an immunoassay to monitor a patient on an opiate prescription for suspected use of another, nonprescribed opiate. If there is a clinical need to know which of the opiates is present in the urine, the provider will have to order definitive testing that is based on analytical methods that can identify the common opiates.

Occurrence of False-Positive Results With Immunoassays

An immunoassay detects, in addition to the target (calibrator) drug compound, all other substances that have immunoreactivity with the assay antibody. Thus, an immunoassay's positive result can be a true positive or a false positive. For example, for the amphetamines immunoassay, the detection of methamphetamine is a true positive because methamphetamine is a member of the target drug class, the amphetamines. If the same assay detects a drug or substance that is not a member of the target drug class, for example, bupropion, then the positive result is a false positive.[23,24] Therefore, in the interpretation of an immunoassay's positive result, it is critically important to treat the positive result as a presumptive positive. Differentiating true and false positives will require a second test, the definitive test.

Analytical Sensitivity

The immunoassay's analytical sensitivity or the detection limit of a drug is determined by the assay's immunoreactivity for that drug. Thus, members of a drug class can have varying immunoreactivities and therefore different detection limits. For example, the opiates immunoassays are designed with morphine as the target. The other opiates—such as the semisynthetic opiates hydromorphone, hydrocodone, oxycodone, and oxymorphone—also exhibit immunoreactivity with the assays and can be detected, although with varying effectiveness.[23] The semisynthetic opiates with lower immunoreactivity relative to that of morphine will have higher detection limits than that of morphine. Consequently, the opiates assay test on a low-reacting semisynthetic opiate may give a negative test because the drug concentration may be below the assay's high detection limit. One study reported that, of the urine samples that tested positive for hydromorphone by mass spectrometry (at a cutoff lower than that of the immunoassay), 70% were negative by the initial opiates immunoassay screen.[25]

Because 6-acetylmorphine (6-AM) is the obligatory intermediate in the metabolic pathway of heroin to morphine, the detection of 6-AM in the urine is indicative of heroin use by the urine donor. Most opiates immunoassays have reactivity for 6-AM, but its specific detection by the opiates immunoassay is generally not possible because of the presence of morphine in the urine of most heroin users. Detection of 6-AM requires an immunoassay that is specifically designed for 6-AM detection. It is interesting that there have been reports of the detection of 6-AM in the absence of morphine.[26,27] In one report, 23% of the urine specimens of pain management patients tested positive for 6-AM in the absence of morphine.[26] In another study of pain clinic urine specimens that were positive for heroin-specific markers (mostly 6-AM, but also diacetylmorphine and 6-acetylcodeine), 23.6% were found to be negative for morphine.[27] Therefore, testing patients suspected of heroin use should include testing for 6-AM in addition to morphine.

Likewise, benzodiazepines immunoassays have varying reactivities, and therefore analytical sensitivities, for some of the commonly prescribed benzodiazepines.[28-30] In one study, benzodiazepines detection frequency by three benzodiazepines immunoassays were compared to the detection findings using liquid chromatography–tandem mass spectrometry (LC-MS/MS). Of the 141 urines that were positive by LC-MS/MS, 22% to 53% were missed by the immunoassays; lorazepam and clonazepam were the most frequently missed.[29] In another study, the benzodiazepines immunoassay failed to detect clonazepam and alprazolam, two of the most prescribed benzodiazepines, in 66% and 53% of urine samples, respectively.[30]

The failure of an immunoassay to detect the presence of a prescription drug because of low immunospecificity (high detection limit) for the drug does have clinical implications. Patients on the lower dose ranges of such drugs (eg, hydrocodone or hydromorphone) may excrete drugs in concentrations that are not measurable by immunoassays at the assay cutoffs (defined for the calibrator drugs) and thus test negative for their medications despite their compliance with their prescriptions. These patients with immunoassay negatives will have clinical false-negative results (in the context of compliance) reported, if no further testing by more sensitive and specific assays is performed.[31,32]

The range of immunoreactivities for drugs within a class can vary widely among immunoassays from different manufacturers. Test results can vary depending on the assay used. A review of the package inserts of six commercial immunoassays shows that the detection limits of hydromorphone vary more than eight-fold and those for hydrocodone more than nine-fold.[23] Thus, a patient's specimen can test positive or negative depending on where the patient goes for testing if laboratories use different assays. The manufacturer's package insert for an assay should be consulted to gain a better understanding of an assay's ability to detect those drugs with low cross-reactivity. The package insert also lists those substances that the manufacturer has tested for possible interference with the assay to cause false-positive results.

Standard Immunoassay Cutoffs May Be Too High

The assay cutoffs of immunoassay test kits are set by the manufacturer and cleared by the FDA. These test kits, although used in the clinical setting, have adopted the cutoffs used in workplace drug testing. Some immunoassays are FDA cleared for more than one cutoff: 1000 and 500 ng/mL cutoffs for the amphetamines assay, 2000 and 300 ng/mL for the opiates assay, and 300 and 150 ng/mL for the cocaine metabolite assay. Choosing to use the lower cutoff will increase the detection rate, but at the risk of a higher false-positive rate. These cutoffs may be inappropriately high for pain management drug testing.[32] In workplace drug testing, the opiates assay cutoff of 2000 ng/mL, rather than 300 ng/mL, is most commonly used because the higher cutoff can minimize positive morphine results due to the consumption of morphine-contaminated poppy seeds. The higher cutoff at 2000 ng/mL, however, is above the detection limits of semisynthetic opiate drugs such as hydromorphone and hydrocodone because of their lower assay immunoreactivity. Consequently, using the higher opiates assay cutoff in pain management drug testing will increase the likelihood of false-negative results.[25] Clinical drug testing for pain management therefore should adopt the lower opiates cutoff of 300 ng/mL.

An FDA-cleared immunoassay can be modified to use with a lower cutoff, which is below that of established thresholds, to further improve assay sensitivity for detection at low drug concentrations to optimize pain management drug testing.[33,34] Any modification of an FDA-cleared test kit, however, will turn it into a laboratory-developed test, and the laboratory will need to conduct extensive validation studies.

Definitive Tests

Definitive assays by mass spectrometry are used for confirmation of immunoassay presumptive positives. Pain management drug testing is clinical testing, and, unlike workplace or forensic testing, confirmation of an initial immunoassay's positive result by definitive testing is neither mandatory nor always necessary. Ordering confirmation testing is a clinical decision; a clinician might forgo definitive testing if the positive result is clinically expected or if the patient is not suspected of aberrant drug behaviors. If definitive testing is not ordered, proper interpretation of immunoassay positive results needs to be based on a solid understanding of immunoassay capabilities and limitations.

Mass spectrometry-based definitive tests are also used to confirm unexpected negative immunoassay results because of their lower detection limits. Studies have shown that when immunoassay testing was compared with LC-MS/MS testing in patients being treated for pain, there was a large number of false-negative results by immunoassays, based on positive results by LC-MS/MS.[35,36] In one study, there were 9.3% false negatives for amphetamines, 22% for benzodiazepines, 10.6% for cannabinoids, 50% for cocaine, 6.1% for methadone, 1.9% for opiates, and 23.4% for propoxyphene.[35] The false negatives by immunoassays could be explained by the low cross-reactivity of some of the drugs for the immunoassays, thus giving negative results, and also could be due to the lower cutoffs used in the LC-MS/MS methods. For example, hydromorphone detection limits by one immunoassay and LC-MS/MS are 1400 ng/mL and 50 ng/mL, respectively. Some laboratories, in order to minimize the false negatives, have opted for bypassing immunoassays to go directly to definitive testing.[36,37] In recent years, some laboratories have explored bypassing immunoassays to perform first-line qualitative and quantitative testing by high-resolution mass spectrometry assays.[38-40]

Details of the advantages of mass spectrometry-based definitive testing, either as a confirmatory test or as first-line qualitative and quantitative testing, can be found in chapter 12, *Approaches to Broad-Spectrum Drug Testing in the Clinical Laboratory.*

Oral Fluid Drug Test Immunoassays

Oral fluid testing for drugs has gained popularity as a reliable alternative to urine-based testing to support pain management. The last few years have witnessed the commercialization of homogeneous and heterogeneous immunoassays for drugs in oral fluids.[18-20] Immunoassays for oral fluid testing in pain management drug testing suffer from the same immunospecificity limitations of the immunoassays for urine, namely, the potential for false-positive and false-negative results. Like urine testing, use of immunoassays for oral fluid pain management drug testing can be effective if definitive testing is employed to eliminate false positives. As with urine immunoassay testing, oral fluid test false negatives can be attributed to an assay cutoff that is set too high or to a lack of immunoreactivity with the prescribed drug. The parent drug–metabolite ratio is generally higher in saliva than urine; therefore, oral fluid assays should not be urine test kits that have been modified for the additional sensitivity necessary for oral fluid screening. Details on immunoassay testing of oral fluids can be found in chapter 14, *Alternate Specimens for Drugs-of-Abuse Testing: Oral Fluid.*

Microarray-Based Immunoassay Testing

Laboratory-based screening assays for drugs of abuse are typically performed using homogeneous immunoassays. These differ from heterogeneous immunoassays, which require a physical separation of antibody-bound and free analytes, and require testing to be performed on more specialized immunoassay analyzers. For homogeneous immunoassays, testing can be conducted using routine clinical chemistry analyzers. These instruments have a limited onboard capacity for reagents. Priority is usually given to groups of tests such as metabolites, proteins, enzymes, some hormones, and therapeutic drugs. After this, reagent space may only be available for seven to 10 drugs-of-abuse assays. In order to detect as many drugs as possible, antibodies are selected such that they cover the families of drugs that have similar chemical structures and medical indications (eg, benzodiazepines, opiates, and barbiturates).

In the design of drugs-of-abuse assays, the selection of assay antibodies is compromised when the criterion is to find as many members of a drug class as possible. Some of the specificity and sensitivity limitations of immunoassays described above are related to these assays being class assays: producing false-positive results with chemical compounds that have similar structures but are themselves not a member of that class and false-negative results due to significant dissimilarity against the target compound (see above section, "Limitations of Urine Drug Test Immunoassays").

If the central laboratory analyzer could accommodate substantially more onboard reagents, it could justify creation of tests directed toward individual drugs rather than a class of compounds. Selecting more-specific antibodies will reduce the problem of false negatives and false positives. Tests for individual drugs overcome the inability of a class assay to give specific identification of the drugs present. For example, there is medical value in differentiating between morphine and hydromorphone use, which cannot be accomplished with the opiate screening assay.[41] The specificity of assays for the benzodiazepines as a class is poor and can be improved through the use of better antibodies.[42]

Table 11-1. Microchip Array for Drugs-of-Abuse Immunoassays*

Novel Panel (Unique Offering)†	
7-Aminoflunitrazepam	Meperidine
Chloral hydrate	Meprobamate
Clonazepam	Naloxone
Escitalopram	Salicyluric acid
Etizolam	Sertraline
Fluoxetine	Tramadol
Ibuprofen	Trazodone
Ketamine	Zaleplon
LSD metabolite	Zolpidem
Designer Drugs and Psychoactive Drugs	
AB-CHMINACA	Salvinorin
AB-PINACA	Synthetic cannabinoids (4 panels)
AH-7921	Synthetic fentanyls (6 panels)
Alpha-PVP	UR-144
Bath salts (2 panels)	U4770
Benzylpiperazine	W-17, W-19, W-16
Mescaline	
NBOMe	
Phenylpiperazine (2 panels)	
Growth Promoters and Steroids	
β-agonists	Nandrolone
Boldenone	Ractopamine
17β-Clostebol	Stanozolol
Corticosteroids	Stilbenes
Ethinyl estradiol	Trenbolone
Gestagens	Zeranol
Methyltestosterone	

* Randox Laboratories Ltd, United Kingdom.
† Available on automated immunoassay analyzers, not including availability as an ELISA.

Increasing onboard capacity will also enable development of new assays for common therapeutic drugs (eg, hypnotics and novel antidepressants). If one includes synthetic analogs such as designer drugs, the menu of possible tests can be large and impractical on current chemistry analyzers.

One approach toward increasing the menu of a drugs-of-abuse screening assay is the use of a multimarker microchip array. A microchip array is a tiny silicon wafer made of semiconductive material. The array contains a collection of antibodies immobilized onto the wafer, enabling the capture of drugs and metabolites. For drugs, there is a competitive reaction between target drugs from the sample and labeled drugs added to the chip. The labeled drug is an indirect measure of the native antibody signal. In a similar manner to the microchip DNA array, the microchip protein array enables detection of dozens (if not hundreds) of analytes.

Construction of a microarray chip will enable simultaneous detection of multiple drugs. In addition to the traditional drugs-of-abuse assays that are widely available, a substantial number of new drugs have been added to these panels.[43] This expanded menu includes therapeutic drugs, synthetic and designer drugs such as "bath salts" and synthetic cannabinoids, and even anabolic steroids (Table 11-1). Specialized instrumentation, however, is required for performing microarray testing. Use of microarray testing does not replace the need for confirmatory analysis using mass spectrometry. It should also be noted that commercial non–FDA-approved assays for these drugs are available using enzyme-linked immunosorbent assay (ELISA) technology. These assays cannot be adapted to commercial chemistry analyzers and require manual or automated ELISA plate readers.

References

1. Nahin RL. Estimates of pain prevalence and severity in adults: United States, 2012. *J Pain.* 2015;16(8):769-780.
2. National Institutes of Health Pathways to Prevention Workshop: The Role of Opioids in the Treatment of Chronic Pain, September 29-30, 2014. Executive Summary. https://prevention.nih.gov/research-priorities/research-needs-and-gaps/pathways-prevention/role-opioids-treatment-chronic-pain. Accessed May 13, 2019.
3. Paulozzi LJ, Jones CM, Mack KA, Rudd RA. Vital signs: overdoses of prescription opioid pain relievers—United States, 1999-2008. *MMWR Morb Mortal Wkly Rep.* 2011;60(43):1487-1492.
4. Levy B, Paulozzi L, Mack KA, Jones CM. Trends in opioid analgesic-prescribing rates by specialty, U.S., 2007-2012. *Am J Prev Med.* 2015;49:409-413.
5. Rudd R, Aleshire N, Zibbell J, Gladden R. Increases in drug and opioid overdose deaths—United States, 2000-2014. *MMWR Morb Mortal Wkly Rep.* 2016;64(50):1378-1382.
6. Seth P, Scholl L, Russ RA, Bacon S. Overdose deaths involving opioids, cocaine, and psychostimulants—United States, 2015-2016. *MMWR Morb Mortal Wkly Rep.* 2018;67(12):349-358.
7. VA/DoD Clinical Practice Guideline for Opioid Therapy for Chronic Pain—Clinician Summary. Version 3.0–2017. Department of Veterans Affairs, Department of Defense. https://www.healthquality.va.gov/guidelines/Pain/cot/VADoDOTCPGProviderSummary022817.pdf. February 2017. Accessed May 17, 2019.
8. Busse J, ed. The 2017 Canadian Guideline for Opioids for Chronic Non-Cancer Pain. National Pain Centre, McMaster University. http://nationalpaincentre.mcmaster.ca/documents/Opioid%20GL%20for%20CMAJ_01may2017.pdf. Accessed May 17, 2019.
9. Simons K, Westlake T, Capodice MJ. Wisconsin Medical Examining Board Opioid Prescribing Guideline–April 19, 2018. Department of Safety and Professional Services, State of Wisconsin. https://dsps.wi.gov/Documents/BoardCouncils/MED/20180321MEBGuidelinesv8.pdf. Accessed May 17, 2019.
10. Interagency Guideline on Prescribing Opioids for Pain. 3rd ed. Washington State Agency Medical Directors' Group. http://www.agencymeddirectors.wa.gov/Files/2015AMDGOpioidGuideline.pdf. Published June 2015. Accessed May 17, 2019.
11. Jarvis M, Williams J, Hurford M, et al. Appropriate use of drug testing in clinical addiction medicine. *J Addict Med.* 2017;11:163-173.
12. Manchikanti L, Abdi S, Atluri S, et al. American Society of Interventional Pain Physicians (ASIPP) guidelines for responsible opioid prescribing in chronic non-cancer pain: part 2--guidance. *Pain Physician.* 2012;15:S67-S116.
13. Sundwall DN, Rolfs RT, Johnson E; Utah Department of Health. Utah Clinical Guidelines on Prescribing Opioids for Treatment of Pain. Utah Department of Health. http://www.health.utah.gov/prescription/pdf/guidelines/final.04.09opioidGuidlines.pdf. Published February 2009. Accessed May 17, 2019.
14. Chou R, Fanciullo GJ, Fine PG, et al. Clinical guidelines for the use of chronic opioid therapy in chronic noncancer pain. *J Pain.* 2009;10:113-130.
15. Using Clinical Laboratory Tests to Monitor Drug Therapy in Pain Management Patients. American Association for Clinical Chemistry. https://www.aacc.org/science-and-practice/practice-guidelines/using-clinical-laboratory-tests-to-monitor-drug-therapy-in-pain-management-patients. January 1, 2017. Accessed May 17, 2019.
16. Dowell D, Haegerich TM, Chou R. CDC guideline for prescribing opioids for chronic pain—United States, 2016. *MMWR Recomm Rep.* 2016;65(1);1-49. Erratum in: *MMWR Recomm Rep.* 2016;65(11):295.
17. Jhingan HP, Jain R, Desai NG, Vaswani M, Tripathi BM, Pandey RM. Validity of self-report of recent opiate use in treatment setting. *Indian J Med Sci.* 2002;56:495-500.
18. Heltsley R, DePriest A, Black DL, et al. Oral fluid drug testing of chronic pain patients, I: positive prevalence rates of licit and illicit drugs. *J Anal Toxicol.* 2011;35(8):529-540.

19. Heltsley R, DePriest A, Black DL, et al. Oral fluid drug testing of chronic pain patients, II: comparison of paired oral fluid and urine specimens. *J Anal Toxicol.* 2012;36(2):75-80.
20. Conermann T, Gosalia AR, Kabazie AJ, et al. Utility of oral fluid in compliance monitoring of opioid medications. *Pain Physician.* 2014;17:63-70.
21. Kwong TC, Magnani BJ. Urine drug testing in opioid therapy for chronic pain management. In: Kwong TC, Magnani B, Rosano TG, Shaw LM, eds. *The Clinical Toxicology Laboratory: Contemporary Practice of Poisoning Evaluation.* 2nd ed. Washington, DC: AACC Press; 2013:447-445.
22. Pesce A, West C, Egan City K, Strickland J. Interpretation of urine drug testing in pain patients. *Pain Med.* 2012;13:868-885.
23. Kwong TC, Dasgupta A, Magnani BJ. Drug screening by immunoassays. In: Kwong TC, Magnani B, Rosano TG, Shaw LM, eds. *The Clinical Toxicology Laboratory: Contemporary Practice of Poisoning Evaluation.* 2nd ed. Washington, DC: AACC Press; 2013:411-422.
24. Saitman A, Park H-D, Fitzgerald RL. False-positive interferences of common urine drug screen immunoassays: a review. *J Anal Toxicol.* 2014;38:387-396.
25. Mikel C, Almazan P, West R, et al. LC-MS/MS extends the range of drug analysis in pain patients. *Ther Drug Monit.* 2009;31:746-748.
26. Crews B, Mikel C, Latyshev S, et al. 6-acetylmorphine detected in the absence of morphine in pain management patients. *Ther Drug Monit.* 2009; 31:749-752.
27. Knight J, Puet BL, DePriest A, et al. Prevalence of heroin markers in urine for pain management patients. *Forensic Sci Int.* 2014;243:79-83
28. Mikel C, Pesce AJ, Rosenthal M, West C. Therapeutic monitoring of benzodiazepines in the management of pain: current limitations of point of care immunoassays suggest testing by mass spectrometry to assure accuracy and improve patient safety. *Clin Chim Acta.* 2012;413:1199-1202.
29. Darragh A, Snyder ML, Ptolemy AS, Melanson S. KIMS, CEDIA, and HS-CEDIA immunoassays are inadequately sensitive for detection of benzodiazepines in urine from patients treated for chronic pain. *Pain Physician.* 2014;17:359-366.
30. West R, Pesce A, West C, et al. Comparison of clonazepam compliance by measurement of urinary concentration by immunoassay and LC-MS/MS in pain management population. *Pain Physician.* 2010;13:71-78.
31. Pyle-Eilola AL, Thornton DJ, Hays HL, Casavant MJ. Is this drug screen really negative?: special investigation of drug screening in pediatrics. *J Appl Lab Med.* 2017;1:437-440.
32. Snyder ML, Fantz CR, Melanson S. Immunoassay-based drug tests are inadequately sensitive for medication compliance monitoring in patients treated for chronic pain. *Pain Physician.* 2017;20(2S):SE1-SE9.
33. Luzzi VI, Saunders AN, Koenig JW, et al. Analytic performance of immunoassays for drugs of abuse below established cutoff values. *Clin Chem.* 2004;50:717-722.
34. Mullins GR, Reeves A, Yu Min, Goldberger BA, Bazydlo LAL. Improved clinical sensitivity of a reflexive algorithm to minimize false-negative test results by a urine benzodiazepine immunoassay screen. *J Appl Lab Med.* 2018;2:555-563
35. Pesce A, Rosenthal M, West R, et al. An evaluation of the diagnostic accuracy of liquid chromatography–tandem mass spectrometry versus immunoassay drug testing in pain patients. *Pain Physician.* 2010;13:273-281.
36. Melanson SEF, Ptolemy AS, Wasan AD. Optimizing urine drug testing for monitoring medication compliance in pain management. *Pain Med.* 2013;14:1813-1820.
37. McMillin GA, Marin SJ, Johnson-Davis KL, Lawlor BG, Strathmann FG. A hybrid approach to urine drug testing using high-resolution mass spectrometry and select immunoassays. *Am J Clin Pathol.* 2015;143:234-240.
38. Rasmussen NN, Barker A, Strathmann FG. Lowering the bar for mass spectrometry: a comparison between immunoassay and rapid time-of-flight for presumptive screening of drugs in urine. *J Clin Lab Med.* 2018;2:535-542.
39. Thoren KL, Colby JM, Shugarts SB, Wu AH, Lynch KL. Comparison of information-dependent acquisition on a tandem quadrupole TOF vs a triple quadrupole linear ion trap mass spectrometer for broad-spectrum drug screening. *Clin Chem.* 2016;62:170-178.
40. Colby JM, Thoren KL, Lynch KL. Suspect screening using LC-QqTOF is a useful tool for detecting drugs in biological samples. *J Anal Toxicol.* 2018;42:207-213.
41. Gingras M, Laberge MH, Lefebvre M. Evaluation of the usefulness of an oxycodone immunoassay in combination with a traditional opiate immunoassay for the screening of opiates in urine. *J Anal Toxicol.* 2010;34:78-83.
42. Koch TR, Raglin RL, Kirk S, Bruni JF. Improved screening for benzodiazepine metabolites in urine using the Triage Panel for Drugs of Abuse. *J Anal Toxicol.* 1994;18:168-172.
43. McLaughlin P, Pounder D, Maskell P, Osselton D. Real-time near-body drug screening during autopsy, I: use of the Randox biochip drugs of abuse DOA I and DOA II immunoassays. *Forensic Toxicol.* 2013;31:113-118.

Chapter 12

Approaches to Broad-Spectrum Drug Testing in the Clinical Laboratory

Kara L. Lynch, PhD

Introduction

Clinical toxicology is defined as the analysis of drugs and chemicals in body fluids for the purpose of patient care. In practice, it is not possible to provide analytical testing for all clinical toxins that may be encountered; however, there are a variety of different analytical approaches used to cover a broad spectrum of potential toxins. The clinical toxicology testing provided by any given laboratory depends on the pattern of local illicit and prescription drug use and the available resources of the institution. Standard clinical toxicology testing usually includes drug screening for common drugs of abuse in urine. This testing includes a panel of tests that is usually referred to as the *urine toxicology screen (utox)*. For urine toxicology screens, immunoassays for classes of abused drugs are routinely used, followed by targeted confirmations for select drug classes (ie, opiates or amphetamines) using chromatographic techniques coupled to mass spectrometry.

Although immunoassay screens are rapid, automated, and readily available, such methods do not exist for all drugs and metabolites of clinical interest. Most immunoassays are designed to detect a drug class and thus have limited specificity for individual drugs or metabolites. Also, some immunoassays have limited sensitivity, and identification is based on detection above a given cutoff. Immunoassays also vary significantly in terms of cross-reactivity with other unrelated compounds. For these reasons, other analytical methods are used for definitive (ie, confirmatory) testing and detection of drugs and metabolites not detected by the currently available immunoassays. Chromatographic techniques coupled to mass spectrometry are the most common methods used for definitive testing after immunoassay screens. Some of the common indications for ordering a urine toxicology screen include (1) workplace drugs testing, (2) to monitor drug use during pregnancy, (3) to evaluate drug exposure or withdrawal in newborns, and (4) to monitor compliance in patients on prescription medications for chronic pain. For these indications, urine is typically the specimen of choice because of the longer detection windows of drugs and metabolites in urine.

The screen-and-confirm two-step approach has limited utility in cases of acute poisoning or overdose and for uncovering public health outbreaks related to illicit drug use. These assays do not cover all potential toxins of interest, and definitive results are often not available in time to influence patient management. There are other routine assays offered in addition to the urine toxicology screen in cases of acute poisoning and overdose. These assays range from specific tests for common intoxicants in serum (eg, acetaminophen, salicylate, ethanol, digoxin) to a broad-spectrum drug test in urine, serum, or plasma that is capable of detecting more than 100 drugs and metabolites. A method or combination of methods designed to detect a large number of drugs and metabolites, including prescription medications, is often referred to as a *broad-spectrum drug test*. There are other terms that are also used to describe this type of testing, including *comprehensive drug screen, general unknown screening,* and *systematic toxicological analysis*. Broad-spectrum drug testing is capable of detecting classes of drugs for which immunoassays have not been developed, which include, but are not limited to, antidepressants, nonbenzodiazepine hypnotics, neuropathic pain medications, muscle relaxants, antipsychotics, β-blockers, calcium-channel blockers, oral antidiabetes drugs, synthetic opioids, and novel psychoactive substances.

The role of broad-spectrum drug testing to aid in the diagnosis of toxicity or drug overdose is somewhat controversial. In cases of toxicity, prompt diagnosis and treatment is essential. Diagnosis is generally made by history and clinical symptoms, and treatment is usually supportive. Similar to urine drug confirmatory testing, results of broad-spectrum drug testing are usually not provided in real time and thus may not have an immediate impact on patient care. In addition, the tests are routinely performed on urine specimens, and the drugs and metabolites detected may not be reflective of the patient's current clinical state. The usefulness of the information acquired from a broad-spectrum drug test is dependent on the time of drug exposure and the window of detection for the drug and/or metabolites of interest. However, the clinical history in cases of drug toxicity and overdose is not always available or reliable, and the symptoms may not be enough to diagnosis drug toxicity. This is especially true in cases of polysubstance use or overdose. If provided in a timely manner, broad-spectrum drug testing results can aid in the rule-in or rule-out of drug toxicity as compared with other suspected causes on the diagnosis differential. The results may also be valuable for clinical follow-up. For example, the presence of a drug that is known to induce seizures may negate the need for a complete epilepsy workup in a case of a patient presenting to the emergency department with a seizure of unknown origin. In the future, broad-spectrum drug testing in serum provided in real time could prove invaluable in cases of drug toxicity or overdose. This chapter will focus on the different analytical approaches that can be used by clinical toxicology laboratories to provide broad-spectrum drug testing results, along with advantages and disadvantages of each analytical approach. The chapter will end with the presentation of cases highlighting the advantages of the use of high-resolution mass spectrometry (HRMS) in the clinical toxicology laboratory.

Poisoning and Overdose Trends

The need for rapid analytical approaches to aid in the diagnosis of poisoning and overdose is stronger than ever before. The rate of overdoses in the United States continues to rise annually. More than 72,000 Americans died from drug overdose in 2017.[1] These deaths resulted from illicit substances and prescribed medications. From 2002 to 2017, there was a three-fold increase in the number of overdose deaths.[1] According to the Annual Report of the American Association of Poison Control Centers' National Poison Data System, there were more than 2 million human exposures reported in 2016.[2] From 2015 to 2016, health care facility human exposure cases increased by 3.6%.[2] Cases with more serious outcomes (moderate, major, or death) have increased by 4.39% per year since 2000.[2] The overdose epidemic shows no signs of slowing in the near future.

The highest rise in overdose deaths has been observed for synthetic opioids other than methadone, with a 22-fold increase from 2012 to 2017.[1] Overdoses resulting from a combination of synthetic opioids and cocaine or benzodiazepines have increased by nearly three-fold and six-fold, respectively.[1] The predominant synthetic opioid responsible is illicit fentanyl, with fentanyl analogues also contributing.[3] This highlights the increased availability of illicitly manufactured synthetic drugs flooding the US drug market. Opioids are not the only class of drugs with readily available illicit novel substances. There has been a significant rise in the number of cases reported involving novel psychoactive substances such as synthetic amines, synthetic cannabinoids, and synthetic benzodiazepines. For example, data from the 2017 Monitoring the Future Survey funded by the National Institutes of Health reported that past-year use of synthetic cannabinoids among 12th graders was 3.7%, higher than classical illicit substances such as cocaine and heroin and second only to marijuana/hashish.[4]

The concerns over the rise in novel or synthetic illicit drugs is not unique to the United States. Between 2009 and 2016, 106 countries and territories reported the emergence of 739 different novel psychoactive substances belonging to diverse chemical groups to the United Nations Office on Drugs and Crime (UNODC).[5] However, the UNODC states that problems in identifying them in laboratories may be a factor in the low level of reporting of these lesser known substances. Also, there is often little clinical or pharmacological data for these compounds that could be used to aid in clinical diagnosis or management of individual cases. If the right diagnostic technologies are used, the clinical toxicology laboratory could play a large role in aiding in the detection of these substances and a better understanding of their toxicity and approaches to clinical management. Traditional toxicology testing approaches, such as immunoassay screens and targeted analytical approaches, are not capable of detecting these new emerging illicit substances. The untargeted analytical approaches that are discussed in this chapter are essential to keep up with the ever-changing drug landscape.

Comprehensive Drug Testing: Analytical Approaches

Clinical laboratories use a variety of different analytical approaches for performing comprehensive drug testing. The choice of analytical technique is often dictated by the resources available in each laboratory. There are several combinations of chromatographic and detection techniques that can be utilized. The three most common instrument combinations include gas chromatography–mass spectrometry (GC-MS), liquid chromatography–tandem mass spectrometry (LC-MS/MS), and liquid chromatography–high-resolution mass spectrometry (LC-HRMS).

Gas Chromatography–Mass Spectrometry

Gas chromatography is widely available and used for qualitative and quantitative drug analysis. Various detectors can be used in combination with GC for drug screening; however, GC-MS and GC-MS/MS offer the greatest sensitivity and specificity. Compounds that are nonpolar, volatile, and have a small molecular weight are suitable for analysis by GC. Electron ionization with full-scan mass detection or selected ion monitoring (SIM) are the most widely used approaches for broad-spectrum drug testing using GC-MS. Full-scan mass detection is an untargeted approach and is capable of potentially detecting all compounds in the sample, which is advantageous for broad-spectrum drug testing. Identification of unknown compounds can be achieved by comparison of their full mass spectrum with a mass spectral library or database. SIM is a targeted approach and will only identify the compounds for which specific acquisition parameters are entered into the analytical method. SIM is considered to be more sensitive compared with full-scan methods for the drugs and metabolites the SIM method is designed to detect.

The major disadvantage of using GC-MS for broad-spectrum drug testing is that GC-MS methods are not capable of directly analyzing drugs that are nonvolatile, polar, or thermally labile. Derivatization is required to increase the volatility and thermal stability of these compounds. This involves derivatizing one or more polar groups on a compound to a less-polar group. Derivatization can also be used to achieve increased sensitivity, selectivity, or specificity for a given chromatographic separation. For broad-spectrum drug testing, lengthy sample preparations, which include hydrolysis and derivatization, are required before GC-MS analysis. This significantly lengthens the time of sample analysis compared with most LC-based methods.

One of the major advantages of GC-MS compared with LC-MS is the high reproducibility of generated mass spectra using electron ionization. The electron impact ionization process, used in GC-MS, is a hard ionization that results in the production of very reproducible mass spectra from one instrument to another. Large transferable electron ionization–mass spectral libraries exist and are available for library searching of acquired spectra from any instrument.[6] Because of the availability of these libraries, individual laboratories do not have to develop their own in-house library, which can be very time consuming and costly. These large commercially available libraries are updated periodically to include emerging illicit drugs and synthetic drugs, which is a major advantage given the ever-changing drug landscape.

Liquid Chromatography–Mass Spectrometry

The use of liquid chromatography–mass spectrometry has become increasingly more prominent in clinical toxicology laboratories for broad-spectrum drug screening. Unlike GC-MS, LC-MS using electrospray ionization can detect nonvolatile, polar, and thermally labile compounds and provides a means of detecting a broad menu of drugs and metabolites without the need for lengthy sample preparations. The sample preparation time is usually significantly reduced for LC-MS methods compared with GC-MS methods because hydrolysis and derivatization are not required. In addition, sample run times can be shorter for broad-spectrum drug tests compared with some GC-MS methods. These features of LC-MS methods are beneficial if results are needed rapidly for patient care. The electrospray ionization process results in a soft ionization, and thus fragmentation is produced by in-source, collision-induced dissociation (CID) for single-MS systems or CID in the collision cell for tandem-MS systems.

One current disadvantage of LC-MS for broad-spectrum drug testing is that product ion spectra produced by CID differ markedly between instruments.[7] This poses a problem for the creation of large product ion spectral libraries utilized by chromatographic deconvolution software for broad-spectrum drug testing. Despite attempts to standardize the production of the product ion spectra, ion relative intensities are highly variable, requiring the need for the development of search algorithms that do not heavily weight ion relative intensities, but rather the absence or presence of ions. Instrument-specific product ion spectral libraries have been created, and vendors are beginning to market predeveloped broad-spectrum drug testing methods, with chromatographic deconvolution software for library searching and compound identification. Some laboratories are capable of developing their own in-house library; however, most laboratories do not have dedicated research and development staff for such undertakings.

Another disadvantage of electrospray ionization LC-MS techniques is ion suppression and matrix effects. Ion suppression results from the presence of less-volatile compounds in a sample matrix that can change the efficiency of droplet formation or evaporation. This affects the amount of charged ions in the gas phase that ultimately reaches the detector. Ion suppression should be extensively evaluated during method development, and sample cleanup and separation should be optimized to eliminate significant ion suppression in clinical toxicology methods. Despite these limitations, LC-MS is the technique of choice for most clinical toxicology laboratories.

LC-MS encompasses a variety of different LC and MS combinations, including LC-MS, LC-MS/MS, and LC-HRMS, to name a few.[8] Mass

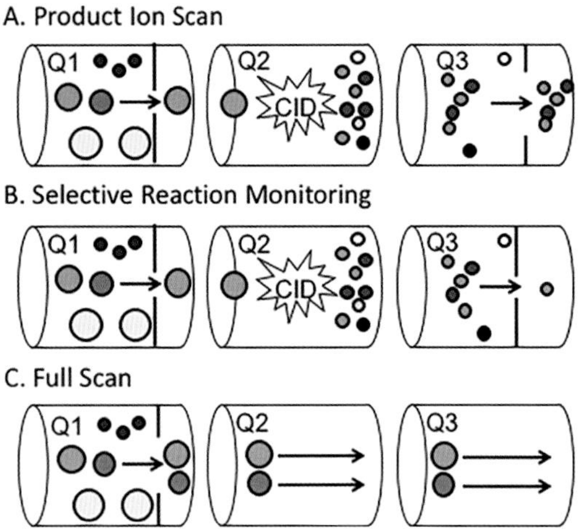

Figure 12-1. Mass spectrometry (MS) scan modes used for broad-spectrum drug testing. The three most common MS scan modes used in broad-spectrum drug testing include (A) product ion scan, (B) selective reaction monitoring, and (C) full scan. CID, collision-induced dissociation; Q, quadrupole.

spectrometry analyzers are classified into two broad groups: beam-type and trapping-type instruments. In *beam-type* instruments, the ions travel through the mass analyzer in a single beam before they strike the detector. The two most common beam-type instruments used for toxicology include quadrupole and time-of-flight (TOF). *Trapping-type* instruments hold the ions in a spatially confined area for a period of time before they travel to the detector. The ion trap is the most common trapping-type instrument used in clinical laboratories. Selection of the best mass analyzer for each laboratory's specific testing needs is very crucial. The remainder of this section will discuss MS/MS and HRMS and their advantages and disadvantages for broad-spectrum drug testing.

Tandem Mass Spectrometry

In MS/MS, two mass analyses occur sequentially to improve selectivity and analytical detection limits. These two mass analysis steps can occur tandem in space or tandem in time. In a tandem-in-space instrument, three quadrupoles are linked sequentially. The first quadrupole (Q1) is used to scan a preset *m/z* (mass/charge) range and select the ions of interest. These ions are called *precursor ions*. The second quadrupole (Q2) functions as a collision cell. The selected ions are accelerated by an electrical potential to high kinetic energy and then collide with neutral gas molecules to fragment the ions. This is called *collision-induced dissociation (CID)*. The ions formed during fragmentation are called *product ions*. The third quadrupole (Q3) analyzes the product ions generated in Q2.

In tandem-in-space instruments, the two mass analysis steps and CID are performed sequentially within the same spectrometer, which is typically an ion trap. Ion trap analyzers are the most common trapping-type instrument used in clinical toxicology laboratories. They are similar to quadrupole analyzers in that they are able to select and filter specific *m/z* values for analysis. Ion traps function by using radio frequency fields to retain and trap ions within a three-dimensional space for a period of time. After the period of ion accumulation, the electric field adjusts, destabilizing the trapped ions and selectively sending them to the detector. All ions initially enter the trap, but only a specific radio frequency will cause ions with a particular *m/z* value to leave. There are two main types of ion traps: quadruple ion traps and linear ion traps. In a quadruple ion trap, the four rods are arranged to form a three-dimensional sphere rather than existing in parallel. A linear ion trap is structurally designed in the same manner as the quadrupole analyzer, with the addition of electrostatic fields applied to the ends to prevent ions from exiting the mass analyzer. The trapping function can be turned on and off to allow the trapped ions to be sent to the detector.

There are several different scan modes that can be used for compound identification in MS/MS (Figure 12-1). The two most common scan modes for broad-spectrum drug screening are product ion (PI) scan and selected reaction monitoring (SRM), both of which are targeted detection methods. LC-MS/MS instruments are also capable of performing a full scan; however, this scan mode in isolation is less common for broad-spectrum drug screening compared with PI scans and SRM. In a PI scan, Q1 is set to select defined precursor ions. The ions are then fragmented in Q2, and all resulting product ions in a specified mass range are detected in Q3, which functions in full-scan mode. A full mass spectrum of the fragmented analyte is acquired (Figure 12-1). The acquired mass spectrum can be compared to mass spectral libraries for compound identification or used for structural elucidation of unknowns. SRM is similar to PI scan except that specific product ions are monitored in Q3 rather than acquiring a mass spectrum of the entire mass range (Figure 12-1). The precursor and product ion pair are referred to as a *transition*. In many clinical applications, two ion transitions are monitored per analyte. The most abundant PI is referred to as the *quantifier ion* and is used for quantification purposes, and the second monitored product ion is referred to as the *qualifier ion* and is used as a second form of identification for the analyte. The ratio of the chromatographic peak area of the more-abundant product ion to the less-abundant product ion can be compared to what is expected for the analyte of interest to further enhance specificity.

SRM and PI scans can be used in the same method, with the instrument alternating between the two different scan modes. A common approach for broad-spectrum drug screening is to perform SRM followed by data-dependent acquisition (DDA) of product ion spectra. DDA allows for specific experimental conditions to be set to allow for the collection of product ion spectra of the compounds of interest. Not all MS/MS analyzers can perform these scan modes simultaneously in the same method. If this functionality is preferred for a clinical toxicology laboratory, they must ensure that the instrument they purchase is not designed solely for SRM-based methods.

Tandem mass spectrometers are the instrument of choice for most clinical toxicology laboratories. For drug confirmation testing, many laboratories utilize SRM-based methods with two transitions monitored per analyte and calculation of the ion ratio between the two most abundant or most selective product ions. However, for broad-spectrum drug testing for more than 100 drugs and metabolites, monitoring two transitions per analyte can be cumbersome. Because of this, many broad-spectrum drug tests utilize SRM-DDA-PI–based methods. The product ions collected are searched against mass spectral libraries. The library match score is used in addition to retention time and SRM for compound identification.

High-Resolution Mass Spectrometry

In recent years there has been an emergence of the use of HRMS methods for drug testing.[8-10] These technologies can achieve high mass accuracy due to their high resolving power, making them ideal technologies for detecting hundreds of compounds simultaneously in complex biological matrices. HRMS technologies can determine the accurate mass of the sample components being analyzed. Some HRMS technologies that can be used for broad-spectrum drug testing include TOF, Orbitrap, and quadrupole TOF (QTOF) mass analyzers.

Time-of-Flight Mass Analyzers

Time-of-flight mass analyzers use an electrical field to pulse gas phase ions through a flight tube toward the detector. The time required for the ion to travel from the pulser to the detector is determined by the *m/z* ratio. Ions with a smaller *m/z* will move faster than larger ions. The ion velocity is inversely related to the square root of the *m/z* value times the voltage. There are different types of TOF analyzers: some contain linear flight tubes, and others make use of reflectrons and ion mirrors to increase the length of the flight path and thus increase the resolution. Unlike quadruple analyzers, TOF analyzers are not capable of filtering out or retaining specific ions. TOF analyzers detect a large mass range and have the advantage of being able to determine the accurate mass and molecular formula of the sample components being analyzed. Although TOF analyzers are very sensitive and have a high mass accuracy and resolution, their dynamic range is limited and thus they are not commonly used for quantitation.

TOF mass analyzers are more expensive than single quadruple-MS analyzers but typically are less expensive than sensitive MS/MS mass analyzers. Compound identification is based on retention time, accurate mass/molecular formula, and isotope pattern. In-source fragmentation is capable with some TOF analyzers, but this is not common. TOF analyzers operate in full-scan mode and therefore are capable of potentially seeing any drug or metabolite in a clinical sample; however, accurate mass, isotope pattern, and retention time are often not adequate for definitive identification of a drug or metabolite. One molecular formula for a small molecule can correspond to several different compounds. For example, morphine and hydromorphone have the same molecular formula and thus the same exact mass. Unless all possible isomers are separated, chromatographically definitive identification is not possible. TOF mass analyzers can be powerful tools for toxicology testing, but confirmation by a different analytical approach is preferred.

Quadrupole Time-of-Flight and Orbitrap

Quadrupole time-of-flight (QTOF) and Orbitrap instruments merge the TOF advantage of high mass resolution and the MS/MS advantage of mass filtering and fragmentation in one instrument. These instruments operate in the same manner as MS/MS instruments, but they provide high-resolution measurements for both precursor and product ions present in the acquired mass spectra. The resolution of a mass spectrometer is defined as the measured mass of an analyte divided by the full width of the corresponding peak at half maximum (FWHM). TOF analyzers typically achieve resolutions of 10,000 to 100,000 FWHM, whereas Orbitrap analyzers can achieve resolutions of 100,000 to 250,000 FWHM. Unlike TOF analyzers, which calculate the time it takes for ions to traverse a flight tube, Orbitrap analyzers measure the stable orbit of an ion. Ions are injected tangentially to an electric field

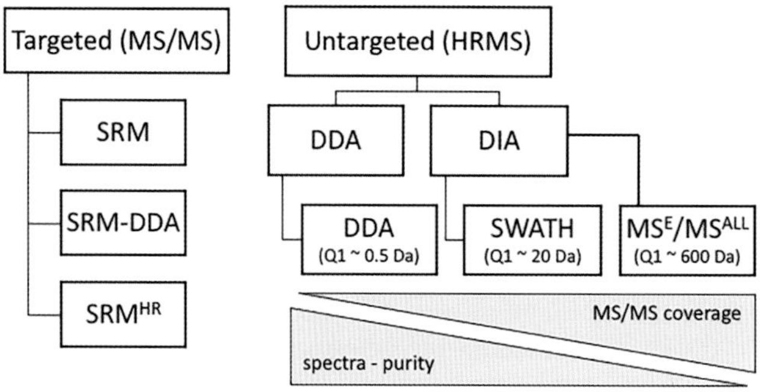

Figure 12-2. Targeted and untargeted approaches to broad-spectrum drug testing. Data can be acquired in a targeted or untargeted manner using tandem mass spectrometry (MS/MS) or high-resolution mass spectrometry (HRMS). Targeted approaches include selected reaction monitoring (SRM), SRM followed by data-dependent acquisition of product ion spectra (SRM-DDA), or SRM using an HRMS (SRM^{HR}). Untargeted approaches can be divided into two main categories: DDA or data-independent acquisition (DIA). Data-independent strategies include MS^E, MS^{ALL}, and Sequential Windowed Acquisition of all Theoretical fragment-ion spectra (SWATH). The Q1 isolation window varies significantly between the different untargeted approaches and will significantly impact the MS/MS spectra coverage and purity.

between an outer barrel and inner spindle-like electrode. The stable orbit achieved by an ion is proportional to the *m/z* ratio. Compound identification using an LC-Orbitrap or LC-QTOF instrument is based on retention time, accurate mass, molecular formula, isotope pattern, and mass spectral matching. The major disadvantage of these technologies in the clinical laboratory is the expense of the instrumentation and the technical expertise required for method development, implementation, and routine use.

Targeted Versus Untargeted Mass Spectral Data Acquisition

Analytical approaches for broad-spectrum drug testing can be classified according to the instrumentation used, as highlighted in the above sections, or by the nature of the mechanism used for data acquisition. There are targeted and untargeted approaches to data acquisition. Targeted approaches require the use of analytical standards for all compounds of interest early in the development of the analytical method. Thus, a list of compounds of interest must be established, and a method must be designed specifically to detect that menu of drugs and metabolites. For LC-MS/MS methods, compound-dependent instrument parameters must be established for each compound of interest. The most common targeted approaches using a tandem mass spectrometer include SRM and SRM-DDA (described above and shown in Figures 12-1 and 12-2). Because of the targeted nature of MS/MS methods, they are usually more sensitive and specific for analytes of interest compared with full-scan untargeted approaches. In addition, most drugs and metabolites of interest for broad-spectrum testing can be incorporated into one MS/MS-based method. However, targeted methods are not capable of detecting all possible intoxicants in broad-spectrum drug testing, thereby presenting a major disadvantage to this approach. Targeted approaches can also be used with HRMS instruments. HRMS methods can be designed to specifically detect specified target masses and acquire product ion spectra only for the designated masses; such methods are often referred to as *SRM-high resolution (SRM^{HR})*. The resulting extracted ion chromatograms for the target precursor mass and one or more resulting product ion masses can be analyzed in a manner similar to SRM data analysis using a nominal mass tandem mass spectrometer. In addition, full high-resolution product ion spectra are still available for identification, if desired. This approach allows for higher sensitivity for the designated compounds, while still providing high-resolution data, however it does not fully capitalize on the power of HRMS instruments for the identification of unknown intoxicants.

All untargeted approaches to data acquisition start with a full scan of all masses in a specified mass range. Untargeted approaches are not limited to high-resolution instruments. For tandem mass spectrometers, a full scan can precede a subsequent data-dependent scan for the acquisition of a product ion spectra (MS-DDA). In this approach, compound identification is based on nominal mass, retention time, and a library match of the acquired product ion spectrum. While this data acquisition approach is untargeted, the ability to identify true unknowns will be limited by the availability of an analytical standard for retention time confirmation and spectral matching to a preexisting mass spectrum in the library used for data analysis. In this regard, the approach is still limited by available data resources. Numerous compounds can have the same nominal mass, and thus nominal mass alone provides limited information for the identification of a compound. Also, product ion spectra are collected on the basis of data-dependent information. For example, a method may be designed to only acquire product ion spectra for the three most abundant ions at any given time throughout the analytical run, which may limit the spectral coverage for all masses present in the sample.

DDA approaches are common for broad-spectrum drug testing using HRMS (HRMS-DDA). In this approach, only a user-defined number of the most abundant precursor ions at a given time in an analytical run (often 10 to 20 per acquisition cycle) are selected for secondary fragmentation and subsequent identification from a spectral library. This approach can have disadvantages for the detection of low-concentration drugs and metabolites in the background of complex biological matrices such as urine and blood. There may be 10 to 20 more-abundant small molecules (endogenous or exogenous) co-eluting with a toxin of interest, precluding the collection of a product ion spectra for identification.

DIA approaches can also be used with HRMS instruments (Figure 12-2). These approaches include MS^E, MS^{ALL}, and Sequential Windowed Acquisition of all Theoretical fragment-ion spectra (SWATH). MS^E and MS^{ALL} data acquisition approaches make use of alternating low-energy CID and high-energy CID, where the former is used to obtain precursor ion accurate mass and the latter is used to obtain the accurate mass of the product ions. The major disadvantage to these approaches is that the precursor mass is not selected and specifically fragmented, but rather all co-eluting masses are fragmented at the same time using high-energy CID. The acquired mass spectra therefore do not correspond to one specified mass, and thus the lack of purity can limit the ability to match acquired spectra with mass spectra in spectral libraries. One advantage is that no mass spectral data are lost because there is no selection of masses for further data acquisition. In theory, for these approaches, fragment information is collected for all masses in the specified mass range providing high MS/MS coverage.

SWATH is a data acquisition approach that allows for the collection of product ion spectra of all masses in a specified mass range like MS^E/MS^{ALL}, but it provides higher purity spectra. Small mass windows (typically approximately 20 Da wide) are specified and selected for subsequent fragmentation. The acquisition method sequentially steps through these windows in one data acquisition cycle covering the entire mass range before it repeats. A data acquisition cycle that steps through all the mass windows is typically only about 1 second in duration, allowing for multiple cycles per analytical run. The resulting product ion spectra that are collected correspond to the cumulative products of all masses in the corresponding mass window at a given time and are therefore less pure than spectra acquired using data-dependent strategies, but more pure than MS^E/MS^{ALL} spectra. The major advantage compared with DDA approaches is that no spectral data are lost.

Recent studies have begun to explore the utility of SWATH for broad-spectrum drug testing in forensic cases and have shown promising results.[11,12] When comparing both SWATH and DDA in the same samples, SWATH was found to identify more unique compounds, with the additional finding that DDA did not trigger the collection of product ion spectra for approximately 10% of substances because of low concentration and/or high matrix background. Despite these promising findings, further studies are needed to determine the utility of SWATH in clinical toxicology laboratories and how it compares to the different approaches of data acquisition described in this section.

High-Resolution Mass Spectrometry Data Analysis

High-resolution mass spectrometry data sets can be analyzed retrospectively using a combination of techniques, which can extend the drug detection capabilities for a broad-spectrum drug test. Most laboratories using HRMS in production settings perform untargeted data collection but analyze data in a targeted manner. To perform targeted data analysis, a laboratory must first analyze a reference standard to determine the expected characteristics of a given compound, specifically retention time and fragmentation pattern. The retention time and product ion spectra for each reference standard are entered into a data analysis database/library for future drug identification in clinical samples. One of the most challenging aspects of implementing an HRMS drug test is establishing appropriate targeted data analysis parameters for compound identification. Unlike other types of mass spectrometry data, guidelines for HRMS data analysis and acceptability criteria have not been established. Although laboratories have published on the utility of HRMS for drug testing, few have included details on how they determined allowable errors and set positivity criteria. One study described a combined scoring approach using a threshold of 70 (out of 100), with 70% weight given to library match and 10% weight given to each of mass error, retention time error, and isotope pattern difference, which provided a drug identification efficiency of 99.2%.[13] The experimental findings from this study demonstrate the importance of library matching in accurately identifying compounds and underscore the utility of robust product ion spectra that contain information on the lineage, mass, and relative abundance of fragments. With careful selection of error limits and positivity criteria for targeted data analysis, HRMS instruments can produce high-quality, high-confidence results that reduce the need for any subsequent testing.

In addition to targeted data analysis of HRMS data, an alternate technique known as *suspect screening* can be used. In suspect screening, compounds can be tentatively identified without the use of reference standards. Instead, predicted or intrinsic characteristics of a compound—such as the accurate mass, isotope pattern, and product ion spectrum—are used to determine its presence in a sample. The fact that reference standards are not required a priori makes this data analysis approach very attractive, especially for the ever-changing landscape of the illicit drug market. Suspect screening using HRMS has been used in several contexts, including analysis of pharmaceuticals, pesticides, and veterinary drug residues in a variety of matrices.[14-19] Most of the literature does not focus on the analytical performance of suspect screening, nor does it address the validation of a suspect screen. Although suspect screening and HRMS have been used for toxicology casework in a handful of laboratories, the technique has not been widely adopted yet, and guidelines for validation do not exist. In one study that evaluated the use of suspect screening in clinical toxicology, a screen using accurate mass, isotope pattern, and product ion library matching was able to identify more than 80% of the drugs that were present in clinical samples.[20] The inclusion of product ion spectral matching produced the largest decrease in false-discovery and false-negative rates as compared with suspect screening using mass alone or using only mass and isotope pattern. Suspect screening shows significant potential promise for clinical toxicology; however, it is imperative that freely available, fully transferable HRMS product ion spectral libraries be developed before widespread adoption.

Finally, HRMS data can be analyzed in an untargeted manner. Data analysis software programs can extract a user-defined number of masses and associated isotope patterns and mass spectra from a data file. The top predicted formulas for a given exact mass are displayed and can be searched using freely available databases. Although this approach is a possibility, it is very time consuming and is not currently used routinely in clinical toxicology laboratories.

Clinical Validation of a Broad-Spectrum Drug Test

There are no specific regulatory guidelines pertaining to qualitative broad-spectrum drug testing in the clinical laboratory. Also, although there are guidelines (eg, Clinical and Laboratory Standards Institute [CLSI] document C62, *Liquid Chromatography-Mass Spectrometry Methods*) pertaining to the development and clinical validation of quantitative targeted LC-MS methods, there are no such guidelines pertaining to broad-spectrum drug testing. In keeping with the theme, there are also no US Food and Drug Administration (FDA)–approved methods for broad-spectrum drug testing, and thus all methods utilized in clinical laboratories are designated *laboratory-developed tests* and must be analytically and clinically validated by each individual laboratory. At a minimum, laboratories should follow standard laboratory guidelines set forth by CLSI on the clinical validation and routine quality assessment of qualitative tests. In the future, guidelines must be established in order to enable widespread implementation of the various analytical approaches for broad-spectrum drug testing.

Advantages of High-Resolution Mass Spectrometry Highlighted in Published Case Series and Reports

The true advantages of HRMS for clinical toxicology are best highlighted in individual clinical cases and case series. This section will highlight the use of HRMS in the author's laboratory through the discussion of published cases. With the emergence of novel psychoactive substances (NPS) and synthetic drugs, targeted mass spectrometric methods are not ideal for their detection. Often a new drug emerges before the availability of an analytical standard for method development. In these situations, an untargeted data acquisition approach followed by targeted and suspect data analysis (described above) is ideal. This approach has been used for several cases involving NPS and other synthetic drugs.

In 2014, an 18-year-old man presented with hallucinations and agitation that progressed to status epilepticus.[21] The urine toxicology screen was positive only for cannabinoids and opioids. Using HRMS with suspect data analysis, a phenylethylamine named 2,5-dimethoxy-4-chloroamphetamine (DOC) was identified and later confirmed by comparison to a reference standard. DOC is a 5-hydroxytryptamine (5-HT2) receptor agonist with hallucinogenic effects. On the basis of chemical similarity of DOC to other epileptogenic amphetamines and a negative workup for other causes of seizures, DOC was determined to be the cause of the patient's status epilepticus. In addition to the detection of DOC, HRMS with suspect data analysis was used for the detection of 4-fluoroamphetamine (4-FA) in another case involving an 18-year-old man presenting to the emergency department with vomiting, shortness of breath, chest tightness, and altered mental status that progressed to cardiogenic shock.[22] This was the first reported case of 4-FA clinical poisoning and allowed for the dissemination of information regarding the risk of life-threatening toxicity—including cardiomyopathy, cardiogenic shock, and pulmonary edema—after recreational use.

HRMS has also been useful for the identification of emerging synthetic drugs and understanding public health outbreaks involving multiple opioid overdoses in specific geographical regions. In late 2015, the California Poison Control System–San Francisco division identified eight patients who experienced adverse effects associated with the ingestion of street-purchased "Xanax" pills.[23] The patients experienced prolonged sedation, unilateral weakness, paresthesias, and, in some cases, death due to severe respiratory depression. Patient serum samples and the pills were analyzed using HRMS and found to contain primarily fentanyl and etizolam, a benzodiazepine analog that is not approved for use in the United States. These findings led to a coordinated response that included the poison control system, clinical toxicology laboratory, state and public health departments, media outlets, and local law enforcement agencies. The analytical testing of these cases in real time, followed by rapid communication with media outlets and health care agencies, led to a prompt end to the outbreak and potentially resulted in lives saved. Subsequently, in early 2016, there was another opioid overdose outbreak in San Francisco involving the use of street-purchased "Norco" (hydrocodone/acetaminophen).[24] The product and samples from seven cases were analyzed by HRMS and found to contain primarily fentanyl and promethazine. Promethazine, a phenothiazine derivative, is routinely prescribed for the treatment of nausea, vomiting, and motion sickness. Promethazine use has been reported to be common among chronic opioid users and is thought to potentiate the "high" from opioids.[25] The use of HRMS allowed for real-time analysis and rapid notification of the outbreak by the public health department.

Subsequent to these outbreaks, another patient was found unconscious, with symptoms of an opioid overdose.[26] His urine drug screen was only positive for benzodiazepines but later did not confirm positive for any benzodiazepines prescribed in the US. Using HRMS, the urine and serum were found to contain the novel synthetic opioid U-47700 and the non–FDA-approved benzodiazepine phenazepam. Phenazepam is a full GABA-A receptor agonist with high abuse potential. It is not currently a controlled substance in the US and can be purchased on the internet as a "research chemical." The patient later confirmed that both were purchased on the darknet using decentralized digital money. This case raised awareness regarding the availability of both synthetic drugs and their potential life-threatening side effects.

In addition to synthetic amines, benzodiazepines, and opioids, synthetic cannabinoids have also emerged in recent years. They produce unpredictable side effects and, in some cases, are life-threatening. In the summer of 2018, a 25-year-old man presented to an emergency department in St Louis with gross hematuria, retroperitoneal hematomas, epistaxis, easy bruising, nausea/vomiting, cramping, and weakness.[27] With high-dose intravenous phytonadione and fresh-frozen plasma, the coagulopathy was corrected. HRMS identified the long-acting vitamin K antagonist brodifacoum and a metabolite of the synthetic cannabinoid AB-FUBINACA in the patient's serum. This case was one of 155 cases identified in the Midwest characterized by unexplained bleeding, high international normalized ratios (INRs; range from 5 to >20 [normal <1/1]), and reported use of synthetic cannabinoids in the previous 3 days.[28] This case highlights the fact that the synthetic cannabinoid supply chain is unregulated, resulting in variable product compositions that can be life-threatening.

Summary

This chapter highlights the different approaches that can be used for comprehensive drug testing in the clinical laboratory. In cases where drug overdose and acute drug toxicity are on the diagnostic differential, supportive care does not have to be the only approach to patient care. Comprehensive drug testing in real time can provide evidence to rule-in or rule-out drug exposure, thereby resulting in the most effective care and, potentially, a shorter hospital stay. It may also eliminate the need for subsequent medical workup and evaluation for other medical conditions. In the case of emerging illicit drugs, HRMS, utilizing untargeted data collection, can be a powerful tool for uncovering emerging drug use trends and raising awareness of ongoing overdose outbreaks.

References

1. Overdose Death Rates. National Institute on Drug Abuse. https://www.drugabuse.gov/related-topics/trends-statistics/overdose-death-rates. Updated January 2019. Accessed June 12, 2019.
2. Gummin DD, Mowry JB, Spyker DA, Brooks DE, Fraser MO, Banner W. 2016 Annual Report of the American Association of Poison Control Centers' National Poison Data System (NPDS): 34th Annual Report. *Clin Toxicol.* 2017;55(10):1072-1252.
3. Armenian P, Vo KT, Barr-Walker J, Lynch KL. Fentanyl, fentanyl analogs and novel synthetic opioids: a comprehensive review. *Neuropharmacology.* 2018;134(Pt A):121-132.
4. Johnston LD, Miech RA, O'Malley PM, Bachman JG, Schulenberg JE, Patrick ME. Monitoring the Future National Survey Results on Drug Use: 1975-2017. 2017 Overview: Key Findings on Adolescent Drug Use. Ann Arbor: Institute for Social Research, University of Michigan; 2018.
5. *World Drug Report 2017: Market Analysis of Synthetic Drugs: Amphetamine-Type Stimulants, New Psychoactive Substances.* United Nations Office on Drugs and Crime. http://www.unodc.org/wdr2017/field/Booklet_4_ATSNPS.pdf. May 2017. Accessed June 12, 2019.
6. Maurer HH, Pfleger K, Weber A. *Mass Spectral and GC-Data of Drugs, Poisons, Pesticides, Pollutants and Their Metabolites.* 3rd rev ed. Weinheim, Germany: Wiley-VHC; 2007.
7. Jansen R, Lachatre G, Marquet P. LC-MS/MS systematic toxicological analysis: comparison of MS/MS spectra obtained with different instruments and settings. *Clin Biochem.* 2005;38:362-372.
8. Ferrer I, Thurman EM. *Liquid Chromatography/Mass Spectrometry, MS/MS and Time of Flight MS.* Cary, NC: Oxford University Press; 2003.
9. Jiwan JL, Wallemacq P, Hérent MF. HPLC-high resolution mass spectrometry in clinical laboratory? *Clin Biochem.* 2011;44(1):136-147.
10. Wu AH, Gerona R, Armenian P, French D, Petrie M, Lynch KL. Role of liquid chromatography–high-resolution mass spectrometry (LC-HR/MS) in clinical toxicology. *Clin Toxicol.* 2012;50(8):733-742.
11. Roemmelt AT, Steuer AE, Poetzsch M, Kraemer T. Liquid chromatography, in combination with a quadrupole time-of-flight instrument (LC QTOF), with sequential window acquisition of all theoretical fragment-ion spectra (SWATH) acquisition: systematic studies on its use for screenings in clinical and forensic toxicology and comparison with information-dependent acquisition (IDA). *Anal Chem.* 2014;86(23):11742-11749.
12. Roemmelt AT, Steuer AE, Kraemer T. Liquid chromatography, in combination with a quadrupole time-of-flight instrument, with sequential window acquisition of all theoretical fragment-ion spectra acquisition: validated quantification of 39 antidepressants in whole blood as part of a simultaneous screening and quantification procedure. *Anal Chem.* 2015;87(18):9294-9301.
13. Colby JM, Thoren KL, Lynch KL. Optimization and validation of high-resolution mass spectrometry data analysis parameters. *J Anal Toxicol.* 2017;41(1):1-5.
14. Bade R, Rousis NI, Bijlsma L, et al. Screening of pharmaceuticals and illicit drugs in wastewater and surface waters of Spain and Italy by high resolution mass spectrometry using UHPLC-QTOF MS and LC-LTQ-Orbitrap MS. *Anal Bioanal Chem.* 2015;407:8979-8988.
15. Moschet C, Piazzoli A, Singer H, Hollender J. Alleviating the reference standard dilemma using a systematic exact mass suspect screening approach with liquid chromatography-high resolution mass spectrometry. *Anal Chem.* 2013;85:10312-10320.
16. González-Mariño I, Gracia-Lor E, Bagnati R, Martins CPB, Zuccato E, Castiglioni S. Screening new psychoactive substances in urban wastewater using high resolution mass spectrometry. *Anal Bioanal Chem.* 2016;408:4297-4309.
17. López A, Yusà V, Millet M, Coscollà C. Retrospective screening of pesticide metabolites in ambient air using liquid chromatography coupled to high-resolution mass spectrometry. *Talanta.* 2016;150:27-36.
18. Solliec M, Roy-Lachapelle A, Sauvé S. Development of a suspect and non-target screening approach to detect veterinary antibiotic residues in a complex biological matrix using liquid chromatography/high-resolution mass spectrometry. *Rapid Commun Mass Spectrom.* 2015;29:2361-2373.
19. Samanipour S, Baz-Lomba JA, Alygizakis NA, Reid MJ, Thomaidis NS, Thomas KV. Two stage algorithm vs commonly used approaches for the suspect screening of complex environmental samples analyzed via liquid chromatography high resolution time of flight mass spectroscopy: a test study. *J Chromatogr A.* 2017;1501:68-78.
20. Colby JM, Thoren KL, Lynch KL. Suspect screening using LC-QqTOF is a useful tool for detecting drugs in biological samples. *J Anal Toxicol.* 2018;42(4):207-213.
21. Burish MJ, Thoren KL, Madou M, Toossi S, Shah M. Hallucinogens causing seizures? A case report of the synthetic amphetamine 2,5-dimethoxy-4-chloroamphetamine. *Neurohospitalist.* 2015;5(1):32-34.

22. Al-Abri S, Meier KH, Colby JM, Smollin CG, Benowitz NL. Cardiogenic shock after use of fluoroamphetamine confirmed with serum and urine levels. *Clin Toxicol.* 2014;52(10):1292-1295.
23. Arens AM, van Wijk XM, Vo KT, Lynch KL, Wu AH, Smollin CG. Adverse effects from counterfeit alprazolam tablets. *JAMA Intern Med.* 2016;176(10):1554-1555.
24. Vo KT, van Wijk XM, Lynch KL, Wu AH, Smollin CG. Counterfeit Norco poisoning outbreak—San Francisco Bay area, California, March 25-April 5, 2016. *MMWR Morb Mortal Wkly Rep.* 2016;65(16):420-423.
25. Lynch KL, Shapiro BJ, Coffa D, Novak SP, Kral AH. Promethazine use among chronic pain patients. *Drug Alcohol Depend.* 2015;150:92–97.
26. Vo KT, van Wijk XM, Wu AH, Lynch KL, Ho RY. Synthetic agents off the darknet: a case of U-47700 and phenazepam abuse. *Clin Toxicol.* 2017;55(1):71-72.
27. Riley SB, Sochat M, Moser K, et al. Case of brodifacoum-contaminated synthetic cannabinoid. *Clin Toxicol (Phila).* 2019;57(2):143-144.
28. Moritz E, Austin C, Wahl M, et al. Notes from the field: outbreak of severe illness linked to the vitamin K antagonist brodifacoum and use of synthetic cannabinoids—Illinois, March-April 2018. *MMWR Morb Mortal Wkly Rep.* 2018;67:607-608.

Chapter 13

Method Validation in Toxicology Testing

Wieslaw Furmaga, MD, MS
Yashpal Agrawal, MD, PhD

Introduction

Laboratory testing is important in the diagnosis, treatment, and monitoring of patients who have used or abused drugs, in a clinical, legal, or forensic setting. Knowledge about test validation is a key component of the College of American Pathologists (CAP) position statement on the ongoing opioid crisis.[1]

This chapter is written with three goals: (1) to help new laboratory directors with responsibilities in directing the clinical toxicology section of the laboratory become aware of special considerations in method validation of toxicology assays and laboratory-developed tests (LDTs); (2) to provide background information with relevant references in a simplified form as it applies to the validation of clinical toxicology assays and, particularly, LDTs; and (3) to clarify method validation concepts listed in the CAP accreditation checklists, emphasizing key requirements for the validation of LDTs. These ideas will be most useful for laboratories that need to validate an occasional LDT. It is not our intention to duplicate the formal Clinical and Laboratory Standards Institute (CLSI) documents that provide detailed guidance on each of the test validation steps, or the forensic toxicology guidelines by the Scientific Working Group for Forensic Toxicology (SWGTOX) group,[2] or the US Food and Drug Administration (FDA) test validation guidance to industry.[3] Workplace drug testing is covered in chapter 6.

Screening Versus a Confirmatory Toxicology Test

In general, toxicology testing comprises a two-step procedure. The initial screening step is usually a qualitative assay, and any presumptive positive results are followed up with a confirmatory step, which may be a qualitative or quantitative test.

Screening Tests

The initial screening test is predominantly an immunoassay for a specific drug or class of drugs. Immunoassays are commonly chosen by clinical laboratories because of their relative simplicity, low cost, potential to provide 24-hour availability, and the highly automated nature of immunoassays when performed on an autoanalyzer. A common example is the urine drugs-of-abuse screening test, which looks for various drug groups (eg, opiates, cocaine, barbiturates, benzodiazepines, amphetamines, tetrahydrocannabinol, methadone, phencyclidine). Any result equal to or above the test cutoff is labeled as a *presumptive positive* and may be followed by a confirmatory test. Immunoassay methods use antibodies for detection of the drug or class of drugs in question. Antibodies can express cross-reactivities with respect to a particular drug or class of drugs, which may cause false-positive and false-negative results with respect to co-administration of prescribed or nonprescribed drugs. For this reason, a positive drug-screening result must be followed with a confirmatory test, especially in situations dealing with legal samples, preemployment testing, before organ transplantation, neonatal testing, and so forth. With the availability of advanced mass spectrometry assays, some large laboratories choose to perform the initial screening of drug compounds using that technology because it provides high accuracy with lower reagent costs.

Confirmatory Testing

Confirmatory testing usually follows screening results, especially when a positive result is unexpected or if such testing is clinically indicated. The rationale behind using a confirmatory test is to use a different physicochemical analysis principle than that used for the initial drug screening. Commonly used confirmatory testing methodologies include high-pressure liquid chromatography (HPLC) using various physicochemical principle–based separation columns, gas chromatography–mass spectrometry (GC-MS), or liquid chromatography–mass spectrometry (LC-MS). Mass spectrometric confirmation is the preferred method for confirmatory testing.

Qualitative Versus Quantitative Testing in Toxicology

Qualitative assays play an important role in clinical and forensic toxicology. They assess the presence or absence of a particular drug or analyte in the specimen and are used when precise measurement of the analyte concentration is not needed. The most popular qualitative toxicology test is urine screening for drugs of abuse, which is reported as negative (below the cutoff concentration) or positive (equal to or above the cutoff concentration) for the presence of tested analyte. Thus, on the basis of the cutoff used and the cross-reactivity of the antibodies, false-positive and false-negative results can occur. According to the CAP Laboratory Accreditation Program, the desirable cutoff separating a positive from a negative result should be established or verified initially during the validation process and needs to be reconfirmed at least every 6 months (*Chemistry and Toxicology Checklist* item CHM.13750) or at changes of reagent lots of analytically critical reagents. It is good laboratory practice to clearly state the test cutoff, instrument platform, and methodology used in the report. For clinical testing, the cutoff should provide the highest possible sensitivity or negative predictive value and, for medicolegal purposes, the highest specificity and positive predictive value.

Quantitative testing gives a numerical value of analyte concentration, and it is used when toxicity is suspected or for therapeutic drug monitoring (see chapter 10, *Pharmacogenomic Testing*).

FDA Terminology and Approval Processes for Commercially Available New Tests

The FDA considers laboratory tests as "medical devices" or "in vitro diagnostic products" (IVDs).[4] The definition of *device* applies equally to IVDs made by conventional device manufacturers and to those produced by laboratories. An IVD therefore meets the device definition, regardless of where and by whom it is manufactured.

In Vitro Diagnostic Products

In vitro diagnostic products are those reagents, instruments, and systems intended for use in diagnosis of disease or other conditions in order to cure, mitigate, treat, or prevent disease or its sequelae. Such products are intended for use in the collection, preparation, and examination of specimens taken from the human body.

The FDA classifies IVD products into Class I, II, or III according to the level of regulatory control that is necessary to assure safety and effectiveness. This classification determines the appropriate premarket process. As device class increases, the regulatory controls also become more stringent, with Class I devices subject to the least stringent and Class III devices subject to the most stringent regulatory control.

Class I (low- to moderate-risk) devices can be monitored using general controls and, unless exempt, require a 510(k) process. Class II (moderate- to high-risk) devices need general controls and special controls and, unless exempt, require a 510(k) process. Class III (high-risk) devices need general controls and premarket approval (PMA). To search the classification of a device or for further details, one can either review the device classification database[5] or the medical specialty panel[6] to which it belongs.

General Controls

General controls does not refer to the quality controls (QC) that laboratories run in relation to tests. The term *general controls* indicates requirements to register the device with the FDA, manufacture of the device under good manufacturing processes, detailed product description on use of the device, and the use of a 510(k) premarket notification process, among other things.

Special Controls

Special controls are used where general controls are insufficient to provide reasonable assurance of the safety and effectiveness of the device. These are usually device specific and may include performance standards, postmarket surveillance, patient registries, special labeling requirements, premarket data requirements, and guidelines for use.

510(k) Process

A 510(k) is a premarket submission made to the FDA to demonstrate that the device to be marketed is at least as safe and effective as—that is, is substantially equivalent to—a legally marketed device (21 CFR 807.92(a)(3)) that is not subject to PMA.[7] Submitters must compare their device to one or more similar legally marketed devices and make and support their substantial equivalence claims.

Premarket Approval

Premarket approval is the FDA process of scientific and regulatory review to evaluate the safety and effectiveness of Class III medical devices.[8] Class III devices are intended to be used in supporting or sustaining human life or preventing impairment of human health. Class III devices may present a potential unreasonable risk of illness or injury for which general controls and special controls are insufficient to provide reasonable assurance of the safety and effectiveness of a device or there is insufficient information to make such a determination of risk.

After a test (IVD) has been approved by the FDA, it is categorized by its complexity[9] as waived or nonwaived.

Waived Versus Nonwaived Toxicology Tests

The Clinical Laboratory Improvement Amendments of 1988 (CLIA '88) regulations include federal standards applicable to all US facilities or sites that test human specimens for health assessment or to diagnose, prevent, or treat disease.

The categorization of tests as waived or nonwaived is done by the FDA after their approval, using criteria indicated in the CLIA regulations. The waived or nonwaived status of a test implies different validation and regulatory requirements. The complexity of a test (waived, moderate complexity, or high complexity) as determined by the FDA is commonly reviewed from a CLIA database,[10] the test package insert, or the FDA site for waived tests.[11]

Waived Tests

According to CLIA, a waived test must possess a low risk for an incorrect result. Waived tests include certain tests listed in the CLIA regulations, tests cleared by the FDA for home use, and tests approved for waiver by the FDA using the CLIA criteria. The CLIA regulations for the laboratories or sites performing waived testing are not as stringent as for the laboratories performing nonwaived assays. Waived-testing laboratories must be CLIA certified and must follow the manufacturer's kit instructions for the testing. Examples of common waived tests in toxicology include the multiple lateral flow immunoassays for urine drugs-of-abuse testing that are available from several manufacturers.

Nonwaived Tests

The term *nonwaived test* describes, collectively, moderate-complexity and high-complexity testing that can be performed by CLIA-certified laboratories and sites. For tests developed by the laboratory or that have been modified from the approved manufacturer's instructions, the complexity category defaults to high complexity per the CLIA regulations.

Nonwaived testing is subject to inspection every 2 years and must meet the CLIA quality system standards, such as those for proficiency testing, quality control, and personnel requirements. The standards for moderate-complexity and high-complexity testing differ only in the personnel requirements and are described in 42 CFR subparts H, J, K, and M.

Exceptions to Applicability of the CLIA Regulations

Exceptions to CLIA '88 regulations exist for certain testing, including employment-related drug testing by Substance Abuse and Mental Health Services Administration (SAMHSA)–certified laboratories, testing performed for forensic purposes (criminal investigations), and research or surveillance testing performed on human specimens in which patient-specific results are not reported (if the results are not used for diagnosis or treatment decisions). These exceptions to CLIA regulations should not be confused with the term *CLIA-exempt*.

CLIA-Exempt

CLIA-exempt refers to a laboratory (not a test system) and means a laboratory that has been licensed or approved by a state where the Centers for Medicare and Medicaid Services (CMS) has determined that the state has enacted laws relating to laboratory requirements that are equal to or more stringent than CLIA requirements, and the state licensure program has been approved by CMS.

Role of the FDA, CMS, and CLIA in Clinical Testing

The appearance of a new test on the market involves interactions between the manufacturer who develops the test, the FDA, CMS, CLIA regulations, and the clinical laboratories who offer the test to the public.

Centers for Medicare and Medicaid Services

CLIA regulates diagnostic laboratories and assures reliable and accurate results of patient testing. CMS oversight through the CLIA program is designed to confirm that a laboratory assesses *analytical validity,* but it does not confirm whether the results from an analytical validity assessment were sufficient to support the clinical claims (clinical validity; see FDA section, below). Analytical validity refers to acceptably demonstrated performance in the measurement or detection characteristics of a test, namely, how well the test measures or identifies something in a person, such as a protein or a gene mutation. CMS also issues laboratory certificates, performs inspections, and enforces regulatory compliance either by itself or by approving private accreditation organizations (grants them deemed status, for example, to the CAP and The Joint Commission), as well as monitors proficiency testing performance.

Food and Drug Administration

The FDA categorizes tests on the basis of their complexity and grants requests for waiver by application. *Clinical validity* is the acceptably demonstrated association of a test result with the presence or absence of the target disease/condition. CLIA regulations do not regulate the clinical validity of laboratory tests, such as their accuracy in diagnosing medical conditions or their efficiency in identification of a patient's predisposition or prognosis. These aspects of laboratory tests (clinical validity) are evaluated by the FDA under the Federal Food, Drug, and Cosmetic Act during the PMA process. During a PMA process, the FDA evaluates whether there is a reasonable assurance of analytical and clinical validities for the test. Under the same act, the FDA regulates manufacturers and ensures that offered "devices" are reasonably safe and effective.

FDA Approval

The practical meaning of FDA approval is that the test has undergone the PMA process and the FDA believes that the test performs at the analytical level claimed by the manufacturers and it can be used safely and efficiently by the clinical laboratory for the purposes stated by the producer. FDA approval does not guarantee analytical performance required by CLIA regulations; it is the laboratory performing the test that must confirm analytical performance required by CLIA.

FDA Cleared

"FDA cleared" means a test system has undergone the 510(k) process by the FDA and has been determined to be substantially equivalent to a test system already legally marketed for the same use. This could apply to waived, moderate-complexity, or high-complexity test systems.

What Constitutes a Laboratory-Developed Test?

Views on the definition and operational validation of laboratory-developed tests are evolving, and, as of 2018, the FDA has not finalized guidance[12,13] on LDTs, nor does it seem that new legislation is imminent from Congress. The text below therefore reflects a definition of LDT that is based on the 2018 CAP accreditation checklists in force at the time of writing this chapter.

Definition of a Laboratory-Developed Test

A laboratory-developed test is one that is used in patient management and has both of the following features: (1) the test is performed by the clinical laboratory in which the test was developed wholly or in part and (2) the test is neither FDA cleared nor FDA approved.

If the laboratory modifies (see the next section) an FDA-approved or FDA-cleared test, it becomes a modified FDA-approved/FDA-cleared test. In such instances, the modification will need to be validated by appropriate matrix studies, or a suitable literature reference may also be used. An example of a modified test is when creatinine is being measured in peritoneal fluid, which is a different matrix. The validation studies performed on serum creatinine can be used as long as accuracy, precision, reportable range, analytical sensitivity, analytical specificity, and reference range are also determined.

What is Modification of a Test?

Any change to the manufacturer's supplied ingredients or modifications to the assay as set forth in the manufacturer's labeling and instructions constitutes modification of a test. It may include a change of specimen type, instrumentation, or procedure that could affect the performance specifications for analytical sensitivity, analytical specificity, accuracy, or precision; or any change to the stated purpose of the test, its approved test population, or any claims related to interpretation of the results. Common examples include changes to the approved sample type (serum vs plasma vs body fluid), sample container (eg, EDTA vs heparin plasma), intended use, and so forth.

Verification Versus Validation of Test Performance

Verification of Test Performance

Verification is defined as a process by which the laboratory provides proof that an FDA-cleared/FDA-approved test performs according to the specifications in the manufacturer's test package insert.

Validation of Test Performance

Validation usually applies to LDTs or non–FDA-approved/non–FDA-cleared tests where the laboratory confirms that the test performs as intended. This chapter is directed toward CAP-accredited laboratories. Table 13-1 shows the minimum requirements for FDA-approved/FDA-cleared tests and LDTs.

Test Validation for Clinical Toxicology Laboratories

A source of user-friendly protocols that we use in our laboratories is the EP Evaluator software[14] from Data Innovations (Datainnovations.com). The suggestions and comments listed below regarding test validation will probably be most useful for CAP-accredited clinical laboratories. For a more comprehensive and formal validation process, the user is advised to refer to CLSI method validation protocols or the FDA Guidance to Industry.[3] Following are some key CAP checklist items for discussion (to avoid unnecessary duplication, not all CAP checklist items have been discussed or referenced).

Table 13-1. Minimum Test Verification/Validation Parameters for FDA-Cleared and FDA-Approved Tests and Laboratory-Developed Tests (LDTs)

Parameter	Minimum Test Verification Requirements for FDA-Approved/Cleared Nonwaived Tests in CAP-Accredited Laboratories	Recommended LDT Validation Requirements for CAP-Accredited Laboratories
Accuracy	X	X
Precision	X	X
AMR or Linearity and Calibration Verification	X	X
Carryover	X	X
Reference Interval/Decision Limit/Cutoffs	X	X
Analytical Sensitivity (LOD/LOQ)		X
Analytical Specificity (Interferences and Cross-Reactivity)		X
Stability (Specimen and Reagent)		X
Clinical Validity (Diagnostic Sensitivity/Diagnostic Specificity)		X

FDA, US Food and Drug Administration; CAP, College of American Pathologists; AMR, analytical measurement range; LOD, limit of detection; LOQ, limit of quantitation.

Test Validation Study and Performance Specifications

Before starting validation, it is strongly recommended that laboratories have a test validation plan (ie, how the individual steps of the validation will be performed, how many samples, what calibrators will be used, etc) and a definition of what will constitute acceptable test performance signed off by the medical director, for example, acceptable accuracy, precision, method comparison parameters (correlation coefficient or r, slope, intercept, etc). In this chapter, the term *analyte* is used interchangeably with the metrological term *measurand.*

Accuracy, precision, and analytical measurement range (AMR) are the first analytical characteristics to be validated for a new method or new instrument.

Accuracy of the assay assesses how close the test result is to the target value. The accuracy is expressed as the difference between the target value and the mean of repeat testing of the same sample. Changes in accuracy affect reference or therapeutic ranges for quantitative tests and cutoffs for qualitative tests. If the mean of the repeat testing of the same sample differs from a true value (eg, reference material), the test is inaccurate and its value is reflected in the bias of the method. If reference material is not available and samples are spiked with analyte, the term *relative recovery* may be used to estimate the bias in the method.

Use five to six specimens over the reportable range.[14] The points (five to six specimens) should also include medically relevant decision points, where possible. The points may be selected at the limit of quantitation (LOQ), as well as at the low, medium, and high parts of the assay range. A minimum of two (ideally three or more) replicates is recommended for each point. The specimen (point) passes accuracy if the observed mean is within the allowable systematic error (usually 25-50% of total error) of its assigned value. Accuracy can also be verified by comparing the results to a known definitive or reference method. For a discussion and list of commonly used total allowable errors and their tables, see Westgard.com or Datainnovations.com. If the laboratory wishes to determine the test's total error, it can be calculated by using the following formula: $\%TE = |\%bias| + 2\ CV$, where TE is total error and CV is coefficient of variation. The FDA suggests that accuracy should be within ±20% at the LOQ and ±15% elsewhere on the AMR.

CAP *All Common Checklist* item COM.40300: Accuracy is verified or established by comparing results to a definitive or reference method, or an established comparative method. Use of matrix-appropriate reference materials, patient specimens (altered or unaltered), or other commutable materials with known concentrations or activities may be used to verify or establish accuracy. The use of routine quality control materials or calibrators that were used to calibrate the method is not appropriate.

CAP *All Common Checklist* item COM.40350 applies to LDTs only and describes the minimum number of samples (minimum of 20) to be used when determining accuracy by comparing to a reference quantitative or qualitative method: For certain methods that test multiple analytes (eg, next-generation sequencing, FISH [fluorescence in situ hybridization], HPLC, GC-MS, MALDI-TOF [matrix-assisted laser desorption/ionization-time-of-flight]), analytic accuracy may be established for each method (not necessarily each analyte), as appropriate.

Precision of the test assesses the width of the spread of the value around the mean of the repeat testing of the same sample, expressed as a standard deviation or as the CV. The CV is calculated as the standard deviation divided by the mean, expressed as a percentage.

Repeatability is a form of precision that measures the agreement among the repeat tests of the same sample within the batch (intraassay, within-day repeatability) or among different batches (interassay, or over several days repeatability). Vendor package inserts use varying terminology, and thus it is important for the laboratory director to be aware of how the terms are used. Thus, one vendor refers to repeatability as the "within-run variation" and refers to interassay repeatability using the older term of "within-lab variation."

The data requirements to establish precision specifications using the CLSI guideline, *User Verification of Precision and Estimation of Bias,* are three replicates per run, one run per day, for a minimum of 5 days.[14,15] Our laboratory runs five replicates each day for 10 days (Monday-Friday), which yields 50 data points at the end of 2 weeks.

CAP *All Common Checklist* item COM.40310: Precision is verified or established by repeat measurement of samples at varying concentrations or activities within-run and between-run over a period of time.

Calibration, Linearity/Analytical Measurement Range, and Reportable Range

Calibration, linearity/AMR, and reportable range are usually reviewed together because they are interrelated. Routine calibration, linearity/AMR, frequency of testing, suitable materials, and so forth are not discussed in detail because these are generally well understood, and we refer the user to the CAP Accreditation Program 2018 *Chemistry and Toxicology Checklist* (CHM.13000, CHM.13100, CHM.13125, CHM.13400, and CHM.13500) and the CAP Calibration Verification/Linearity Survey Users' Guide,[16] which is extensively illustrated and well documented. Some salient issues regarding these terms are addressed below.

Calibration in Toxicology

Calibration establishes the relationship between instrument responses and concentrations. Linearity is a special case of such a relationship. The calibration material can be prepared in the laboratory by spiking a blank matrix with different amounts of analyte (drug or substance of interest), such that the final concentrations are close to the medically important decision points or they are evenly spaced through an entire AMR. The recommendation on the number of specimens and number of replicas per testing level varies, but it is better to use fewer concentrations (minimum of four) and higher replicates per concentration (minimum of five) than more concentrations with fewer repeats. If the AMR is over a three-log concentration, a minimum of six calibrators is suggested.

Linearity

Linearity is defined as the ability (within a given range) to provide results that are directly proportional to the concentration (amount) of the analyte in the tested sample. The linearity of a system is measured by testing individual levels of an analyte of known concentrations by formulation or through dilution of a single stock solution of known concentrations.[17] When the results are plotted against these values, the degree to which the plotted curve conforms to a straight line is a measure of the test system's linearity.

The results of the linearity experiment are charted using a mathematical model describing the relationship between analyte concentration and instrument-reagent system response.[16,17] The most common situation is to use a simple model, such as the linear regression model, but in a significant number of assays, a linear relationship may not be seen. In such cases, it is better not to force linearity, but rather to use the more appropriate second-order or third-order polynomial regression. A first-order polynomial gives a straight line ($y = a + bx$), the standard linear regression used by laboratories (Figure 13-1). The second-order polynomial (quadratic polynomial) describes a relationship where there is a curved response (up or down), and

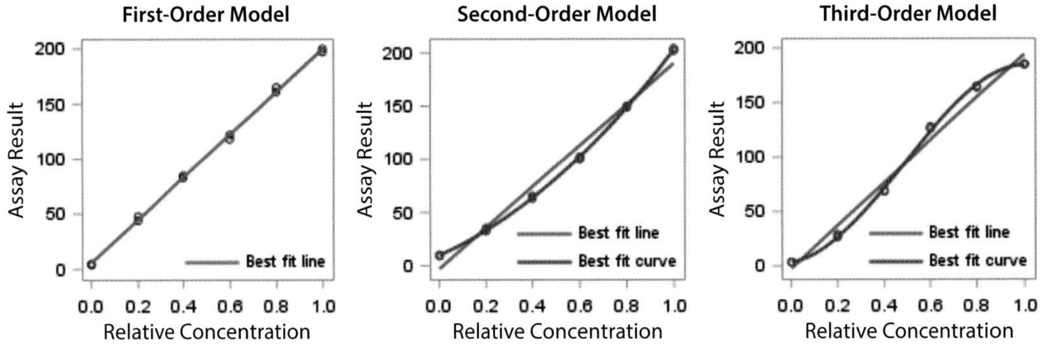

Figure 13-1. Regression models for calibration curves. The appropriate use of a linear regression model is shown in the first graph. In the second graph, the data points may result in an upward or downward curve, and a second-order polynomial (quadratic polynomial) fit should be used. In the third graph, when the data points show an S-shaped curve, a third-order polynomial (cubic polynomial) best fits the data. (Data kindly provided by R. Souers, College of American Pathologists.)

a third-order polynomial (cubic polynomial) fits situations where the response is changing across the levels (eg, a sigmoid response). In practice, users use commercially available software to do these calculations. Appendix 4 of the CAP Calibration Verification/Linearity Survey Users' Guide[16] provides a technical guide to linearity evaluation.

Analytical Measurement Range

The AMR is the range of analyte values that a method can directly measure on the specimen without any dilution, concentration, or other pretreatment that is not part of the usual assay process. Consequently, the reportable range can be wider than the AMR because, in addition to the AMR, it may combine a span of concentrations obtained by acceptable dilution or concentration procedures. When dilution of a high-concentration sample is performed, care must be taken to avoid matrix effects, such as by using analyte-free matrix to dilute the sample, when possible. The key 2018 CAP All Common and Chemistry and Toxicology checklist items are COM.40600 and CHM.13600, CHM.13710, CHM.13720, and CHM.13730.

Carryover

Carryover is defined as the contamination of a sample by the sample or reagent used immediately in the analysis before it. With advances in technology leading to the progressively lower volumes that are used for testing, carryover testing becomes particularly important.

CAP *Chemistry and Toxicology Checklist* items CHM.16800, CHM.21200, CHM.24400: There is a procedure for detection and evaluation of potential carryover. There are written procedures to minimize and detect contamination of results obtained by ICP [inductively coupled plasma]/MS. The laboratory evaluates its automatic pipetting systems for carryover.

Carryover studies are a part of the initial evaluation of the instruments and methods. The data from the studies performed by manufacturers may be used, but it still must be verified in a laboratory setting. In addition, carryover studies are recommended after major maintenance or repair of the pipetting assembly of the instrument. Carryover studies are not required if the instrument uses disposable pipette tips.

Rigorous designs of a carryover protocol have been described.[14] The proposed experiment (Figure 13-2) tests the transfer (carryover) of an analyte from a tube with high to low concentration and the transfer of a diluent from a tube with low to high concentration of analyte. A carryover of diluent or analyte may have a significant effect on the measured concentration of analyte when the instrument uses a small sample volume for analysis.

A less rigorous and simpler protocol for routine validations using three low samples and three high samples can also be used and is described in the CAP Serum Carryover (SCO) survey.[18]

Reference Intervals, Decision Limits, and Cutoffs

In toxicology, with respect to drugs, the use of therapeutic ranges and cutoffs is more relevant than the use of reference intervals. When reference intervals are needed, three approaches can be used by laboratories. These involve determination of the reference interval, transference of the reference interval, and verification of the manufacturer's reference interval. The applicable 2018 CAP *All Common Checklist* items are COM.50000 and COM.50100. We describe these principles below, but the reader is encouraged to refer to the CLSI guideline, *Defining,*

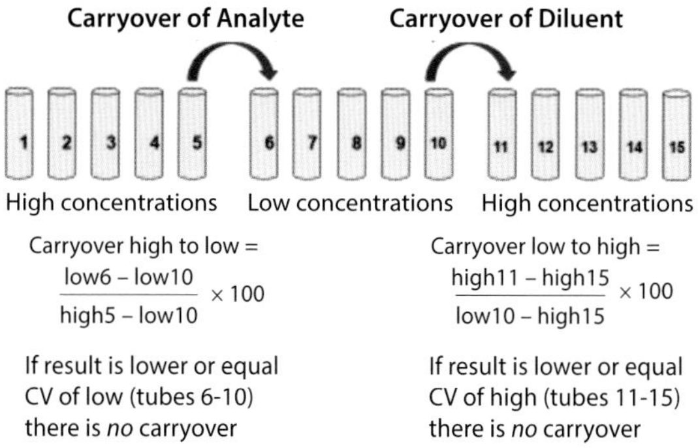

Figure 13-2. Example of a carryover experiment. The experiment is designed such that a series of five runs of a high-concentration specimen is followed by five runs of a low-concentration specimen and a final five runs of a high-concentration specimen. The carryover of analyte is identified when the calculated high-to-low carryover is larger than the imprecision (coefficient of variation [CV]) calculated for the low concentrations. The carryover of diluent is identified when the calculated low-to-high carryover is larger than the imprecision (CV) calculated for the high concentrations.

Establishing and Verifying Reference Intervals in the Clinical Laboratory, as a useful reference on reference intervals.[19]

Reference Intervals

The reference interval, more commonly termed the *reference range,* defines the central 95% distribution of analyte values in a population of apparently healthy men and women.[19] Reference interval determination is the process used in creating a reference interval de novo, encompassing all of the steps from selection of reference intervals, through exact details of the analytical methods, and concluding with data collection and analysis.

How measured. In brief, the standard recommendation is to use at least 120 individuals to perform a reference interval determination from a carefully selected reference population.[19] The lower and upper reference limits are at the 2.5th and 97.5th percentiles of a reference distribution of values. The outliers are excluded from the data by using the Dixon test or Tukey method as described in the CLSI guideline.[19] A less rigorous option of outlier removal is to use the Chauvenet's criterion, available widely online. The criterion for an outlier in a distribution with 20 values is any value beyond 2.24 SD of the mean and any value beyond 3.00 SD of the mean for 100 values. This approach can be used when the distribution of values is bell shaped (Gaussian, parametric distribution). If the distribution is not bell shaped—in other words, it is skewed to the left or right (a non-Gaussian or nonparametric distribution)—the data are usually logarithmically transformed before determination of the 2.5th and 97.5th percentiles.

When 120 individuals are selected as the reference population, the lower limit of the 2.5th percentile and the upper limit of the 97.5th percentile reflect a 90% confidence interval (CI). To obtain a CI of 95% for these same percentiles, 146 individuals need to be studied, and 210 individuals studied if a 99% CI is desired.

Transferring a Reference Interval

Transferring a reference interval is the process by which one may be able to adapt a previously established reference interval to a new analytical method or instrument.

As discussed above, the determination of a reference interval can be a daunting task for resource-limited laboratories. Thus, in many cases, the best solution would be to transfer the reference interval from one laboratory or instrument to another. In general, if the instrumentation is the same or of comparable accuracy and the patient population is similar, one could transfer a previously established reference interval to the new assay.

As an example, when two assays are compared and a regression equation is obtained that is:

$y = 1.002x - 0.520$, with $r = 0.999$.

In this equation, the correlation coefficient r is very high (0.999), the slope is a near-perfect 1.002, and the intercept is small, at -0.520.[19] If the studied populations are similar, this is a good example where transference of a reference interval is justified. The new reference ranges are calculated by substitution for x in the equation, where x represents the upper and lower reference limits, for example, 50 and 100. In this example, the new reference range would be 49.58 to 99.68, which could be rounded off to 50 to 100.

In case of a higher or lower slope (1.002 in the example), the equation can still be used, as long as the correlation coefficient is acceptably high. The significance of the absolute value of the intercept should be evaluated in relation to the reference interval. Thus, an intercept of 0.52 is small when compared to the reference interval of 50 to 100 and is not likely to be problematic. On the other hand, a potential intercept of 10 or 15 is relatively high and of concern in relation to the reference interval of 50 to 100 provided in this example. In such a case, the reference interval should be determined or verified. It is good laboratory practice to verify the reference range, even if transferring a reference interval is scientifically sound.

Regression Equations

To compare two laboratory methods, it is traditional to plot the values from the old method on the x-axis and the values from the new method on the y-axis. Typically, one of three regression equations are used. Regular or standard linear regression assumes that the x-axis method values were determined without error (ie, this is the "gold standard" method) as compared with the y-axis method. Deming regression on the other hand assumes that neither the x-axis nor y-axis data were obtained without errors. The disadvantage of Deming regression is that it assumes that the ratio of the analytical variances is constant over the range of values studied. The third method, Passing-Bablok regression, is the most statistically robust method, but its calculation is complicated and is not available on all software programs. Compared with the previous regression methods, Passing-Bablok regression does not make any special assumptions regarding the variances of the samples (x or y), and the results do not depend on the assignment of the methods (or instruments) to x-axis or y-axis. Statistical texts should be consulted for more details on these equations.

Verifying a Reference Interval[19]

Verification of a reference interval is the process by which a laboratory ensures, with reasonable confidence and using a relatively small number of individuals, that a reference interval established elsewhere or transferred from another study can be used locally.

How performed. To verify a transferred or published reference interval, the laboratory identifies 20 reference individuals that are similar to the population studied in the original reference interval determination. After the outliers have been excluded, and if the results of no more than two of the 20 individuals lie within the original reference interval, the reference interval is considered verified. If results from three to four individuals lie outside the reference interval, the study must be repeated with another 20 reference individuals. Again, after the outliers have been excluded, and no more than two results from these additional 20 individuals lie outside the reference interval, the reference interval is considered verified. If a repeat verification study fails, a laboratory must either determine a new reference interval or evaluate whether the populations being studied are similar.

Decision Limits

Decision limits for an assay are usually determined by expert consensus/opinion and not used commonly in toxicology. When available, decision limits can be used in lieu of reference intervals. Thus, as an example, on the basis of expert opinion, a decision limit for cholesterol of less than 200 mg/dL could be desirable.

Therapeutic Ranges

Therapeutic ranges are not usually determined by the laboratory, nor is there a CAP requirement to do so. For this reason, it is best to obtain therapeutic ranges from the drug's package insert or derive them from the institution's clinical experience.

CAP *Chemistry and Toxicology Checklist* item CHM.29025: For the reporting of immunosuppressive drug results, the patient report contains all of the following:

1. Appropriate therapeutic ranges based on the test method used
2. Analytical method (all tests) and method platform (immunoassays only)
3. Elements required in GEN.41096

This is important in view of the variation in cross-reactivity of the drugs and their in vivo metabolites in immunoassays.

Cutoffs

A cutoff is defined as the test response point below which a qualitative or quantitative result is determined to be negative and at or above which the result is determined to be positive.[20]

The cutoff concentration is expressed relative to the calibrator used in the assay. A negative result does not exclude the presence of the drug in the sample but simply indicates that no drug is detectable by the assay. Cutoffs are selected on the basis of the purpose of the testing. For clinical use, a low cutoff (high sensitivity) is generally desirable because it prolongs the detection window of the drug being tested. In some situations, a laboratory may use more than one cutoff for different clinical applications (eg, to accommodate workplace drug testing).

CAP *Chemistry and Toxicology Checklist* item CHM.13750: For qualitative tests that use a quantitative cutoff value to distinguish positive from negative results, the analytic performance around the cutoff value is verified or established initially and reverified at least every six months thereafter.

Appropriate materials for validation of cutoffs are the same as those recommended by the CAP for calibration verification. In our laboratory, the samples used for cutoff testing contain concentrations that are about 25% above and 25% below the cutoffs being tested. This is done so as to account for the imprecision of the device at the cutoff level. This requirement does not apply to qualitative tests for which the laboratory is not able to access an actual numerical result from the instrument.

Analytical sensitivity is commonly referred to as the *lower limit of detection (LOD)*. The CAP *All Common Checklist* item COM.40400 applies. LOD is defined as the lowest concentration of analyte that can be differentiated from zero (blank matrix) in a testing system. There are two related terms, the *limit of blank* (LOB[21]) and the *limit of quantitation* (LOQ,[21] functional sensitivity). Of these, the LOB[22] is the highest measurement result that is likely to be observed when analyzing many replicates ($n = 10$ or more) of a blank sample (LOB = mean + 1.645 SD of blank sample). When establishing the LOB, the raw analytical signal value is preferred, if available, because many analyzers may automatically convert signal values up to a certain limit to a "zero concentration." The LOQ represents the lowest analyte concentration that can be measured with respect to predefined accuracy and precision goals and is also known as the functional sensitivity.

LOD. Usually 10 or more zero samples (blank matrix samples) and three nonzero samples (lowest value of calibrator) are run. The LOD is the lowest concentration[14,22] that corresponds to the LOB + 1.645 SD of the nonzero calibrator (LOD = LOB + 1.645 SD of nonzero calibrator).

LOQ. One option is to select the LOD or the lowest calibrator concentration as the LOQ if accuracy and precision are acceptable at that level.[2,14,22] Another option is to select a clinically relevant concentration at which accuracy and precision are acceptable. The third, most labor-intensive option is to perform a precision profile experiment (Figure 13-3) at low concentrations (see below). Five to 10 samples are prepared such that the concentration of the analyte increases logarithmically (as opposed to arithmetically) by a factor of 2 (eg, concentrations of 1, 2, 5, 10, 20, etc). Twenty aliquots at each concentration are made and frozen. Subsequently, one aliquot per day is tested, and the experiment continues for 20 days if 20 aliquots were frozen. The results are evaluated by plotting the precision (CV) against the concentrations of the analyte. The LOQ is the lowest concentration of analyte that can be measured with an acceptable CV. In toxicology, the acceptable CV at the LOQ level is usually 20%. LOD/LOQ is an important parameter, particularly in forensic toxicology, workplace testing, or doping applications.

Analytical specificity can be described as a freedom from interference or the ability of the assay to measure the targeted analyte and not structurally related components, such as chemically related drugs or metabolites of the parent drug. In other words, it involves examination of interference factors and cross-reactivity in the assay.

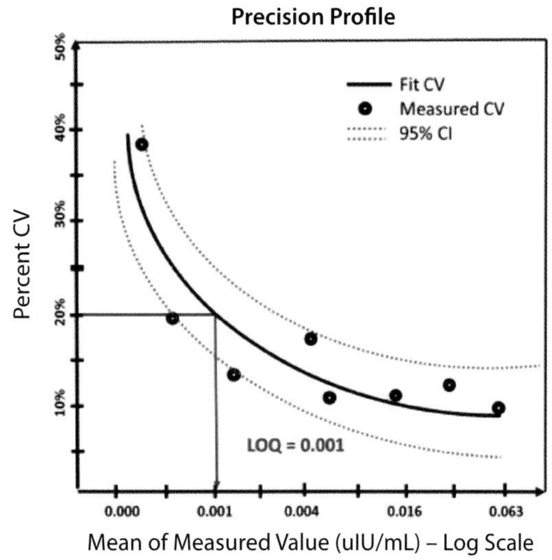

Figure 13-3. Precision profile experiment to determine the limit of quantitation (LOQ). Low concentrations of analyte are plotted against the observed precision (percent coefficient of variation [CV%]). The LOQ is the concentration at which an acceptable precision and accuracy are observed. In the figure, the lowest concentration of analyte with acceptable precision (CV of 20%) is approximately 0.001 uIU/mL.

CAP *All Common Checklist* item COM.40450: The analytical specificity refers to the ability of a test or procedure to correctly identify or quantify an entity in the presence of interfering or cross-reactive substances that might be expected to be present. Laboratories are encouraged to review the published literature for guidance and provided confidence intervals to estimated analytical specificity.

CAP *All Common Checklist* item COM.40500: Interfering substances may pose a significant problem for the clinical laboratory and health care providers who may be misled by laboratory results that do not reflect patient clinical status. The laboratory must be aware of common interferences by performing studies or referencing studies performed elsewhere (such as by the instrument-reagent manufacturer).

Interference

Interference is a cause of medically significant difference in analyte test result due to the effect of another component or property of the sample.[22] It may result from nonselectivity of the detection system, suppression of an indicator reaction, or some other cause of specimen-dependent difference.

For measurement of interference, the CLSI provides formal guidance in their documents,[23-25] including a list of interferents and the concentrations at which they should be tested. Simplified protocols based on the CLSI document, *Interference Testing in Clinical Chemistry,*[23] are available in EP Evaluator[14] or from Sun Diagnostics (New Gloucester, ME; sundiagnostics.us), which provides kits for testing common exogenous and endogenous interferents.

Cross-Reactivity

In toxicology, cross-reactivity usually refers to an interferent drug that is structurally similar to the analyte (drug) being measured and "cross-reacts" in the immunoassay.[23] The degree of cross-reactivity is regarded as a measure of selectivity of the assay. Cross-reactivity studies are designed to define the analytical specificity of the immunoassay for the specific analyte the assay is designed to detect.

How measured.[14,26] Ideally, cross-reactivity of an interferent should be tested both in the absence and presence of analyte, at a concentration near the upper limit of the concentration expected to be found in the patient's serum: % cross-reactivity = 100 (measured value − true value) / (concentration of cross-reactant).

However, the package inserts for many urine tests for drugs of abuse indicate determination of cross-reactivity by adding cross-reactive drugs to a negative urine so as to obtain a similar reaction at the cutoff of the assay using the assay calibrator. As an example, one urine drugs-of-abuse screening assay for benzodiazepines uses lormetazepam as the calibrator, with a 200-ng/mL cutoff value for a positive result. The assay cross-reacts with alprazolam and shows that an alprazolam concentration of 65 ng/mL has reactivity similar to 200 ng/mL lormetazepam. Cross-reactivity to various drugs is tested by adding these compounds, one at a time, to a negative urine specimen and determining the minimum concentration of the cross-reactive drug that provides a positive result similar to lormetazepam using the 200 ng/mL cutoff. If a low concentration of cross-reactive drug gives a positive result, that implies high cross-reactivity. If a high concentration of the cross-reactive drug is needed to turn the result positive, that implies low cross-reactivity to that particular drug. Therefore, if the laboratory were to use this assay to screen for a drug with low cross-reactivity, that particular drug must be specifically documented in the validation. Another common example is that very high concentrations of oxycodone are needed in urine to yield a positive result in the opiate drugs-of-abuse assay, which, in practice, may mean that the particular opiate assay is unsuitable for screening for oxycodone in most cases.

Stability of Analytes and Reagents

Analyte stability is the ability of the analyte to remain unchanged over a period of time, under varying storage conditions, and prior to the extraction or analysis. The required duration of stability that needs to be verified depends on the clinical setting of that assay. Thus, if a laboratory is required to add tests for up to 5 days after receiving the original sample, then the analyte stability should be tested for at least that period of time. Analyte stability is usually examined using different storage conditions (room temperature, 4°C, freeze-thaw, etc) and different specimen types and containers (serum, plasma, with EDTA, etc). CAP *All Common Checklist* item COM.40000 refers to the need for validating stability, particularly for LDTs and modified FDA-approved/FDA-cleared tests.

Reagent stability is the ability of an in vitro diagnostic (IVD) reagent to maintain its performance characteristics over time.[27] Reagent stability can be examined for different storage and transportation conditions, including its stability when loaded on to the instrument.

How measured.[14,27] If analyte stability at room temperature is being assessed, a sufficient number of aliquots for daily testing over the period of the study (eg, days 0, 1, 3, 5, and 7), with several replicates (usually three to five for each day of testing), must be prepared. The results are plotted with days of testing on the x-axis and the measured analyte values on the y-axis. The drift in analyte recovery over time is monitored by using regression of y-axis over x-axis. The allowable drift is predetermined, and usually it is around ±15%, or about 25% to 50% of the total allowable error for that analyte. If software is being used, confidence interval limits are plotted on the regression line at the level of 95%. Usually, only points outside the lower 95% confidence interval are significant (because many analytes decline with time). Alternatively and more simply, the observed drift and allowable bias at every time point can be compared to the analyte concentration at time zero.

Clinical Claims Validation

All clinical claims made by the laboratory need to be validated for LDTs or for FDA-cleared/FDA-approved tests for which the laboratory claims extend beyond what is indicated in the package insert. *Clinical claims* generally refers to the terms *clinical sensitivity* and *clinical specificity,* but it may also include *clinical utility* (effects of environment, economy, and patient outcomes), which is not discussed further in this publication.

Clinical sensitivity (diagnostic sensitivity) is defined as the proportion of patients with a well-defined clinical disorder whose test values are positive or above a decision limit. It refers to the assay's ability to detect subjects with the condition or disease.

Clinical specificity (diagnostic specificity) is defined as the proportion of patients without a specified clinical disorder whose test results are negative or below the decision limit. It refers to the assay's ability to distinguish subjects who do not have the condition or disease from those who have the condition or disease.

CAP *All Common Checklist* item COM.40640: Clinical claims include statements about a test's diagnostic sensitivity and specificity, ability to predict the risk of a disease or condition, clinical usefulness, or cost-effectiveness. Clinical claims may be found on the test report or in other information distributed by the laboratory (websites, test catalogs, newsletters, memoranda, advertisements, etc). Laboratories are not required to make clinical claims about a test, but any claims made by the laboratory must be validated. In order to adequately support a claim about diagnostic sensitivity, diagnostic specificity, and/or ability to predict risk of a disease or condition, the laboratory must perform a clinical validation study, unless the clinical validity of the test is documented in peer-reviewed literature or textbooks. The clinical validation study must include at least 20 samples and must include both positive and negative samples. If the laboratory uses fewer samples, the laboratory director must record the criteria used to determine the appropriateness of the sample size.

The usual method of determining clinical sensitivity and clinical specificity is by the use of ROC (receiver operator characteristics) curves using suitable software.[14] To make an ROC curve (Figure 13-4), one needs the patient's result and a gold-standard diagnostic test, which indicates whether the patient has or does not have the disease or condition.

The advantage of an ROC curve is that the clinical sensitivity and specificity at any cutoff can be read off the curve. The ROC curve can also be used to compare different assays, and the assay curve closest to the upper left corner of the plot is the one with the highest sensitivity and specificity. Similar information can also be gained by reviewing the assay's area under the curve (AUC), which is expressed as a number between 0.5 to 1.0, where 0.5 suggests the test is no better than a coin flip and 1.0 reflects a perfect test (100% sensitivity and specificity).

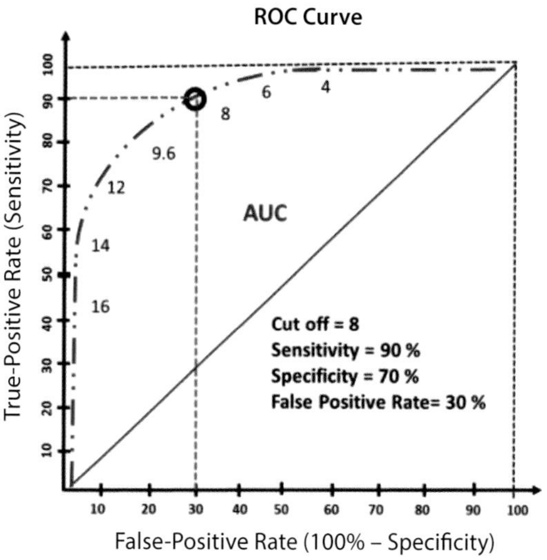

Figure 13-4. A typical receiver operator characteristics (ROC) curve. The analyte concentrations are plotted on the red line, and after selection of a cutoff concentration (eg, 8), the sensitivity and specificity can be read off the y-axis and x-axis, which, in this case, are 90% and 70%, respectively. AUC, area under the curve.

Liquid Chromatography–Mass Spectrometry Method Validation[28]

Chromatography refers to a number of techniques that separate components present in the sample on the basis of their physicochemical properties. During the process of separation, the sample is suspended in the mobile phase and is moved through or around a liquid or solid stationary phase. The mobile phase determines classification as either liquid or gas chromatography. Liquid chromatography predominates in today's market, and it can be subcategorized as high-performance/pressure liquid chromatography (HPLC) or ultra-high-pressure liquid chromatography (UHPLC). UHPLC generally refers to the ability to perform liquid chromatographic separations at high pressures (>600 bar using sub–2-micron-particle size columns). The type of columns used with HPLC/UHPLC vary, and examples include reverse phase columns, ion exchange chromatography, and size exclusion chromatography. Performance of thin-layer chromatography (TLC) on solid media–coated glass plates or on special paper dipped in solvents is an outdated technique and is used infrequently because of its low resolution.

Mass spectrometers are available in a wide variety of chromatography and mass spectrometer configurations.[29,30] In mass spectrometry, the specimen or analyte is first ionized using one of many possible mechanisms (electrospray ionization [ESI], atmospheric pressure chemical ionization [APCI], etc). During the second step, the precursor ion/product ion pairs are detected using various types of mass detectors (quadrupoles, tandem quadrupole, time of flight, etc). Currently, there are only a few FDA-approved LC-MS/MS tests (tacrolimus, vitamin D, and testing for inborn errors of metabolism as part of newborn screening), and most mass spectrometry–based assays in the toxicology laboratory are LDTs. It is beyond the scope of this chapter to discuss the details of mass spectrometric LDT assay validation. Accordingly, only aspects of LC-MS assay validation as they relate to key CAP checklist items are discussed. For details of LC-MS validations, the reader is referred to two recent publications.[31,32]

Sample Preparation for Mass Spectrometry

In some cases (eg, urine specimens), samples may be diluted and injected straight onto an HPLC column. In other cases, excess proteins, lipids, and so forth need to be removed (eg, vitamin D assay from blood) so that the mass spectrometer remains clean and interferences can be minimized. One of the important considerations in sample preparation is the possibility that the analyte may adhere to the sides of the tube, pipette tips, and so forth, which may produce significant inaccuracy in reported results. To minimize such error, an internal standard is used (discussed below). Samples in a complex matrix (eg, serum) need preparation, which can be done using one of many approaches, such as protein precipitation, liquid-liquid extraction, solid-phase extraction, and direct online injection of a diluted sample, or online solid-phase extraction followed by injection onto the main HPLC column. When using these sample preparation techniques, the aim is to use "orthogonal techniques," in other words, to use different principles of protein purification in the initial sample preparation step, followed by the analyte separation step.

CAP *Chemistry and Toxicology Checklist* Item CHM.16650: Appropriate controls are extracted and run through the entire procedure on each day of patient testing.

Controls used in chromatographic procedures must evaluate as much of the complete testing process as is technically feasible. The control process includes any pretreatment, prepurification, or extraction steps, unless nonpretreated control material is inappropriate. For qualitative assays, the negative and positive controls should be at concentrations that meaningfully confirm performance below and above the decision threshold for the analyte. For quantitative assays, appropriate controls must include at least one normal sample and at least one sample reflecting a disease range. For some assays, an additional control concentration may be useful to confirm performance near the assay's LOD, LOQ, or cutoff, if appropriate, or at a concentration consistent with highly abnormal levels that test the AMR. If a hydrolysis step is required in the assay, the laboratory includes a control (when available) with each batch to evaluate the effectiveness of hydrolysis.

Role of the Internal Standard

The addition of a stable isotope-labeled internal standard (IS) to all samples (calibrators, quality QC, patient samples) before extracting or processing the samples is important for monitoring loss of analyte during the sample preparation, studying matrix effects, or determining ionization efficiency during the mass spectrometric sample analysis. 13C-labeled and 15N-labeled forms are more stable than the deuterated 2H. A good IS meets several criteria,[28] and when added at a fixed concentration to all samples, it acts as a normalization factor in the normalization process.[28] The normalization process adjusts for the variability in extraction efficiency, ionization, and so forth and is calculated by dividing the area under the analyte peak by the area under the peak of the IS.

CAP *Chemistry and Toxicology Checklist* items related to chromatography state that column performance (CP) parameters must be established during validation and be used during the testing (CHM.16770, CHM.16850). CP can be assessed by monitoring retention time (time at which the relevant peak elutes from the column), which should remain within ±2.5% of the target location. Chromatographic resolution (RS) is another monitoring parameter (defined as the distance between two peak centers divided by the average peak width) for which the desirable value should be larger than 1.25. RS is affected by the pH (mainly for ion exchange columns) and composition of the mobile phase, as well as by the type and the temperature of the column. Modification of these parameters improves RS.

Other parameters that laboratories commonly review are peak shape, peak width, peak area, and any peak broadening or asymmetry of peaks.

Measurement Range

For quantitative clinical mass spectrometry assays, establishing the LOB and the LOD may not be necessary if the LOQ has been determined. Instead, the upper and lower limits of the AMR are verified, which in the CLSI literature are referred to as the upper and lower limits of the measuring interval (ULMI, LLMI).[27] In quantitative LC-MS, the extreme AMR peaks should have their signal-to-noise

(S/N) ratio measured by detectors at a minimum of 10:1 or even 20:1 if a more specific measurement is desired (CHM.16950).

Evaluation of Matrix Effects in Body Fluids

If an FDA-approved assay intended for blood testing is offered as a routine orderable test for measuring the analyte in another nonapproved specimen (fluid) type, it must be validated as a modified FDA-approved/FDA-cleared test. As described in the note to *All Common Checklist* item COM.40620, there are several options that the laboratory director may consider.[30] If upon review of COM.40620 it is decided that spiking and dilution assays will need to be performed on body fluids, simplified protocols are available.[30]

Evaluation of Matrix Effects in Mass Spectrometry Assays

Ion suppression (or *ion enhancement*) is a matrix effect in LC-MS that results in a decrease (or increase) of analytical signal, independent of the selectivity or sensitivity of the mass analyzer. Common causes of ion suppression could include hemolysis, lipemia, icterus, as well as drugs and certain other endogenous compounds. When ion suppression/enhancement exceeds ±25% or when the percentage of the CV of the ion suppression/enhancement exceeds ±15%, a matrix effect cannot be excluded, and additional study must be performed to show that the accuracy of the assay is not affected (*Chemistry and Toxicology Checklist* item CHM.18825).

The CAP checklist item refers to two methods of looking at ion suppression: (1) the postcolumn infusion method[2,28] and (2) the postcolumn extraction and spiking approach, as described in the Scientific Working Group for Forensic Toxicology (SWGTOX) article.[2] A minimum of 10 samples should be used, of which five should be abnormal (eg, hemolysis, lipemia, icterus, potential interfering drugs).

CAP *Chemistry and Toxicology Checklist* item CHM.18850 notes that ion suppression/enhancement studies are part of an LC-MS method validation, but it is also important to be aware of the possibility of ion suppression when running any individual patient sample. CHM.18850 (see Note) gives important pointers for detecting this.

CAP *Chemistry and Toxicology Checklist* item CHM.18850: The laboratory LC-MS assay procedure includes an evaluation for possible ion-suppression or enhancement in patient samples during routine testing.

Note: Ion suppression (or, less frequently, ion enhancement) is a recognized analytical anomaly in LC-MS assays. Such suppression can lead to false-negative results or poor quantitative analyses (especially near the assay LOQ). While difficult to predict and observe from specimen to specimen, certain precautions should be used to try to recognize when ion suppression or enhancement occurs. Routine monitoring of the signal intensity of internal standard(s) is an effective way to recognize signal suppression in a single patient sample, due to unexpected interfering components of the matrix. Internal standards to be used are those that cover the areas of the elution profile where matrix effects are most pronounced, and that the suitability of these internal standards has been determined (ie, with acceptance limits) during assay development and validation. Internal standard abundance acceptance criteria may be based on signal-to-noise ratio or may be compared to internal standard abundance in QC samples. As an example, for isotopically labeled internal standards, if there is poor recovery of the internal standard, a signal-to-noise ratio greater than 3:1 should still suffice for acceptance of the specimen in question. If recovery of the isotopically labeled internal standard is considered poor, then an alternate analysis should be considered, eg, the method of standard addition. For analogue-type internal standards, internal standard recovery may be used as a guide for identification of ion suppression/enhancement, although another option, such as the method of standard addition, would be a reasonable alternative. It should be noted that even isotopically labeled internal standards do not always readily identify ion suppression or enhancement.

The CAP checklist has two items related to compound identification criteria in mass spectrometry.

CAP *Chemistry and Toxicology Checklist* item CHM.18700: The identification criteria for single-stage mass spectrometry (ie, GC-MS, LC-MS) are in compliance with recommendations.

Typically, this refers to GC-MS applications because single-stage quadrupole mass analyzers (LC-MS) are rarely used. The ratio of the chromatographic peak area of the abundant fragment to the peak area of the less abundant fragment produces an ion ratio of the two m/z transitions.[28] A precursor/product pair is called a *transition* and is usually written as (Precursor m/z / Product m/z). For component identification, usually two ion ratios are required, but one ion ratio may suffice if combined with other characteristics, such as retention time.

CAP *Chemistry and Toxicology Checklist* item CHM.18800: In tandem mass spectrometry using multiple reaction monitoring (MRM) there is at least one transition monitored for the internal standard and another for the analyte.

This item refers to tandem mass spectrometry where the first quadrupole [Q1] and the third quadrupole [Q3] are used as mass filters. In Q1 the precursor ion is isolated, in Q2 it is dissociated with collision gas, and in Q3 the product ion generated from the collision in Q2 is isolated. In high specificity MRM mode, multiple precursor/product transitions are measured, of which at least one transition must be monitored for the IS.

At time of this writing, the CAP checklist criteria for identification of compounds by high-resolution accurate mass spectrometry have not yet been released, and the reader is referred to chapter 12, *Approaches to Broad-Spectrum Drug Testing in the Clinical Laboratory.*

Reporting of Laboratory-Developed Test Results

Last, once the method has been validated, the CAP requires that a suitable statement be added to the result of the LDT. CAP *All Common Checklist* item COM.40850 requires that reports for laboratory-developed tests contain a statement that the assay was developed by the laboratory: "This test was developed and its performance characteristics determined by <insert laboratory/company name>. It has not been cleared or approved by the US Food and Drug Administration." The CAP also recommends including the following: The FDA does not require this test to go through premarket FDA review; the test is used for clinical purposes and should not be regarded as investigational or for research; and that the laboratory is certified under CLIA as qualified to perform high-complexity clinical laboratory testing.

The report should also contain a brief description of the method and any performance characteristics needed for clinical use, unless the information is readily available to the clinician in an equivalent form (eg, test catalog).

Reporting of Results

After the test method has been validated, there are a still a few requirements (see below) that must be met.

CAP *All Common Checklist* item COM.40000: For each nonwaived test, there is an evaluation of the test method validation or verification study (accuracy, precision, etc) signed by the laboratory director, or designee meeting CAP director qualifications, prior to use in patient testing to confirm the acceptability of the data and approve each nonwaived test for clinical use.

The evaluation must include (1) a written assessment of each component of the validation or verification study, including the acceptability of the data; (2) a signed approval statement, such as, "I have reviewed the verification (or validation) data for accuracy, precision, reportable range, and reference interval studies (insert other components, as required) for the (insert instrument/test name), and the performance of the method is considered acceptable for patient testing." If data include discordant results, there must be a record of the discordance and investigation of any impact on the approval of the test for clinical use.

If a validation or verification study (accuracy, precision, reportable range, etc) was not performed or is missing required components, the appropriate, related checklist requirements must also be cited (eg, COM.40300, COM.40350, COM.40400).

For an FDA-cleared/FDA-approved test, an evaluation of the verification data must address analytical performance specifications, including analytical accuracy, precision, interferences, and reportable range, as applicable. In addition, for modified FDA-cleared/FDA-approved tests or LDTs, the evaluation must address analytical sensitivity, analytical specificity, and any other parameter that is considered important, to assure the analytical performance of a test (eg, specimen stability, reagent stability, linearity, carryover, cross-contamination, etc as appropriate and applicable). If the laboratory makes clinical claims about its tests, the evaluation must address the validation of these claims.

Conclusions

To facilitate review, it is desirable to have a validation plan and performance specifications signed by the medical director before the validation process is started. When the validation is finished, it should be signed off by the laboratory director with necessary statements (COM.40000, COM.40630), and a summary of the validation results should be prepared for review by the inspectors.

References

1. CAP Position Statement on the Opioid Crisis. 2018. https://www.cap.org/news/2018/pathologists-confront-the-opioid-crisis. Accessed May 13, 2019.
2. Scientific Working Group for Forensic Toxicology. Scientific Working Group for Forensic Toxicology (SWGTOX) standard practices for method validation in forensic toxicology. *J Anal Toxicol.* 2013;37:452-474

3. Office of Clinical Pharmacology, in the Center for Drug Evaluation and Research and the Center for Veterinary Medicine. *Bioanalytical Method Validation: Guidance for Industry.* Silver Spring, MD: Food and Drug Administration, US Dept of Health and Human Services; May 2018.
4. Overview of IVD Regulation. US Food and Drug Administration. https://www.fda.gov/MedicalDevices/DeviceRegulationandGuidance/IVDRegulatoryAssistance/ucm123682.htm. Updated July 9, 2018. Accessed May 13, 2019.
5. Product Classification. US food and Drug Administration. https://www.accessdata.fda.gov/scripts/cdrh/cfdocs/cfpcd/classification.cfm. Updated February 11, 2019. Accessed May 13, 2019.
6. Device Classification Panels. US Food and Drug Administration. https://www.fda.gov/MedicalDevices/DeviceRegulationandGuidance/Overview/ClassifyYourDevice/ucm051530.htm. Updated September 19, 2018. Accessed May 13, 2019.
7. Premarket Notification 510(k). US Food and Drug Administration. https://www.fda.gov/medicaldevices/deviceregulationandguidance/howtomarketyourdevice/premarketsubmissions/premarketnotification510k/default.htm. Updated September 27, 2018. Accessed May 13, 2019.
8. Premarket Approval (PMA). US Food and Drug Administration. https://www.fda.gov/MedicalDevices/DeviceRegulationandGuidance/HowtoMarketYourDevice/PremarketSubmissions/PremarketApprovalPMA/default.htm. Updated February 4, 2019. Accessed May 13, 2019.
9. Test Complexities. Centers for Disease Control and Prevention. https://wwwn.cdc.gov/CLIA/Resources/TestComplexities.aspx. Updated June 11, 2018. Accessed May 13, 2019.
10. List of cleared and approved tests. US Food and Drug Administration. https://www.accessdata.fda.gov/scripts/cdrh/cfdocs/cfCLIA/search.cfm. Updated February 11, 2019. Accessed May 13, 2019.
11. CLIA—Clinical Laboratory Improvement Amendments—Currently Waived Analytes. US Food and Drug Administration. https://www.accessdata.fda.gov/scripts/cdrh/cfdocs/cfClia/analyteswaived.cfm. Updated February 11, 2019. Accessed May 13, 2019.
12. Laboratory developed tests. US Food and Drug Administration. https://www.fda.gov/medicaldevices/productsandmedicalprocedures/invitrodiagnostics/laboratorydevelopedtests/default.htm. Updated October 12, 2018. Accessed May 13, 2019.
13. Center for Biologics Evaluation and Research, Office of In Vitro Diagnostics and Radiological Health, Center for Devices and Radiological Health. *Draft Guidance for Industry, Food and Drug Administration Staff, and Clinical Laboratories. Framework for Regulatory Oversight of Laboratory Developed Tests (LDTs).* Silver Spring, MD: Food and Drug Administration, US Dept of Health and Human Services; October 3, 2014. Document no. 1739.
14. EP-Evaluator v.12 user guide. Datainnovations.com/EP-Evaluator. https://datainnovations.com/sites/default/files/webinar_archive/EE%2012.0%20whats%20new.pdf. Accessed May 13, 2019.
15. *User Verification of Precision and Estimation of Bias. Approved Guideline.* 3rd ed. Wayne, PA: Clinical and Laboratory Standards Institute; 2014. CLSI document EP15-A3.
16. Calibration Verification/Linearity Users' Guide. Northfield, IL: College of American Pathologists; 2016.
17. *Evaluation of the Linearity of Quantitative Measurement Procedures: A Statistical Approach. Approved Guideline.* Wayne, PA: Clinical and Laboratory Standards Institute; 2003. CLSI document EP06-A.
18. College of American Pathologists. Serum Carryover Survey. https://www.cap.org/laboratory-improvement/catalogs-ordering-and-shipping. Accessed May 14, 2019.
19. *Defining, Establishing and Verifying Reference Intervals in the Clinical Laboratory. Approved Guideline.* 3rd ed. Wayne, PA: Clinical and Laboratory Standards Institute; 2010. CLSI document EP28-A3c.
20. *Toxicology and Drug Testing in the Medical Laboratory.* 3rd ed. Wayne, PA: Clinical and Laboratory Standards Institute; 2017. CLSI document C52.
21. *Evaluation of Detection Capability of Clinical Laboratory Measurement Procedures. Approved Guideline.* 2nd ed. Wayne, PA: Clinical and Laboratory Standards Institute; 2012. CLSI document EP17-A2.
22. Armbruster DA, Pry T. Limit of blank, limit of detection and limit of quantitation. *Clin Biochem Rev.* 2008;29(Suppl 1):S49-S52.
23. *Interference Testing in Clinical Chemistry.* 3rd ed. Wayne, PA: Clinical and Laboratory Standards Institute; 2018. CLSI document EP07-Ed3.
24. *Supplemental Tables for Interference Testing in Clinical Chemistry.* Wayne, PA: Clinical and Laboratory Standards Institute; 2018. CLSI document EP37.

25. *Hemolysis, Icterus, Lipemia/Turbidity Indices as Indicators of Interference in Clinical Laboratory Analysis. Approved Guideline.* Wayne, PA: Clinical and Laboratory Standards Institute; 2012. CLSI document C56-A.
26. *Clinical Evaluation of Immunoassays. Approved Guideline.* 2nd ed. Wayne, PA: Clinical and Laboratory Standards Institute; 2008. CLSI document I/LA21-A2.
27. *Evaluation of Stability of In Vitro Diagnostic Reagents. Approved Guideline.* Wayne, PA: Clinical and Laboratory Standards Institute; 2009. CLSI document EP25-A.
28. *Liquid Chromatography–Mass Spectrometry Methods. Approved Guideline.* CLSI document C62-A. Wayne, PA: Clinical and Laboratory Standards Institute; 2014.
29. Strathmann FG, Hoofnagle AN. Current and future applications of mass spectrometry to the clinical laboratory. *Am J Clin Pathol.* 2011;136:609-616.
30. Block DR, Franke DDH. *Quick Guide To Body Fluid Testing.* Washington, DC: AACC Press; 2015.
31. Nair H, Clarke W. *Mass Spectrometry for the Clinical Laboratory.* Cambridge, MA: Academic Press; 2016.
32. Grant RP, Rappold BA. Development and validation of small molecule analytes by liquid chromatography–tandem mass spectrometry. In: Rifai N, Horvath AR, Wittwer CT, eds. *Tietz Textbook of Clinical Chemistry and Molecular Diagnostics.* 6th ed. St. Louis, MO: Elsevier; 2018.

Chapter 14

Alternate Specimens for Drugs-of-Abuse Testing: Oral Fluid

Jennifer A. Collins, PhD

Introduction

Saliva has been used for many years in therapeutic drug monitoring and, more recently, has been proposed as a diagnostic sample to screen for a variety of disease states and conditions because of its accessibility and abundance of biomarkers and proteins.[1,2] Although testing for prescribed and abused drugs in compliance and workplace settings has traditionally been performed using urine, interest in use of saliva in those contexts has also been growing.

Performing drug testing as a component and condition of employment in the United States has been common since the 1990s when the Mandatory Guidelines for Federal Workplace Drug Testing were first implemented.[3] Collection and testing of urine specimens for this purpose is required for federal agencies/employers, and similar paradigms are utilized in nonregulated drug-free workplace programs. Likewise, guidance on laboratory testing in support of pain management testing often recommends use of urine drug testing to monitor compliance and detect potential abuse or diversion of medications used in treatment of chronic pain.[4] However, interest in use of alternate specimen types, such as oral fluid, has been growing for a variety of reasons, including ongoing concerns about attempts by the donor (patient) to subvert the urine specimen collection process by substitution or use of adulteration products.

Although urine remains the most commonly utilized drug testing specimen matrix in clinical, workplace, drug treatment, and criminal justice settings, oral fluid has become the most common alternative matrix in these testing programs. Many nonregulated workplace drug testing policies have incorporated oral fluid as a matrix, and the Substance Abuse and Mental Health Services Administration (SAMHSA) has recently finalized revisions to the federal workplace drug testing guidelines to include oral fluid.[5] The effective date of the HHS guidelines for oral fluid testing is January 1, 2020; however, implementation is expected to take 12 to 18 months while stakeholders prepare to meet the requirements.

Among the potential advantages of oral fluid over other specimen types is the ability to collect a sample under direct supervision without the need for a special collection facility. Oral fluid can also be an indicator of more recent drug use and may provide better correlation with concentrations of drugs in blood.[6]

Oral Fluid as an Analytical Specimen

In the literature, the terms *oral fluid* and *saliva* are often used interchangeably; however, *oral fluid* is the preferred term because it better represents the collected analytical specimen. Oral fluid contains saliva secreted from major and minor salivary glands, as well as mucosal transudate and crevicular fluid.[7,8] Although oral fluid composition can change with secretion rates, it contains approximately 90% water and 10% solutes, such as electrolytes, amylase, glucose, and urea. Under normal healthy conditions, adults produce 0.5 L to 1.5 L of oral fluid per day; however, production can be altered by mechanical stimulation, such as chewing, as well as by disease states, including diabetes, alcoholism, and drug use.[9] Drugs enter the oral fluid primarily by passive diffusion from the blood; however, ultrafiltration and secretion may be contributing factors.[6,10] Drugs are also deposited in the oral cavity during active drug use by oral, transmucosal, smoked, and inhaled or intranasal routes of administration. The movement of drugs from blood into oral fluid depends on physiochemical properties of the drug, such as lipid solubility, degree of ionization, and binding with plasma proteins.[11] Lipid-soluble, unbound (free), and un-ionized drugs move more freely into oral fluid than do water-soluble or highly bound compounds. As parent drugs tend to be more lipid soluble, the unmetabolized drug is often the predominant analyte in oral fluid and generally reflects the free, unbound drug concentration in plasma.[9,10] The pH of the oral fluid also plays a role in oral fluid drug concentrations. Unstimulated saliva is slightly acidic to neutral, with a pH of approximately 6.2 to 7.0. Because the pH of oral fluid is usually lower than that of plasma, weakly basic drugs (such as cocaine and amphetamines) tend to concentrate in oral fluid as a result of "ion trapping" and therefore have higher oral fluid concentrations relative to plasma.[12] Weakly acidic and more highly protein-bound drugs are present in oral fluid in lower concentrations. This partitioning of a drug between oral fluid and plasma is often expressed as the saliva/plasma ratio

Table 14-1. Average Saliva/Plasma (S/P) Ratios[10]

Drug	Average S/P Ratio
Ethyl alcohol	1.07
Barbiturates	0.3
Buprenorphine	1.0
Codeine	4.0
Methamphetamine	2.0
3,4-Methylenedioxymethamphetamine (MDMA)	7.0
Cocaine	3.0
Diazepam	0.02
Methadone	1.6
Morphine	0.8
Δ^9-Tetrahydrocannabinol (THC)	1.2
Tramadol	9.0

(S/P ratio). Average S/P ratios of some commonly measured drugs are shown in Table 14-1.

As a filtrate of plasma, oral fluid is generally considered to represent more recent drug use compared to urine. The following are common prescription medications and drugs of abuse that have been measured in oral fluid: amphetamines, cocaine, cannabinoids, opiates and opioids, phencyclidine (PCP), barbiturates, benzodiazepines, ethanol, gamma-hydroxybutyrate, and nicotine. Detection of designer drugs, such as synthetic cannabinoids (K2/Spice), has also been reported.[13]

Applications of Oral Fluid Testing

Outside of clinical diagnostic applications, the primary interest in oral fluid has been as an alternative matrix to urine or blood in drugs-of-abuse testing. The most common applications are as an alternative specimen in workplace and criminal justice drug testing programs, in identifying impaired drivers at the roadside, and to monitor compliance with treatment programs such as substance abuse, pain management, and smoking cessation.

Workplace Testing

Workplace drug testing generally falls into one of two categories: testing performed under the Mandatory Guidelines for Federal Workplace Drug Testing Programs or testing performed for public and private employers not subject to the federal rules. As testing for employment purposes has evolved since the early 1990s, efforts by donors to subvert the testing process have become a concern. The ability to perform an observed collection is one of the primary reasons for using oral fluid in workplace drug testing programs.

Although somewhat dependent on state employment law and other regulatory considerations, oral fluid is currently in use in many nonregulated workplace drug testing programs. Incorporation of oral fluid into the Mandatory Guidelines for Federal Workplace Drug Testing Programs was first proposed in 2004, along with hair and sweat as alternative matrices.[14] At that time, however, there were sufficient scientific, legal, and public policy concerns about the alternative matrices such that the US Department of Health and Human Services determined that the best path forward was to address each matrix independently. Since 2004, there has been significant growth in the body of published scientific data regarding drugs in oral fluid and analytical methodologies used for testing. The proposed Mandatory Guidelines for Federal Workplace Drug Testing Programs—Oral Fluid (OFMG) were published for public comment in the *Federal Register* on May 15, 2015, and the final version was published on October 25, 2019.[5] When implemented, the OFMG will allow federal agencies to collect and test oral fluid either as a primary test specimen or as an alternative when a donor cannot provide a urine specimen.

Criminal Justice

Drug testing in the criminal justice system is used primarily as a tool to monitor offenders for compliance with conditions of pretrial release or probation and parole.[15] Participation in a drug testing program may also be offered as an alternative to incarceration for individuals with identified substance-abuse disorders and appearing in drug courts. Routine testing in the criminal justice system is based on data linking frequent drug use to crime and behaviors strongly linked to recidivism.[16] Most of the testing utilizes urine as the primary specimen; however, use of oral fluid, particularly as a specimen that is collected under direct observation, is increasing.

Driving Under the Influence of Drugs

For traffic safety purposes, blood has traditionally been the specimen of choice in order to determine whether drivers are under the influence of drugs or alcohol, although urine has also been used. There is significant interest in the use of oral fluid and, more specifically, oral fluid point-of-collection (POC) or on-site test devices to be able to assess a driver at the roadside. The relative ease of collection by nonmedical personnel and the potential for correlation with impairment are benefits. Studies such as the Roadside Testing Assessment (ROSITA) project undertaken in eight European countries between 1999 and 2000 have included oral fluid devices as potential tools for assessment of drug use in drivers.[17] Results have revealed issues with inconsistent specimen volumes, test device failures, and lack of sufficient sensitivity for some drug classes. Although more recent studies have shown improved performance,[18,19] the utility of oral fluid for this purpose continues to be device dependent.

Compliance Testing

Testing for compliance with a prescribed treatment program is applicable to patients in both substance abuse and chronic pain treatment programs. In the case of substance use disorders, drug testing is utilized to monitor compliance with medication-assisted treatment regimens, such as methadone maintenance or buprenorphine, as well as abstinence from drugs of abuse. In chronic pain patients, treating physicians monitor use of prescribed medications that have addiction potential, as well as potential diversion of controlled substances and concomitant use of illicit and nonprescribed prescription medications. Concerns about the integrity of the urine collection process similar to those in workplace drug testing programs are driving additional interest in the use of oral fluid as an alternative. Several studies have been performed in substance abuse treatment and pain patients that show acceptable equivalence to urine tests, providing evidence for the utility of oral fluid in these programs.[20-22]

Preanalytical Considerations in Oral Fluid Drug Testing

Specimen Collection

Specimen collection is a very important consideration in the use of oral fluid as a test matrix. There are multiple techniques that can be used for oral fluid specimen collection and, as a result, the collection process is a major variable in oral fluid testing.[23] One technique involves collection of undiluted (neat) oral fluid by expectoration or spitting; however, viscosity, stability, and frothing of the saliva can be problematic. Expectoration may produce more froth than actual liquid, resulting in a viscous and small sample size that may be insufficient for drug analyses. Furthermore, the sample may be contaminated with food and other debris. Because of these limitations, commercial collection devices are more commonly used for oral fluid collection. These collection devices range from a simple cotton pad (eg, Salivette) to devices consisting of an absorbent pad with a transport tube containing a stabilization buffer (eg, Quantisal, Intercept, OralEze, StatSure). Samples collected using these devices are generally cleaner, provide a more stable sample, and have higher volume compared with samples obtained via direct spitting. However, depending on the device, collected specimen volume and recovery of drug from the absorbent pad may vary, and these variables become critical when evaluating the accuracy and scientific validity of test results for oral fluid specimens. Because the collection method and device can affect test results, oral fluid collection devices are considered Class II devices and require US Food and Drug Administration (FDA) 510(k) clearance with the specified oral fluid test(s).[24] In the guidelines for use of oral fluid in federal workplace drug testing programs, SAMHSA establishes performance requirements for collection devices that include quantitative sample collection, stability, and minimum drug recovery criteria.[5]

Before sample collection, it is recommended that a waiting period be observed, with the donor in the presence of the collector, during which time the donor is not allowed to put anything in his or her mouth for 10 to 20 minutes. For collection purposes, oral fluid production can be stimulated by use of citric acid candy, chewing gum, or mechanical stimulation such as chewing on a rubber band; however, these processes can change the pH and resulting drug concentrations in oral fluid.[10] When using commercial collection devices, there is generally no need for stimulation of oral fluid secretion by the aforementioned methods because the absorbent pads provide sufficient stimulation.

There may be significant variation in oral fluid secretion within an individual and among individuals, depending on the collection technique used, individual physiology, and the influence of factors such as the presence of therapeutic or abused drugs. At times, a donor may not be able to produce an adequate sample for testing, which may be due to dry mouth, known as *xerostomia*. Many conditions—such as diabetes, alcoholism, and use of anticholinergic drugs—may result in decreased oral fluid formation.[9] Hormonal changes, stress, smoking, and use of analgesics, anticonvulsants, amphetamines, cannabis, and tranquilizers can also decrease production of oral fluid. Under those circumstances, collection times may be extended. Although use of a stimulant such as citric acid candy or chewing on inert material may be useful in these situations, enhanced secretion by these techniques may produce dilute samples, which can lead to false-negative results.

After the sample is collected, it may be tested using a POC on-site testing device or transported to the laboratory. Depending on the collection methodology and/or device, the specimen is placed in a transport tube with a buffer solution before shipping, or it may be sent directly without any pretreatment. Specimen stability during transport is an important variable for consideration. Several studies have shown that most of the drugs are stable for several days at 4°C or room temperature when stored in a buffered solution; however, unpreserved specimens (ie, neat oral fluid) may show losses for drugs such as cocaine and 6-acetylmorphine (6-AM).[25,26] Manufacturers of collection devices that have been cleared by the FDA should have stability data available for review.

Recovery of drugs of interest from the collection device should also be considered. In a study published in 2005, Crouch reported that drug recoveries from a group of oral fluid collection devices varied significantly.[23] The drug recoveries ranged from 16% to 57% for amphetamines, 15% to 59% for methamphetamine, 61% to 97% for cocaine, 9% to 56% for PCP, 33% to 50% for morphine, and there was very poor recovery for Δ^9-tetrahydrocannabinol (THC). Since that time, new and reformulated devices have been introduced by manufacturers that demonstrate improved performance, particularly for THC.[27,28] As indicated previously, the SAMHSA guidelines for oral fluid establish performance criteria for collection devices, including drug recovery of 80% to 120% at the initial test cutoff.

When using an oral fluid collection device that incorporates a buffer into the transport tube, the reproducibility of the neat oral fluid specimen volume collected by the pad is also an important consideration. Analysis of specimens collected in this manner requires incorporation of a dilution factor into the analytical procedure, and variations in collected sample volume or device buffer content can have a significant impact on the accuracy and reliability of reported results. Buffer volume varies by device, but volumes of 1 mL to 3 mL are common. As seen in the recovery studies, earlier devices demonstrated some inconsistencies both in collected specimen volumes and in device buffer volumes.[27] Most newer devices incorporate volume sufficiency indicators, and the SAMHSA guidelines specify collection of 1.0 mL oral fluid with an accuracy of +/−10%.

A final consideration in oral fluid collection procedures is how to collect a "split" specimen. It is common practice in workplace urine drug testing programs to collect a single specimen and split it into two vials, one of which is retained for retesting if results are challenged. The relatively small volumes of oral fluid collected present a challenge in this regard. The OFMG require a split-specimen collection protocol, which can be achieved by any of the following three methods: (1) simultaneous collection with two separate devices, (2) serial collections with two separate devices, or (3) simultaneous collection into a single device that directs the oral fluid into two separate collection tubes or is subdivided subsequent to the collection.[5] There are collection devices available that meet the requirements for simultaneous collection into a single device that separates the oral fluid into two separate tubes. The most basic devices incorporate a single mouthpiece that directs expectorated neat oral fluid into separate collection tubes (eg, Oasis Diagnostics UltraSal-2, Scitek Split Collector). A more elegant solution using a buffered collection device has recently been cleared by the FDA for split oral fluid specimen collections (Quantisal II). Minimum oral fluid specimen volume required in each tube is 1.0 mL.

Specimen Validity Testing

Even though oral fluid is collected under direct supervision and the chances of adulteration are fairly low, questions have been raised about the possibility of sample adulteration. As with urine drug testing, there are many products available on the internet that claim to thwart drug testing of oral fluid. In addition, the impact of ingestion of food, beverages, oral hygiene products, and smoking on drug levels in oral fluid should be considered. Wong et al[29] investigated the effect of various foods, beverages, food ingredients, cosmetics, and hygiene products on a device and found that the products did not interfere with the testing. Two commercial adulterant products, Clear Choice Fizzy Flush and Kleen Mouthwash, were also tested with similar results. In another study, ingestion of hard candy, gum, coffee, tea, orange juice, and other foodstuffs did not affect test results using an enzyme immunoassay for opiates.[30] As has been true in urine testing, it is anticipated that products designed to negate oral fluid drug tests will proliferate as oral fluid testing is more widely incorporated into drug testing programs. A recent search of the internet produced a suite of products "frequently bought together," including Oral Clear Gum, Stinger Detox Mouthwash, and a five-panel oral fluid drug test device.[31]

There are currently no universally accepted oral fluid specimen validity tests that are the equivalent of specimen temperature, creatinine, pH, and oxidant tests utilized as validity markers in urine. Measurement of IgG has been proposed and is cur-

Table 14-2. Food and Drug Administration (FDA)-Cleared Oral Fluid Immunoassay Cutoffs

Test	Cutoffs for FDA-Cleared Tests (ng/mL)*	SAMHSA Cutoffs (ng/mL); Effective 01/01/2020
Amphetamine	50, 120, 150, 300	50
Methamphetamine	50, 120	50
3,4-Methylenedioxymethamphetamine (MDMA), MDA	50	50
Δ^9-Tetrahydrocannabinol (THC)	3, 4	4
Cocaine	9, 15, 20	15**
Opiates/opioids	30, 40	30†
6-Acetylmorphine (6-AM)	4	4
Phencyclidine (PCP)	3, 6, 10	10

SAMHSA, Substance Abuse and Mental Health Services Administration; MDA, methelenedioxyamphetamine.

* Derived from the FDA searchable 510(k) database at www.fda.gov.[90]

** Cocaine and benzoylecgonine are both target analytes.

† Codeine, morphine, hydrocodone, hydromorphone, oxycodone, oxymorphone are required analytes in this category.

rently utilized in some workplace testing programs. However, some data indicate that IgG is not an effective marker for in vitro and in vivo dilution of oral fluid and may also be an inappropriate marker in donors who are immunocompromised or are taking immunosuppressant medications for a medical condition.[23] Albumin has been proposed as an alternative marker, but there are few data available to verify its efficacy. The final version of the OFMG permits but does not require specimen validity testing; options include IgG, albumin, or other relevant biomarkers as they are identified.

Analytical Methods for Drug Testing in Oral Fluid

After the specimen is collected, analysis may be performed on site or may be transported to a laboratory for testing.

Point-of-Collection Testing Devices

Depending on the reason for the test, POC or on-site testing may be highly desirable, particularly in situations of driving under the influence of drugs. However, performance of on-site testing devices has been variable with respect to sensitivity and specificity for different drugs.[32-35] First-generation devices demonstrated problems with insufficient sample volumes, device failures, and poor sensitivity and specificity for cannabinoids, amphetamines, and benzodiazepines.[36] In a large-scale study performed in Europe and the United States to evaluate on-site oral fluid test devices under field conditions in 2003 to 2005 (Roadside Testing Assessment, ROSITA-2), none of the devices met the proposed criteria of sensitivity and specificity greater than 90% and accuracy of greater than 95% for all drugs tested.[37] Another large-scale study conducted as a part of the Driving Under the Influence of Drugs, Alcohol and Medicines (DRUID) project in Europe evaluated eight on-site testing devices. Although the results were improved as compared with earlier studies, sensitivity and specificity did not meet the study's target values.[38] Oral fluid screening technology has continued to evolve, and more recent studies demonstrate significant improvement in sensitivity and specificity, with few device failures[39-41]; however, overall performance of these technologies and assigned assay cutoffs continue to vary across devices.

Laboratory-Based Testing

Specimens transported to the laboratory for testing may be tested by routine analytical methods adapted for the oral fluid matrix, lower drug concentrations, and limited sample volume. As with the testing paradigm utilized in urine drug testing programs, an initial test may be performed to identify negative samples, followed by a second, confirmatory test for nonnegative specimens. Initial tests are often performed using immunoassay methodology; however, direct chromatographic methods, such as liquid chromatography with tandem mass spectrometry (LC-MS/MS), are becoming more common in practice, particularly if monitoring of multiple compounds is desired.

Immunoassays

Both heterogeneous and homogeneous immunoassays are currently available for oral fluid testing applications. Although similar to those used for drugs of abuse in urine, assays have been modified to improve cross-reactivity with parent drugs commonly present in oral fluid. As indicated previously, the FDA has required clearance of reagents with the collection device to ensure that device components do not alter performance of the reagent system. There are a number of FDA-cleared oral fluid tests for screening of routine drugs such as amphetamine, methamphetamine, cocaine, opiates, cannabinoids, and PCP; however, cutoffs for some compounds are quite variable, as shown in Table 14-2. Assays that are not FDA cleared but marketed as *Forensic Use Only (FUO)* or *Research Use Only (RUO)* are also available. Use of such test kits requires validation as laboratory-developed tests on the site where they will be used. The variability in cutoffs is due in large part to the lack of a regulatory standard for workplace oral fluid drug testing programs as well as to methodological differences between enzyme-linked immunosorbent assays (ELISAs) and homogeneous enzyme immunoassays (HEIAs). Thus, it is important for the laboratory decision makers to evaluate and ensure that the selected test provides sufficient sensitivity as well as selectivity for the intended use.

Procedures for implementation of oral fluid immunoassays in the laboratory are similar to those for urine. The earliest FDA-cleared kits were ELISAs modified for use with oral fluid. As interest in oral fluid has grown, however, the demand for more automated testing platforms has led to development of homogeneous immunoassays that can be run on automated chemistry analyzers. Reagents should be optimized for lower cutoffs and for parent drugs as indicated. For specimens collected in devices containing a transport buffer, calibrators and controls must also incorporate a dilution factor for accurate assessment of drug concentration in the collected sample. As an example, a device that collects 1.0 mL of sample into 3.0 mL of buffer represents a 4x dilution of the neat oral fluid. To accurately measure drug concentration, the calibrator(s) must incorporate the same dilution factor.

Chromatographic Tests

Challenges of oral fluid testing related to limited specimen volumes and low drug concentrations can be overcome by use of directed chromatographic methods with high sensitivity and high specificity, such as gas chromatography with mass spectrometry (GC-MS) or LC-MS/MS. These methods are widely used for confirmation of initial immunoassay results, but they are also increasingly being employed as initial test methodology, particularly when a more comprehensive test panel is desired.[42-45]

Sample preparation techniques required for oral fluid analysis depend on the sample collected (ie, neat or buffered) and on the analytical methodology. The protein content of oral fluid as well as the presence of salts, surfactants, and other components of stabilization buffers must be considered. For LC-MS/MS analysis, direct injection[46] and dilute-and-shoot[47] methods have been published; however, use of techniques providing additional sample cleanup—such as protein precipitation, liquid-liquid extraction, or solid phase extraction—are also common. Additional sample preparation can be particularly important for analysis of oral fluid specimens collected in buffered collection devices where the buffers can cause matrix effects in LC-MS/MS analysis. In addition, because the composition of buffers used in specimen collection differs from device to device, laboratory validation protocols must incorporate the appropriate buffered matrix into the validation experiments. Analytical methods have been developed for individual analytes[48-51] and for multiple analytes for comprehensive test panels often used in pain management programs.[52,53]

Proficiency Testing

As is true for other matrices used for toxicology testing, participation in proficiency testing programs is required for accreditation and licensure. There are at least two programs currently available in the US, and the National Laboratory Certification Program will require a separate program for laboratories certified to perform oral fluid testing under the SAMHSA guidelines. The program offered by the Center for Forensic Sciences at RTI International consists of three shipments, each with five samples, over a 12-month period.[54] This survey is ungraded but provides overall statistics for laboratories to evaluate their performance against other participants. The College of American Pathologists Oral Fluid for Drugs of Abuse (OFD) proficiency testing program consists of four shipments per year, each shipment consisting of five samples.[55] This survey is graded against peer group mean data, and results are sent to participating laboratories. Both surveys are provided as neat oral fluid, permitting laboratories to prepare samples in appropriate collection devices, if applicable, for analysis using routine laboratory methods. Initial testing (screening) and confirmatory test results are submitted for evaluation.

Oral Fluid Testing of Specific Drug Classes

Detailed information for individual drugs in oral fluid is beyond the scope of this chapter; however, a brief synopsis of compounds commonly tested in oral fluid is provided below.

Alcohol

Ethanol is distributed throughout body fluids after ingestion, including into oral fluid. The strong correlation between blood alcohol concentrations and oral fluid levels was first reported in the 1930s and has been verified in multiple studies under various conditions since that time, with saliva/plasma (S/P) ratios ranging from 0.88 to 1.36.[56-58] The use of POC saliva alcohol test devices is approved as an initial test in the US Department of Transportation drug and alcohol testing program, provided confirmatory testing is performed using an evidential breath testing device.[59]

Amphetamines

Amphetamine and methamphetamine appear rapidly in oral fluid after administration, with peak concentrations measured 2 to 12 hours after dosing.[60] Levels generally parallel those measured in plasma; however, actual concentrations of amphetamine and methamphetamine may be higher in oral fluid because of ion trapping of weak bases in the more acidic oral fluid matrix. Oral fluid/plasma ratios of 2.0 or greater have been reported, although the ratio exhibits significant interindividual variability.[36] Detection periods of approximately 24 hours have been reported in controlled dosing studies; however, detection of up to 48 hours was reported with higher doses.[1]

3,4-Methylenedioxymethamphetamine (MDMA) demonstrates a similar profile to the amphetamines, with peak oral fluid concentrations appearing 1.5 hours after drug intake.[6] Concentrations of MDMA in oral fluid were also higher compared with concentrations in plasma. 3,4-Methylenedioxyamphetamine (MDA) and *N*-ethyl-3,4-methylenedioxyamphetamine (MDEA) have also been reported in oral fluid of recreational drug users.[61]

Benzodiazepines

Monitoring benzodiazepines in oral fluid is challenging because of the wide range of available compounds and potencies. S/P ratios are very low (0.04-0.07), probably resulting from the high protein binding and weakly acidic properties of these drugs.[36] Instability of some compounds within the class has also been reported. Detection periods vary depending on the compound and dosing patterns. As an example, detection periods of up to 50 hours have been reported for diazepam,[6] whereas detection periods for 7-aminoflunitrazepam are generally 6 hours or less.[62]

Cocaine

Cocaine is the predominant analyte in oral fluid and can be detected along with other metabolites and related products, including benzoylecgonine, cocaethylene, norcocaine, ecgonine methyl ester, and anhydroecgonine methyl ester, a pyrolysis product of cocaine.[63] Reported S/P ratios are generally greater than 1.0 for cocaine but less than 1.0 for benzoylecgonine because of its more polar nature. Half-lives for cocaine and benzoylecgonine in oral fluid are almost twice as long as in plasma, with reported detection periods of 1 to 2 days.[64]

Opiates and Opioids

Many opioid compounds have been measured in oral fluid, including heroin, 6-AM, codeine, morphine, hydrocodone, oxycodone, methadone, propoxyphene, tramadol, meperidine, fentanyl, and buprenorphine. Detection periods of most opioids in oral fluid parallel those in plasma; however, concentrations are often higher in oral fluid because of ion trapping of weak bases.[36]

6-Acetylmorphine

Oral fluid appears to be a superior matrix for detecting heroin use because the heroin metabolite 6-acetylmorphine has been shown to exhibit higher prevalence in oral fluid than in plasma and urine.[63,65] Heroin and 6-AM appear in oral fluid within 2 minutes of smoking or intravenous (IV) administration, with peak concentrations observed within 2 to 5 minutes.[66] Heroin and 6-AM are detectable for 2 to 24 hours after smoking and for 5 to 30 minutes after IV administration.

Codeine and Morphine

Codeine is detected in oral fluid after controlled dosing, and concentrations in oral fluid positively correlate with those in plasma, although concentrations in oral fluid are generally higher (S/P ratio of approximately 4.0).[67] Mean detection times of 21 hours have been reported; however, reported detection periods have varied depending on assay reporting limits used in the studies. Norcodeine is also detected, whereas morphine and normorphine metabolites have not been reported in oral fluid. Morphine is detected in oral fluid after morphine administration, heroin use, and poppyseed ingestion.[66,68] Detection periods are similar to those for codeine.

Oxycodone

Oxycodone is detected in oral fluid within 30 minutes of dosing and is present in higher concentrations than in plasma. S/P ratios greater than 5.0 have been reported.[69,70] Noroxycodone is also present, with concentrations approximating those in plasma. In general, oxymorphone is detectable only in very low concentrations in oral fluid after single-dose studies and may never exceed the reporting threshold. Detection periods in oral fluid of 24 to 34 hours have been reported.

Hydrocodone

Hydrocodone appears in oral fluid within 15 minutes of an oral dose and may be detectable for up to 30 hours. The mean S/P ratio reported in one study was 3.2.[71] Hydrocodone metabolites norhydrocodone and dihydrocodeine are also present, whereas hydromorphone, a prevalent metabolite in urine, is generally not observed in oral fluid after hydrocodone administration. Reported detection periods range from 8 to 48 hours.

Other Pain Management Drugs: Methadone, Tramadol, and Buprenorphine

Methadone and the metabolite 2-ethylidene-1,5-dimethyl-3,3-diphenylpyrrolidine (EDDP) have both been detected in oral fluid after dosing; however, methadone is the primary marker of methadone use in this matrix.[72,73] Detection periods of approximately 24 hours have been reported.

Detection of tramadol and its metabolites in oral fluid have been reported in several studies.[22,51] S/P ratios for parent drug and the primary metabolites *O*-desmethyltramadol and *N*-desmethyltramadol are generally high, reported as 9.0, 1.6, and 12.3, respectively, in one study.[74]

Buprenorphine concentrations in oral fluid are highly dependent on route of administration. Concentrations measured in oral fluid after intramuscular administration are substantially lower than in plasma, which is probably due to the high percentage of protein binding. Oral fluid concentrations measured after sublingual administration are much higher than plasma concentrations, which is attributed to oral contamination and depoting of the drug in the oral mucosa.[75]

Cannabinoids

Cannabinoids are the most common analyte found in most drug screens, regardless of matrix. The primary psychoactive component of cannabis, THC, is detected in oral fluid, but transfer from the blood to oral fluid appears to be minimal. Rather, the primary source of detected THC in oral fluid is from drug deposited in the oral cavity during smoking, inhaling, or consuming the drug in foodstuffs.[76] As a result, very high concentrations are detected in specimens collected soon after exposure, with levels declining as the buccal contamination is eliminated. Levels generally decline below analytical cutoffs within 12 hours of use; however, low levels of THC may be detected for several days after use in chronic users, similar to what has been observed in blood.[77,78] The THC acid metabolite, 9-carboxy-11-nor-Δ^9-tetrahydrocannabinol (carboxy-THC, THC-COOH), is detectable in oral fluid as a result of hepatic metabolism and transfer from plasma; however, the metabolite is often present in very low concentrations, exhibits large interindividual variability, and varies considerably with route of administration, making it challenging to detect and use to interpret results. When present, THC-COOH exhibits longer elimination times compared with THC and may also be detectable in chronic users for an extended period. It has been proposed as a marker for distinguishing active cannabinoid use versus passive exposure because studies have not documented the presence of THC-COOH in oral fluid of nonsmokers during passive exposure studies[79,80]; however, its utility as a biomarker may be limited by the variable pharmacokinetics observed in exposure studies. In a study evaluating pharmacokinetic profiles of cannabinoids after oral ingestion, THC levels were lower than those observed for smoked cannabis, and it was eliminated over a longer period of time. Detection of the THC-COOH metabolite was erratic and was never detected in some donors during the study period, regardless of the ingested dose.[81] In general, S/P ratios for THC vary from study to study, ranging from 1.2 to 8.2, and are dependent on route of administration and elapsed time from dosing.[76]

Interpretation of Results: Correlation of Drug Concentrations and Positivity Rates Between Oral Fluid and Urine or Blood

Interpretation of drug testing results in oral fluid can be dependent on the purpose and context of the testing.[6] In workplace drug testing, results are generally interpreted with respect to an established cutoff, and actions may be taken based solely on the presence or absence of drugs, without evaluation of other factors. For substance abuse treatment and pain management programs for which compliance with prescription medications and abstinence from illicit and/or nonprescribed medications are the goals, reporting thresholds may be lower, and the presence or absence of a drug is interpreted in the context of program conditions and medical history. Testing in legal settings—for example, involving probation, parole, or driving under the influence—is used to document program violations, compliance, and evidence of impairment. It is widely accepted that while detection of drugs and drug metabolites in urine provides an indication of drug use or exposure, it provides little or no definitive information related to dose, time of use, or impairment. Oral fluid can provide the same information regarding drug exposure and is a better indicator of more recent drug use, reflected in detection periods more similar to those in plasma (Table 14-3).[82] There is also interest in whether plasma drug levels and related behavioral effects can be inferred from drug concentrations measured in oral fluid. Most studies have demonstrated a temporal correlation between drug

Table 14-3. Reported Detection Times of Drugs in Oral Fluid[36,82]

Drug	Detection Time (h)
Amphetamine/methamphetamine	20-48
MDMA	24
Barbiturates	50
Benzodiazepines	5-50
Cocaine/benzoylecgonine	12-48
THC	2-24
Codeine/morphine/hydrocodone/ oxycodone	12-24
6-AM	0.52-24
Methadone	24
Buprenorphine	13-28

MDMA, 3,4-methylenedioxymethamphetamine; THC, Δ^9-tetrahydrocannabinol; 6-AM, 6-acetylmorphine.

in plasma and drug in oral fluid, while actual concentrations can differ depending on the lipophilicity, degree of protein binding, and the pK_a of the drug and the pH of the oral fluid.[9-12] Concentrations of weakly basic drugs are higher in oral fluid, and drug concentrations overall may be higher during recent use and in the absorptive phase, depending on the route of administration. Several publications have attempted to interpret oral fluid drug concentrations on the basis of reported S/P ratios or other parameters, with mixed results.

In a study of paired oral fluid and blood specimens collected during a national roadside survey, 23 pairs of samples positive for oxycodone were evaluated to determine whether a therapeutic level in oral fluid could be proposed.[70] Results were promising, suggesting that additional controlled studies would be informative. In contrast, a second study of oxycodone in oral fluid and plasma found poor correlation between the matrices.[83] Poor correlation and high variability were also observed in comparison studies of benzodiazepines,[84] whereas a positive correlation has been reported for many antiepileptic drugs, suggestive of value in therapeutic drug monitoring for these patients.[85] In studies where poor correlations are observed, significant variability in S/P ratios were reported for the study subjects. If sources of this variability can be identified and controlled, more relevant oral fluid–plasma interpretation models may be developed.

Table 14-4. Urine and Oral Fluid Positivity Rates in the US General Workforce, 2013-2017*

Year	Oral Fluid (% Positive)	Urine (% Positive)
2013	6.7	4.3
2014	7.7	4.7
2015	9.1	4.8
2016	10.5	4.9
2017	10.4	5.0

* Data derived from the 2018 Quest Diagnostics Drug Testing Index.[87]

Although the concordance between oral fluid and plasma drug concentrations has not been fully elucidated, prevalence studies provide insight into the relative equivalence of oral fluid to more established matrices in monitoring drug exposure. Several large-scale prevalence studies have provided comparison data for urine and oral fluid. One large study evaluating workplace drug testing data tabulated results for 77,218 positive oral fluid specimens tested for amphetamines, cannabinoids, cocaine, opiates, and PCP. The overall positive rate was 5.06%, which is similar to the positive rate of 4.46% for contemporaneous urine data from more than 5.2 million specimens.[86] In both matrices, marijuana and cocaine were the most common findings, and the prevalence of amphetamines and cocaine was approximately 60% higher in oral fluid than in urine. 6-AM was detected in 67% of the morphine-positive oral fluid samples. A limitation of this study was that the oral fluid and urine samples were not collected from the same individuals, and therefore these data do not provide direct correlation between the matrices. Urine and oral fluid prevalence rates in workplace populations are also available from the Quest Diagnostics Drug Testing Index, which monitors positivity rates from their laboratory testing data by workplace sector and by matrix.[87] As shown in Table 14-4, positive rates between urine and oral fluid in the general workforce population are similar and are increasingly higher in oral fluid over time. On the basis of individual drug data provided in the 2018 report, the positive rate of THC in oral fluid is 2.6 times higher than that detected in urine, which is somewhat unexpected, considering the difference in detection periods between the two matrices. As in the study noted above, these data are population based and do not represent paired specimens. A study using paired oral fluid and urine specimens collected from individuals in a workplace random drug testing program detected positive findings in 3.7% of urine samples and in 0.5% of oral fluid samples out of 1500 collections.[88] Some of the discrepancies identified in this study were due to the presence of one or more metabolites in urine that are not generally present in oral fluid, such as morphine after codeine ingestion. Also, application of a 10-ng/mL cutoff for THC in oral fluid probably reduced the observed incidence of this drug. Therefore, it is important to keep in mind that prevalence data can be influenced by measured analytes, use of different cutoffs, and different analytical methods, and thus should be interpreted carefully.

Studies have also been performed in patient populations in treatment for chronic pain and substance use disorders. One study reported positive prevalence rates in urine and oral fluid from more than 6000 patient samples submitted from 231 pain clinics in the United States. The overall positive rate for oral fluid was 83.9%, compared to 78% for urine, and the prevalence of drug analytes was similar. Illicit or nonprescribed drug use was identified in 11.5% of oral fluid samples, compared to 10.9% in urine donors.[21] In a second study of 133 chronic pain patients, paired oral fluid and urine specimens were collected over the study period, providing 1544 paired results.[22] The overall qualitative agreement was 85%. Of the discordant sample pairs, 5.4% had a positive finding in oral fluid and negative in urine, and 9.6% had a positive finding in urine with a negative oral fluid result. Another study using paired samples was performed in a population of patients in a medication-assisted treatment program for opioid use disorder.[89] In 126 paired oral fluid and urine specimens, 7% were positive for a drug in both specimen types and 91% were negative, demonstrating an overall agreement of 98%. Of the discrepant samples, marijuana and benzodiazepines were detected more often in urine than in oral fluid. The authors note that the high degree of agreement may be impacted by the lower overall positive rate, resulting in fewer positive result comparisons; however, they conclude that oral fluid is a reliable alternative matrix for monitoring compliance in these programs.

Thus, although use of oral fluid drug concentrations to infer drug concentrations in plasma requires further study, prevalence data have shown good correlation overall, demonstrating the utility of oral fluid in workplace and compliance programs. However, as mentioned previously, differences in study paradigms and a lack of verified equivalence between cutoffs used in oral fluid and urine should be considered in evaluation of these studies.

Summary

Urine and blood are the traditional matrices used for toxicology testing, and while urine remains the most common matrix used for detecting drug abuse, oral fluid has gained in popularity as analytical advances have facilitated testing specimens with limited volume and low analyte concentrations. Immunoassays specific for use with oral fluid and chromatographic methods optimized for oral fluid are available and are commonly used for testing. Oral fluid has current and potential applications in workplace drug testing, criminal justice, driving under the influence, and compliance monitoring for substance use disorders and pain management programs. Of keen interest in workplace and compliance programs is the ability to perform a noninvasive, observed oral fluid specimen collection, minimizing the opportunity for a donor to subvert the process by adulteration or substitution. Oral fluid can also offer a unique perspective on drug exposure because it more closely mirrors plasma levels. However, the specimen collection process and procedures as well as the physiochemical characteristics of individual drugs in oral fluid affect drug concentrations and kinetics, making contextual interpretations challenging. As with other matrices used for substance use and abuse testing, practitioners should understand both the strengths and limitations of oral fluid testing as one of multiple assessment tools.

Author's note: The HHS Mandatory Guidelines for Federal Workplace Drug Testing Programs – Oral Fluid were published in final form on October 25, 2019, with an effective date of January 1, 2020. While it was possible to include some updates to this chapter, the author recommends review of the full document available at https://www.federalregister.gov/documents/2019/10/25/2019-22684/mandatory-guidelines-for-federal-workplace-drug-testing-programs-oralfluid. It should be noted that at the time of publication, revisions to the procedures governing drug testing in the transportation industry, 49 CFR Part 40, have not been proposed but would be expected to follow most of the technical aspects of the HHS guidelines.

References

1. Choo RE, Huestis MA. Oral fluid as a diagnostic tool. *Clin Chem Lab Med.* 2004;42(11):1273-1287.
2. Kaczor-Urbanowicz KE, Martin Carreras-Presas C, Aro K, Tu M, Garcia-Godoy F, Wong DT. Saliva diagnostics: current views and directions. *Exp Biol Med (Maywood).* 2017;242(5):459-472.
3. Mandatory guidelines for federal workplace drug testing programs, 53 *Federal Register* 11979 (1988).

4. Jannetto PJ, Bratanow N, Clark WA, et al, eds. *Using Clinical Laboratory Tests to Monitor Drug Therapy in Pain Management Patients: The National Academy of Clinical Biochemistry Laboratory Medicine Practice Guidelines.* Washington, DC: American Association for Clinical Chemistry; 2017.
5. Mandatory guidelines for federal workplace drug testing programs - oral fluid. 84 *Federal Register* 57554 (2019).
6. Cone EJ, Huestis MA. Interpretation of oral fluid tests for drugs of abuse. *Ann N Y Acad Sci.* 2007; 1098:51-103.
7. Atkinson JC, Dawes C, Ericson T, et al. Guidelines for saliva nomenclature and collection. *Ann N Y Acad Sci.* 1993;694: xi-xii.
8. Schramm W, Smith RH, Craig PA. Methods of simplified saliva collection for the measurement of drugs of abuse, therapeutic drugs and other molecules. *Ann N Y Acad Sci.* 1993;694:311-313.
9. Aps JKM, Martens, LC. Review: the physiology of saliva and transfer of drugs into saliva. *Forensic Sci Int.* 2005;150:119-131.
10. Drummer OH. Drug testing in oral fluid. *Clin Biochem Rev.* 2006;27:147-159.
11. Jusko WJ, Milsap RL. Pharmacokinetic principles of drug distribution in saliva. *Ann N Y Acad Sci.* 1993;694:36-47.
12. Cone EJ. Saliva testing for drugs of abuse. *Ann N Y Acad Sci.* 1993;694:91-127.
13. Rodrigues WC, Catbagan P, Rana S, Wang G, Moore C. Detection of synthetic cannabinoids in oral fluid using ELISA and LC-MS-MS. *J Anal Toxicol.* 2013;37(8):526-533.
14. Proposed revisions to mandatory guidelines for federal workplace drug testing programs. 69 *Federal Register* 19673 (2004).
15. Timrots A. *Fact Sheet: Drug Testing in the Criminal Justice System.* Rockville, MD: Drugs & Crime Data Center & Clearinghouse; March 1992.
16. Harrell A, Kleiman M. Drug testing in criminal justice settings. In: Leukefeld CG, Tims F, Farabee D, eds. *Treatment of Drug Offenders: Policies and Issues.* New York, NY: Springer; 2002.
17. Verstraete AG. Oral fluid testing for driving under the influence of drugs: history, recent progress and remaining challenges. *Forensic Sci Int.* 2005;150(2-3):143-150.
18. Veitenheimer AM, Wagner JR. Evaluation of oral fluid as a specimen for DUID. *J Anal Toxicol.* 2017; 41(6):517-522.
19. Rohrig TP, Moore CM, Stephens K, et al. Roadside drug testing: an evaluation of the Alere DDS® 2 mobile test system. *Drug Test Anal.* 2018; 10(4):663-670.
20. Vindenes V, Yttredal B, Oiestad EL, et al. Oral fluid is a viable alternative for monitoring drug abuse: detection of drugs in oral fluid by liquid chromatography-tandem mass spectrometry and comparison to the results from urine samples from patients treated with methadone or buprenorphine. *J Anal Toxicol.* 2011;35(1):32-39.
21. Heltsley R, DePriest A, Black D, et al. Oral fluid drug testing of chronic pain patients, I: positive prevalence rates of licit and illicit drugs. *J Anal Toxicol.* 2011;35(8):529-540.
22. Heltsley R, DePriest A, Black D, et al. Oral fluid drug testing of chronic pain patients, II: comparison of paired oral fluid and urine specimens. *J Anal Toxicol.* 2012;36:75-80.
23. Crouch DJ. Oral fluid collection: the neglected variable in oral fluid testing. *Forensic Sci Int.* 2005;150:165-173.
24. Lias CH. FDA Regulation of Drugs of Abuse Tests: SAMHSA DTAB Meeting, July 26, 2016. Substance Abuse and Mental Health Services Administration. https://www.samhsa.gov/sites/default/files/meeting/documents/dtab-fda-regulation-drugs-abuse-tests-clearance.pdf. Accessed May 17, 2019.
25. Cone EJ, Menchen SL. Stability of cocaine in saliva. *Clin Chem.* 1988;34(7):1508.
26. Ventura M, Pichini S, Ventura R, Zuccaro P, Pacifici R, de la Torre R. Stability studies of principal illicit drugs in oral fluid: preparation of reference materials for external quality assessment schemes. *Ther Drug Monit.* 2007;29:662-665.
27. Langel K, Engblom C, Pehrsson A, Gunnar T, Ariniemi K, Lillsunde P. Drug testing in oral fluid: evaluation of sample collection devices. *J Anal Toxicol.* 2008;32:393-401.
28. Quintela O, Crouch DJ, Andrenyak D. Recovery of drugs of abuse from the Immunalysis Quantisal oral fluid collection device. *J Anal Toxicol.* 2006; 30(8):614-616.
29. Wong RC, Tran M, Tung JK. Oral fluid drug tests: effects of adulterants and foodstuffs. *Forensic Sci Int.* 2005;150:175-180.
30. Cooper G, Wilson L, Reid C, Baldwin D, Hand C, Spiehler V. Validation of the Cozart microplate EIA for analysis of opiates in oral fluid. *Forensic Sci Int.* 2005;154:240-246.
31. Clear Choice Oral Clear Saliva Neutralizing Gum. https://www.testnegative.com/saliva-testing/oral-clear. Accessed May 17, 2019.
32. Barrett C, Good C, Moore C. Comparison of point-of-collection screening of drugs of abuse in oral fluid with a laboratory-based urine screen. *Forensic Sci Int.* 2001;122:163-166.
33. Walsh JM, Flegel R, Crouch DJ, Cangianelli L, Baudys J. An evaluation of rapid point-of-collection oral fluid drug-testing devices. *J Anal Toxicol.* 2003;27:429-439.
34. Walsh JM, Crouch DJ, Danaceau JP, Cangianelli L, Liddicoat L, Adkins R. Evaluation of ten oral fluid point-of-collection drug-testing devices. *J Anal Toxicol.* 2007;31:44-54.
35. Pehrsson A, Blencowe T, Vimpari K, Langel K, Engblom C, Lillsunde P. An evaluation of on-site oral fluid drug screening devices DrugWipe® 5+ and Rapid STAT® using oral fluid for confirmation analysis. *J Anal Toxicol.* 2011;35(4):211-218.

36. Bosker WM, Huestis MA. Oral fluid testing for drugs of abuse. *Clin Chem.* 2009;55:1910-1931.
37. Verstraete AG, Raes E, eds. ROSITA-2 Project: Final Report. European Commission. https://ec.europa.eu/transport/road_safety/sites/roadsafety/files/pdf/projects_sources/rosita2_final_report.pdf. March 2006. Accessed May 10, 2019.
38. Blencowe T, Pehrsson A, Lillsunde P, eds. Analytical Evaluation of Oral Fluid Screening Devices and Preceding Selection Procedures. 2010. DRUID Deliverable D 3.2.2. Revision 2.0.
39. Beirness DJ, Smith DR. An assessment of oral fluid drug screening devices. *Can Soc Forensic Sci J.* 2017;50(2):55-63.
40. Logan BK, Mohr AL, Talpins SK. Detection and prevalence of drug use in arrested drivers using the Drager Drug Test 5000 and Affiniton DrugWipe oral fluid drug screening devices. *J Anal Toxicol.* 2014;38(7):444-450.
41. Ellefsen K, Concheiro M, Pirard S, Gorelick D, Huestis M. Cocaine and benzoylecgonine oral fluid on-site screening and confirmation. *Drug Test Anal.* 2016;8(3-4):296-303.
42. Gunnar T, Ariniemi K, Lillsunde P. Validated toxicological determination of 30 drugs of abuse as optimized derivatives in oral fluid by long column fast gas chromatography/electron impact mass spectrometry. *J Mass Spectrom.* 2005;40:739-753.
43. Concheiro M, de Castro A, Quintela O, Cruz A, Lopez-Rivadulla M. Determination of illicit and medicinal drugs and their metabolites in oral fluid and preserved oral fluid by liquid chromatography-tandem mass spectrometry. *Anal Bioanal Chem.* 2008;391:2329-2338.
44. Oiestad EL, Johansen U, Christophersen AS. Drug screening of preserved oral fluid by liquid chromatography-tandem mass spectrometry. *Clin Chem.* 2007;53:300-309.
45. Allen KR, Azad R, Field HP, Blake DK. Replacement of immunoassay by LC tandem mass spectrometry for the routine measurement of drugs of abuse in oral fluid. *Ann Clin Biochem.* 2005;42:277-284.
46. Liu H, Lee H, Hsu Y, et al. Direct injection LC-MSMS analysis of opiates, methamphetamine, buprenorphine, methadone and their metabolites in oral fluid from substitution therapy patients. *J Anal Toxicol.* 2015;39(6):472-480.
47. Enders JR, McIntire GL. A dilute-and-shoot LC-MS method for quantitating opioids in oral fluid. *J Anal Toxicol.* 2015;39(8):662-667.
48. Moore C, Coulter C, Crompton K, Zumwalt M. Determination of benzodiazepines in oral fluid using LC-MS-MS. *J Anal Toxicol.* 2007; 31(9):596-600.
49. Coulter C, Garnier M, Moore C. Analysis of tetrahydrocannabinol and its metabolite, 11-nor-9-tetrahydrocannabinol-9-carboxylic acid, in oral fluid using liquid chromatography with tandem mass spectrometry. *J Anal Toxicol.* 2012;36(6):413-417.
50. Kala SV, Harris SE, Freijo TD, Gerlich S. Validation of analysis of amphetamines, opiates, phencyclidine, cocaine, and benzoylecgonine in oral fluids by liquid chromatography-tandem mass spectrometry. *J Anal Toxicol.* 2008;32(8):605-611.
51. Moore C, Rana S, Coulter C. Determination of meperidine, tramadol and oxycodone in human oral fluid using solid phase extraction and gas chromatography-mass spectrometry. *J Chromatogr B Analyt Technol Biomed Life Sci.* 2007;850(1-2):370-375.
52. Badawi N, Simonsen KW, Steentoft A, Bernhoft IM, Linnet K. Simultaneous screening and quantification of 29 drugs of abuse in oral fluid by solid-phase extraction and ultraperformance LC-MS/MS. *Clin Chem.* 2009;55(11):2004-2018.
53. Valen A, Leere Oiestad AM, Strand DH, Skari R, Berg T. Determination of 21 drugs in oral fluid using fully automated supported liquid extraction and UHPLC-MS/MS. *Drug Test Anal.* 2017;9(5):808-823.
54. Proficiency testing program for alcohol and drugs in oral fluid. RTI International. https://www.rti.org/sites/default/files/brochures/rti-brochure-file-4c114ded-f166-4339-8225-a46c5798fccb.pdf. Accessed May 17, 2019.
55. College of American Pathologists. 2019 Surveys and Anatomic Pathology Education Programs [catalog]. Oral Fluid for Drugs of Abuse OFD. https://www.cap.org/laboratory-improvement/catalogs-ordering-and-shipping. Accessed May 17, 2019.
56. Haeckel R. Factors influencing the saliva/plasma ratio of drugs. *Ann N Y Acad Sci.* 1993;694:128-142.
57. Jones AW. Inter- and intra-individual variations in the saliva/blood alcohol ratio during ethanol metabolism in man. *Clin Chem.* 1979;25:1394-1398.
58. Gubala W, Zuba D. Comparison of ethanol concentrations in saliva and blood. *Can Soc Forensic Sci J.* 2002;35:229-235.
59. Procedures for Transportation Workplace Drug and Alcohol Testing Programs. US Department of Transportation. https://www.ecfr.gov/cgi-bin/text-idx?SID=44edbc0e557a4cc5ff03365810ee5b1c&mc=true&node=pt49.1.40&rgn=div5#sp49.1.40.a. Title 49 CFR Part 40. Updated February 8, 2019. Accessed May 20, 2019.
60. Schepers RF, Oyler JM, Joseph RE, Cone EJ, Moolchan ET, Huestis MA. Methamphetamine and amphetamine pharmacokinetics in oral fluid and plasma after controlled oral methamphetamine administration to human volunteers. *Clin Chem.* 2003;49:121-132.
61. Samyn N, De Boeck G, Wood M, et al. Plasma, oral fluid and sweat wipe ecstasy concentrations in controlled and real life conditions. *Forensic Sci Int.* 2002;128:90-97.

62. Samyn N, DeBoeck G, Cirimele V, Verstraete A, Kintz P. Detection of flunitrazepam and 7-aminoflunitrazepam in oral fluid after controlled administration of rohypnol. *J Anal Toxicol.* 2002; 26:211-215.
63. Dams R, Choo RE, Lambert WE, Jones H, Huestis MA. Oral fluid as an alternative matrix to monitor opiate and cocaine use in substance-abuse treatment patients. *Drug Alcohol Depend.* 2007; 87(2-3):258-267.
64. Moolchan ET, Cone EJ, Wstadik A, Huestis MA, Preston KL. Cocaine and metabolite elimination patterns in chronic cocaine users during cessation: plasma and saliva analysis. *J Anal Toxicol.* 2000;24:458-466.
65. Presley L, Lehrer M, Seiter W, et al. High prevalence of 6-acetylmorphine in morphine-positive oral fluid specimens. *Forensic Sci Int.* 2003;133:22-25.
66. Jenkins AJ, Oyler JM, Cone EJ. Comparison of heroin and cocaine concentrations in saliva with concentrations in blood and plasma. *J Anal Toxicol.* 1995;19(6):359-374.
67. Kim I, Barnes AJ, Oyler JM, et al. Plasma and oral fluid pharmacokinetics and pharmacodynamics after oral codeine administration. *Clin Chem.* 2002;48(9):1486-1496.
68. Rohrig T, Moore C. The determination of morphine in urine and oral fluid following ingestion of poppy seeds. *J Anal Toxicol.* 2003;27(7):449-452.
69. Cone EJ, DePriest AZ, Heltsley R, et al. Prescription opioids. III. Disposition of oxycodone in oral fluid and blood following controlled single-dose administration. *J Anal Toxicol.* 2015;39(3):192-202.
70. Moore C, Kelley-Baker T, Lacey J. Interpretation of oxycodone concentrations in oral fluid. *J Opioid Manag.* 2012;8(3):161-166.
71. Cone EJ, DePriest AZ, Heltsley R, et al. Prescription opioids, IV: disposition of hydrocodone in oral fluid and blood following single-dose administration. *J Anal Toxicol.* 2015;39(7):510-518.
72. Cone EJ, Clarke J, Tsanaclis L. Prevalence and disposition of drugs of abuse and opioid treatment drugs in oral fluid. *J Anal Toxicol.* 2007; 31(8):424-433.
73. Gray TR, Dams R, Choo RE, et al. Methadone disposition in oral fluid during pharmacotherapy for opioid-dependence. *Forensic Sci Int.* 2011;206(1-3): 98-102.
74. Ardakani YH, Rouini MR. Pharmacokinetic study of tramadol and its three metabolites in plasma, saliva and urine. *DARU: J Faculty Pharm.* 2009;17(4):245-255.
75. Cone EJ, Dickerson SL, Darwin WD, Fudala P, Johnson RE. Elevated drug saliva levels suggest a "depot-like" effect in subjects treated with sublingual buprenorphine. *NIDA Res Monogr.* 1991; 105:569.
76. Lee D, Huestis MA. Current knowledge on cannabinoids in oral fluid. *Drug Test Anal.* 2014; 6(1-2):88-111.
77. Huestis MA, Cone EJ. Relationship of delta 9-tetrahydrocannabinol concentrations in oral fluid and plasma after controlled administration of smoked cannabis. *J Anal Toxicol.* 2004;28(6):394-399.
78. Lee D, Milman G, Barnes AJ, Goodwin RS, Hirvonen J, Huestis MA. Oral fluid cannabinoids in chronic, daily cannabis smokers during sustained, monitored abstinence. *Clin Chem.* 2011;57:1127-1136.
79. Moore C, Coulter C, Uges D, et al. Cannabinoids in oral fluid following passive exposure to marijuana smoke. *Forensic Sci Int.* 2011;212:227-230.
80. Cone EJ, Bigelow GC, Herrmann ES, et al. Nonsmoker exposure to secondhand cannabis smoke, III: oral fluid and blood drug concentrations and corresponding subjective effects. *J Anal Toxicol.* 2015;39(7):497-509.
81. Vandrey R, Herrmann E, Mitchell J, et al. Pharmacokinetic profile of oral cannabis in humans: blood and oral fluid disposition and relation to pharmacodynamic outcomes. *J Anal Toxicol.* 2017;41(2):83-99.
82. Verstraete AG. Detection times of drugs of abuse in blood, urine, and oral fluid. *Ther Drug Monit.* 2004;26(2):200-205.
83. Hardy J, Norris R, Anderson H, O'Shea A, Charles B. Is saliva a valid substitute for plasma in pharmacokinetic studies of oxycodone and its metabolites in patients with cancer? *Support Care Cancer.* 2012;20(4):767-772.
84. Gjerde H, Langel K, Favretto D, Verstraete AG. Detection of 4 benzodiazepines in oral fluid as biomarker for presence in blood. *Ther Drug Monit.* 2014;36(2):252-256.
85. Patsalos PN, Berry DJ. Therapeutic drug monitoring of antiepileptic drugs by use of saliva. *Ther Drug Monit.* 2013;35(1):4-29.
86. Cone EJ, Presley L, Lehrer M, et al. Oral fluid testing for drugs of abuse: positive prevalence rates by Intercept immunoassay screening and GC-MS-MS confirmation and suggested cutoff concentrations. *J Anal Toxicol.* 2002;26(8):541-546.
87. Drug Testing Index. Quest Diagnostics. https://www.questdiagnostics.com/home/companies/employer/drug-screening.html. Accessed May 20, 2019.
88. Casolin A. Comparison of urine and oral fluid for workplace drug testing. *J Anal Toxicol.* 2016; 40(7):479-485.
89. Miller KL, Puet BL, Roberts A, Hild C, Carter J, Black DL. Urine drug testing results and paired oral fluid comparison from patients enrolled in long-term medication-assisted treatment in Tennessee. *J Subst Abuse Treat.* 2017;76:36-42.
90. US Food and Drug Administration. 510(k) Premarket Notification. http://www.accessdata.fda.gov/scripts/cdrh/cfdocs/cfpmn/pmn.cfm. Accessed May 20, 2019.

Chapter 15

Drug Testing in Hair, Sweat, Meconium, Cord Tissue, and Breast Milk

Uttam Garg, PhD
Gwendolyn A. McMillin, PhD

Introduction

Substance abuse leads to tens of thousands of deaths each year in the United States and around the world. It is estimated that more than 25 million Americans abuse illicit or prescription drugs, costing more than $400 billion annually in health care costs and lost productivity. Patient counseling and drug testing are widely used in the prevention and deterrence of drug abuse. Because patient questioning and counseling are very subjective and less reliable, drug testing is frequently used for detection and prevention of drug abuse.

Although urine is the most commonly used specimen for drug testing, alternate samples—such as oral fluid, sweat, meconium, hair, nail, and cord tissue—are increasingly being used. These specimens offer many advantages, such as easy sample collection without a need for a special collection facility or personnel, supervised sample collection, and reduced potential for sample adulteration. However, these specimens pose unique preanalytical, analytical, and interpretive challenges.

The US Substance Abuse and Mental Health Services Administration (SAMHSA) and European Workplace Drug Testing Society (EWDTS) proposed guidelines for oral fluid, hair, and sweat,[1] but, because of concerns raised by the public and federal agencies in 2008, SAMHSA concluded that there was insufficient information to include these alternate samples in Federal Workplace Drug Testing Programs.[2] SAMHSA remains committed to monitoring the developments in alternative specimen testing. In 2017 guidelines, SAMHSA allows oral fluid as an alternate specimen if the donor is unable to provide a urine specimen.[3]

Hair

In the 1960s, hair samples were used for the evaluation of heavy metal exposure. At that time, it was believed that drugs accumulate in hair. In 1979, Baumgartner et al[4] reported the presence of morphine in hair. Baumgartner et al[4] also reported that the presence of morphine along the hair shaft can be correlated with the time of drug use. Further studies on the patients from rehabilitation treatment centers showed higher drug concentration in terminal parts and lower drug concentration in proximal parts of hair.[5-7]

Hair testing can detect long-term drug use, making hair a good specimen for preemployment, random, return-to-duty, or follow-up testing. Because it takes 4 to 10 days for a drug to appear in hair, it is not a good specimen for evaluation of postaccident or reasonable suspicion testing. Hair drug analysis has been used in the determination of compliance, alcohol abuse, prenatal drug exposure, doping practices, traffic violations, and the reissuance of a driver's license.[8] Fetal hair has been used to detect maternal drug use during pregnancy. Fetal hair grows in the last trimester, indicating maternal drug use in the last trimester of pregnancy.[9,10]

Hair consists of the hair follicle and hair shaft. At the base of the hair follicle are matrix cells in the dermis of the skin. Circulating drugs in blood capillaries first incorporate in hair follicles and then get entrapped in the core of the shaft as the hair grows out of the follicle. Once in the hair shaft, under good conditions such as protection from light, heat, and moisture, the drugs are very stable. For example, cocaine metabolites have been detected in the hair of mummies more than 4000 years old.[11,12] In hair, drugs can also incorporate from sweat and sebum and from the external environment. The physiochemical properties of a drug greatly influence its incorporation into the hair. Neutral and basic lipophilic drugs incorporate into the hair more easily than acidic hydrophilic drugs.[13]

Hair Collection and Analysis

Hair sample collection is not well standardized and varies significantly among collection facilities. An ideal sample would come from the area at the back of the head called the *vertex posterior,* ie, there is less variability in hair growth, and the hair is less influenced by age, sex, climate, and health.[14,15] Sample size also varies significantly among laboratories, from a few milligrams to several hundred milligrams. Hair should be cut close to the root as the distance from the hair root reflects the time elapsed since drug use, and the root end must be clearly indicated. SAMHSA proposed the use of 1.5 inches of hair. This corresponds to an approximately 3-month time period because hair grows at a rate of 0.5 ± 0.2 inch/month. A 100-mg sample contains approximately 100 hair strands. Because hair collection is done under direct supervision, it is less

Table 15-1. US Substance Abuse and Mental Health Services Administration (SAMHSA) Proposed Initial Screening and Confirmatory Cutoffs for Hair Testing

Analyte	Concentration (pg/mg)	
	Initial Screening	Confirmatory Cutoffs
Cannabinoids		
Tetrahydrocannabinol (THC) metabolites	1	—
11-nor-Δ^9-carboxy-THC (THC-COOH)	—	0.05
Cocaine		
Cocaine metabolites	500	—
Cocaine*	—	500
Cocaine metabolites*	—	50
Opiates/Opioids		
Opiate metabolites†	200	—
Morphine	—	200
Codeine	—	200
6-Monoacetylmorphine (6-MAM)	200	—
6-MAM (specimen must also contain morphine at a concentration ≥200 pg/mg)	—	200
Phencyclidine (PCP)	300	300
Amphetamines		
Amphetamines (target analyte: methamphetamine)	500	—
Amphetamine	—	300
Methamphetamine (specimen must also contain amphetamine at ≥50 pg/mg)	—	300
3,4-Methylenedioxymethamphetamine (MDMA)	500	300
3,4-Methylenedioxyamphetamine (MDA)	—	300
3,4-Methylenedioxyethylamphetamine (MDEA)	—	300

* A positive cocaine concentration is greater than or equal to the confirmatory cutoff and benzoylecgonine/cocaine ratio is ≥0.05, cocaethylene is ≥50 pg/mg, or norcocaine ≥50 pg/mg.

† Laboratories are permitted to initial test all specimens for 6-acetylmorphine (6-AM) using a cutoff of 200 pg/mg.

invasive and less prone to adulteration; however, hair collection can be invasive if samples have to be collected from other body sites.

After a hair sample is collected, it is thoroughly washed to remove any external drug contamination before analysis. Washed hairs are dried, cut or grinded into small pieces, and drugs are extracted using organic solvents. The decontamination step to remove external contamination is an important step in hair drug analysis. Hair washing should not be so gentle that it does not remove contamination or too harsh such that it removes drugs that are incorporated into the hair. Although there is no consensus on a specific procedure, various aqueous and organic solvents have been used for decontaminating hair. These washing solvents include methanol, ethanol, dichloromethane, dichloromethane/water, 2-propanol, and 2-propanol/phosphate buffer. Despite the most comprehensive and complex decontamination procedures, measurable concentrations of some drugs have been reported.[15,16] After the hair is washed, drugs are extracted using various extraction solvents and buffers.[16,17]

Two major techniques, immunoassays and chromatography, are used for the analysis of hair. Immunoassay techniques include radioimmunoassays (RIAs), enzyme immunoassays (EIAs), and fluorescent immunoassays. Commonly used chromatographic techniques are gas chromatography-mass spectrometry (GC-MS) and high-performance liquid chromatography-tandem mass spectrometry (HPLC-MS/MS).[13,17] Immunoassays are generally used for screening, followed by confirmation with GC-MS or HPLC-MS/MS. Tandem mass spectrometry is becoming the method of choice for hair drug analysis because of its higher sensitivity, higher specificity, and easier sample preparation than GC-MS. The SAMHSA and EWDTS proposed screening and confirmatory cutoffs for hair drug testing are shown in Tables 15-1 and 15-2, respectively.[1,15]

Table 15-2. European Workplace Drug Testing Society (EWDTS) Recommended Initial Screening and Confirmatory Cutoffs for Hair Testing

Analyte	Concentration (pg/mg)	
	Initial Screening	Confirmatory Cutoffs
Alcohol (segment 0-3)	—	EtG: 30; FAEE: 500
Cannabinoids		
Tetrahydrocannabinol (THC)	100	50
11-nor-Δ^9-carboxy-THC (THC-COOH)	—	0.2
Cocaine	500	500
Benzoylecgonine	—	50
Cocaethylene	—	50
Norcocaine	—	50
Opiates/Opioids	200	—
Morphine	—	200
Codeine	—	200
6-Monoacetylmorphine (6-MAM)	—	200
Amphetamines	200	—
Amphetamines	—	200
Methamphetamine	—	200
3,4-Methylenedioxymethamphetamine (MDMA)	—	200
3,4-Methylenedioxyamphetamine (MDA)	—	200
3,4-Methylenedioxyethylamphetamine (MDEA)	—	200
Methadone	200	200
2-Ethylidene-1,5-dimethyl-3,3-diphenylpyrrolidine (EDDP)	—	50
Buprenorphine	10	10
Norbuprenorphine	—	10
Ketamine	500	500
Norketamine	—	100
Benzodiazepines/Z-drugs	50	50

ETG, ethylglucuronide; FAEE, fatty acid ethyl esters.

Drug Detection in Hair

A number of drugs of abuse have been detected in hair, including amphetamines, cocaine, cannabinoids, phencyclidine (PCP), and opioids. In addition, many other drugs have been found in hair, including barbiturates, benzodiazepines, buprenorphine, cotinine, ethanol metabolites, fentanyl, γ-hydroxybutyrate, ketamine, methadone, methylphenidate, nicotine, quetiapine, tramadol, and Z-drugs.[8,14,16,18]

Opioids were the earliest drugs detected in hair. Baumgartner et al[4] used RIAs for the assay of morphine and heroin in hair samples collected from heroin addicts. When the hair and urine results were compared, strikingly, the positivity rate in urine samples was only 30% compared with 100% in hair. This was probably due to chronic versus acute use. They also noted a good correlation between hair drug concentration and duration of drug use. A study of 20 participants in a heroin maintenance program who received drug doses of 30 mg/day to 800 mg/day found no significant correlation between the heroin dose and the concentration.[19] Later studies reported many other opioids in hair, including codeine, hydrocodone, hydromorphone, oxycodone, 6-acetylmorphine, and buprenorphine. Various methods have been used for the assay of opioids, including RIA, EIAs, GC-MS, and LC-MS/MS. Cooper et al[20] collected 164 hair specimens from volunteers and drug-related postmortem cases. Cozart EIA and GC-MS were used in the hair analyses. Using a cutoff of 200 pg/mg hair, Cozart EIA had a sensitivity and specificity of 98% and 93%, respectively. For GC-MS analysis, drugs were extracted in methanol at 60°C and derivatized with *N,O*-bis(trimethylsilyl)trifluoroacetamide (BSTFA).

Lachenmeier et al[21] evaluated an oral fluid microplate EIA for hair opiate testing and compared the results with GC-MS. There was a good correlation between EIAs and GC-MS. Jones et al[22] described a GC-MS method for the simultaneous determination of several opioids in hair, including codeine, morphine, hydrocodone, hydromorphone, 6-acetylmorphine, and oxycodone. Their method involved hair grinding using stainless steel balls, solid phase extraction, and sample derivation with methoxime/BSTFA. In recent years, LC-MS/MS use has increased in hair analysis. Fernandez Mdel et al[23] described an LC-MS/MS method for a simultaneous analysis of 33 drugs, including opiates, opioids, and their metabolites.

Various stimulants have been detected in hair, including amphetamines, methamphetamine, cocaine, methylenedioxyamphetamine (MDA), methylenedioxymethamphetamine (MDMA), and methylenedioxyethylamphetamine (MDEA). Immunoassays, GC-MS, and LC-MS/MS are the most commonly used methods for the detection of stimulants in hair.[20,24-28] Cooper et al[27] analyzed amphetamine, methamphetamine, MDA, MDMA, and MDEA in hair samples collected from 100 participants who were recruited from the "dance scene" in and around Glasgow, Scotland. The hair samples were analyzed in two 6-cm segments or in full, ranging from 1.5 cm to 12 cm, depending on the length of the hair. Of 139 segments analyzed, 77 (52.5%) were positive for amphetamines. Despite more than 50% concordance between the drugs consumed and the drugs detected in hair, there was no correlation between the drug concentrations and drug doses. In one study, seven volunteers with a history of stimulant use received four doses of 10 mg of sustained-release methamphetamine within 1 week. Weekly head hair samples were collected by shaving. After 3 weeks, four volunteers received four doses of 20 mg, followed by weekly sample collections. The maximum concentration of methamphetamine occurred from 1 to 2 weeks after both dosing regimens. The amphetamine:methamphetamine ratio ranged from 0.07 to 0.37.[29]

Both cocaine and its major metabolite, benzoylecgonine, have been detected in persons using cocaine.[30,31] The measurement of cocaine metabolites is preferred to rule out external contamination. Baumgartner et al[32] used RIA for analysis of the cocaine metabolite benzoylecgonine in hair collected from patients undergoing drug rehabilitation. A highly sensitive GC-MS/MS method for the simultaneous determination of cocaine and three of its metabolites—anhydroecgonine methylester, ecgonine methylester, and cocaethylene—has been reported. The limit of detection for these compounds was 0.005, 0.050, 0.025, and 0.005 ng/mg of hair, respectively.[31] Studies have been performed to correlate the amount of cocaine consumed with the cocaine concentration in hair. Despite large variation, there is a correlation between the concentration of cocaine in hair and the amount of cocaine consumed. Graham et al[33] reported a benzoylecgonine concentration of 0.64 ng/mg to 29.1 ng/mg of hair in heavy users and 0.032 ng/mg to 1.21 ng/mg of hair in occasional users. Also, correlation between the time elapsed after use and the cocaine concentration has been reported. In one study, seven participants were tested for benzoylecgonine after 2 to 12 months of cocaine use and after 2 months of abstinence. Benzoylecgonine concentrations estimated by RIA were 0.6 ng/mg to 6.4 ng/mg and 0.3 ng/mg to 0.5 ng/mg of hair after cocaine use and after abstinence, respectively. Hair samples from infants born to mothers who used cocaine during pregnancy had benzoylecgonine concentrations of 0.2 ng/mg to 2.75 ng/mg of hair.[33] The drug was not detected after 10 weeks, which corresponded to the loss of fetal hair. A study on maternal urine and neonatal hair testing for cocaine showed hair analysis for gestational cocaine exposure had a sensitivity of 88%, specificity of 100%, and positive and negative predictive values of 100% and 85%, respectively.[34] In another study, median cocaine concentration was 10-fold higher in hair of the mothers compared with hair of the neonates (3.56 vs 0.31 ng/mg of hair). A segmental analysis was used and correlated with the timing of drug use. A study on a cocaine abuser showed the disappearance of cocaine in the hair sections closest to the root after 3 months of abstinence.[5]

Δ^9-tetrahydrocannabinol (THC) and its major metabolite, 11-nor-Δ^9-carboxy-9-tetrahydrocannabinol (THC-COOH), have been detected in hair. Unlike in urine, the concentration of THC in hair is much higher than the concentration of THC-COOH. Detection of THC-COOH is preferred because it provides a better proof of active drug use. It is not present in the smoke or dust and is produced in vivo. Immunoassays for screening and chromatographic methods for confirmation are widely used for the assay of THC and THC-COOH in hair. GC-MS is a commonly used method for the confirmation of THC and THC-COOH in hair.[35,36] In a GC-MS/MS method described by Han et al,[36] hair samples were pulverized in sodium hydroxide for 30 minutes at 85°C. THC and THC-COOH were extracted with hexane:ethyl acetate and a derivatization with pentafluoropropionic anhydride/pentafluoropropanol (PFPA/PFP-OH). This method was used on hair samples collected from known cannabis users. THC and THC-COOH concentrations ranged from 7.52 to 60.4 ng/mg and 0.1 to 11.7 pg/mg of hair, respectively. LC-MS/MS methods are available for the determination of cannabinoids.[37,38]

Baumgartner et al[39] used RIA for the detection of PCP in hair from participants admitting PCP use. PCP concentrations in these individuals ranged from 0.3 ng/mg to 5.2 ng/mg and 0.3 ng/mg to 2.8 ng/mg in unwashed and washed hair samples and correlated with the duration of drug use. In another study on psychiatric patients, hair analysis detected PCP in 11 of 47 patients. Strikingly, blood and urine were negative in all of these patients.[40] These studies demonstrate the longer stability and wider window of detection for PCP in hair samples.

Hair has also been used to detect chronic ethanol consumption. In addition to oxidative metabolism, a small amount of ethanol is converted to ethyl glucuronide (EtG), ethyl sulfate (EtS), and fatty acid ethyl esters (FAEEs). These minor ethanol metabolites have been used as long-term biomarkers of ethanol intake. Concentrations of EtG and FAEEs in hair have been correlated with amount of ethanol consumption.[41] EtG levels less than 7 pg/mg of hair are indicative of abstinence of ethanol use. An EtG level greater than 30 pg/mg of hair is indicative of chronic, excessive use of ethanol. EtG levels between 7 and 30 pg/mg of hair are indicative of regular ethanol consumption.[42,43]

Interpretive Considerations in Hair Drug Analysis

Environmental or External Contamination

Because hair is in direct contact with the environment, external contamination remains a significant concern in hair drug testing. Questions about the external contamination are raised, particularly by the individuals who test positive for drugs. Generally speaking, there is little concern of external contamination by the drugs that are consumed orally and not smoked; however, external contamination can be a significant issue for the drugs that are smoked, such as marijuana, cocaine, and methamphetamine. Therefore, the removal of external drug contamination is an important step in hair drug analysis. Various methods have been used to remove external drug contamination, but they show significant variability. One study investigated the effect of different wash solutions on the removal of cocaine and its metabolites benzoylecgonine, norcocaine, ecgonine methylester, and cocaethylene. There were significant differences among different wash solutions.[44] Some studies have even shown that despite extensive hair washing, external contamination for certain drugs cannot be completely removed. In two studies involving the external contamination of hair, extensive washings did not completely remove the cocaine contamination.[45,46] In another study, volunteers' hair was contaminated with a small amount of heroin hydrochloride and acetylcodeine hydrochloride for 5 consecutive days. Despite extensive washings, in this study, external contamination could not be completely removed. In fact, hair from the study participants tested positive for heroin, 6-monoacetylmorphine (6-MAM), morphine, acetylcodeine, and codeine for at least 3 months.[47] In a study in New Zealand, hair samples were collected from children removed from nonsanctioned (clandestine) laboratories and were tested for methamphetamine and amphetamine; 38 (73%) and 34 (65%) of 52 hair samples tested positive for methamphetamine and amphetamine, respectively. Amphetamine was not detected in any case without the presence of methamphetamine.[48] The presence of PCP in hair has also been reported in external contamination.

To address issues of external contamination, the detection of drug metabolites has been proposed. The presence of drug metabolites is a better indicator of active drug use than are the parent drugs. Koren et al[49] showed that pyrolysis of crack cocaine results in the accumulation of cocaine in hair, but not of its metabolite benzoylecgonine. On the other hand, in cocaine users, both cocaine and benzoylecgonine are detectable in hair. Likewise, detection of THC-COOH, the major metabolite of THC, can rule out the external contamination. Uhl and Sachs[50] tested for marijuana and its metabolites in hair samples from a couple. The couple tested positive for parent drugs THC and cannabinol (CBN); however, only the hair sample from the man, who used marijuana, tested positive for THC-COOH. The hair from the woman, who did not use marijuana, tested negative for THC-COOH (limit of quantitation, 0.1 pg/mg of hair). SAMHSA guidelines proposed the use of THC-COOH in hair analysis. Nakahara et al[51] proposed the analysis of PCP and its metabolites 1-(1-phenylcyclohexyl)-4-hydroxypiperidine (PCHP) and trans-1-(1-phenyl-4-hydroxycyclohexyl)-4'-hydroxypiperidine (t-PCPdiol) to rule out external contamination and passive exposure. The authors recommend that the detection of t-PCPdiol be an indicator of active PCP use. Despite the use of metabolites as an indicator of active drug use, many studies have shown the presence of drug metabolites in hair after external contamination.[16,52,53] Romano et al[52] showed the presence of benzoylecgonine in cocaine-contaminated hair; however, the amount of benzoylecgonine was less than 0.5 ng/mg of hair.

Another approach has been proposed to address the issue of external contamination. In this approach, both the wash solution and the hair are tested and compared for drug concentrations. If the ratio of wash residue to hair is less than a specific cutoff, then environmental contamination is unlikely.[54]

Certain products have been implicated as a source of external contamination. For example, certain shampoos contain a significant amount of cannabinoids (1-3%). In one study, an analysis of a Cannabio shampoo revealed the presence of THC, cannabidiol (CBD), and CBN at concentrations of 412 ng/mg, 4079 ng/mg, and 380 ng/mL, respectively.[55] In the same study, hair samples were collected from three volunteers who used this shampoo for 2 weeks. None of the participants tested positive for THC, CBD, or CBN. Also, in this study the hairs were incubated in water:Cannabio shampoo (20:1, v/v) for 30 minutes, 2 hours, and 5 hours, and analyzed for THC, CBD, and CBN. The samples that were incubated for 30 minutes tested negative for all three compounds; however, the samples that were incubated for 2 hours and 5 hours tested positive for CBD and CBN, but not for THC.[55] Therefore, it is highly unlikely that the use of Cannabio shampoo will result in false-positive results.

On the basis of these studies, it seems that questions regarding external hair contamination are valid. The use of effective wash procedures, appropriate cutoffs, metabolite ratios, and metabolite analyses can help distinguish external drug contamination from active drug use.

Hair Color and Drug Incorporation

Hair color has been a concern since the 1980s when the Navy tried to use hair specimens in its drug testing program. Navy research and many other studies demonstrated that different-colored natural hair incorporates drugs to different degrees. Because of the fear of color bias and racial disparity, the military decided not to use hair in its drug testing programs. It has been shown that darker hair retains significantly higher amounts of drug compared with lighter colored hair. This has been attributed to the higher concentration of melanin that determines the hair color. It is a polyanionic polymer of eumelanin and pheomelanin. Eumelanin concentration is the highest in natural black hair, whereas pheomelanin is highest in natural red hair. White hair has little to no melanin. Because different drugs have different affinities for these pigments, this results in differences in drug concentrations in different colors of hair. This effect has been studied in both animals and humans (see below).

The Long-Evans rat, which produces both white and black hairs, provides a good model for studying the effects of hair color on the incorporation of different drugs. Borges et al[56] dosed Long-Evans rats with amphetamine or its nonbasic analogue *N*-acetylamphetamine. The black hair had approximately three times higher concentration of amphetamine than the white hair (6.44 vs 2.04 ng/mg); however, *N*-acetylamphetamine concentrations were not different in white and black hairs. Another study used Long-Evans rats to study the incorporation of PCP into different hair colors. In this study, the animals received 12 mg PCP/kg of rat body weight by intraperitoneal injection daily for 5 days. After 14 days, the hair samples were collected and analyzed for PCP. Concentrations of PCP in pigmented hair were significantly higher than in nonpigmented hair: 14.33 ± 1.43 versus 0.47 ± 0.04 ng/mg of hair, respectively.[57] In a recent study, Long-Evans rats were administered 25B-, 25C- or 25I-NBOMe, new psychoactive substances derived from phenethylamines. The drug doses ranged from 30 μg/kg to 300 μg/kg of rat body weight over a period of 10 days. Rats were shaved before their first dose and reshaved after the 10-day period. Black and white hairs were separated and analyzed using LC-MS/MS. A dose-dependent concentration increase was observed in the black hair, whereas in white hair only 25B- and 25C-NBOMe were quantifiable at higher doses.[58] Using a black-hooded rat model, Kulaga et al[59] studied the effect of hair color on the incorporation of FAEEs, the markers of ethanol intake. The rats received ethanol intraperitoneally. Total FAEE levels were significantly higher in posttreatment hair compared with the baseline, but no significant difference was found between black and white hairs.

Human studies have also shown influence of different-colored hair on the incorporation of different drugs. Kronstrand et al[60] analyzed methamphetamine and amphetamine in hair from patients with Parkinson disease who were receiving selegiline, a drug that metabolizes to methamphetamine and amphetamine. The drugs were analyzed on pigmented and nonpigmented hair from gray-haired patients. Pigmented hair had a higher concentration of drugs compared with nonpigmented hair. The authors also performed segmental hair analysis and found that some patients were not compliant with their medication. In another study on self-reported cocaine users, 37 of 38 (95%) hair samples were positive for cocaine. There was significantly more cocaine in black hair than in brown or blond hair per milligram of cocaine reported to have been consumed.[61] Goldberger et al[7] found higher concentrations of cocaine in the Africoid group than in the Caucasoid group. There was significantly more cocaine in black hair than in brown or blonde hair per milligram of cocaine dosed.[61] Codeine incorporation in different colors of hair has also been studied. In one study, the volunteers with different hair color received 30 mg codeine three times a day for 5 consecutive days (total dose of 450 mg).[62] Codeine concentrations in black, brown, blond, and red hair were 1429 ± 249, 208 ± 17, 99 ± 10, and 69 ± 11 pg/mg of hair (mean ± SE), respectively. Plasma codeine concentrations were also measured to rule out the differences in bioavailability and metabolism. Interestingly, codeine concentrations in black hair from Asians and Caucasians were significantly different: 2564 ± 170 versus 865 ± 162, respectively. Another observation in this paper was that with the SAMHSA proposed cutoff of 200 pg/mg of hair, 100% of the participants with black hair would have tested positive for codeine as compared with only 50% of those with brown hair. These differences were attributed to differences in melanin concentrations; when the results were normalized with respect to melanin concentrations, these differences attenuated. The effect of hair color on cocaine incorporation has also been studied in vitro. Incubation of hair with cocaine and benzoylecgonine resulted in higher concentration of benzoylecgonine in darker colored hair as compared with blonde hair. The concentration of benzoylecgonine with respect to hair color was black greater than brown greater than blond hair.[63]

In contrast to the above-mentioned studies, a number of studies did not find a significant difference in drug concentrations among different hair colors, races, or ethnic groups. Schaffer et al[64] did not find a difference in cocaine incorporation among blond, auburn, brown, and black hair; however, when the hair was permed, there was an increase in cocaine uptake. These authors postulated that porosity, not hair color, was responsible for the observed differences. In another study, 1852 preemployment applicants classified themselves as black or white. Hair and urine drug testing in these individuals did not show a significant difference in drug positivity rates.[65] In another study that involved 4000 urine samples and 1000 hair samples, the drug positivity rates for cannabinoids, cocaine, and amphetamine were comparable among various ethnic and racial groups.[66]

In addition to hair color, many other factors can influence drug concentrations in hair, including hair permeability, cosmetic hair treatments, hair care habits, drug removal during personal hygiene, and manner and route of drug administration.[67] For example, very black hair from Asians and Caucasians incorporates much less cocaine and morphine compared with black hair from African Americans.[68]

Hair Adulteration Issues

Because hair samples are collected under direct supervision, the chances of sample adulteration at the site of sample collection are minimal, but the donor may adulterate the sample at home before the sample collection. A number of products that guarantee to foil hair drug testing can be found online. Many of these products claim to work 100%, but there is little scientific evidence to back up this claim. Ultra Clean shampoo is one of these products. The website for Ultra Clean Shampoo claims, "Hair purifying shampoo is designed for extremely swift yet elegant removal of all toxin residues. Within 10 minutes, you will be in the 'Clean Zone' for up to 4 hours. It is safe for the scalp and all hair types." Using postmortem hair samples from known drug addicts, Rohrich et al[28] investigated the effect of Ultra Clean shampoo on removing THC, cocaine, amphetamine, MDA, MDMA, MDEA, heroin, 6-MAM, morphine, codeine, dihydrocodeine, and methadone. The samples were tested for various drugs with and without the Ultra Clean shampoo treatment. The hair samples washed with Ultra Clean shampoo showed a slight decrease in concentrations of certain drugs. In treated hair, concentrations of cocaine, 6-MAM, morphine, and THC decreased by 5% (n = 10), 9% (n = 12), 26% (n = 12), and 36% (n = 4), respectively. The authors concluded that a single use of Ultra Clean shampoo did not sufficiently remove these drugs enough to cause negative results.

Pritchett and Phinney[69] looked at the effect of chemical straightening products (Silk Elements) on the removal of cocaine and its metabolites. Only a single use of the product caused a 70% to 95% decrease in cocaine, benzoylecgonine, and cocaethylene. The authors speculated that the high pH of the product could cause hydrolysis or decomposition of the drugs.

Sweat

Interest in sweat drug testing is increasing because of reliable and less-invasive sample collection and the development of sensitive analytical methods. Sweat drug testing is more cost effective than urine drug testing because one sample can provide drug exposure information for 1 to 4 weeks versus only a few days for urine. Sweat drug testing is currently used to monitor drug abstinence in drug rehabilitation and criminal justice programs.

Sweat is produced through two types of mechanisms: insensible (consisting of diffusion) or sensible (caused by activity). Sweat is slightly acidic, with an average pH of 5.8. Many factors can affect sweat pH—such as exercise, temperature, hydration, diet, and presence of other drugs—and thus the diffusion and concentration of drugs. Passive diffusion is thought to be the major mechanism of drug transport in sweat.

Sweat Collection and Analysis

Sweat may be collected as liquid perspiration on sweat wipes or with a commercially available sweat patch. In the US, sweat is almost always collected by sweat patch. Sample collection with a sweat patch is more consistent and provides long-term sample collection because the patch can stay in contact with skin for days to weeks. The patch is affixed to the upper arm or torso, similar to a Band-Aid. It consists of an adsorbent pad sandwiched between a porous inner layer and a semipermeable outer layer that allows oxygen, carbon dioxide, and water vapor to pass while larger, nonvolatile molecules adhere to the pad. The patches are waterproof, tamper-evident, comfortable to wear, and are well accepted by the donor. Several commercially available devices are available for sweat collection. One such device approved by the US Food and Drug Administration (FDA) that has been used in multiple studies is PharmChek (PharmChem Inc, Haltom City, Texas). Before application of a sweat patch, the skin should be thoroughly cleaned with an organic solvent (such as isopropyl alcohol) to remove any dirt or skin products, which also helps in the removal of any external drug contamination. Once the patch is in place, it is difficult to adulterate because the outer polyurethane layer is impermeable to molecules larger than water.[70]

When the sweat collection is complete, the patch is removed, observed for any possible tampering, and sent to a laboratory for analysis. In the laboratory, the adsorbent pad is removed, and the drugs are eluted into a buffer. The eluent is tested for drugs using immunoassays or chromatographic techniques, such as GC-MS or LC-MS/MS.[71,72] Various drugs have been detected in sweat, including amphetamines, cannabinoids, cocaine, opiates, and PCP. There is no point-of-collection device available for sweat testing. The SAMHSA proposed screening and confirmation cutoffs in sweat for various drugs of abuse are shown in Table 15-3. Of note, the cutoffs are significantly lower for sweat than for urine.

Drug Detection in Sweat

A number of commonly abused drugs have been detected in sweat, including amphetamines, cannabinoids, cocaine, opiates, PCP, and ethanol. In addition, many other drugs and their metabolites have been reported in sweat, including atomoxetine, barbiturates, benzodiazepines, buprenorphine, bupropion, carbamazepine, clozapine, methadone, methadone metabolite 2-ethylidene-1,5-dimethyl-3,3-diphenylpyrrolidine (EDDP), 6-MAM, nicotine, phenytoin, and phenobarbital.[71-73] In contrast to urine, which has higher concentrations of drug metabolites, sweat generally has higher concentrations of parent drugs.

Stimulants—including amphetamine, methamphetamine, cocaine, and MDMA—have been detected in sweat. Fay et al[74] collected sweat from volunteers who were given 10, 20, and 25 mg methamphetamine. The sweat samples were collected by PharmChek sweat patch and analyzed using EIA and GC-MS. The samples primarily contained the parent drug methamphetamine, although amphetamine was also detected. In another study, 180 sweat samples collected from drivers who failed a field sobriety test were tested by GC-MS. The positive predictive value of sweat wipe analysis was greater than 90% for cocaine and amphetamines.[75] Samyn et al[76] collected sweat samples from MDMA users after 75 mg of MDMA administration. The average MDMA concentration was 25 ng per wipe. Other studies involving human volunteers and the disposition of MDMA in sweat have also been done.[75,77] MDMA and MDA were detected in sweat, but metabolites 4-hydroxy-3-methoxyamphetamine (HMA) and 4-hydroxy-3-methoxymethamphetamine (HMMA) were not detected.

Cocaine and its major metabolites ecgonine methyl ester and benzoylecgonine have been detected in sweat. Like many other drugs, sweat primarily contains the parent drug cocaine, although cocaine metabolites were also detected.[78,79] Kacinko et al[79] carried out a detailed study on cocaine disposition in 15 volunteers with a history of cocaine use. The study was carried out for 12 weeks in a closed research unit. The first 3 weeks were used as a washout period to excrete any previously self-administered drug. On the 4th week, the participants received three subcutaneous injections of cocaine hydrochloride (75 mg/70 kg of body weight). Three weeks later, the participants received three additional doses of cocaine hydrochloride (150 mg/70 kg of body weight). In total, 1390 samples were collected before, during, and after cocaine administration. Sweat collection was performed using PharmChek sweat collection devices. Sweat

Table 15-3. US Substance Abuse and Mental Health Services Administration (SAMHSA) Proposed Initial Screening and Confirmatory Cutoffs for Sweat Patch Testing

Analyte	Concentration (ng/patch)	
	Initial Screening	Confirmatory Cutoffs
Cannabinoids		
Tetrahydrocannabinol (THC) metabolites	4	—
THC	—	1
Cocaine		
Cocaine metabolites	25	—
Cocaine or benzoylecgonine	—	25
Opiates/Opioids		
Opioid metabolites*	25	—
Morphine	—	25
Codeine	—	25
6-Monoacetylmorphine (6-MAM)	—	25
Phencyclidine (PCP)	20	20
Amphetamines		
Amphetamines (target analyte: methamphetamine)	25	—
Amphetamine	—	25
Methamphetamine (specimen must also contain amphetamine)	—	25
3,4-Methylenedioxymethamphetamine (MDMA)	25	25
3,4-Methylenedioxyamphetamine (MDA)	—	25
3,4-Methylenedioxyethylamphetamine (MDEA)	—	25
Benzodiazepines/Z-drugs	50	50

* Laboratories are permitted to initial test all specimens for 6-acetylmorphine (6-AM) at 2.5 ng/patch.

analysis was performed on GC-MS. In this study, 24% and 7% of patches were positive at a cutoff of 2.5 and 25 ng/patch, respectively. Cocaine metabolites were also studied; ecgonine methyl ester was detected more often and at generally higher concentrations than benzoylecgonine. Cocaine and ecgonine methyl ester appear in sweat after 2 hours of ingestion, whereas benzoylecgonine appears after 4 hours.[78]

THC and its metabolites have also been studied in sweat. Using cosmetic wipes, Kintz et al[80] collected sweat from 198 injured drivers. The samples were analyzed for THC and its major metabolite THC-COOH; 16 samples were positive for THC, and 22 samples were positive for THC-COOH. Sweat can stay positive for THC long after cessation of drug use. A recent study of 11 marijuana users investigated THC disposition after marijuana use was stopped. All the samples tested positive after 1 week, three tested positive after 2 weeks, and one tested positive 4 weeks after cessation of drug use.[81]

Opioids that have been reported in sweat include morphine, codeine, and hydrocodone. Fogerson et al[70] studied codeine and heroin disposition in sweat. In their study, the samples were collected using PharmChek and analyzed by EIA and GC-MS. Sweat primarily contained the parent opiates, heroin and codeine, and the lipophilic metabolite 6-MAM. The antibody used in the EIA method had a cross-reactivity with morphine, codeine, hydrocodone, diacetylmorphine, and 6-MAM of 100%, 588%, 143%, 28%, and 30%, respectively. Using 215 patches from 95 participants and receiver operator characteristics curves, the optimal cutoff was 10 ng/mL morphine equivalents. At this cutoff concentration, the assay had a diagnostic sensitivity and specificity rate of 86.9% and 92.8%, respectively. The positive predictive value was 85% at a prevalence rate of 50%.

Sweat Adulteration and Contamination Issues

Because sweat patches can be worn for several days without being overseen, questions about sweat patch adulteration have been raised. It is difficult to tamper with and contaminate the patch because the outer polyurethane layer is impermeable to molecules larger than water. Various studies have shown that the contaminants applied to the outer layer of the sweat patch do not reach the collection pad. Fogerson et al[70] added 18 different adulterants to sweat patches and allowed them to air dry. The patches were then spiked with heroin, codeine, or morphine and incubated for 7 days at 37°C. Most of the adulterants had no effect on drug detection. In addition, the adulterants caused visible irritation to the skin, which would increase suspicion of tampering. Injecting adulterant with a hypodermic needle is a possible means of tampering, and thus it is recommended that the outside layer of the patch be examined for punctures before analysis. Rarely, some individuals can develop an allergic reaction to a sweat patch.

Biological Testing Relevant to the Newborn

Many chemical compounds that a pregnant woman ingests or is otherwise exposed to are known to pass through the placenta and, consequently, into the unborn child. Drugs and drug metabolites are also known to pass from a woman's circulation into the breast milk. *Neonatal abstinence syndrome (NAS),* a characteristic drug withdrawal syndrome originally called *congenital morphinism,* has been a recognized consequence of maternal opioid use during pregnancy for more than 100 years. Signs typically occur within 72 hours of birth and may include a range of neurological symptoms (eg, tremor, high-pitched cry), gastrointestinal manifestations (eg, diarrhea, uncoordinated suckling), and autonomic sequelae (eg, fever, rapid respirations). NAS may also occur after birth from maternal use of other classes of drugs. Symptoms may be masked if the newborn is breastfed and the mother is continuing to use drugs. Newborns are classically diagnosed with NAS on the basis of clinical presentation and maternal history. The opioid epidemic in the US has increased awareness that pregnant women are a vulnerable population when drug abuse, misuse, and addiction occur before a woman recognizes she is pregnant. For those women who seek care during pregnancy, medication-assisted therapy, such as opioid substitution coupled with supportive care and addiction management, may help minimize the adverse effects on the newborn.[82-84]

Among pregnant women, substance misuse varies depending on age and the trimester of pregnancy. In the US, it is estimated that 10% to 11% of all births (400,000-440,000 newborns) are affected by prenatal alcohol or illicit drug exposure and that 75% to 90% of them go undetected.[85,86] In a survey conducted by the Centers for Disease Control and Prevention, the overall incidence of NAS among the 28 states that participated increased by 300% from 1999 to 2013.[87] Because self-report of drug use during pregnancy is known to be poor, biological testing of specimens from newborns is an important tool for identification of drug-exposed newborns who may require medical or social management or both. Health care facilities may collect specimens based on risk of the pregnancy or birth scenario, or based on universal collection. In the case of universal collection, specimens would be stored for a period of time (eg, 1 week) and sent for drug testing only if signs and symptoms of drug withdrawal or related concerns arise. Examples of maternal risk factors that have been best correlated with illicit drug use include past history of substance use disorder or abuse (including nicotine and alcohol), lack of regular prenatal care, unexplained obstetric events (including premature birth), and newborn risk factors, such as growth restriction, symptoms of NAS, and unexplained complications.[88-90]

The most common newborn specimens used today are meconium and umbilical cord tissue. Both specimens are thought to reflect drug exposures occurring over approximately the last trimester of a full-term birth; however, neither specimen accumulates drugs in a linear fashion, and neither is 100% sensitive or 100% specific. Pros and cons of these two specimen types are compared in Table 15-4 and described in detail within this section, followed by a brief discussion of using breast milk to detect and evaluate drug exposures during nursing.

Neonate Specimens

Meconium is the fetal stool formed during gestation and is typically passed in the first few days of an infant's life. Meconium starts to form at approximately the 12th to 16th week of gestation and accumulates throughout pregnancy. Drugs, along with cells, waste products, and other components, are deposited in the meconium as a consequence of placental transfer and through swallowing of amniotic fluid. More than two thirds of meconium is formed during the last weeks of gestation, so it is most likely that third-trimester exposures (vs second trimester) will be detected. Meconium is regarded as the "gold standard" for newborn drug exposure detection, backed by more than 30 years of research and clinical experience.[91-95] Meconium is typically collected from a newborn's diaper, taking care not to collect milk stool or urine, a process that can be laborious. Because meconium passage often occurs over multiple days, collections are combined, often in a standard urine cup, and stored in a refrigerator between collections. The contents of all collections are mixed thoroughly before testing to homogenize the specimen. Ideally, meconium should be collected before administration of any

Table 15-4. Characteristics of Meconium, Umbilical Cord Tissue, and Breast Milk for Detection and Management of a Drug-Exposed Newborn

	Meconium	Umbilical Cord	Breast Milk
Collection available at birth	Not likely	Likely	Not likely
Multiple collections required	Likely	Not likely	Likely
Collection after newborn becomes symptomatic	Likely	Not likely	Likely
Time frame for detection	Weeks to months	Weeks to months	Hours to days
Typical range of drug concentrations observed	ng to mg/g	pg to ng/g	ng to μg/mL
Detects drugs administered during labor and delivery	Likely	Likely	Not likely
Detects drugs administered directly to the newborn after birth	Likely	Not likely	Likely
Subject to external contamination	Possible: infant urine, milk stool, adulteration	Possible: maternal blood, collection conditions, adulteration	Possible: adulteration

drugs directly to the newborn to assure that drug testing results reflect drug exposure in utero rather than drug exposure after birth.

The umbilical cord is formed early in pregnancy (at approximately the 5th week of gestation), connecting the developing embryo or fetus to the placenta during pregnancy and protecting the fetal blood vessels within the Wharton's jelly.[96] The Wharton's jelly consists of mucopolysaccharides and other components and is thought to be the site of deposition for drugs that have passed through the placenta. Drug testing of umbilical cord tissue is thought to reflect fetal exposure because it is located on the fetal side of the placenta and is physically attached to the fetus. Unlike meconium, which can be passed in utero or delayed for several days after birth, umbilical cord tissue is available immediately after birth for easy collection. In addition, utilizing umbilical cord tissue avoids the detection of drugs administered to the newborn after birth. It is for these reasons that umbilical cord testing has become popular in recent years as an alternative to meconium, although it may not be as sensitive as meconium for some drugs.[97-101] The portion of umbilical cord tissue that is analyzed does not appear relevant because segmental analysis of umbilical cord shows consistent drug concentrations throughout the specimen.[102,103] However, care should be taken to rinse the cord of obvious maternal blood to minimize the contamination of maternal blood on the results.

Both meconium and umbilical cord tissue may detect drugs administered during labor and delivery. The actual detection window for drugs in these specimens will depend on the timing of drug administration relative to specimen collection. Detection window is also affected by the maternal drug use patterns, efficiency of drug deposition in the specimen, the handling and storage of the specimen, the quality of the specimen submitted for testing, and the performance of the analytical method used. Drug concentrations in umbilical cord tissue are lower than in meconium for most drugs, sometimes in the picograms-per-gram range. Methods that target multiple metabolites are likely to improve detection of drug use, although the source drug cannot always be determined from metabolite patterns. In addition, some drugs and drug metabolites may be preferentially deposited in meconium or in umbilical cord tissue. Whereas umbilical cord tissue patterns have not been extensively studied to date, there are some unique drug metabolites that are detected primarily in meconium as compared with urine, such as *para*-hydroxymethamphetamine for methamphetamine, *meta*-hydroxybenzoylecgonine for cocaine, and 11-hydroxytetracannabinol for cannabis products.[104-106] The value of quantitative testing in predicting neonatal outcome is limited, suggesting that qualitative analysis may be sufficient.

Breast Milk

The first mammary secretion produced shortly after birth is colostrum, which is replaced with transition milk within the first few days and mature milk starting approximately 2 weeks after birth.[107,108] Most drug substances are transferred into breast milk to a certain extent. The rate of drug excretion into breast milk is determined by the physicochemical properties of the drug (eg, ionizability, lipophilicity, molecular weight, volume of distribution, lipid solubility, maternal plasma protein, and lipid binding) and by the blood flow and circulation in the mammary glands. Resources are available to guide breastfeeding decisions when drug use is known.[109-110] Guidelines for opioid treatment in lactation are also published.[83] Essentially, if drugs in breast milk are not expected to harm the child, breastfeeding is encouraged. For example, breastfeeding is encouraged for mothers who are treated with buprenorphine or methadone because concentrations of these drugs in breast milk are low.[111] Conversely, breastfeeding is discouraged for mothers who use cannabis products because THC becomes concentrated in breast milk.[112] Pharmacogenetics may also influence the proportion of drugs and drug metabolites in breast milk. As such, mothers who do not know their metabolic phenotype for cytochrome P450 isozyme 2D6 (CYP2D6) should not breastfeed while taking codeine because ultrarapid metabolizers could inadvertently expose a child to very high doses of morphine.[113] Determination of breast milk concentrations of drugs and drug metabolites may, however, provide only an estimate of the newborn's acute exposure to drugs excreted in breast milk (newborn dose) because the window of detection in breast milk is short (hours to days). Furthermore, concentrations may vary during a feeding, such that the entire feeding may need to be collected and mixed before submitting a specimen for drug testing.

Analytical Methods for Testing

Because commercial methods for drug testing with meconium, umbilical cord tissue, and breast milk are not currently available, testing is limited to laboratory-developed tests, which may include immunoassays, but typically is performed using a chromatographic separation and mass spectrometric detection. Meconium and umbilical cord tissue require extensive preanalytical processing to homogenize, digest, or otherwise prepare the sample for analysis. Homogenized samples are generally centrifuged to obtain a liquid supernatant, followed by sample extraction to purify and potentially concentrate the sample. Extraction is critical because of the high complexity of these matrices. Removal of lipids and proteins is particularly important for mass spectrometry because they may produce ion suppression that can compromise detection of drug analytes. In breast milk, natural emulsifying agents with detergent-like activity can also affect the detection threshold.

Summary

In summary, alternate samples, including hair and sweat, provide unique opportunities in the detection of drug abuse. Although urine remains the most widely used matrix, interest in alternate matrices is growing. At the same time, alternative samples pose a number of preanalytical, analytical, and interpretive challenges.

References

1. Proposed revisions to mandatory guidelines for federal workplace drug testing programs. 69 *Federal Register* 19673 (2004).
2. Mandatory guidelines for federal workplace drug testing programs. 80 *Federal Register* 28054 (2015).
3. Mandatory guidelines for federal workplace drug testing programs. 82 *Federal Register* 7920 (2017).
4. Baumgartner AM, Jones PF, Baumgartner WA, Black CT. Radioimmunoassay of hair for determining opiate-abuse histories. *J Nucl Med.* 1979;20:748-752.
5. Felli M, Martello S, Marsili R, Chiarotti M. Disappearance of cocaine from human hair after abstinence. *Forensic Sci Int.* 2005;154:96-98.
6. Musshoff F, Lachenmeier K, Wollersen H, Lichtermann D, Madea B. Opiate concentrations in hair from subjects in a controlled heroin-maintenance program and from opiate-associated fatalities. *J Anal Toxicol.* 2005;29:345-352.
7. Goldberger BA, Darraj AG, Caplan YH, Cone EJ. Detection of methadone, methadone metabolites, and other illicit drugs of abuse in hair of methadone-treatment subjects. *J Anal Toxicol.* 1998;22:526-530.
8. Villain M, Cirimele V, Kintz P. Hair analysis in toxicology. *Clin Chem Lab Med.* 2004;42:1265-1272.
9. Garcia-Bournissen F, Rokach B, Karaskov T, Koren G. Methamphetamine detection in maternal and neonatal hair: implications for fetal safety. *Arch Dis Child Fetal Neonatal Ed.* 2007;92:F351-F355.
10. Garcia-Bournissen F, Rokach B, Karaskov T, Koren G. Cocaine detection in maternal and neonatal hair: implications to fetal toxicology. *Ther Drug Monit.* 2007;29:71-76.

11. Rivera MA, Aufderheide AC, Cartmell LW, Torres CM, Langsjoen O. Antiquity of coca-leaf chewing in the south central Andes: a 3,000 year archaeological record of coca-leaf chewing from northern Chile. *J Psychoactive Drugs.* 2005;37:455-458.
12. Cartmell LW, Aufderhide A, Weems C. Cocaine metabolites in pre-Columbian mummy hair. *J Okla State Med Assoc.* 1991;84:11-12.
13. Vogliardi S, Tucci M, Stocchero G, Ferrara SD, Favretto D. Sample preparation methods for determination of drugs of abuse in hair samples: a review. *Anal Chim Acta.* 2015;857:1-27.
14. Kintz P. Value of hair analysis in postmortem toxicology. *Forensic Sci Int.* 2004;142:127-134.
15. Salomone A, Tsanaclis L, Agius R, Kintz P, Baumgartner MR. European guidelines for workplace drug and alcohol testing in hair. *Drug Test Anal.* 2016;8:996-1004.
16. Cuypers E, Flanagan RJ. The interpretation of hair analysis for drugs and drug metabolites. *Clin Toxicol (Phila).* 2017:1-11.
17. Restolho J, Barroso M, Saramago B, Dias M, Afonso CA. Development, optimization, and validation of a novel extraction procedure for the removal of opiates from human hair's surface. *Drug Test Anal.* 2015;7:385-392.
18. White RM. Drugs in hair, part I: metabolisms of major drug classes. *Forensic Sci Rev.* 2017;29:23-55.
19. Kintz P, Bundeli P, Brenneisen R, Ludes B. Dose-concentration relationships in hair from subjects in a controlled heroin-maintenance program. *J Anal Toxicol.* 1998;22:231-236.
20. Cooper G, Wilson L, Reid C, Baldwin D, Hand C, Spiehler V. Validation of the Cozart microplate ELISA for detection of opiates in hair. *J Anal Toxicol.* 2003;27:581-586.
21. Lachenmeier K, Musshoff F, Madea B. Determination of opiates and cocaine in hair using automated enzyme immunoassay screening methodologies followed by gas chromatographic-mass spectrometric (GC-MS) confirmation. *Forensic Sci Int.* 2006;159:189-199.
22. Jones J, Tomlinson K, Moore C. The simultaneous determination of codeine, morphine, hydrocodone, hydromorphone, 6-acetylmorphine, and oxycodone in hair and oral fluid. *J Anal Toxicol.* 2002;26:171-175.
23. Fernandez Mdel M, Di Fazio V, Wille SM, Kummer N, Samyn N. A quantitative, selective and fast ultra-high performance liquid chromatography tandem mass spectrometry method for the simultaneous analysis of 33 basic drugs in hair (amphetamines, cocaine, opiates, opioids and metabolites). *J Chromatogr B Analyt Technol Biomed Life Sci.* 2014;965:7-18.
24. Takayama N, Iio R, Tanaka S, Chinaka S, Hayakawa K. Analysis of methamphetamine and its metabolites in hair. *Biomed Chromatogr.* 2003;17:74-82.
25. Miki A, Katagi M, Tsuchihashi H. Application of EMIT d.a.u. for the semiquantitative screening of methamphetamine incorporated in hair. *J Anal Toxicol.* 2002;26:274-279.
26. Lendoiro E, Jimenez-Morigosa C, Cruz A, Paramo M, Lopez-Rivadulla M, de Castro A. An LC-MS/MS methodological approach to the analysis of hair for amphetamine-type-stimulant (ATS) drugs, including selected synthetic cathinones and piperazines. *Drug Test Anal.* 2017;9:96-105.
27. Cooper GA, Allen DL, Scott KS, Oliver JS, Ditton J, Smith ID. Hair analysis: self-reported use of "speed" and "ecstasy" compared with laboratory findings. *J Forensic Sci.* 2000;45:400-406.
28. Rohrich J, Zorntlein S, Potsch L, Skopp G, Becker J. Effect of the shampoo Ultra Clean on drug concentrations in human hair. *Int J Legal Med.* 2000;113:102-106.
29. Polettini A, Cone EJ, Gorelick DA, Huestis MA. Incorporation of methamphetamine and amphetamine in human hair following controlled oral methamphetamine administration. *Anal Chim Acta.* 2012;726:35-43.
30. Bermejo AM, Lopez P, Alvarez I, Tabernero MJ, Fernandez P. Solid-phase microextraction for the determination of cocaine and cocaethylene in human hair by gas chromatography-mass spectrometry. *Forensic Sci Int.* 2006;156:2-8.
31. Cognard E, Rudaz S, Bouchonnet S, Staub C. Analysis of cocaine and three of its metabolites in hair by gas chromatography-mass spectrometry using ion-trap detection for CI/MS/MS. *J Chromatogr B Analyt Technol Biomed Life Sci.* 2005;826:17-25.
32. Baumgartner WA, Black CT, Jones PF, Blahd WH. Radioimmunoassay of cocaine in hair: concise communication. *J Nucl Med.* 1982;23:790-792.
33. Graham K, Koren G, Klein J, Schneiderman J, Greenwald M. Determination of gestational cocaine exposure by hair analysis. *JAMA.* 1989;262:3328-3330.
34. Katikaneni LD, Salle FR, Hulsey TC. Neonatal hair analysis for benzoylecgonine: a sensitive and semiquantitative biological marker for chronic gestational cocaine exposure. *Biol Neonate.* 2002;81:29-37.
35. Tassoni G, Cippitelli M, Ottaviani G, Froldi R, Cingolani M. Detection of cannabinoids by ELISA and GC-MS methods in a hair sample previously used to detect other drugs of abuse. *J Anal Toxicol.* 2016;40:408-413.

36. Han E, Park Y, Kim E, et al. Simultaneous analysis of Δ(9)-tetrahydrocannabinol and 11-nor-9-carboxy-tetrahydrocannabinol in hair without different sample preparation and derivatization by gas chromatography-tandem mass spectrometry. *J Pharm Biomed Anal.* 2011;55:1096-1103.
37. Wu F, Scroggin TL, Metz TD, McMillin GA. Development of a liquid chromatography-tandem mass spectrometry method for the simultaneous determination of four cannabinoids in umbilical cord tissue. *J Anal Toxicol.* 2017:1-7.
38. Prego-Meleiro P, Lendoiro E, Concheiro M, Cruz A, Lopez-Rivadulla M, de Castro A. Development and validation of a liquid chromatography tandem mass spectrometry method for the determination of cannabinoids and phase I and II metabolites in meconium. *J Chromatogr A.* 2017;1497:118-126.
39. Baumgartner AM, Jones PF, Black CT. Detection of phencyclidine in hair. *J Forensic Sci.* 1981; 26:576-581.
40. Sramek JJ, Baumgartner WA, Tallos JA, Ahrens TN, Heiser JF, Blahd WH. Hair analysis for detection of phencyclidine in newly admitted psychiatric patients. *Am J Psychiatry.* 1985;142:950-953.
41. Politi L, Morini L, Leone F, Polettini A. Ethyl glucuronide in hair: is it a reliable marker of chronic high levels of alcohol consumption? *Addiction.* 2006;101:1408-1412.
42. Andresen-Streichert H, Muller A, Glahn A, Skopp G, Sterneck M. Alcohol biomarkers in clinical and forensic contexts. *Dtsch Arztebl Int.* 2018;115:309-315.
43. Oppolzer D, Barroso M, Gallardo E. Determination of ethyl glucuronide in hair to assess excessive alcohol consumption in a student population. *Anal Bioanal Chem.* 2016; 408:2027-2034.
44. Paulsen RB, Wilkins DG, Slawson MH, Shaw K, Rollins DE. Effect of four laboratory decontamination procedures on the quantitative determination of cocaine and metabolites in hair by HPLC-MS. *J Anal Toxicol.* 2001;25:490-496.
45. Blank DL, Kidwell DA. External contamination of hair by cocaine: an issue in forensic interpretation. *Forensic Sci Int.* 1993;63:145-56; discussion, 157-160.
46. Stout PR, Ropero-Miller JD, Baylor MR, Mitchell JM. External contamination of hair with cocaine: evaluation of external cocaine contamination and development of performance-testing materials. *J Anal Toxicol.* 2006;30:490-500.
47. Romano G, Barbera N, Spadaro G, Valenti V. Determination of drugs of abuse in hair: evaluation of external heroin contamination and risk of false positives. *Forensic Sci Int.* 2003;131:98-102.
48. Bassindale T. Quantitative analysis of methamphetamine in hair of children removed from clandestine laboratories—evidence of passive exposure? *Forensic Sci Int.* 2012;219:179-182.
49. Koren G, Klein J, Forman R, Graham K. Hair analysis of cocaine: differentiation between systemic exposure and external contamination. *J Clin Pharmacol.* 1992;32:671-675.
50. Uhl M, Sachs H. Cannabinoids in hair: strategy to prove marijuana/hashish consumption. *Forensic Sci Int.* 2004;145:143-147.
51. Nakahara Y, Takahashi K, Sakamoto T, Tanaka A, Hill VA, Baumgartner WA. Hair analysis for drugs of abuse, XVII: simultaneous detection of PCP, PCHP, and PCPdiol in human hair for confirmation of PCP use. *J Anal Toxicol.* 1997;21:356-362.
52. Romano G, Barbera N, Lombardo I. Hair testing for drugs of abuse: evaluation of external cocaine contamination and risk of false positives. *Forensic Sci Int.* 2001;123:119-129.
53. Wang X, Drummer OH. Review: interpretation of drug presence in the hair of children. *Forensic Sci Int.* 2015;257:458-472.
54. Tsanaclis L, Wicks JF. Differentiation between drug use and environmental contamination when testing for drugs in hair. *Forensic Sci Int.* 2008;176:19-22.
55. Cirimele V, Kintz P, Jamey C, Ludes B. Are cannabinoids detected in hair after washing with Cannabio shampoo? *J Anal Toxicol.* 1999;23:349-351.
56. Borges CR, Wilkins DG, Rollins DE. Amphetamine and N-acetylamphetamine incorporation into hair: an investigation of the potential role of drug basicity in hair color bias. *J Anal Toxicol.* 2001;25:221-227.
57. Slawson MH, Wilkins DG, Foltz RL, Rollins DE. Quantitative determination of phencyclidine in pigmented and nonpigmented hair by ion-trap mass spectrometry. *J Anal Toxicol.* 1996; 20:350-354.
58. Nisbet LA, Venson R, Wylie FM, Scott KS. Application of a urine and hair validated LC-MS-MS method to determine the effect of hair color on the incorporation of 25B-NBOMe, 25C-NBOMe and 25I-NBOMe into hair in the rat. *J Anal Toxicol.* 2017;41:559-565.
59. Kulaga V, Velazquez-Armenta Y, Aleksa K, Vergee Z, Koren G. The effect of hair pigment on the incorporation of fatty acid ethyl esters (FAEE). *Alcohol Alcohol.* 2009;44:287-292.
60. Kronstrand R, Ahlner J, Dizdar N, Larson G. Quantitative analysis of desmethylselegiline, methamphetamine, and amphetamine in hair and plasma from Parkinson patients on long-term selegiline medication. *J Anal Toxicol.* 2003;27:135-141.

61. Ursitti F, Klein J, Sellers E, Koren G. Use of hair analysis for confirmation of self-reported cocaine use in users with negative urine tests. *J Toxicol Clin Toxicol.* 2001;39:361-366.
62. Rollins DE, Wilkins DG, Krueger GG, et al. The effect of hair color on the incorporation of codeine into human hair. *J Anal Toxicol.* 2003;27:545-551.
63. Reid RW, O'Connor FL, Crayton JW. The in vitro differential binding of benzoylecgonine to pigmented human hair samples. *J Toxicol Clin Toxicol.* 1994;32:405-410.
64. Schaffer M, Hill V, Cairns T. Hair analysis for cocaine: the requirement for effective wash procedures and effects of drug concentration and hair porosity in contamination and decontamination. *J Anal Toxicol.* 2005;29:319-326.
65. Hoffman BH. Analysis of race effects on drug-test results. *J Occup Environ Med.* 1999;41:612-614.
66. Kelly RC, Mieczkowski T, Sweeney SA, Bourland JA. Hair analysis for drugs of abuse: hair color and race differentials or systematic differences in drug preferences? *Forensic Sci Int.* 2000;107:63-86.
67. Kidwell DA, Lee EH, DeLauder SF. Evidence for bias in hair testing and procedures to correct bias. *Forensic Sci Int.* 2000;107:39-61.
68. Shults TF. Hair testing: the conceptual and practical challenge of hair testing. In: Shults TF, ed. *Medical Review Officer Handbook.* 9th ed. Research Triangle Park, NC: Quadrangle Research; 2009:78-90.
69. Pritchett JS, Phinney KW. Influence of chemical straightening on the stability of drugs of abuse in hair. *J Anal Toxicol.* 2015;39:13-16.
70. Fogerson R, Schoendorfer D, Fay J, Spiehler V. Qualitative detection of opiates in sweat by EIA and GC-MS. *J Anal Toxicol.* 1997;21:451-458.
71. Gentili S, Mortali C, Mastrobattista L, Berretta P, Zaami S. Determination of different recreational drugs in sweat by headspace solid-phase microextraction gas chromatography mass spectrometry (HS-SPME GC/MS): application to drugged drivers. *J Pharm Biomed Anal.* 2016;129:282-287.
72. Koster RA, Alffenaar JW, Greijdanus B, VanDerNagel JE, Uges DR. Application of sweat patch screening for 16 drugs and metabolites using a fast and highly selective LC-MS/MS method. *Ther Drug Monit.* 2014;36:35-45.
73. De Giovanni N, Fucci N. The current status of sweat testing for drugs of abuse: a review. *Curr Med Chem.* 2013;20:545-561.
74. Fay J, Fogerson R, Schoendorfer D, Niedbala RS, Spiehler V. Detection of methamphetamine in sweat by EIA and GC-MS. *J Anal Toxicol.* 1996;20:398-403.
75. Samyn N, De Boeck G, Verstraete AG. The use of oral fluid and sweat wipes for the detection of drugs of abuse in drivers. *J Forensic Sci.* 2002;47:1380-1387.
76. Samyn N, De Boeck G, Wood M, et al. Plasma, oral fluid and sweat wipe ecstasy concentrations in controlled and real life conditions. *Forensic Sci Int.* 2002;128:90-97.
77. Barnes AJ, De Martinis BS, Gorelick DA, Goodwin RS, Kolbrich EA, Huestis MA. Disposition of MDMA and metabolites in human sweat following controlled MDMA administration. *Clin Chem.* 2009;55:454-462.
78. Liberty HJ, Johnson BD, Fortner N. Detecting cocaine use through sweat testing: multilevel modeling of sweat patch length-of-wear data. *J Anal Toxicol.* 2004;28:667-673.
79. Kacinko SL, Barnes AJ, Schwilke EW, Cone EJ, Moolchan ET, Huestis MA. Disposition of cocaine and its metabolites in human sweat after controlled cocaine administration. *Clin Chem.* 2005;51:2085-2094.
80. Kintz P, Cirimele V, Ludes B. Detection of cannabis in oral fluid (saliva) and forehead wipes (sweat) from impaired drivers. *J Anal Toxicol.* 2000;24:557-561.
81. Huestis MA, Scheidweiler KB, Saito T, et al. Excretion of delta9-tetrahydrocannabinol in sweat. *Forensic Sci Int.* 2008;174:173-177.
82. Gomez-Pomar E, Finnegan LP. The epidemic of neonatal abstinence syndrome, historical references of its origin, assessment, and management. *Front Pediatr.* 2018;6:33.
83. Reddy UM, Davis JM, Ren Z, Green MF. Opioid Use in Pregnancy, Neonatal Abstinence Syndrome, and Childhood Outcomes Workshop Invited Speakers. Opioid use in pregnancy, neonatal abstinence syndrome, and childhood outcomes: executive summary of a joint workshop by the Eunice Kennedy Shriver National Institute of Child Health and Human Development, American College of Obstetricians and Gynecologists, American Academy of Pediatrics, Society for Maternal-Fetal Medicine, Centers for Disease Control and Prevention, and the March of Dimes Foundation. *Obstet Gynecol.* 2017;130:10-28.
84. Coluzzi F, Valensise H, Sacco M, Allegri M. Chronic pain management in pregnancy and lactation. *Minerva Anestesiologica.* 2014;80:211-224.
85. Infants with Prenatal Substance Exposure. National Center on Substance Abuse and Child Welfare. https://ncsacw.samhsa.gov/resources/substance-exposed-infants.aspx. Accessed May 22, 2019.
86. National Survey on Drug Use and Health (NSDUH-2016). Substance Abuse and Mental Health Services Administration (SAMHSA). https://www.datafiles.samhsa.gov/study/national-survey-drug-use-and-health-nsduh-2016-nid17184. Accessed May 22, 2019.

87. Ko JY, Patrick SW, Tong VT, Patel R, Lind JN, Barfield WD. Incidence of neonatal abstinence syndrome: 28 states, 1999-2013. *MMWR Morb Mortal Wkly Rep.* 2016;65:799-802.
88. Lester BM, ElSohly M, Wright LL, et al. The Maternal Lifestyle Study: drug use by meconium toxicology and maternal self-report. *Pediatrics.* 2001;107:309-317.
89. Chiandetti A, Hernandez G, Mercadal-Hally M, et al. Prevalence of prenatal exposure to substances of abuse: questionnaire versus biomarkers. *Reprod Health.* 2017;14:137.
90. Wood KE, Sinclair LL, Rysgaard CD, et al. Retrospective analysis of the diagnostic yield of newborn drug testing. *BMC Pregnancy Childbirth.* 2014;14:250.
91. Gareri J, Klein J, Koren G. Drugs of abuse testing in meconium. *Clin Chim Acta.* 2006;366:101-111.
92. Himes SK, Tassiopoulos K, Yogev R, et al. Antiretroviral drugs in meconium: detection for different gestational periods of exposure. *J Pediatr.* 2015;167:305-311.
93. Gray TR, Shakleya DM, Huestis MA. A liquid chromatography tandem mass spectrometry method for the simultaneous quantification of 20 drugs of abuse and metabolites in human meconium. *Anal Bioanal Chem.* 2009;393:1977-1990.
94. Ostrea EM Jr, Brady M, Gause S, et al. Drug screening of newborns by meconium analysis: a large-scale, prospective, epidemiologic study. *Pediatrics.* 1992;89:107-113.
95. Wabuyele SL, Colby JM, McMillin GA. Detection of drug-exposed newborns. *Ther Drug Monit.* 2018;40:166-185.
96. Wang Y, Zhao S. *Vascular Biology of the Placenta.* San Rafael, CA: Morgan & Claypool Life Sciences; 2010.
97. Wright TE. Biochemical screening for in utero drug exposure. *Drug Metab Lett.* 2015;9:65-71.
98. Montgomery D, Plate C, Alder SC, et al. Testing for fetal exposure to illicit drugs using umbilical cord tissue vs meconium. *J Perinatol.* 2006;26:11-14.
99. Colby JM. Comparison of umbilical cord tissue and meconium for the confirmation of in utero drug exposure. *Clin Biochem.* 2017;50:784-790.
100. Palmer KL, Wood KE, Krasowski MD. Evaluating a switch from meconium to umbilical cord tissue for newborn drug testing: a retrospective study at an academic medical center. *Clin Biochem.* 2017;50:255-261.
101. Labardee RM, Swatzweider JR, Gebhardt KE, et al. *Clin Biochem.* 2017;50:1093-1097.
102. Marin SJ, Metcalf A, Krasowski MD, et al. Detection of neonatal drug exposure using umbilical cord tissue and liquid chromatography time-of-flight mass spectrometry. *Ther Drug Monit.* 2014;36:119-124.
103. Jones J, Jones M, Plate C, Lewis D. The detection of 1-palmitoyl-2-oleoyl-sn-glycero-3-phosphoethanol and ethyl glucuronide in human umbilical cord. *Am J Anal Chem.* 2012;3:800-810.
104. Gray TR, Kelly T, LaGasse LL, et al. Novel biomarkers of prenatal methamphetamine exposure in human meconium. *Ther Drug Monit.* 2009;31:70-75.
105. McMillin GA, Wood KE, Strathmann FG, et al. Patterns of drugs and drug metabolites observed in meconium: what do they mean? *Ther Drug Monit.* 2015;37:568-580.
106. Kelly T, Gray TR, Huestis MA. Development and validation of a liquid chromatography-atmospheric pressure chemical ionization-tandem mass spectrometry method for simultaneous analysis of 10 amphetamine-, methamphetamine- and 3,4-methylenedioxymethamphetamine-related (MDMA) analytes in human meconium. *J Chromatogr B Analyt Technol Biomed Life Sci.* 2008;867:194-204.
107. Godhia ML, Patel N. Colostrum: its composition, benefits as a nutraceutical: a review. *Curr Res Nutr Food Sci.* 2013;1:37-47.
108. Ballard O, Morrow AL. Human milk composition: nutrients and bioactive factors. *Pediatr Clin North Am.* 2013;60:49-74.
109. Reece-Stremtan S, Marinelli KA. ABM Clinical Protocol #21: guidelines for breastfeeding and substance use or substance use disorder, revised 2015. *Breastfeed Med.* 2015;10:135-141.
110. LactMed: a TOXNET database. Drugs and Lactation Database. US National Library of Medicine: Toxicology Data Network. https://www.toxnet.nlm.nih.gov/newtoxnet/lactmed.htm. Accessed May 22, 2019.
111. Jansson LM, Spencer N, McConnell K, et al. Maternal buprenorphine maintenance and lactation. *J Hum Lact.* 2016;32:675-681.
112. Jansson LM, Bunik M, Bogen DL. Lactation and the marijuana-using mother. *Breastfeed Med.* 2015;10:342-343.
113. Madadi P, Avard D, Koren G. Pharmacogenetics of opioids for the treament of acute maternal pain during pregnancy and lactation. *Curr Drug Metab.* 2012;13(6):721-727.

Section III

Specific Analytes

Tai C. Kwong, PhD, and Gwendolyn A. McMillin, PhD, Editors

Chapter 16. Ethanol
Graham R. Jones, PhD

Chapter 17. Non-Ethanol Volatiles and Ethylene Glycol
Graham R. Jones, PhD

Chapter 18. Cannabis
Paul J. Jannetto, PhD

Chapter 19. Club Drugs
Matthew D. Krasowski, MD, PhD, and Christine L.H. Snozek, PhD

Chapter 20. Cocaine
Daniel S. Isenschmid, PhD

Chapter 21. Amphetamines
Matthew D. Krasowski, MD, PhD, Christine L.H. Snozek, PhD, and Stacy E.F. Melanson, MD, PhD

Chapter 22. Barbiturates
Matthew D. Krasowski, MD, PhD, Christine L.H. Snozek, PhD, and Stacy E.F. Melanson, MD, PhD

Chapter 23. Benzodiazepines
Christine L.H. Snozek, PhD, Matthew D. Krasowski, MD, PhD, and Stacy E.F. Melanson, MD, PhD

Chapter 24. Opioids I: Opiates and Semisynthetic Opioids
Matthew D. Krasowski, MD, PhD, and Gwendolyn A. McMillin, PhD

Chapter 25. Opioids II: Synthetic Opioids
Hoi-Ying Elsie Yu, PhD, and Nicholas Heger, PhD

Chapter 26. Novel Psychoactive Substances
Donna Papsun, MS

Chapter 27. Over-the-Counter Analgesics
Hoi-Ying Elsie Yu, PhD, and Gary L. Horowitz, MD

Chapter 28. Lead and Other Toxic Metals
Robert A. Middleberg, PhD

Chapter 29. Common Household and Environmental Toxicants
Christine L.H. Snozek, PhD, and Leland B. Baskin, MD

Chapter 16

Ethanol

Graham R. Jones, PhD

Introduction[1]

Origin

Ethanol is the natural product of fermentation of sugars present in a wide variety of fruits, grains, and other foodstuffs, which may be distilled to produce "spirits" in which much higher concentrations are achieved than occur naturally. Alcoholic beverages (beer, ale, mead, wine, whiskey, etc) thus cover a very wide range of ethanol concentrations (2-60% vol/vol).[2]

Descriptive Chemistry

Ethanol is the two-carbon aliphatic mono-alcohol.

Ethanol

Synonyms: Ethyl alcohol, ethan-1-ol, hydroxy-ethane, grain alcohol, and most commonly simply "alcohol"

Formula: CH_3CH_2OH

Molecular mass = 46.0684 Daltons

CAS-64-17-5

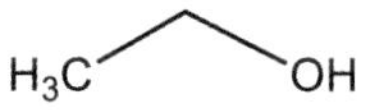

Pharmacology

Type of Agent

Alcohol is primarily a central nervous system (CNS) depressant but also causes many peripheral and local effects. The initial effects of alcohol are mild stimulation and euphoria, caused by inhibition of inhibitory central mechanisms.[3]

Context of Human Use

Ethanol has been used socially for millennia. The ancient Sumerians are said to have invented beer, and wine has been celebrated as "the fruit of the vine" since at least biblical times. Alcohol is undoubtedly the most widely available and consumed drug in the world. It is so widely available and relatively inexpensive that, other than home-based beer or wine making, large-scale illicit synthesis and distribution has become all but nonexistent in the Western world since prohibition ended.

Abuse Potential and Characteristics

Individuals partaking of alcoholic beverages become more sociable and talkative, with generally decreased inhibitions. Frequent high-dose intake can lead to physical dependence, or alcoholism, evidenced by increasing tolerance and an unpleasant withdrawal reaction when intake ends. Alcoholics may go to considerable lengths to maintain high alcohol intake in order to prevent the withdrawal reaction, often despite adverse consequences.[2]

Adverse Effects

The wide-scale availability and use of alcohol has meant that it is associated with a large number of deaths annually, mostly due to motor vehicle accidents, drug-alcohol intoxications, and drug-induced natural illness such as liver and cardiac disease. In 2016, The National Highway Traffic Safety Administration (NHTSA) reported that in 2015, there were 10,265 fatalities in motor vehicle traffic crashes involving drivers with blood alcohol concentrations (BACs) of 0.08 g/100 mL or higher, totaling 29% of all traffic fatalities for the year.[4] The costs to health care of alcohol-related disease is estimated to be in the billions annually.[5] Moderate alcohol consumption is regarded as having a minimal detrimental effect on long-term health, but chronic consumption of large amounts has been associated with a variety of serious health effects. The Centers for Disease Control and Prevention lists the following diseases as the most common for causing alcohol-attributable nonaccidental deaths: alcoholic liver disease, liver cirrhosis, hemorrhagic stroke, hypertension, ischemic heart disease, ischemic stroke, liver cancer, alcoholic psychosis, acute and chronic pancreatitis, cardiomyopathy, esophageal and oropharyngeal cancer, laryngeal cancer, prostate cancer, esophageal varices, and esophageal hemorrhage.[6] Chronic alcohol abuse can lead to other adverse effects, such as malnutrition (including vitamin deficiency) and alcoholic withdrawal seizures as well as fetal alcohol syndrome.

Overdose and Toxicity

At BACs above 0.08 g/100 mL, judgment and reaction time are adversely affected. At still higher concentrations, balance, coordination, speech, and vision are affected. Ultimately, depression of the CNS leads to the depression of reflexes, reduced level of consciousness, incontinence, sleep, coma, and impaired circulation and respiration, leading to death. A comprehensive description of the pharmacology of alcohol is beyond the scope of this chapter, and the reader is referred elsewhere for more detail.[7]

Toxic Dose

No toxic dose has been generally established for ethanol, although 500 mL of 50% spirit ingested within 1 hour has been cited as a minimum.[2] Toxicity is dose related, but it is subject to much interindividual variability. BACs around 0.40 g/100 mL are often cited as being potentially fatal in the absence of another reasonable cause in an otherwise healthy person; however, sometimes alcoholics can tolerate concentrations of 0.60 g/100 mL or so without fatal outcome. Medical and physical factors such as severe natural disease, positional asphyxia, or the presence of drugs that depress the CNS or have cardiotoxic properties can combine to cause death at lower alcohol concentrations.[8]

Pharmacokinetics, Metabolism, and Excretion

Pharmacokinetics

Gastrointestinal absorption of ethanol is a passive process beginning with ingestion.[9] It is absorbed in the stomach, but small intestine absorption is much more rapid because of the larger surface area. Because food in the stomach causes a delay in passage of ethanol into the small intestine, it will decrease the overall rate of absorption; ethanol will continue to be absorbed from the stomach but at a slower rate. Peak blood ethanol concentrations are generally reached 20 to 60 minutes after ingestion, depending on the amount and concentration ingested and whether or not food is present in the stomach.[2]

Metabolism and Excretion

Less than 2% alcohol is excreted unchanged in the urine.[9] Approximately 94% of alcohol is cleared from the body by liver alcohol dehydrogenase (ADH). The initial product is acetaldehyde, which is rapidly metabolized to acetate, which enters the Krebs cycle. Metabolism of alcohol in the body is a remarkably robust process that appears to be minimally affected by damage to the liver caused by alcohol abuse.[10,11] In most of the population, ADH starts to become saturated above 0.01 g/100 mL; for this reason, alcohol clearance approximates to zero-order kinetics. However, at low BACs, the rate of metabolism and clearance is better defined by Michaelis-Menten kinetics.[12-15] In most of the population, alcohol is cleared from the blood at a rate between 0.01 g/100 mL/h and 0.02 g/100 mL/h, with an average of 0.015 g/100 mL/h to 0.018 g/100 mL/h.[16] Of course, true alcohol clearance rates can only be measured after all alcohol has been absorbed by the body. Alcohol clearance rates may appear to be lower when alcohol absorption from the gut is incomplete (ie, continued absorption of alcohol is partially offsetting clearance from the blood). Alcohol clearance rates greater than 0.03 g/100 mL/h have been reported, although usually in chronic alcoholics with high blood concentrations.[17-20] The presence of food in the stomach will significantly reduce the absorption of alcohol from the gut, leading to a lower peak BAC and a lower area under the curve.[21] It is also useful to bear in mind that near-fatal concentrations may be cleared from the body in less than 24 hours. For example, a person with a BAC of 0.40 g/100 mL and a clearance rate of 0.02 g/100 mL/h will clear most or all of the alcohol from the body in about 20 hours. Such estimates can be used to explain why someone found dead in the morning with a low or negligible BAC reading may have had a corroborated history that he or she was drinking heavily the evening before.

Analysis

Analytical Parameters[2]

Dissociation constant: pK_a 15.9 (25°C).
Partition coefficient: Log *P* (octanol/water): -0.3.

Specimen Types, Requirements, and Characteristics

Plasma/Serum Versus Blood

Most jurisdictions state their per se drunk driving laws in terms of whole blood and/or breath alcohol equivalent. This is done because most of the original research into intoxication, measurement, and interpretation was performed on whole blood; however, most clinical laboratories measure alcohol in serum or plasma, not whole blood, primarily because the methods commonly used in clinical laboratories (eg, enzymatic assays) are best suited to serum or plasma. Alcohol is distributed in the body in direct proportion to the water content of the fluid or tissue; alcohol has very poor solubility in fat. Serum and plasma have an almost identical water content of about 92%, and therefore, at equilibrium, serum alcohol concentration and plasma alcohol concentration are virtually the same. However, whole blood has a water content of only about 80%. Therefore, serum and plasma alcohol concentrations typically average about 15% higher than the alcohol concentration in whole blood. Obviously, there will be some variability due to differing hematocrit and lipid content, and therefore this is not a precise mathematical conversion. The larger studies have reported mean serum alcohol–whole blood alcohol ratios of 1.14 to 1.16, with a range of approximately 1.04 to 1.25.[22-24]

Urine

The relationship between whole blood alcohol and urine alcohol concentrations is even more variable, mainly because urine is not a circulating fluid but a reservoir of fluid reflecting an average of alcohol concentration in the kidney filtrate since the last void. Blood alcohol–urine alcohol ratios average about 1:1.3, although the actual ratio for any given person at any specific time will depend on the drinking history relative to the last void.[25,26] Some circumstances will, however, lead to extreme blood-urine ratios. The occurrence of relatively high urine alcohol concentrations compared with the BAC is typically caused by the consumption of alcohol followed by a period of abstinence for several hours during which the bladder is not voided. Although people tend to void their bladder at regular intervals while they are awake, this will usually not happen if they are asleep or in a coma. The BAC continues to fall due to normal metabolic activity, but the urine alcohol concentration will only fall slowly in proportion to the accumulation of newly formed urine. It should also be borne in mind that in poorly controlled diabetics, high urine alcohol concentrations can be readily attained due to fermentation of glucose in the bladder or in vitro (ie, after collection) if a bladder infection exists or the urine becomes contaminated with yeast or other ethanol-forming microorganisms. Alcohol formation in urine of greater than 500 mg/100 mL has been reported.[27-29]

Postmortem Considerations

It is well documented that alcohol can be formed in postmortem blood and other tissues as a result of bacteria or other microorganism activity, either in vivo or in vitro. Although not common, alcohol concentrations due to so-called "postmortem fermentation" can exceed the common "legal limit" for operation of a motor vehicle of 0.08 g/100 mL. Whether or not alcohol is formed—and, if so, the resulting concentration—depends on the specific microorganisms present and on other conditions, such as the degree of tissue breakdown, source of a suitable substrate (such as glucose), and temperature. It is also important to recognize that postmortem formation of alcohol is not a linear process; it can take up to 24 hours after death for significant amounts of alcohol to be formed. Moreover, once formed, alcohol itself can be metabolized as the growth cycle continues. However, although rare, apparent BACs of up to 0.40 g/100 mL have been reported.[30-32] Sodium fluoride (1-2%) can be added to blood at the time of collection to retard or eliminate the possibility of in vitro formation of alcohol, although obviously the possibility of prior in vivo formation before collection must be considered.

Analysis of Vitreous Fluid

Unless damaged, the vitreous humor in the eye remains sterile for a period of 2 to 4 days after death. Therefore, the presence of significant concentrations of alcohol in the eye is usually considered proof of consumption before death. It is a common practice in forensic laboratories to screen blood for alcohol first and, if those results are positive, to then analyze vitreous fluid for confirmation of consumption before death. On average, vitreous alcohol concentrations are 10% to 15% higher than the corresponding blood concentration because of the higher water content of that fluid, although there can be significant case-to-case variation due to such factors as the state of alcohol absorption (ascending or descending) and the presence or absence of alcohol in blood from postmortem formation.[33,34]

Other Specimens

Bile can be used for the measurement of alcohol; however, it may not always be a reliable indicator of the BAC because of its proximity to the liver and stomach and the possibility of postmortem diffusion or neoformation.[35,36] Like vitreous fluid, cerebrospinal fluid may provide a valuable corroboration of a BAC; however, cerebrospinal fluid is more difficult to collect than vitreous fluid and may be more susceptible to postmortem processes. Although organ tissues and muscle may be used to measure alcohol concentrations, the measurements are often not reliable because of postmortem neoformation.

Modes of Analysis

Colorimetric

Classically, alcohol has been measured spectrophotometrically by monitoring the change in color of potassium dichromate (orange color) as it is reduced to potassium chromate (green color). This is the chemical basis for the classic Breathalyzer breath alcohol device. This reaction was also used for decades in the laboratory using Conway diffusion plates or Widmark flasks. However, this manual headspace method is not well suited to producing rapid results or for a busy clinical laboratory.

Enzymatic

Enzymatic methods have been used for years and continue to be the primary basis for measuring alcohol in serum, plasma, or urine in clinical practice. The basis of the method is monitoring the change in absorbance at 340 nm caused by the reduction of NAD+ to NADH that accompanies oxidation of alcohol to acetaldehyde (and further to acetate) by ADH.

Gas Chromatography

A properly designed gas chromatography (GC) method will be able to detect and measure ethanol specifically and accurately. A well-chosen GC column will be able to separate acetaldehyde, methanol, ethanol, isopropanol, and acetone, which can be particularly valuable for intoxications involving methanol or isopropanol. There are two ways in which GC can be used for ethanol measurement. For clinical purposes, a single column with direct on-column injection may be adequate. With such a system, serum, plasma, or urine is typically diluted up to 1 in 10 with water and injected directly into the injection port via a manual syringe or an autoinjector. The disadvantage is that thermally degraded proteins can build up on the injection port liner and GC column, requiring frequent maintenance. However, with care, such systems can work well, and even with diluted whole blood, especially if samples are injected in "split" mode with a fairly high split ratio. For high-volume applications, use of a headspace sampler is preferred, which allows only the volatile alcohol and water vapor to pass into the GC system, thereby avoiding the nonvolatile buildup that can degrade column performance and chromatographic separation. For forensic purposes, use of a second GC column is preferred. The second column should have a different stationary phase and a different order of elution for at least acetone and isopropanol. In some forensic laboratories, that second column is used on a second system or it can be run in parallel in the same GC system with both columns connected to the same injection port (directly or via a splitter) but with the end of each column connected to separate flame ionization detectors. Some forensic laboratories are starting to use mass spectrometry as the detector for GC/headspace blood alcohol measurement, although this has not yet been widely adopted and is probably not necessary for most clinical applications.

Known Analytical Issues and Problems

Although well suited for clinical purposes, there are two caveats regarding robustness of the enzymatic ethanol methodology. Because of the similarity in structures, some enzymatic assays have a degree of cross-reactivity with isopropanol. The other, potentially more serious, problem is elevated concentrations of lactate and lactate dehydrogenase causing "apparent" false alcohol readings. The basis of the problem is that the metabolism of lactate to pyruvate by lactate dehydrogenase (LDH) also involves the conversion of NAD+ to NADH, the same reaction that is involved in the metabolism of ethanol to acetaldehyde by ADH. However, because lactate itself is not a substrate for ADH, the presence of significant amounts of both lactate and LDH would be a prerequisite for interference in an enzymatic ethanol assay.[37,38] Although elevated lactate concentrations may not be uncommon, elevated LDH would typically occur after hepatic injury and also as a result of postcollection hemolysis. Such injury could be inferred from elevated hepatic enzymes such as aspartate aminotransferase (ASAT) and alanine aminotransferase (ALAT); but in the absence of elevated liver enzymes, the presence of elevated LDH in the general circulation of a living patient would seem to be unlikely. However, the presence of elevated lactate and LDH in postmortem blood is much more likely and perhaps even to be expected. For these reasons, ethanol results generated using enzymatic methods have to be interpreted cautiously for forensic applications, especially involving postmortem blood. Most of the time, the only volatiles seen in GC methods in blood are methanol, ethanol, acetone, and isopropanol. In addition, some other volatiles associated with solvent abuse do elute in the same general region of the chromatogram (eg, difluoroethane [Dust-Off], methyl ethyl ketone, ether, chloroform, and acetonitrile).

Clinical Issues

Clinical Interpretation of Analytical Findings

Most experienced emergency department physicians will be able to recall events such as uncooperative patients discharging themselves and walking out with serum alcohol concentrations of 300 mg/100 mL or higher. Doubtless they will also be able to recall incidents in which someone at a party, whose blood alcohol level would have been barely up to the "legal limit," was practically passed out. This can be due to differences in the degree of tolerance to alcohol, although other factors also play a role. The literature describes three types of tolerance: acute, chronic, and metabolic. *Acute tolerance* is perhaps best characterized by noting that if the "feeling" of intoxication is plotted against time, the resulting curve displays hysteresis. In other words, people tend to feel less intoxicated at the same BAC of the descending curve than on the ascending part of the curve. This is short-term acquisition of tolerance and is sometimes referred to as the *Mellanby effect*.[39,40] *Chronic* or *long-term tolerance* is best characterized by the ability to behave and function well beyond that expected for the BAC attained. There can be no doubt that some degree of physiological tolerance is attained; however, alcoholics learn, at least partially, to mask the typical effects of intoxication (eg, speaking slowly and deliberately to avoid slurring words, walking carefully, and holding on to stationary objects to aid balance). *Metabolic tolerance* typically occurs in chronic alcoholics and describes the ability of an individual to tolerate higher rates of alcohol consumption because of a higher rate of metabolic clearance. Several reports describe the difficulty of estimating BAC just by observation, even by professionals, such as emergency physicians and police, who are accustomed to dealing with intoxicated people.[41-45] Remarkably, many people with BACs approaching or even greater than 200 mg/100 mL show little in the way of outward signs of intoxication, although they may perform poorly on field sobriety tests. Because of the variability in the way intoxication with alcohol is manifested, virtually all jurisdictions in the world have instituted statutory limits for BAC. Up until a few years ago, many states had a per se limit of 100 mg/100 mL; many states have since lowered that to 80 mg/100 mL, and some are considering even lower limits—either as a criminal limit or to determine temporary suspension of driving privileges (eg, 24 hours).

Back-Extrapolation of Blood Alcohol Concentration

In legal cases such as motor vehicle accidents, there is usually a desire to know what the BAC of a driver was at the time of an accident. However, in practice, a blood sample for alcohol measurement might not be drawn for 1 to 3 hours or more after the accident took place. If the alcohol clearance rate for that individual is known, an estimation of the BAC at the time of the accident may be attempted. The problem is that the actual clearance rate for that person will not be known unless multiple blood alcohol measurements were made in the hours after the accident. In the absence of such measurements, estimates of the BAC can be made using a series of hypothetical clearance rates (eg, 0.01, 0.015, 0.02 g/100 mL/h). Even then, the validity of such estimates is only true if alcohol absorption was complete by the time of the accident. If it were not, the analytically measured BAC would be overestimated because of continued absorption after the accident (and therefore the BAC at the time of the accident overestimated). It is also clear that back-extrapolations of dose become increasingly unreliable the further back in time they are attempted.

Estimation of Dose

The total dose of alcohol in a person may be estimated, given the weight of that individual, the BAC, and the volume of distribution (V_d) of alcohol for that person.

$$\text{Dose (g)} = \text{Body weight (kg)} \times \text{BAC (g/L)} \times V_d \text{ (L/kg)}$$

While the V_d for that person will almost never be known, estimates from the forensic literature may be used, typically based on sex and body type (eg, lean, normal, obese) and are generally in the range of 0.6 L/kg to 0.8 L/kg. Such estimates are not precise but may serve a useful purpose in some circumstances. For example, a claim that someone consumed only "two beers" can be disproved clearly if the dose estimation indicates the presence of the equivalent of six beers in the body at the time the BAC measurement was made. If the dose estimation is attempted, care must be taken to use whole-blood alcohol values, not serum or plasma concentrations. "Dose" is also commonly expressed in terms of the number of "beers" (330 mL of 5% vol/vol alcohol) or the equivalent in spirits (1.5 fluid ounces of 40% vol/vol alcohol) or wine (150 mL of 12% vol/vol alcohol).

Other Sources of Alcohol

It is normal practice to sterilize the skin before a venipuncture procedure, and this is sometimes done with iodine-based formations (eg, Betadine), although the use of alcohol-based pads is still common. Ethanol was used in these pads, but because of the legal implication in driving under the influence of alcohol cases, it has mostly been replaced with isopropanol. Earlier studies on the potential for ethanol-based skin sterilization to cause positive blood alcohol results demonstrated that this was not likely unless sloppy practice allowed pooled alcohol to be present on the skin during venipuncture.[46]

Urine specimens from diabetics with high glucose content and yeast contamination can give rise to ethanol within the specimen as a fermentation product.[46]

Treatment and Rehabilitation for Overdose and Toxicity

Diagnosing an acutely intoxicated individual at an emergency room may be fairly straightforward. The person will usually have a strong odor of alcohol on their breath, slurred speech, reduced coordination, bloodshot eyes, and a reduced level of consciousness. If vital signs are within normal limits, simple observation may be all that is needed—and indeed the person might be released to police to sober-up in the local "drunk tank." Active medical treatment may not be needed. However, careful evaluation is warranted if there is a possibility that alcohol intoxication may be masking a brain injury (eg, resulting from a fall or a motor vehicle accident) or toxicity due to co-ingested depressant drugs or hepatotoxins such as acetaminophen. Caution is also advised if methanol or ethylene glycol is present, but toxicity is temporarily delayed because of the preferential metabolism of the ethanol. In these circumstances, measurement of the BAC can be useful to estimate whether the apparent degree of intoxication is consistent. The presence of mild CNS-depressant drugs, such as the benzodiazepines or older style antihistamines (eg, diphenhydramine), may cause simple additive CNS depression that results in a reduced level of consciousness. However, the presence of more potent narcotics, such as morphine or methadone, carries a much more serious risk of life-threatening respiratory depression. In these circumstances, rapid medical intervention may be vital. BAC measurement and other clinical tests may be the best way to determine if the patient's symptoms can be accounted for by alcohol alone or whether undiagnosed injuries or drug intoxication may be present.

Ethanol Biomarkers

Ethanol is easy to detect and quantify in serum or blood as a measure of acute impairment, but clinical monitoring of ethanol abuse is problematic because ethanol is rapidly cleared from the body. Even potentially fatal concentrations of ethanol can be cleared from the body in less than 24 hours. For example, an individual who metabolizes ethanol at an average rate of 18 mg/100 mL/h will clear 400 mg/100 mL in just over 22 hours. Chronic alcoholics clear ethanol from blood faster than nonalcoholics, shortening the window of detection even more. Therefore, measurement of blood ethanol is not a useful indicator as to whether or not a recovering alcoholic is indeed abstaining from ethanol consumption. However, several potential biomarkers of ethanol consumption have been explored, the most common of which are ethyl glucuronide (EtG) and ethyl sulfate (EtS). These ethanol metabolites persist in urine for approximately 1 to 4 days after ethanol consumption and are sensitive enough to detect consumption of a single drink.[48] Urine is the most commonly used specimen. Serum and whole blood are not useful matrices as EtG and EtS are cleared much more quickly than from urine. EtG has a half-life in blood of 2 to 3 hours.[48] The following cutoffs have been suggested for EtG: >1000 ng/mL (high positive) may indicate heavy drinking within the previous day or two or light drinking the same day; a low positive (500-1000 ng/mL) may indicate heavy drinking within the previous 2 to 3 days or recent light drinking (eg, past 24 hours) or recent intense extraneous exposure (within 24 hours or less).[49,50]

Urine EtG and EtS are usually measured by tandem liquid chromatography-mass spectrometry (LC-MS/MS) methods using the corresponding deuterated internal standards. While direct analysis of urine is possible, a solid phase extraction (SPE) clean-up step will minimize potential interference. The sensitivity of these methods is usually well below the suggested cutoffs for clinical or forensic use (eg, <50 ng/mL).[51-55] A commercial immunoassay for EtG has also been developed, although as of September 2018 is not FDA approved.[56,57]

References

1. Moffat AC, Osselton MD, Widdop B, Watts J, eds. *Clarke's Analysis of Drugs and Poisons.* 4th ed. London, UK: Pharmaceutical Press; 2011:1357-1358.
2. Wills S. *Drugs of Abuse.* 2nd ed. London, UK: Pharmaceutical Press; 2005:303-323.
3. Levine B, Caplan YH. Pharmacology and toxicology of ethyl alcohol. In: Caplan YH, Goldberger BA, eds. *Garriott's Medicolegal Aspects of Alcohol.* 6th ed. Tucson, AZ: Lawyers & Judges Publishing Company Inc; 2015:25-48.
4. Traffic Safety Facts, 2015 Data. Alcohol-Impaired Driving. Washington, DC: NHTSA's National Center for Statistics and Analysis; 2016 Publication DOT HS 812350. US Department of Transportation, National Highway Traffic Safety Administration (NHTSA), National Center for Statistics and Analysis. https://crashstats.nhtsa.dot.gov/Api/Public/ViewPublication/812350. Accessed May 23, 2019.
5. Alcohol-Related Disease Impact Data Portal. Centers for Disease Control and Prevention. https://chronicdata.cdc.gov/browse?category=Alcohol-Related+Disease+Impact. Accessed May 23, 2019.
6. Alcohol and Public Health. Fact Sheets - Alcohol Use and Your Health. Centers for Disease Control and Prevention. https://www.cdc.gov/alcohol/fact-sheets/alcohol-use.htm. Accessed May 23, 2019.
7. Caplan YH, Goldberger BA, eds. *Garriott's Medicolegal Aspects of Alcohol.* 6th ed. Tucson, AZ: Lawyers & Judges Publishing Company Inc; 2015.
8. Davis AR, Lipson AH. Central nervous system tolerance to high blood alcohol levels. *Med J Aust.* 1986;144:9-12.
9. Kalant H. Pharmacokinetics of ethanol: absorption, distribution, and elimination. In: Begleiter H, Kissin B, eds. *The Pharmacology of Alcohol and Alcohol Dependence.* Oxford, UK: Oxford University Press; 1996:15-58.

10. Jokipii SG. Experimental studies on blood alcohol in healthy subjects and in some diseases. *Ann Med Exp Biol Fenn.* 1951;29:1-99.
11. Jones AW. Ethanol metabolism in patients with liver cirrhosis. *J Clin Forensic Med.* 2000;7:48-51.
12. Rangno RE, Kreeft JH, Sitar DS. Ethanol 'dose-dependent' elimination: Michaelis-Menten v classical kinetic analysis. *Br J Clin Pharmacol.* 1981; 12:667-673.
13. Lewis MJ. Blood alcohol: the concentration-time curve and retrospective estimation of level. *J Forensic Sci Soc.* 1986;26:95-113.
14. Forrest AR. Non-linear kinetics of ethyl alcohol metabolism. *J Forensic Sci Soc.* 1986;26:121-123.
15. Holford NH. Clinical pharmacokinetics of ethanol. *Clin Pharmacokinet.* 1987;13:273-292.
16. Holzbecher MD, Wells AE. Elimination of alcohol in humans. *Can Soc Forensic Sci J.* 1984;17:197-208.
17. Bogusz M, Pach J, Stasko W. Comparative studies on the rate of ethanol elimination in acute poisoning and in controlled conditions. *J Forensic Sci.* 1977;22:446-451.
18. Gershman H, Steeper J. Rate of clearance of ethanol from the blood of intoxicated patients in the emergency department. *J Emerg Med.* 1991; 9:307-311.
19. Jones AW, Sternebring B. Kinetics of ethanol and methanol in alcoholics during detoxification. *Alcohol.* 1992;27:641-647.
20. Jones AW. Disappearance rate of ethanol from the blood of human subjects: implications in forensic toxicology. *J Forensic Sci.* 1993;38:104-118.
21. Jones AW, Jonsson KA. Food-induced lowering of blood-ethanol profiles and increased rate of elimination immediately after a meal. *J Forensic Sci.* 1994;39:1084-1093.
22. Hak EA, Gerlitz BJ, Dermont PM, Bowthorpe WD. Determination of serum alcohol:blood alcohol ratios. *Can Soc Forensic Sci J.* 1995;28:123-126.
23. Charlebois RC, Corbett MR, Wigmore JG. Comparison of ethanol concentrations in blood, serum, and blood cells for forensic application. *J Anal Toxicol.* 1996;20:171-178.
24. Winek CL, Carfagna M. Comparison of plasma, serum, and whole blood ethanol concentrations. *J Anal Toxicol.* 1987;11:267-268.
25. Jones AW. Reference limits for urine/blood ratios of ethanol in two successive voids from drinking drivers. *J Anal Toxicol.* 2002;26:333-339.
26. Jones AW. Time-adjusted urine/blood ratios of ethanol in drinking drivers. *J Anal Toxicol.* 2003;27:167-168.
27. Alexander WD, Wills PD, Eldred N. Urinary ethanol and diabetes mellitus. *Diabet Med.* 1988; 5:463-464.
28. Saady JJ, Poklis A, Dalton HP. Production of urinary ethanol after sample collection. *J Forensic Sci.* 1993;38:1467-1471.
29. Jones AW, Eklund A, Helander A. Misleading results of ethanol analysis in urine specimens from rape victims suffering from diabetes. *J Clin Forensic Med.* 2000;7:144-146.
30. Blackmore DJ. The bacterial production of ethyl alcohol. *J Forensic Sci Soc.* 1968;8:73-78.
31. Corry JE. A review: possible sources of ethanol ante- and post-mortem: its relationship to the biochemistry and microbiology of decomposition. *J Appl Bacteriol.* 1978;44:1-6.
32. Petkovic SM, Simic MA, Vujic DN. Postmortem production of ethanol in different tissues under controlled experimental conditions. *J Forensic Sci.* 2005;50:204-208.
33. Pounder DJ, Kuroda N. Vitreous alcohol is of limited value in predicting blood alcohol. *Forensic Sci Int.* 1994;65:73-80.
34. Jones AW, Holmgren P. Uncertainty in estimating blood ethanol concentrations by analysis of vitreous humour. *J Clin Pathol.* 2001;54:699-702.
35. Pleuckhahn VD, Ballard B. Diffusion of stomach alcohol and heart blood alcohol concentration at autopsy. *J Forensic Sci.* 1967;12:463-470.
36. Pounder DJ, Smith DR. Postmortem diffusion of alcohol from the stomach. *Am J Forensic Med Pathol.* 1995;16:89-96.
37. Nine JS, Moraca M, Virji MA, Rao KN. Serum-ethanol determination: comparison of lactate and lactate dehydrogenase interference in three enzymatic assays. *J Anal Toxicol.* 1995;19:192-196.
38. Powers RH, Dean DE. Evaluation of potential lactate/lactate dehydrogenase interference with an enzymatic alcohol analysis. *J Anal Toxicol.* 2009;33:561-563.
39. Nicholson ME, Wang M, Airhihenbuwa CO, Mahoney BS, Christina R, Maney DW. Variability in behavioral impairment involved in the rising and falling BAC curve. *J Stud Alcohol.* 1992; 53:349-356.
40. Bennett RH, Cherek DR, Spiga R. Acute and chronic alcohol tolerance in humans: effects of dose and consecutive days of exposure. *Alcohol Clin Exp Res.* 1993;17:740-745.
41. Picton WR, Bowthorpe WD. *Roadside Screening for Impaired Drivers in Canada.* Morton Grove, IL: American Association for Automotive Medicine; 1977:241-250.
42. Urso T, Gavaler JS, Van Thiel DH. Blood ethanol levels in sober alcohol users seen in an emergency room. *Life Sci.* 1981;28:1053-1056.
43. Perper JA, Twerski A, Wienand JW. Tolerance at high blood alcohol concentrations: a study of 110 cases and review of the literature. *J Forensic Sci.* 1986;31:212-221.
44. Davis AR, Lipson AH. Central nervous system tolerance to high blood alcohol levels. *Med J Aust.* 1986;144:9-12.

45. Sullivan JB Jr, Hauptman M, Bronstein AC. Lack of observable intoxication in humans with high plasma alcohol concentrations. *J Forensic Sci.* 1987;32:1660-1665.
46. Ryder KW, Glick MR. The effect of skin cleansing agents on ethanol results measured with the Du Pont automatic clinical analyzer. *J Forensic Sci.* 1986;31:574-579.
47. Haverstick DM, Bruns DE. Unexpected ethanol in urine: increasing proof. *Clin Chem.* 2010;56:146-147.
48. Allen JP, Sillanaukee P, Strid N, Raye Z. Litten RZ. Biomarkers of Heavy Drinking. National Institute on Alcohol Abuse and Alcoholism. https://pubs.niaaa.nih.gov/publications/AssessingAlcohol/biomarkers.htm. Prepared August 2004. Accessed May 23, 2019.
49. SAMHSA Advisory. The Role of Biomarkers in the Treatment of Alcohol Use Disorders, 2012 Revision. https://etg.weebly.com/uploads/7/4/7/5/74751/samsha_biomarker_advisory_may_2012.pdf. Accessed May 23, 2019.
50. Jatlow P, O'Malley SS. Clinical (nonforensic) application of ethyl glucuronide measurement: are we ready? *Alcohol Clin Exp Res.* 2010;34(6):968-75.
51. Dresen S, Weinmann W, Wurst FM. Forensic confirmatory analysis of ethyl sulfate-a new marker for alcohol consumption-by liquid-chromatography/electrospray ionization/tandem mass spectrometry. *J Am Soc Mass Spectrom.* 2004; 15:1644-1648.
52. Bicker W, Lämmerhofer M, Keller T, Schuhmacher R, Krska R, Lindner W. Validated method for the determination of the ethanol consumption markers ethyl glucuronide, ethyl phosphate, and ethyl sulfate in human urine by reversed-phase/weak anion exchange liquid chromatography-tandem mass spectrometry. *Anal Chem.* 2006; 78(16):5884-5892.
53. Favretto D, Nalesso A, Frison G, Viel G, Traldi P, Ferrara SD. A novel and an effective analytical approach for the LC-MS determination of ethyl glucuronide and ethyl sulfate in urine. *Int J Legal Med.* 2010;124(2):161-164.
54. Albermann E, Musshoff F, Madea B. A high performance liquid chromatographic-tandem mass spectrometric method for the determination of ethyl glucuronide and ethyl sulfate in urine validated according to forensic guidelines. *J Chromatogr Sci.* 2012 50(1):51-56.
55. Côté L. Determination of urinary ethyl glucuronide and ethyl sulfate by LC/MS/MS for clinical research. Poster A-386, AACC Conference Chicago, IL, 2014. https://www.agilent.com/cs/library/posters/public/AACC2014_Poster_Urinary-EtG-EtS_Fe2514_LC_km_dn%20RR.pdf. Accessed May 23, 2019.
56. Böttcher M, Beck O, Helander A. Evaluation of a new immunoassay for urinary ethyl glucuronide testing. *Alcohol Alcohol.* 2008;43(1):46-48.
57. DRI® Ethyl Glucuronide Assay Product Insert. ThermoScientific. October 2012.

Chapter 17

Non-Ethanol Volatiles and Ethylene Glycol

Graham R. Jones, PhD

Introduction[1-6]

Origin

Methanol, acetone, and ethylene glycol are the simplest possible organic compounds in their respective classes, and isopropanol is one of the two possible isomers of the 3-carbon aliphatic mono-alcohol.

Descriptive Chemistry

Acetone

Acetone is a ketone that is a clear, colorless, highly flammable liquid at room temperature, with a distinctive sharp aromatic odor that has been variously described as "fruity" or "mint-like" and a pungent sweetish taste. It is miscible with water, ethanol, chloroform, ether, dimethylformamide, and most oils.

Synonyms: β-ketopropane, cetona, dimethylformaldehyde, dimethyl-ketone, 2-propanone, pyroacetic ether

Formula: C_3H_6O

Molecular mass = 58.0791 Daltons

CAS-67-64-1

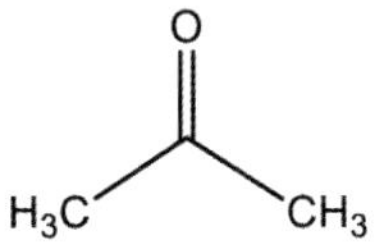

Methanol

Methanol is a mono-alcohol that is a clear, colorless, highly flammable liquid at room temperature, with a slight alcoholic odor in the pure state (crude material may have a repulsive pungent odor). It is miscible with water, ethanol, chloroform, ether, benzene, ketones, and most other organic solvents, and forms azeotropes (constant boiling mixtures) with many compounds.

Synonyms: Carbinol, colonial spirit, methylol, monohydroxymethane, wood alcohol, wood naphtha, wood spirit

Formula: CH_4O

Molecular mass = 32.0419 Daltons

CAS-67-56-1

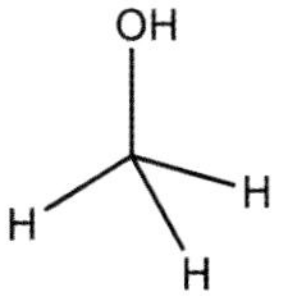

Isopropanol

Isopropanol is a mono-alcohol that is a clear, colorless, flammable liquid at room temperature, with a slight odor resembling a mixture of ethanol and acetone and a slightly bitter taste. It is miscible with water, ethanol, chloroform, and ether, and is insoluble in salt solutions. It forms an azeotrope with water.

Synonyms: Dimethyl carbinol, isolol, isopropyl alcohol, petrohol, 2-propanol, propan-2-ol, secondary propyl alcohol

Formula: C_3H_8O

Molecular mass = 60.0950 Daltons

CAS-67-63-0

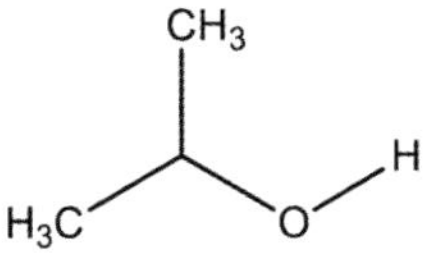

Ethylene Glycol

Ethylene glycol is a 1,2-diol or glycol that is a colorless, slightly viscous, syrupy liquid at room temperature, with little odor and a sweet taste. It is highly hygroscopic, absorbing twice its weight in water at 100% relative humidity, and is miscible with water, alcohols, glycerol, acetic acid, acetone and similar ketones, aldehydes, pyridine, and coal tar bases. It is slightly soluble in ether and nearly insoluble in benzene, petroleum ether, and oils.

Synonyms: 1,2-dihydroxyethane; 1,2-ethanediol; ethylene alcohol, ethylene dihydrate, glycol, glycol alcohol, monoethylene glycol

Formula: $C_2H_6O_2$

Molecular mass = 62.0678 Daltons

CAS-107-21-1

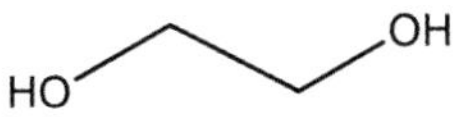

Pharmacology

Context of Human Use

Acetone

Acetone is sold as nail polish remover and as a general solvent. It is frequently employed as a solvent for fats, oils, waxes, resins, rubber, paints, varnishes, plastics, and adhesives like rubber cement, and is a chemical intermediate in the manufacture of many other organic chemicals (including drugs of abuse). It is formed endogenously in vivo in various forms of ketosis and is a major metabolite of isopropanol. It is a common laboratory chemical.

Methanol

Methanol is a better solvent than ethanol, dissolving many inorganic compounds, and is therefore widely used commercially as such, especially in paints and varnishes as well as pharmaceuticals and natural products. It is found in a variety of automotive products, including some antifreeze solutions, windshield de-icers, and gasoline additives, as well as in fuel for picnic stoves and soldering torches; is used as an intermediate in the commercial synthesis of formaldehyde and other organic chemicals; and is used to denature ethanol. It is also found in trace amounts as an endogenous secondary constituent in a variety of alcoholic beverages, especially fortified wines. It is a common laboratory chemical.

Isopropanol

Isopropanol is found in isopropyl rubbing alcohol (as 70% aqueous solution), hand lotions, after-shave lotions and similar cosmetics, and quick-drying inks, and has been used as a topical antiseptic. Isopropanol is also used in some antifreeze mixtures, industrially in the extraction of alkaloids, and as a solvent for gums, shellacs, essential oils, resins, and creosote. It is a common laboratory chemical.

Ethylene Glycol

Ethylene glycol is found as a major constituent in automotive antifreeze, de-icers, hydraulic brake fluid, and industrial drying agents. It is used as a solvent in the paint and plastics industries, a softening agent for cellophane, and a stabilizer for the foam in certain fire extinguishers. It is used as an intermediate in the formulation of inks, synthetic fibers (eg, Dacron), and synthetic waxes.

Exposure

All of these compounds are readily absorbed through the lungs and skin, as well as after oral administration, and they are rapidly distributed into body compartments according to the water content of tissues.

Airborne and Workplace Exposures: Hazardous Material (Hazmat) Considerations[7]

The American Conference of Governmental Industrial Hygienists (ACGIH) Threshold Limit Value–Time-Weighted Average (TLV-TWA) air concentration is meant to represent the level of an airborne contaminant that nearly all workers can be exposed to during a 40-hour work week without ill effect, including mere discomfort. The National Institute of Occupational Safety and Health (NIOSH) immediately dangerous to life or health (IDLH) level represents "a maximum air concentration from which one could escape within 30 minutes without any escape-impairing symptoms or any irreversible health effects."

The National Fire Protection Association (NFPA) codes represent an identification and ranking of potential fire hazards of materials, and includes three categories of hazard rating: health (H), flammability (F), and reactivity (R). Within each of these, hazards are graded from zero (0), indicating no hazard, to four (4), indicating a severe hazard. The system is intended to provide basic information to fire-fighting and emergency-response personnel and includes both the intrinsic toxicity of the parent material and its thermal breakdown products. These hazmat parameters are summarized in Table 17-1.

Exposure by Ingestion: Epidemiology[8]

The 2016 annual report of the American Association of Poison Control Centers' National Poisoning and Exposure Database lists 28,684 recorded US exposures to non-ethanol volatiles and ethylene glycol in that year. The largest number of these exposures (56%) involved ingestion of isopropanol, followed by ethylene glycol (25%), acetone (12%), and methanol (7%). The majority of isopropanol ingestions involved products labeled as "isopropyl rubbing alcohol," followed by those labeled with the chemical name. All ethylene glycol ingestions involved products labeled as "antifreeze." Acetone exposures most frequently involved products labeled as "nail polish remover," followed by those labeled with the chemical name. Methanol ingestions most frequently involved material labeled as automotive products, followed by those labeled with the chemical name.

For all four compounds, the majority of exposures involved two patient age groups: infants (≤5 years old) and adults (≥20 years old). Isopropanol and acetone were ingested more frequently by infants, while methanol and ethylene glycol predominated among adults. For all four, the majority of exposures were recorded as "unintentional"

Table 17-1. Hazardous Materials (Hazmat) Parameters

Compound	ACGIH TLV-TWA	NIOSH IDLH	National Fire Protection Association (NFPA) Codes		
			Health (H)	Flammability (F)	Reactivity (R)
Acetone	500 ppm	2500 ppm*	1	3	0
Methanol	200 ppm	6000 ppm	1	3	0
Isopropanol	400 ppm	2000 ppm*	1	3	0
Ethylene glycol	100 mg/m^3**	Not established	1	1	0

ACGIH TLV-TWA, American Conference of Governmental Industrial Hygienists Threshold Limit Value–Time-Weighted Average; NIOSH IDLH, National Institute of Occupational Safety and Health, immediately dangerous to life or health level.

* For this substance, IDLH is set at 10% of the lower explosive limit (LEL).

** This is the ceiling air concentration (TLV-C) that should not be exceeded at any time.

Table 17-2. Mortality and Morbidity[8]

Compound	Exposures	Medical Facility Treated	Mortality Rate	
			Deaths/10^5 Exposures	Percentage of Exposures
Acetone	3483	600	0	0
Methanol	2017	676	793	0.79
Isopropanol	16,099	2880	12	0.01
Ethylene glycol	7085	2672	240	0.24

Table 17-3. Toxicokinetic Parameters

Compound	Elimination Half-Life ($t_{½}$, h)	Volume of Distribution (V_d, L/kg))	Usual Clearance (mL/min)
Acetone	3–6	0.8	—
Methanol	2–24	0.6	40–60
Isopropanol	2.5–3.0	0.6	30
Ethylene glycol	2–5	0.5–0.8	200

(n = 22,034) versus "intentional" (n = 3,134). Presumably, the intentional category includes documented suicide attempts as well as intentional abuse, such as "sniffing" or "huffing" glue or acetone. The unintentional category includes both accidental exposures as well as misuse due to substitution of one or more of these substances for ethanol among alcoholics in withdrawal.

The rate of treatment in a health care facility resulting from these exposures varied by compound (methanol = 34%, ethylene glycol = 38%, isopropanol = 18%, acetone = 17%). These rates reflect the relative frequency of moderate to major injury and/or death as outcomes of exposure. The specific mortality rates calculated from the 2016 data are shown in Table 17-2.

Toxicokinetics, Metabolism, and Excretion[1,3,5,14]

Toxicokinetic parameters are shown in Table 17-3.

Metabolism and Excretion

Acetone

In high concentrations, acetone is predominantly excreted unchanged in the breath and (~3%) in urine. The average breath/blood concentration ratio has been estimated as 330, and the average urine/blood ratio, 1.34. It is also metabolized by enzymatic oxidation to acetate, lactate, and pyruvate (and ultimately to CO_2) at a slow constant rate of 1 to 3 mg/kg/h by various dehydrogenase and oxidase enzyme systems including alcohol dehydrogenase. Acetone is one of the endogenous metabolic intermediates known as "ketone bodies" and, as such, can be present in poorly controlled diabetics in concentrations up to 80 mg/dL or more. It may also be present at lower concentrations (<10 mg/dL) in chronic alcoholics and the malnourished. There is also a minor pathway by which it can be reduced to isopropanol. A retrospective review of deaths due to diabetic ketoacidosis (175) and alcoholic ketoacidosis (79) found that isopropanol was present in 77% of diabetic ketoacidosis deaths (averaging 15.1 ± 13.0 mg/dL in blood) and 52% of alcoholic ketoacidosis deaths (averaging 18.5 ± 22.1 mg/dL).

Isopropanol

Isopropanol is an alternate substrate for alcohol dehydrogenase, which metabolizes it (more slowly than ethanol) to acetone. Both isopropanol and acetone are eliminated in breath and urine, where some of the urinary isopropanol may be in the form of the glucuronide conjugate, particularly after large doses. Isopropanol elimination follows first-order kinetics in man, although that may change to zero-order with sufficient dose.

Methanol

Like isopropanol, methanol is an alternative substrate for alcohol dehydrogenase, being oxidized at a rate approximately one-tenth that of ethanol. It is oxidized to formaldehyde, which, however, does not accumulate but is further oxidized to formic acid by aldehyde dehydrogenase and then to CO_2 to a very limited extent in humans, likely via a folate-dependent mechanism. Up to 60% of a dose is oxidized, and urinary formic acid may account for 2% to 5% of total elimination for a 4- to 10-day period. The average urine/blood ratio is the same as ethanol, 1.30. Via the lungs, 10% to 20% of a dose is eliminated unchanged, and 3% is eliminated via the kidneys. Methanol exhibits zero-order elimination kinetics in man. Low levels of methanol are generated by endogenous metabolism, blood methanol levels normally being around 0.15 mg/dL, and urine formic acid levels 1.2 mg/dL to 1.7 mg/dL.

Ethylene Glycol

The toxic metabolism of ethylene glycol in humans is less completely understood than that of the non-ethanol volatiles, but it does generally appear to undergo extensive alcohol dehydrogenase catalyzed oxidation analogous to that of ethanol, giving rise to glycoaldehyde, then to glycolic acid, glyoxylic acid, and oxalic acid. Related pathways give rise to glyoxal, formic acid, and ultimately CO_2. Calcium oxalate crystals are deposited in the kidneys, and some oxalate may be excreted in the urine along with unchanged ethylene glycol. In experiments with animals, ethylene glycol toxicity appears to correlate with the amount of oxalate formed by different species.

Toxicity[1-5,7,9]

Acetone

Acetone, while considered overall to show relatively low toxicity, is a definite central nervous system (CNS) depressant. Diabetic patients in ketoacidosis may have blood acetone levels of 15 mg/dL to 75 mg/dL associated with CNS symptoms of confusion, drowsiness, and hyperventilation. Well-controlled diabetics normally have blood acetone levels <3 mg/dL.

Oral: CNS narcosis and sometimes coma have been seen in significant acetone ingestions (eg, 800 mL), and hyperglycemia is a frequent finding.

Inhalation: Vapors cause mild eye and respiratory tract irritation, moderate overexposure (air concentration = 1000-6000 ppm) has been associated with eye irritation and headache as common symptoms, and CNS depression occurs at high exposure levels (>10,000 ppm), accompanied by electroencephalogram changes, dizziness, muscle weakness, nausea and vomiting, and hyperglycemia. Acetone is abused in "glue-sniffing," with toxic effects at blood concentrations of 20 mg/dL to 30 mg/dL, and a report of 55 mg/dL in a fatality.

Topical: Prolonged or repeated topical use may cause erythema, dryness.

Methanol

Methanol is sometimes used as a substitute for ethanol by alcoholics. Although methanol itself produces mainly inebriation, its toxic metabolites, formaldehyde and formic acid, cause metabolic acidosis, blindness, coma, and death after a latent period of typically 6 to 30 hours. Methanol is slowly oxidized to formaldehyde by alcohol dehydrogenase and then to formic acid by aldehyde dehydrogenase. Humans have limited metabolic capacity to oxidize formic acid. The metabolic acidosis is caused by the combination of formic acid and lactic acid (the latter appears late and is likely due to tissue hypoxia resulting from anaerobic glycolysis). The blindness is caused by the formic acid acting as a mitochondrial poison and inhibiting cytochrome oxidase (and thus oxidative phosphorylation) in photoreceptors, Muller glial cells, and the optic nerve.

Oral: Reported lethal doses of methanol show considerable variation, with reports of fatalities typically due to ingestion of 100 mL to 200 mL and survival with as much as 500 mL, with an overall average estimate of ~1 g/kg. Much lower amounts (eg, 10-30 mL) can result in permanent blindness. The lethal blood level left untreated has been estimated at 80 mg/dL.

Inhalation: Vapors are mildly irritating to eyes and skin; systemic toxicity may result from absorption by all routes. Due to slow elimination, daily exposure to fumes (>3000 ppm) may result in accumulation to toxic levels, but very-long-term exposures to lower levels (800-1000 ppm) may also result in serious eye injury.

Topical: Skin and eye irritant.

Isopropanol

Unlike the other common alcohol substitutes, methanol and ethylene glycol, isopropanol is not metabolized to highly toxic organic acids and therefore doesn't give rise to a profound anion gap acidosis. Isopropanol, however, is a potent CNS depressant, with about two to three times the depressant potency of ethanol.

Oral: By ingestion, isopropanol produces an ethanol-like intoxication that may progress through ataxia, dysarthria, confusion, and stupor to coma and respiratory arrest at higher doses. Such doses may also cause hypotension secondary to vasodilation and possibly myocardial depression. The alcohol is irritating to the gastrointestinal (GI) tract and commonly causes gastritis. Toxic oral doses have been variously reported as ~0.5 mL/kg to 1.0 mL/kg and 2 mL/kg to 4 mL/kg of rubbing alcohol (70% isopropanol), and fatalities have been reported at ingestions as low as 240 mL.

Inhalation: Vapors produce mild eye and respiratory tract irritation (400-800 ppm). High exposures can produce CNS depression, headache, dizziness, hallucinations, dyspnea, flushing, pulse rate increase, hypotension, anesthesia (~10,000 ppm), and coma.

Topical: Skin and eye irritant (corneal burns and eye damage). Poisonings have been reported in infants following sponge baths with isopropanol.

Ethylene Glycol

Ethylene glycol itself is relatively nontoxic, but each of the acidic metabolites is much more toxic than the parent compound. These, along with excess lactic acid produced by tissue hypoxia, are responsible for causing a characteristic positive anion gap metabolic acidosis. Tissue injury is believed to be due to the combination of widespread deposition of calcium oxalate crystals coupled with the toxic effects of glycolic and glyoxylic acids.

Oral: Ethylene glycol intoxication by ingestion classically involves three stages. The CNS phase (1-12 hours post ingestion) involves ataxia, nystagmus, myoclonic jerks, coma, and focal and/or generalized seizures. Cerebral edema may develop, and GI complaints of nausea, vomiting, and abdominal pain may occur. The cardiovascular phase (12-72 hours post ingestion) involves mild hypertension, tachycardia, tachypnea, and hyperthermia. Up to a third of patients may become hypocalcemic secondary to the formation of calcium oxalate crystals and exhibit electrocardiogram symptoms of prolonged QT interval and muscle tetany. At higher doses, pulmonary edema, pneumonitis, and congestive heart failure or shock may develop. The renal toxicity phase (24-72 hours post ingestion) involves flank pain, costovertebral angle tenderness, and oliguric renal failure, which may present with hyperkalemia. Without proper intervention, renal failure may become permanent. The lethal dose in adults has been listed as 100 mL (1.0-1.5 mL/kg); however, survival has been reported with an ingestion of 2 L treated within 1 hour of ingestion.

Inhalation: The aerosolized particulate form is very toxic on inhalation, associated with lacrimation, headache, cough, nausea, and vomiting; pulmonary, renal, and liver changes; agitation; loss of consciousness; and lymphocytosis. Threshold limit value is 100 mg/m^3.

Analysis[10,11,15]

Specimen Types, Requirements, and Characteristics

These compounds have been measured in blood, serum, and urine.

Modes of Analysis

For acetone, methanol, and isopropanol, gas chromatographic (GC) techniques with flame ionization detection (FID) utilizing either direct injection or headspace analysis are in widespread use and perform well. Typically these volatiles are combined in GC assays that also measure ethanol. Gas chromatography-mass spectrometry (GC-MS) methods can also be used. Ethylene glycol can be screened for using commercial enzymatic methods, although none appear to be Food and Drug Administration (FDA) approved for clinical use at this time. Enzymatic assays have the potential to cross-react to propylene glycol, which can be problematic if the apparent concentration of ethylene glycol is low and propylene glycol-containing

Table 17-4. Selected Analytical Parameters (in Order of Decreasing Volatility)

	Acetone	Methanol	Isopropanol	Ethylene glycol
Class	Ketone	Mono-alcohol	Mono-alcohol	1,2-diol (glycol)
Volatility: boiling point/ vapor pressure at 25°C	56.5°C/ 231 mmHg	64.6°C/ 127 mmHg	82.5°C/ 45 mm Hg	197.5°C/ 0.08 mmHg
Dissociation constant, pK_a	NA	15.3	17.1	15.0
Partition coefficient, log *P* (octanol/water)	-0.2	0.8	0	-1.4

injectable solutions have been administered. In larger clinical or forensic laboratories, determination of ethylene glycol in serum or urine is most commonly determined by dilution with water and direct injection onto a GC-FID system. Some GC-based methods use derivatization to improve chromatographic peak shape. High-performance liquid chromatography and GC-MS have also been used for determination of ethylene glycol, other glycols, and the acidic metabolites of ethylene glycol. Determination of glycolic acid can be important in the later stages of poisoning where ethylene glycol is present at only a very low concentration due to metabolism and clearance. Ethylene glycol can also be determined by colorimetric or fluorometric methods after oxidation to formaldehyde, although these methods are seldom used now. Selected analytical parameters are shown in Table 17-4.

Known Analytical Issues/Problems

Enzymatic screening methods for ethanol involving alcohol dehydrogenase are not satisfactory for the determination of the non-ethanol volatiles compounds and ethylene glycol due to the lack of substrate discrimination of this enzyme among this family of compounds. False-positive or apparent elevated concentrations of ethylene glycol can occur in the presence of severe lactic acidosis or severe ketosis using enzymatic assays. Colorimetric or fluorometric methods for ethylene glycol exhibit a number of interferences by propylene glycol in pharmaceuticals and other compounds like elevated triglycerides and 2,3-butanediol in alcoholics.

Caution must be exercised in interpreting apparent low concentrations of ethylene glycol in GC-based assays using flame ionization detection. Interfering substances can sometimes elute at a similar retention time as ethylene glycol.

Clinical Issues[7,9,12,13]

Clinical Interpretation of Analytical Findings

Patients typically present in the emergency department acutely intoxicated or unconscious, with or without a history of ingestion of one of these substances. The initial laboratory workup should include arterial blood gases, acid/base parameters, electrolytes, glucose, BUN, creatinine, ketones, lactate, and a stat blood ethanol level if available. Critical to the workup of poisoning in these cases is calculation of the two "gaps."

The anion gap (AG) is best calculated from the formula that does not use [K]:

$$\text{AG} = [\text{Na}] - ([\text{Cl}] + [\textbf{bicarbonate}])$$

(typical normal <12-16)

The osmolal gap (OG) is the difference between the serum osmolality measured in the laboratory by freezing point depression or heat of vaporization and the osmolarity calculated from the major, independently measured, osmotically active molecules in serum (Na, Cl, glucose, and urea), according to the formula:

$$\text{OG} = \textbf{Measured osmolality} - \textbf{Calculated osmolarity}$$

where

$$\text{Calculated osmolarity} = (1.86\,[\text{Na}]) + ([\text{glucose}]/18) + ([\text{BUN}]/2.8) + ([\text{ethanol}]/4.6)$$

Generally, an osmolal gap >10 indicates the presence of unaccounted-for low-molecular-weight osmotically active substance(s), like the non-ethanol volatiles or ethylene glycol in serum.

The results of the two "gaps" determinations, in the context of other laboratory test values, can give insight into the likelihood of ingestion of non-ethanol volatiles compounds or ethylene glycol, as follows.

Acetone and Isopropanol

If the acidosis is low to nonexistent, but there is a significant ketosis and an osmolal gap, acetone or isopropanol are the more likely ingestants. The ketosis is due to acetone, and both compounds contribute to the increased osmolality. Note that acetone can be associated with spuriously increased creatinine, so an increased creatinine with normal

BUN can also be a clue. Specific levels of isopropanol and acetone should be obtained if available.

Methanol and Ethylene Glycol

A significant metabolic acidosis with a large anion gap not accounted for by lactate and without ketosis, but accompanied by a positive osmolal gap, is consistent with methanol or ethylene glycol as the ingestant. Note that if ethanol is co-ingested, it may competitively inhibit the alcohol dehydrogenase-catalyzed conversion of methanol to formate or of ethylene glycol to its acidic metabolites, but the osmolal gap will remain significant in either case. When methanol poisoning is suspected, specific methanol levels should be obtained if available. Formate levels are considered confirmatory and a better measure of toxicity but are even less commonly available than are methanol levels. When ethylene glycol poisoning is suspected, examination of the urine may be extremely helpful. Most antifreezes have fluorescein present as an additive, so examining urine for fluorescence with a Wood's lamp may provide a clue. Crystalluria on microscopic urinalysis can be diagnostic. Though not universally present in all cases, crystals that are birefringent, octahedral, envelope-shaped, needle-shaped, or dumbbell-shaped are consistent with calcium oxalate. Additional findings may include hematuria, epithelial cells, and proteinuria. Specific levels of ethylene glycol should be obtained if available. Specific levels of glycolic acid are considered a better measure of toxicity but are very rarely available.

In the absence of symptoms and of elevated osmolal and anion gaps, serious ingestion is not likely to have occurred. Combined osmolal and anion gap elevation, however, may also be seen with severe alcoholic ketoacidosis or diabetic ketoacidosis due to accumulation of unmeasured anions (beta-hydroxybutyrate) and osmotically active substances (acetone, glycerol, and amino acids). Serum beta-hydroxybutyrate levels may distinguish ethylene glycol poisoning from alcoholic ketoacidosis. Chronic renal failure, lactic acidosis, hyperlipidemia, hyperproteinemia, and several drugs and other chemicals can give rise to an elevated osmolal gap.

Serum levels of the non-ethanol volatiles compounds and ethylene glycol are typically only available at larger hospitals and regional centers, and are frequently not available stat. Empirical formulas allow the crude estimation of the serum concentration of a suspected compound by multiplying the osmolal gap by a molecular-weight–based factor (note that reporting units are mg/dL, which must be corrected to mmol/L to be used in the osmolal gap calculations).

Treatment and Management[7,9,13]

For patients who arrive in the emergency department acutely debilitated, emergency supportive measures are necessary, including maintaining an open airway, assisting ventilation, administering supplemental oxygen, and treating coma, seizures, cardiac arrhythmias, and hypocalcemia. Fluid intake and output should be monitored, and intravenous fluids should be provided to maintain good urine output. Loop diuretics may be used to maintain urine output once volume replacement has been accomplished.

GI decontamination has relatively little value. All these compounds are relatively rapidly absorbed from the gastric mucosa, making lavage impractical except in cases of immediate ingestion. Activated charcoal absorbs alcohols and glycols poorly, and the early onset of CNS symptoms, including seizures, are relative contraindications to the use of ipecac. Specific and antidotal therapy varies by compound.

Acetone

Generally, acetone exposures/ingestions require only supportive care. No more toxic metabolites are formed, and acetone is excreted unchanged, for the most part, by the kidneys and lungs. Observation and monitoring are usually sufficient.

Isopropanol

Isopropanol, like acetone, usually requires only supportive care. There is no specific antidote for isopropanol poisoning; no toxic metabolites are produced. Some authors recommend the use of activated charcoal in these cases. Hemodialysis will effectively remove both isopropanol and acetone from the system, but it is rarely indicated since the majority of patients can be managed supportively. Dialysis should be considered only when levels are extremely high (>500-600 mg/dL) or if there is a degree of hypotension that does not respond to fluid replacement and vasopressors.

Methanol

Methanol does give rise to a toxic metabolite, formate, and so antidotal therapy involving the competitive inhibition of alcohol dehydrogenase is indicated in cases in which there is a significant history of ingestion, metabolic acidosis, and a serum osmolal gap >10 mOsm/L not accounted for by ethanol and/or serum methanol levels (if available) of >20 mg/dL. The drug 4-methylpyrazole (4-MP; also known under the trade names Fomepizole and Antizol) is FDA approved for this indication. It has predictable pharmacokinetics, ease of use, and lack of adverse side effects. The alternative is the use of an intravenous 5% or 10% ethanol infusion to maintain blood ethanol levels at 100 mg/dL to 150 mg/dL, with close monitoring of blood ethanol and glucose levels. Folic or folinic acid or intravenous leukovorin may be added. This is used to promote the elimination of formate by its enzymatic conversion to CO_2 and water. Gastric aspiration is advocated by some authors if initiated within 30 to 60 minutes post ingestion. Hemodialysis is effective at removing both methanol and formate from the system, and the indications are the same as for antidotal therapy.

Methanol is overall the most lethal of these compounds, and despite aggressive treatment, mortalities of 20% have been reported. Among survivors of this form of poisoning, 20% to 25% are left with permanent visual defects, ranging from loss of visual acuity to complete blindness, and the course of this appears to correlate with the severity of the acidosis, blood formate levels, and delays in the institution of therapy. Other neurologic sequelae are also common and include cerebral edema (in 10% of cases), pseudobulbar palsy, seizures, primitive reflexes, intellectual deficits, transverse myelitis, and persistent vegetative state.

Ethylene Glycol

Ethylene glycol gives rise to its toxic acidic metabolites via an alcohol dehydrogenase enzymatic mechanism, and therefore antidotal therapy, directly analogous to that used in methanol poisoning, is also used with this compound. Indications for antidotal therapy include a significant history of ingestion accompanied by two or more of the following: a serum osmolal gap >10 mOsm/L not accounted for by ethanol, serum bicarbonate <20 meq/L, arterial pH <7.3, presence of oxalate crystals in the urine, or a serum ethylene glycol level (if available) of >20 mg/dL. Pyridoxine, folate, and thiamine may be added to the regimen to promote the enzymatic conversion of glyoxylic acid to less-toxic compounds. Gastric aspiration is advocated by some authors if initiated within 30 to 60 minutes post ingestion. Hemodialysis is effective at removing both ethylene glycol and its metabolites from the system, and the indications are the same as for antidotal therapy

References

1. Klaassen CD, ed. *Casarett and Doull's Toxicology: The Basic Science of Poisons.* 6th ed. New York, NY: McGraw-Hill; 2001:1119.
2. Lewis RJ, ed. *Sax's Dangerous Properties of Industrial Materials.* 8th ed. New York, NY: Van Nostrand Reinhold; 1992.
3. Moffat AC, Osselton MD, Widdop B, Watts J, eds. *Clarke's Analysis of Drugs and Poisons.* 4th ed. London, UK: Pharmaceutical Press; 2011.
4. Budvavari S, ed. *The Merck Index: An Encyclopedia of Chemicals and Drugs.* 12th ed. Rahway, NJ: Merck and Co; 1996.
5. Baselt RC. *Disposition of Toxic Drugs and Chemicals in Man.* 10th ed. Seal Beach City, CA: Biomedical Publications; 2014.
6. Rumble JR, ed. *CRC Handbook of Chemistry and Physics.* 99th ed. Boca Raton, FL: CRC Press; 2018.
7. Olson KR, ed. *Poisoning and Drug Overdose.* 6th ed. New York, NY: Lange Medical Books, McGraw-Hill; 2012.
8. Gummin DD, Mowry JB, Spyker DA, Brooks DE, Fraser MO, Banner W. 2016 Annual Report of the American Association of Poison Control Centers' National Poison Data System (NPDS): 34th Annual Report. *Clin Toxicol (Phila).* 2017;55(10):1072-1254, 2017.
9. Ling LJ, Clark RF, Erickson TB, Trestrail JH. *Toxicology Secrets.* Philadelphia, PA: Henley and Belfus; 2001.
10. Burtis CA, Ashwood ER, Bruns DE, eds. *Tietz Textbook of Clinical Chemistry and Molecular Diagnostics.* 4th ed. St. Louis, MO: Elsevier Saunders; 2006.
11. Wu AHB, ed. *Tietz Clinical Guide to Laboratory Tests.* 4th ed. St. Louis, MO: Elsevier Saunders; 2006.
12. Holstege CP, Rusnyiak DE, eds. *Medical Toxicology: Medical Clinics of North America.* Vol. 89, No. 6, November 2005. Philadelphia, PA: Elsevier Saunders; 2005.
13. Linden CH, Rippe JM, Irwin RS, eds. *Manual of Overdoses and Poisonings.* Philadelphia, PA: Lippincott, Williams, and Wilkins; 2006.
14. Petersen TH, Williams T, Nuwayhid N, Harruff R. Postmortem detection of isopropanol in ketoacidosis. *J Forensic Sci.* 2012;57(3):674-678.
15. Boissier F, Weiss N, Faisy C. False positive ethylene glycol determination by spectrophotometry in the presence of severe lactic acidosis and ketosis. *Ann Emerg Med.* 2010;56(1):75-76.

Acknowledgment

The author would like to acknowledge Michael G. Bissell, MD, PhD, MPH, for his original version of this manuscript published in the first edition of this book.

Chapter 18

Cannabis

Paul J. Jannetto, PhD

Introduction[1-4]

Origin

Cannabis resin is secreted specifically by glandular hair structures, or trichromes, most thickly clustered on the surfaces of flowering heads and adjacent grey-green leaves of the hemp plant. The plant's resin content depends on several variables: growing conditions, time of harvest, plant sex (female plants have more resin than male), and genetics. Samples of wild cannabis strains have traditionally contained low to moderate THC concentrations, but improved cultivation techniques and plant selection have led to significant increases. For example, it has been reported that the mean THC content in seized US cannabis specimens increased nearly three-fold during the decades of the 1980s and 1990s, such that whereas an average 1970's "joint" contained only about 10 mg of THC, its late 1990's counterpart may frequently have contained six-to10-fold more. The three main types of cannabis sold at street level are marijuana, hashish, and hash oil. *Marijuana* (or marihuana) refers to the dried and crushed flower heads and small leaves of the cannabis plant, but it is also sometimes used to refer to the cannabis plant itself (as is the term *hash plant*). Slang synonyms include grass, dope, blow, skunk, weed, pot, hemp, bhang, and ganja, among many others. Marijuana typically contains up to 5% THC. Hashish (derived from the Arabic *hashish al kief* [dried herb of pleasure], otherwise known as *hash*) refers to the cannabis resin alone, sans plant. Pure hashish is typically a brown malleable semi-solid, but depending on its origin and purity, it can vary from soft and gooey to brittle or hard, and its color varies from brown to black, red, or yellow. Hashish can contain up to 20% THC (sinsemilla, made from unfertilized female plants, being the strongest variety). Hash oil, the most potent form of cannabis, is a concentrated, greenish black, viscous liquid extract of the resin that may contain greater than 60% THC.

Descriptive Chemistry

Cannabis refers to the flowering tops of the hemp plant, *Cannabis sativa,* which originated on the Indian subcontinent but is now widely cultivated. Hemp is composed of many different compounds. Cannabis resin contains more than 60 pharmacologically active derivatives of 2-(2-isopropyl-5-methylphenyl)-5-pentylresorcinol, known collectively as *cannabinoids.* The most abundant cannabinoids are (-)-*trans*-Δ^9-tetrahydrocannabinol (Δ^9-THC, Δ^1-THC), (-)-*trans*-Δ^8-tetrahydrocannabinol (Δ^8-THC [Δ^1-6-THC]), cannabinol (CBN), cannabidiol (CBD), and Δ^9-tetrahydrocannabinolic acid.* Of these, Δ^9-tetrahydrocannabinol has the most psychoactive potency, nearly 20-fold greater than that of Δ^8-THC. Cannabinol and cannabidiol, although present in large amounts, likewise have low activity. Δ^9-tetrahydrocannabinolic acid is inactive but is converted by smoking into active Δ^9-THC.

Δ^9-Tetrahydrocannabinol

Synonyms: (-)-*trans*-Δ^9-tetrahydrocannabinol, Δ^1-THC, Δ^9-THC

Formula: $C_{21}H_{30}O_2$

Molecular mass = 314.4617 Daltons

CAS-1972-08-3

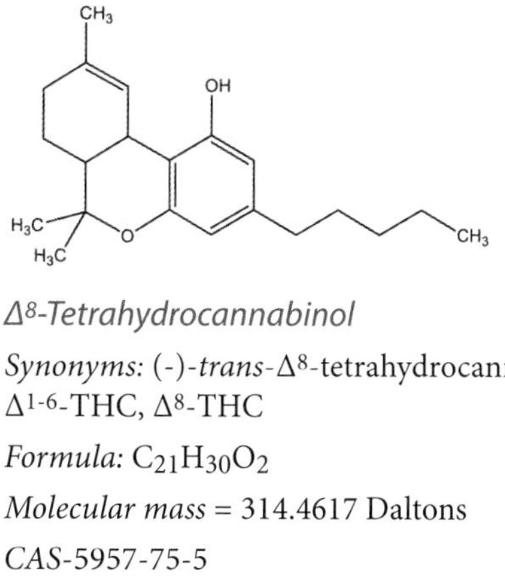

Δ^8-Tetrahydrocannabinol

Synonyms: (-)-*trans*-Δ^8-tetrahydrocannabinol, $\Delta^{1\text{-}6}$-THC, Δ^8-THC

Formula: $C_{21}H_{30}O_2$

Molecular mass = 314.4617 Daltons

CAS-5957-75-5

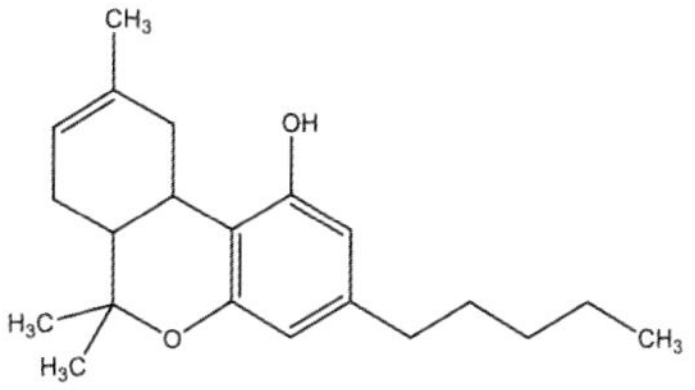

* Note that cannabinoid nomenclature is complicated by the fact that cannabinoids can be described as either substituted monoterpene (Δ^1) or dibenzopyran (Δ^9) compounds, giving rise to two different molecular numbering systems. We will conform to the dibenzopyran (Δ^9) system here.

Cannabinol

Synonym: CBN; 6,6,9-trimethyl-3-pentyl-6H-dibenzo[b,d]pyran-1-ol

Formula: $C_{21}H_{26}O_2$

Molecular mass = 310.4299 Daltons

CAS-521-35-7

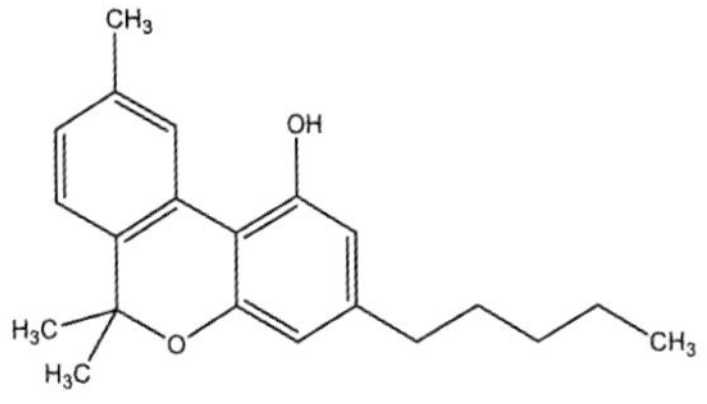

Cannabidiol

Synonyms: CBD; 2-[3-methyl-6-(l-methylethenyl)-2-cyclohexen-l-yl]-5-pentyl-1,3-benzenediol

Formula: $C_{21}H_{30}O_2$

Molecular mass = 314.4617 Daltons

CAS-13956-29-1

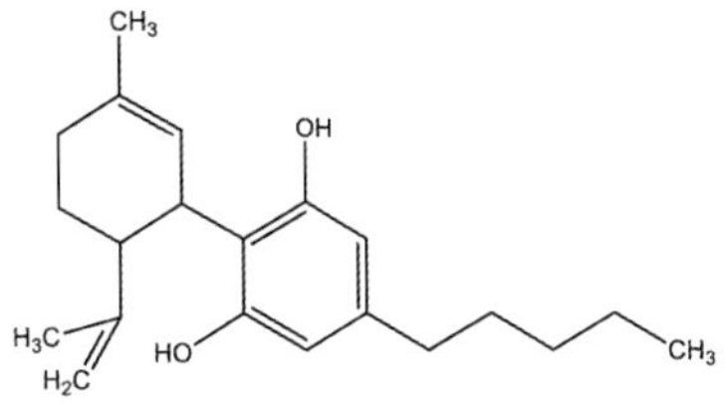

Δ⁹-Tetrahydrocannabinolic acid

Formula: $C_{22}H_{30}O_4$

Molecular mass = 358.4712 Daltons

CAS-23978-85-0

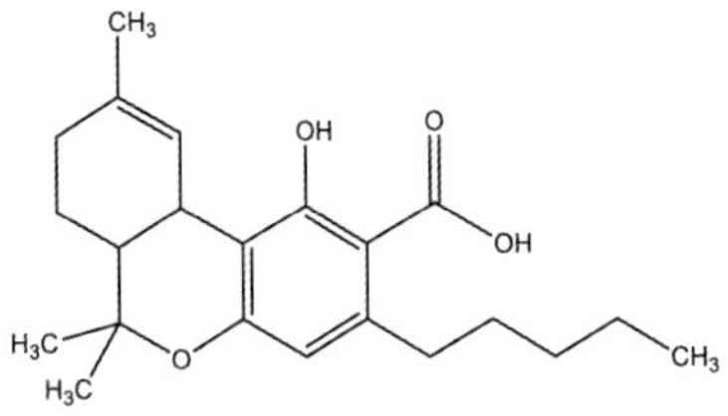

Pharmacology

Intended Use/Medical Use[1,3,5-7]

Hemp was known and used by the Chinese, Egyptians, Greeks, and Romans from ancient times as a source of fiber in rope and textiles, seeds in lamp oil and food, and resin as a medicinal. These cultures are not known to have developed a tradition of using it for intoxication, whereas India, the Middle East, and Eastern Europe did use it as an intoxicant. Although the recreational use of cannabis in Western Europe and the United States is said to date from the mid-19th century, it achieved real popularity beginning in the 1960s. Today, cannabis is the most common, most widely cultivated, and most broadly distributed illicit substance worldwide; it was used, according to United Nations estimates, by as many as 192 million people in the year 2016. Marijuana has been characterized as "the number one cash crop in the US," with earnings estimated at more than $500 billion a year. Cannabis has potential medical uses, including as an appetite stimulant in, for example, anorexia related to AIDS or cancer; as an antiemetic treatment for vomiting associated with cancer chemotherapy; and in the treatment of glaucoma and multiple sclerosis. Table 18-1 lists various formulations of medical cannabis. Two cannabis pharmaceutical preparations in capsule form (2.5-10 mg; daily adult oral doses ranging from 2.5 to 20 mg) are dronabinol (Marinol), which is identical to natural THC (synthetic Δ^9-tetrahydrocannabinol in sesame oil), and nabilone (Cesamet), which is a synthetic analog similar to Δ^9-tetrahydrocannabinol. Another standardized cannabis pharmaceutical preparation, Sativex (THC plus CBD in approximately equal ratios), is a mouth spray used to treat neuropathic pain in patients with multiple sclerosis. (Each spray delivers a fixed dose of 2.7 mg THC and 2.5 mg CBD.) Under federal workplace drug testing regulations, the use of one of these approved pharmaceutical forms of cannabis is an acceptable alternative medical explanation for a finding of positive THC in a preemployment or "for cause" urine drug screen, whereas use of "medical marijuana" is not.

At the time of this writing, 29 states, the District of Columbia, Guam, and Puerto Rico have all enacted laws that permit the use of medical cannabis.[8] With the exception of the District of Columbia, each state has limited the conditions for which cannabis can be prescribed. Examples of acceptable medical indications for cannabis include chronic pain, nausea, seizures, epilepsy, muscle spasms, cachexia, cancer, glaucoma, and anorexia in AIDS patients.[9] However, broader use is allowed in some states for other "debilitating medical conditions" of the same kind or class as those listed previously where the potential benefits outweigh the health risks.[10] In order to prescribe medical cannabis, states typically require physicians to have an established relationship with the patient, register with the state, and possibly complete a medical education program. The prescribed cannabis can then be obtained at specified state dispensaries.

Despite many states decriminalizing the use of medical marijuana and some even decriminalizing the possession of small amounts of the drug, marijuana remains listed as a Schedule I drug under the

Table 18-1. Formulations of Medical Cannabis

Formulation	Description	Composition	FDA Approved
Dronabinol	Oral medication (capsules/liquid) for relief of chemotherapy-induced nausea and vomiting; treatment of anorexia associated with weight loss in adults with AIDS	Synthetic Δ^9–THC	Yes
Nabilone	Oral medication (capsules) for relief of chemotherapy-induced nausea and vomiting	Synthetic analog of Δ^9–THC	Yes
Nabiximols	Botanical cannabis oromucosal spray for relief of spasticity in multiple sclerosis	Δ^9–THC/CBD*	No
Epidiolex	Liquid formulation of plant-derived CBD for severe infantile-onset, drug-resistant pediatric epilepsy	CBD	Yes

FDA, Food and Drug Administration; THC, Δ^9-tetrahydrocannabinol; CBD, cannabidiol.

* Nabiximols (Sativex) contains approximately equal ratios of Δ^9-tetrahydrocannabinol (Δ^9-THC) and cannabidiol (CBD) along with other cannabinoids, terpenoids, and flavonoids flavored with peppermint oil.

federal Controlled Substances Act. While strong feelings prevail in the debate over legalization of marijuana, thus far an employer's legal rights to prohibit use of marijuana as a condition of employment have been unaffected, and cannabis continues to be included in state statutes regarding driving under the influence of drugs (DUID, or per se laws). "Recreational" cannabis is most frequently smoked: marijuana rolled into pure cigarettes or mixed with tobacco in what are called "joints," "reefers," or "spliffs," or smoked in a pipe; hashish or hash oil is often mixed with tobacco to add volume and promote burning of the resin or oil. Another technique is called "hot knifing," where a hot knife is cut through a block of resin, causing some to adhere to it and vaporize as it is subsequently held under the nose. Smoking is also commonly accomplished with bongs, water pipes, or hookahs. In these devices, part-filled with water, the cannabis, ignited in a separate container, emits smoke that is drawn through the water before being inhaled, thus cooling the smoke and "filtering" out some of the tars and carcinogens (or so it is commonly believed). Cannabis ingested in food or tea is also pharmacologically active, and such use has been a longstanding tradition in India, the Middle East, and North Africa; but oral cannabis has not been as popular elsewhere because the drug effects come on more slowly, may be less pronounced, and last much longer than with smoked drug.

Mechanism of Action[3,5]

Cannabis, though often characterized as a depressant, is hard to classify pharmacologically because it causes a variety of effects. Both endogenous and exogenous cannabinoids act on G-protein–coupled cannabinoid binding receptors (CB) known as CB1 and CB2. CB1 receptors are primarily concentrated in the basal ganglia, cerebellum, hippocampus, association cortices, spinal cord, and peripheral nerves, while CB2 receptors are mainly found on the cells (eg, leukocytes) in the immune system.[11]

Depending on the location of the CB and the specific G-protein involved, the stimulation of CB1 may result in the inhibition or stimulation of various neurotransmitters (eg, acetylcholine, L-glutamate, dopamine, norepinephrine, and 5-hydroxytryptamine), which contributes to the central and peripheral effects observed.[12] THC is only a partial agonist and binds to brain anandamide receptors causing dose-dependent and time-dependent stimulant, sedative/hypnotic, or hallucinogenic central nervous system (CNS) effects, accompanied by peripheral catecholamine release, tachycardia and/or sympathetic antagonism, and orthostatic hypotension. Other side effects include analgesia, muscle relaxation, antiemesis, appetite stimulation, and the reduction of intraocular pressure. On the other hand, synthetic cannabinoids are full agonists and have a much higher affinity for the CB receptors, thus increasing the physiological and toxicological effects.

Pharmacokinetics[1,2,4,5,13,14]

Route of drug administration and drug formulation determine the rate of drug absorption. Smoking or vaporization provides extremely rapid absorption of THC, dissolving rapidly in pulmonary surfactant upon entering the lungs, entering the bloodstream in seconds, and achieving peak CNS levels within

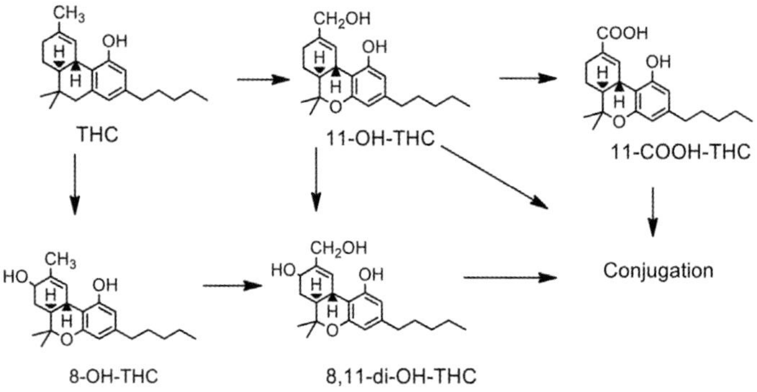

Figure 18-1. Principal metabolites of tetrahydrocannabinol.

a few minutes because of high lipid solubility (the high THC octanol/water coefficient being variously estimated in the range of 6×10^3 to 9×10^6). Only a relatively small proportion of the dose crosses the blood-brain barrier, because blood THC is so lipophilic that it is 95% to 99% bound to plasma lipoproteins. Bioavailability of smoked drug ranges from 2% to 56% because of variability in smoking technique, which allows the user to effectively titrate the dose. More recently, vaporization (ie, vaping) as route of cannabis administration has grown in both medical and recreational users. The duration of action lasts approximately 2 to 3 hours. Another alternative method of cannabis use growing in popularity is the inhalation of highly concentrated THC extract known as "dabbing." Butane hash oil "dabs" may contain THC concentrations of 70% to 90% compared to traditional flower concentrations of 3% to 6%. The creation of the extract and process of inhalation involves using a solvent (eg, butane), resulting in a sticky oil which is then placed on the end of a hot surface (eg, nail), typically heated with a blow torch, and inhaled through a dab rig. While producing rapid effects, the higher THC concentrations and risk of burns leads to more toxicity and drug dependence.

THC can also be ingested. It is absorbed from the gastrointestinal tract more slowly and irregularly, with oral bioavailability estimated at 4% to 20% (10-20% for ingested dronabinol). Onset of effects may take 30 to 60 minutes, with peak THC absorption at 2 to 4 hours, and lower peak concentrations than when cannabis is inhaled. Among factors accounting for these differences between the smoked route and the oral route are marked effects of drug dose and vehicle on absorption rate, as well as gastric degradation of ingested drug.

After absorption by either route, THC blood levels quickly decline because of rapid redistribution from blood to tissues and subsequent extensive first-pass liver metabolism. Drug is initially taken up by highly vascular tissues, such as brain, lung, heart, and liver; it builds up more slowly during redistribution in tissues with lower rates of perfusion, such as fat. It has been estimated that a pseudo-equilibrium between plasma and tissue drug levels occurs approximately 6 hours after intravenous dose. The rate-limiting step in the overall metabolism of THC appears to be its redistribution from fat into the blood, and after longer periods of exposure, the drug is concentrated in fat, where its retention may be lengthy, possibly caused by formation of fatty acid conjugates of THC and 11-OH-THC, increasing their fat stability. Chronic cannabis use does not appear to cause major alterations in its initial pharmacokinetics, suggesting that the observed tolerance seen with such use is more likely due to altered pharmacodynamics.

Metabolism[2,4,5,15]

The principal routes of THC metabolism are shown in Figure 18-1. THC is metabolized in the liver via oxidation by the cytochrome P450 system (principally by CYP2C9, CYP2C19, and CYP3A4) to many different compounds (more than 100 minor oxidative metabolites have been identified, including hydroxyl derivatives, ketones, aldehydes, and carboxylic acids). The principal route of metabolism, however, appears to be via hydroxylation by CYP2C9 to 11-OH-THC, which is pharmacologically active, and to a lesser extent to the less active 8Δ- and 8Δ-OH-THC. These three compounds, in turn, are subject to further hydroxylation to 8,11-diOH-THC. Route of drug administration has a major impact on the rate of these reactions, such that 10 to 15 minutes after the onset of smoking cannabis, plasma 11-OH-THC levels peak at only about 10% of THC concentration, which is much lower than after cannabis ingestion. 11-OH-THC is also majorly subject to oxidation to the inactive metabolite 11-nor-9-carboxy-Δ^9-THC (THCCOOH), levels of which increase steadily and exceed those of THC by 30 minutes or so after smoking. The final phase of THC metabolism involves derivatization of the hydroxyl groups of THCCOOH, 11-OH-THC, and 8,11-diOH-THC, principally by glucuronidation, making them more water soluble, although they remain extensively protein bound in plasma. Enterohepatic circulation of metabolites may occur.

(It should be noted that drug-drug interactions between THC and other legal or illicit drugs may affect its metabolism and those of the other agents. Such interactions have been described for atropine, barbiturates, cocaine, disulfiram, fluoxetine, HIV medications, lithium, neuroleptics, opioids, sildanifil, theophylline, and tricyclic antidepressants, among others. For more details on this topic, see *Drugs of Abuse* by Wills.[1])

Excretion[1,2,4,6,15]

The principal routes of excretion for the broad range of cannabinoid metabolites are feces (60-70%) and urine (30-40%). The primary fecal THC excretion product is conjugated 11-OH-THC, and the predominant urinary THC metabolite is conjugated THCCOOH (conjugated parent drug and 11-OH-THC are only minor constituents of urine, typically undetectable; note that there is significant renal tubular reabsorption of THC and its metabolites). Altogether, anywhere from 70% to 90% of a THC dose is normally excreted within 3 to 5 days by both routes, but the terminal elimination half-life may be significantly prolonged in chronic users, due to prolonged redistribution of cannabinoids stored in body fat. In one reported case in an individual who had used cannabis for more 10 years, the urine was positive by immunoassay (at >20 ng/mL) for 67 days after drug exposure.[16]

Volume of Distribution[2,4,15]

The standard volume of distribution (V_d) for THC is reported at about 10 L/kg (range 4-14 L/kg) in spite of the fact that the drug is heavily protein bound. Taking this into account, dynamic estimates of the steady-state V_d are in the range of 3 L/kg to 4 L/kg.[17]

Half-Life[2, 4, 6]

Plasma half-lives ($t_{1/2}$) for THC have been estimated at 1.5 hours in occasional users and 2 hours in chronic users, and for THCCOOH, 120 hours and 144 hours, respectively. Estimates of THCCOOH urinary excretion half-lives range from 9 to 27 hours, whereas terminal urinary THCCOOH elimination $t_{1/2}$ estimates have ranged from 3 to 4 days in occasional users to 12 days or more in frequent users. Detection of cannabinoids in urine is indicative of prior cannabis exposure, but the long excretion half-life of THCCOOH in the body, especially in chronic cannabis users, makes it difficult to predict the timing of past drug use.

Abuse Potential and Characteristics[1,3,4,6]

As with most other drugs of abuse, the recreational experience with cannabis is partly conditioned by surroundings, mood, and prior expectations of the user. First-time users sometimes report little or no effect, possibly because of inadequate dosage but also possibly attributable to lack of a placebo effect (experienced users frequently asserting that one must have some familiarity with the cannabis "high" in order to enjoy it fully). This high typically consists of initial elation, followed by relaxation, social disinhibition, heightened imagination, increased sensory awareness of colors, textures, and sounds, and increased appetite (the "munchies"). There may also be a pleasant perception of time passing more slowly. At high doses, illusions or hallucinations may appear. As users "come down" from the high, they not infrequently become drowsy and sleep. Smoking, the principal route of administration, delivers drug rapidly and efficiently from the lungs to the brain, contributing to the abuse potential of cannabis, with the strong reinforcement produced by the almost immediate drug exposure to the CNS. In spite of reports of chronic cannabis use leading to tolerance and psychological dependence, major degrees of physical dependence have not definitively been shown to occur. Withdrawal symptoms that have been described are nonspecific and may include such things as anorexia, anxiety, insomnia, irritability, restlessness, sweating, headache, and mild gastrointestinal upsets.

Analysis

Analytical Parameters[2]

Dissociation constant: Δ^9-THC: pK_a 10.6.
Partition coefficient: Δ^9-THC: Log *P* (octanol/water): 7.6.

Specimen Types, Requirements, and Characteristics[2,4,15]

Cannabinoids and metabolites have been reported as measured in many specimens such as urine, whole blood, serum, plasma, hair, sweat, meconium, umbilical cord tissue, breast milk, and postmortem tissues.

Plasma THC specimens collected in glass are reportedly stable for 4 to 6 months at 5°C or -20°C, but whole blood specimens are said to be stable for only 2 weeks at -20°C, requiring lower freezer temperatures for longer periods. Specimens should never be collected or stored in plastic or at room temperature because THC binds readily to plastic, reducing recoveries during analytical procedures. This THC adsorption can be reduced by storing the compound in organic solvents or in basic solution in amber silylated glassware.

Urine specimens for THCCOOH are not stable, even when frozen, for periods beyond 4 weeks, especially if pipetted or stored in plastic. Urine specimens reportedly lost 11% of their original THCCOOH content after 45 days at -18°C.[18] The effects of potassium nitrite used as a urine adulterant can reportedly be countered by the addition of bisulfite or sulfamic acid to the specimen.[19,20] Specimen preparation for confirmatory cannabinoid testing often includes hydrolysis (either enzymatic using β-glucuronidase or alkaline with sodium hydroxide [NaOH]) to remove glucuronide conjugates.

Modes of Analysis[2,15]

A number of immunoassays are available for detection of cannabinoids in body fluids, and a variety of chemical methods are used for confirmation, including separation and identification methods. Given the range of compounds encountered both in cannabis drug specimens and in vivo, high degrees of analytical specificity are required.

Known Analytical Issues and Problems[4,6]

Over the years, cannabinoid immunoassays have been optimized for the detection of THCCOOH, the principal urinary THC metabolite, at the expense of decreasing cross-reactivity with other cannabinoid metabolites. This has necessarily represented a trade-off between analytical specificity and overall clinical sensitivity, but it has increased the reliability (eg, likelihood of confirmation) of positive THCCOOH screens. Cannabinoid immunoassays have been reported to be subject to analytical interferences from prescription drugs. For a period of time, the Syva EMIT assay for THCCOOH was subject to false-positive interference by the nonsteroidal anti-inflammatory drug ibuprofen (Advil), but this was corrected in a reformulation of the kit by the manufacturer some years ago. No other immunoassays have shown this problem. In 2002, the antacid pantoprazole (Protonix), a proton pump inhibitor, was found to cause false-positive immunoassay results for marijuana metabolites; however, these screening results do not confirm with gas chromatography-mass spectrometry confirmatory testing. Another common inquiry from patients is regarding the ability of passive cannabinoid smoke inhalation to give a "positive" immunoassay result for THC. However, passive exposure has not been demonstrated to reliably produce concentrations high enough (eg, >50 ng/mL; common immunoassay cutoff) to be detected in most urine drug screens.[12]

Clinical Issues

Clinical Interpretation of Analytical Findings[4,6,7]

For medicolegal (workplace or forensic) purposes, administrative regulatory cutoffs have been established by the Department of Health and Human Services for declaring positivity of urine screening immunoassays (50 ng/mL) and gas chromatography-mass spectrometry confirmatory assays (15 ng/mL). These cutoffs do not challenge the limits of detection of most assay methodologies and differ from one another because of the analytical difference between quantitating THCCOOH glucuronide and other cross-reacting cannabinoids and metabolites in the screen versus a single analyte—free THCCOOH posthydrolysis—in the confirmation. Historically, a number of considerations entered into the federal government's determination of these cutoffs, including the necessity for the cutoffs to be applicable across multiple different immunoassay platforms with different specificities and cross-reactivities, the desire to eliminate potential false positives due to passive inhalation of sidestream marijuana smoke, and so forth. Studies comparing clinical sensitivity, specificity, and efficiency of a variety of commercial immunoassays at 20, 50, and 100 ng/mL urinary cutoff levels in experimental subjects after exposure to measured inhaled doses of cannabis showed that lowering the cutoff concentration to 50 ng/mL increased sensitivity in all immunoassays (range, 57.0-79.5%), while specificity decreased slightly (with false-positive results increasing 1.0-2.6%), with all assays being highly efficient (increasing from 91.4% to 94.7%) at both cutoff concentrations.[21] At this cutoff, a naïve or infrequent user smoking a single joint may test positive for 1 to 3 days, whereas a frequent, chronic user's urine may continue at detectable levels below the cutoff values for a month or longer (estimates ranging from 3 to 8 weeks). In addition, there is considerable interindividual variation in mean detection times in urine after smoking, even in controlled-dose studies. Given all of this, a positive urine cannabinoid test can really only be interpreted as indicating the occurrence of drug exposure and does not provide information about how much, when, how, if significant impairment resulted, or whether the urine positivity was due to residual excretion of drug redistributed from body fat or from new drug use. In drug treatment settings, this latter issue may be important to differentiate; some have utilized urine creatinine normalization of THCCOOH concentrations to address this.[22] Others have suggested that urinary THC parent drug and 11-OH-THC, although present as alkaline-resistant glucuronides in low concentrations, might nonetheless be useful as biomarkers of recent cannabis use, but this has been shown not to be the case.[23] In this study, the authors showed extended urinary excretion of both THC and 11-OH-THC for at least 24 days, which demonstrated it couldn't be used as a biomarker for recent cannabis exposure.[23]

Cannabinoid testing in alternative matrix specimens (oral fluid, sweat, and hair) is also being continuously developed and is in used in a variety of settings. In 2015, the Substance Abuse and Mental Health Services Administration introduced guidelines for oral fluid testing for workplace testing, with initial THC screening cutoffs of 4 ng/mL and confirmatory testing cutoffs of 2 ng/mL. Lastly, as the legalization and decriminalization of recreational cannabis and approval of medical cannabis continues, a single blood THC laboratory-based concentration for a legal per se limit or zero tolerance concentration that is always associated with impairment in all users (eg, occasional or frequent) is desired but very unlikely to exist.[24] While studies continue, the reality of a single cannabinoid concentration that would consistently indicate impairment fades.

Overdose and Toxicity[2,5,25]

Severe cannabis intoxication may result in confusion, dizziness, weakness, malaise, visual impairment, short-term memory deficit, depersonalization, visual hallucinations, and occasional episodes of acute paranoid psychosis or panic reaction. Nausea and vomiting may be seen with oral use of cannabis. The manufacturers' warnings for Marinol include not engaging in any hazardous activity until tolerance is established and avoiding use of alcohol or other CNS depressants, which could potentially cause additive effects with THC (*Physicians' Desk Reference,* 1997). On physical examination, patients with THC intoxication may exhibit tachycardia, orthostatic hypotension, conjunctival injection, incoordination, dry mouth, slurred speech, ataxia, fine tremor, and stupor. THC intoxication has been reported to result in coma in children. In adults, the principal risk of fatality relates to impaired judgment and motor incoordination in driving or operating machinery while under the influence; however, there are rare reports of loss of consciousness or even death directly from cannabis, such as in very infrequent instances of intravenous injections of marijuana extract or hash oil causing dyspnea, abdominal pain, fever, shock, disseminated intravascular coagulation, acute renal failure, and death. Cannabis may also be used in combination with other drugs that increase the risk of lethality, for example, phencyclidine (PCP) combined with marijuana in so-called "superweed" or "wicky stick" to obtain a more intense high. Cannabis toxicity is typically diagnosed on the basis of history of use accompanied by altered mood or cognitive function and typical physical findings, such as tachycardia and conjunctival injection. Useful routine laboratory results may include electrolytes and glucose.

Adverse Effects and Complications

Central Nervous System[1]

Effects of chronic cannabis use on the CNS are poorly understood. Early reports of CNS structural changes have not been confirmed, and reported associations with chronic schizophrenia remain unproven. Flashbacks (eg, reruns of the intoxication experience) have been reported with cannabis, but they are both milder and less frequent than with the major hallucinogens like lysergic acid diethylamide (LSD). Findings regarding increased incidence of anxiety, depression, and deficits in learning and short-term memory are conflicting. Chronic drug abuse in general often coincides with tendencies toward social isolation and poor personal performance. In the case of heavy chronic cannabis use, this has been characterized as the so-called *amotivational syndrome,* in which users seem deficient in goal-oriented behavior, have short attention spans, and have increased tendencies toward introversion and apathy. To what extent such tendencies may result from any CNS changes due specifically to cannabis use is unclear.

Cardiovascular[1,26]

Activation of CB1 by endocannabinoids or synthetic ligands mediates acute hemodynamic effects and might contribute to pathology in cardiovascular disease. Cannabis use is associated acutely with increased cardiac output and decreased oxygen-carrying capacity of the blood, in turn associated with tachycardia. This may increase the frequency of angina on exertion in patients with ischemic heart disease, but the incidence of myocardial infarction does not appear to be increased. Although cardiac palpitations are sometimes reported, they are not generally accompanied by arrhythmias. Dilation of peripheral veins associated with local impairment of cerebral blood flow results in postural hypotension, with dizziness and fainting upon standing. Desensitization or tachyphylaxis may lead to both orthostatic hypotension and tachycardia in frequent users.

Respiratory[1,5]

It may be useful to compare the smoking of cannabis to tobacco cigarette smoking. Marijuana joints are homemade, loosely wrapped cylinders, without filters, that are usually smoked down to the very end, with the final draws being of smoke that is hotter and denser with particulates, tar, and carbon monoxide than those of a cigarette, and they are inhaled much more deeply, with the breath commonly being held for a few seconds after inhaling (unlike with cigarettes). All of this, plus the higher tar content of cannabis smoke, puts the airways at greater risk of damage and allows cannabis particulates to permeate the lower airways more completely and deposit more tar than tobacco smoke typically does. Acute inhalation of cannabis smoke causes bronchodilation in normal individuals, but the irritant smoke stimulates bronchoconstriction in people with asthma, and chronic use increases large-airway resistance, unlike tobacco. On the other hand, cannabis smoking, like tobacco, commonly causes chronic productive cough and/or sore throat and inhibits pulmonary defense mechanisms, increasing the risk of infection or allergy. Fungal spores (typically *Aspergillus*) often found in dried cannabis have been reported to cause infection (in immunocompromised persons) or hypersensitivity pneumonitis (in people who are allergic to the fungus). Likewise, cannabis pollen may be allergenic. Rare instances of pneumomediastinum, secondary to alveolar overdistention and rupture associated with deep inhalation, have been described during marijuana smoking. Chronic cannabis smoking has not been definitively associated with lung cancer, primarily because studies of its epidemiology have been confounded by the frequency with which chronic cannabis smokers also use tobacco. Nonetheless, expert consensus remains that such a link is likely. Although risk might be thought to be mitigated among chronic cannabis smokers (who usually smoke less often than do tobacco smokers), studies of the prevalence of precancerous airway lesions have shown higher rates in exclusive cannabis smokers than in exclusive tobacco smokers, and the highest rates in those who smoke both.[9] Anecdotal reports of cancer of the head, neck, mouth, jaw, and tongue in young adults have been attributed to chronic cannabis use.

Reproductive[1,27]

Reported associations between chronic cannabis use and gynecomastia, oligospermia, decreased testosterone in males, and decreased libido in both sexes are unconfirmed, and no effect on fertility has ever been described. The US National Birth Defects Prevention Study found that fetuses with marijuana exposure within their first month of gestation were at significant risk for anencephaly.[28] Reports of behavioral alterations among the infants of women who smoked marijuana during pregnancy are inconclusive, and most epidemiological studies of infants from cannabis-exposed pregnancies are confounded by alcohol and tobacco use, race, and socioeconomic status. THC and metabolites are excreted in breast milk, but the few studies of its effects on breastfed infants are inconclusive; nonetheless, the American Academy of Pediatrics regards marijuana use as contraindicated in breastfeeding mothers (Committee on Drugs, American Academy of Pediatrics, 1994).

Toxic Dose[2,5,15]

No toxic dose has been generally established for THC, given the rarity of cannabis dosage fatalities. Toxicity is dose related but subject to much interindividual variability. An admission radioimmunoassay cannabinoid blood level of 180 ng/mL was reported in a comatose 19-year-old user of cannabis who recovered.[29] Postmortem THC blood levels ranging from 3 ng/mL to 22 ng/mL were recorded in six cases of presumed fatal cardiovascular drug toxicity; postmortem THC tissue concentrations in another presumed THC fatality were 3.75 μg/100 g in liver, 4.2 μg/100 g in kidney, and 1.2 μg/100 g in spleen.[30]

Treatment and Rehabilitation for Overdose and Toxicity[5,7]

Treatment of toxicity includes the following emergency and supportive measures. Psychological disturbances—such as anxiety or panic reactions or transient psychosis—may be managed by a combination of reassurance and benzodiazepines. Sinus tachycardia is usually self limited but may require beta blockers. Orthostatic hypotension usually responds to the head-down position plus fluids (intravenous, if necessary). If stat detoxification is necessary after a large oral ingestion, for example by children in the home, ipecac-induced vomiting may be of benefit if instituted immediately; otherwise, prompt administration of activated charcoal without gastric emptying is the treatment of choice. The V_d of cannabinoids is so large that enhanced elimination is ineffective in dealing with acute oral overdose.

References

1. Wills S. *Drugs of Abuse.* 2nd ed. London, UK: Pharmaceutical Press; 2005.
2. Moffat AC, Osselton MD, Widdop B, eds. *Clarke's Analysis of Drugs and Poisons.* 34th ed. London, UK: Pharmaceutical Press; 2011.
3. *Martindale: The Complete Drug Reference.* 38th ed. London, UK: Pharmaceutical Press; 2014.
4. Huestis MA. Cannabinoids. In: Ropero-Miller JD, Goldberger BA, eds. *Handbook of Workplace Drug Testing.* 2nd ed. Washington, DC: AACC Press; 2009:355-382.

5. Olson KR. *Poisoning and Drug Overdose.* 7th ed. New York, NY: McGraw-Hill Education; 2017.
6. Shults TF. *Medical Review Officer Handbook.* Research Triangle Park, NC: Quadrangle Research, LLC; 2009.
7. Ling LJ CR, Erickson TB, Trestrail JH. *Toxicology Secrets.* Philadelphia, PA: Hanley and Belfus; 2001.
8. Klieger SB, Gutman A, Allen L, Pacula RL, Ibrahim JK, Burris S. Mapping medical marijuana: state laws regulating patients, product safety, supply chains and dispensaries, 2017. *Addiction.* 2017;112:2206-2216.
9. Bestrashniy J, Winters KC. Variability in medical marijuana laws in the United States. *Psychol Addict Behav.* 2015;29:639-642.
10. Abuhasira R, Shbiro L, Landschaft Y. Medical use of cannabis and cannabinoids containing products: regulations in Europe and North America. *Eur J Intern Med.* 2018;49:2-6.
11. Hill KP. Medical marijuana for treatment of chronic pain and other medical and psychiatric problems: a clinical review. *JAMA.* 2015; 313:2474-2483.
12. Kelly BF, Nappe TM. *Cannabinoid Toxicity.* Treasure Island, FL: Stat Pearls Publishing; 2019.
13. Pacula RL, Jacobson M, Maksabedian EJ. In the weeds: a baseline view of cannabis use among legalizing states and their neighbours. *Addiction.* 2016;111:973-980.
14. Loflin M, Earleywine M. A new method of cannabis ingestion: the dangers of dabs? *Addict Behav.* 2014;39:1430-1433.
15. Baselt R. *Disposition of Toxic Drugs and Chemicals in Man.* 8th ed. Foster City, CA: Biomedical Publications; 2008.
16. Ellis GM Jr, Mann MA, Judson BA, Schramm NT, Tashchian A. Excretion patterns of cannabinoid metabolites after last use in a group of chronic users. *Clin Pharmacol Ther.* 1985;38:572-578.
17. Grotenhermen F. Pharmacokinetics and pharmacodynamics of cannabinoids. *Clin Pharmacokinet.* 2003;42:327-360.
18. Paul BD, McKinley RM, Walsh JK Jr, Jamir TS, Past MR. Effect of freezing on the concentration of drugs of abuse in urine. *J Anal Toxicol.* 1993;17:378-380.
19. El Sohly MA, Feng S, Kopycki WJ, et al. A procedure to overcome interferences caused by the adulterant "Klear" in the GC-MS analysis of 11-nor-delta9-THC-9-COOH. *J Anal Toxicol.* 1997;21:240-242.
20. Frederick DL. Improved procedure for overcoming nitrite interferences in GC-MS procedures for cannabinoids. *J Anal Toxicol.* 1998;22:255-256.
21. Huestis MA, Mitchell JM, Cone EJ. Detection times of marijuana metabolites in urine by immunoassay and GC-MS. *J Anal Toxicol.* 1995; 19:443-449.
22. Smith ML, Barnes AJ, Huestis MA. Identifying new cannabis use with urine creatinine-normalized THCCOOH concentrations and time intervals between specimen collections. *J Anal Toxicol.* 2009;33:185-189.
23. Lowe RH, Abraham TT, Darwin WD, Herning R, Cadet JL, Huestis MA. Extended urinary delta9-tetrahydrocannabinol excretion in chronic cannabis users precludes use as a biomarker of new drug exposure. *Drug Alcohol Depend.* 2009;105:24-32.
24. Huestis MA. Cannabis-impaired driving: a public health and safety concern. *Clin Chem.* 2015;61:1223-1225.
25. Baselt R. *Drug Effects on Psychomotor Performance.* Foster City, CA: Biomedical Publications; 2001.
26. Pacher P, Steffens S, Hasko G, Schindler TH, Kunos G. Cardiovascular effects of marijuana and synthetic cannabinoids: the good, the bad, and the ugly. *Nat Rev Cardiol.* 2018;15:151-166.
27. Friedman JM, Polifka JE. *The Effects of Drugs on the Fetus and Nursing Infant: A Handbook for Healthcare Professionals.* Baltimore, MD: Johns Hopkins University Press; 1996.
28. van Gelder MM, Reefhuis J, Caton AR, Werler MM, Druschel CM, Roeleveld N; National Birth Defects Prevention Study. Maternal periconceptional illicit drug use and the risk of congenital malformations. *Epidemiology.* 2009;20:60-66.
29. Garrett CP, Braithwaite RA, Teale JD. Unusual case of tetrahydrocannabinol intoxication confirmed by radioimmunoassay. *Br Med J.* 1977;2:166.
30. Tewari SN, Sharma JD. Detection of delta-9-tetrahydrocannabinol in the organs of a suspected case of cannabis poisoning. *Toxicol Lett.* 1980;5:279-281.

Chapter 19

Club Drugs

Matthew D. Krasowski, MD, PhD
Christine L.H. Snozek, PhD

Introduction

There have been many drugs that have been designated as "club drugs" because they have been associated with "rave" parties or other social gatherings where drugs are used by teenagers and young adults, and there is a group culture that promotes their use.[1,2] The term *club drug* also can group substances that show more restricted use patterns in society than more commonly abused drugs such as ethanol, cannabis, cocaine, and opioids. The drugs covered in this chapter include γ-hydroxybutyric acid (GHB), dextromethorphan (DXM), 3,4-methylenedioxymethamphetamine (MDMA), ketamine, and phencyclidine (PCP). γ-Butyrolactone (GBL) and 1,4-butanediol (1,4BD), two compounds that are converted by metabolism to GHB, are also discussed together with GHB. Novel designer drugs including synthetic cannabinoids and opioids, which may also be abused on the club scene, are covered in chapter 26, *Novel Psychoactive Substances.*

GHB, GBL, and 1,4BD

Origin

GHB is an endogenous substance found in the mammalian central nervous system (CNS) and peripheral tissues with as yet unknown biological functions.[3-5] GHB is also found in small amounts in certain foods and beverages. GHB is a minor metabolite of γ-aminobutyric acid (GABA), the major inhibitory neurotransmitter in the mammalian CNS. GHB was first synthesized in 1960 as an experimental GABA analog for possible treatment of seizure disorders and later abandoned for this clinical purpose.[6,7] GHB now has limited clinical use as a treatment for the sleep disorder narcolepsy and is sometimes used off label for other clinical indications.[8] Two compounds with widespread industrial application, GBL and 1,4BD, are structurally related to GHB and are metabolized to GHB in humans. GHB, GBL, and 1,4BD have all seen use as recreational drugs and further may be used surreptitiously for drug-facilitated crimes, including sexual assault.[9-11]

Descriptive Chemistry[12]

γ-Hydroxybutyric Acid (GHB)

GHB is structurally related to the neurotransmitter GABA. GHB is sold illicitly as a white powder or a colorless liquid with a salty or soapy taste that can be masked in an alcoholic beverage.

Synonyms: Gamma hydroxybutyrate, BRN-1720582, liquid ecstasy, liquid X, liquid XE, Georgia home boy, grievous bodily harm, scoop, fantasy, 4-hydroxybutanoic acid

Trade name: Xyrem

Formula: $C_4H_8O_3$

Molecular mass = 104.1045 Daltons

CAS-591-81-1

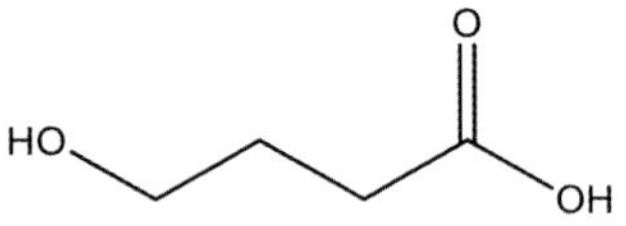

γ -Butyrolactone (GBL)

GBL is widely used for commercial and industrial applications and is metabolized to GHB in humans. GBL is produced industrially by dehydrogenation of 1,4BD. Pure GBL is a hygroscopic liquid miscible in water and has a weak odor and unpleasant taste.

Synonyms: Blue nitro, gamma G, blue nitro vitality, firewater, G3

Formula: $C_4H_6O_2$

Molecular mass = 86.0891 Daltons

CAS-96-48-0

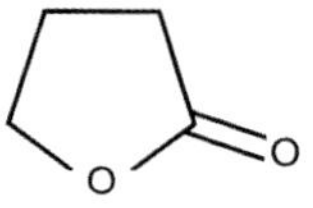

1,4-Butanediol (1,4BD)

1,4BD is produced commercially starting with the reaction of acetylene with formaldehyde. Pure 1,4BD is an odorless and colorless viscous liquid miscible in water and soluble in ethanol. The distinct bitter taste of 1,4BD can be masked by ethanol.

Synonyms: BD, BlueRaine, dream on, fubar, pine needle oil, rejuv @nite, thunder, cleaner, enliven, inner G, one comma four, one four bee, one four B-D-O

Formula: $C_4H_{10}O_2$

Molecular mass = 90.1210 Daltons

CAS-110-63-4

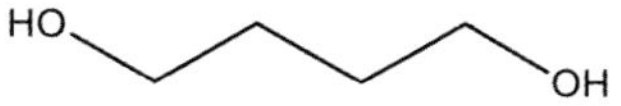

Pharmacology

Intended Uses

GHB is an anesthetic agent that causes CNS depression.[7] GHB has been evaluated experimentally as a general anesthetic and to treat conditions such as insomnia, clinical depression, narcolepsy, and alcoholism.[5,6] Although GHB is an endogenous compound, the amounts present in body fluids are normally near or below the detection limits of analytical methods, but urine levels as high as 14 μg/mL have been reported.[3,13-15] GHB was evaluated for the treatment of narcolepsy beginning in the 1970s and is now available today as Xyrem.[8]

GBL, the metabolic precursor of GHB, is used as a food additive and found in many food items such as soups, cheeses, and breakfast cereal. GBL is also an industrial solvent and can be found in myriad products such as glue remover, drilling oils, and paint removers.[10,16] 1,4BD is used industrially as a solvent and for the manufacture of elastic fibers and plastics.[10,17] Neither GBL nor 1,4BD has any clinical applications.

Mechanism of Action

GHB is a naturally occurring neurotransmitter whose endogenous function is still not fully understood.[18-20] GHB is a metabolic precursor to the neurotransmitters GABA, glutamate, and glycine in certain brain regions. GHB binds to the excitatory GHB receptor in the brain and is also a weak agonist of the inhibitory $GABA_B$ receptor. GHB may be synthesized from GABA. GHB is also produced as a result of fermentation and is thus found in small quantities in some alcoholic beverages (especially beers and wines), meat, and citrus fruits. GBL and 1,4BD have no known endogenous functions and are considered prodrugs of GHB.

Pharmacokinetics

GHB is rapidly absorbed, with onset of action within 15 minutes. Bioavailability is approximately 65%, with a short half-life in blood of approximately 25 minutes with oral dosing. The drug is not protein bound in the plasma. Half-life increases with increasing doses. The nonlinear kinetics may be a result of saturation of metabolic pathways or a capacity-limited absorption process.

Volume of distribution and half-life information for GHB is summarized in Table 19-1.

Table 19-1. Volume of Distribution (V_d) and Half-Life ($t_{1/2}$)[117]

Drug	V_d (L/kg)	Plasma $t_{1/2}$ (h)
GHB	0.5	0.3-1.0
Dextromethorphan	255-316	3.2-3.6
MDMA	5-8	~6-7
Ketamine	3	2-3
Phencyclidine	6.2	7-46

GHB, gamma-hydroxybutyric acid; MDMA, 3,4-methylenedioxymethamphetamine.

For GHB, the predominant metabolic pathway is oxidation to succinic semialdehyde by a cytosolic GHB dehydrogenase.[21] The second step in the metabolism is oxidation of the succinic semialdehyde to succinic acid via succinic semialdehyde dehydrogenase. The succinic acid then enters the Krebs cycle for complete metabolism to carbon dioxide and water. Less than 2% of GHB is eliminated unchanged in the urine, resulting in short detection times for urine screening programs of generally only 8 to 12 hours.

GBL is rapidly converted by blood paraoxonase enzymes to GHB.[9,10] GBL is more lipophilic than GHB and is absorbed faster with higher bioavailability. 1,4BD is converted to GHB by the sequential action of alcohol dehydrogenase and aldehyde dehydrogenase.[9,10] Interindividual differences in levels of these enzymes can influence response and adverse effects of 1,4BD. Co-ingestion of ethanol and 1,4BD can be especially dangerous, since each drug impacts the metabolism of the other.

Abuse Potential and Characteristics

Beginning in the 1980s, GHB was misleadingly sold in health food stores as an enhancer for growth hormone, during which time abuse occurred by weight-lifters and body-builders who thought the drug would aid in building muscle mass.[7] During the 1990s, increasing reports of abuse and toxic reactions caused the US Drug Enforcement Agency (DEA) to restrict GHB as a Schedule I drug in March 2000. The specific formulation of GHB used for treatment of narcolepsy (marketed as Xyrem) is DEA Schedule III. Most of the GHB available in the US is manufactured clandestinely.

GBL and 1,4BD are readily available because of their widespread use in industry. GBL and 1,4BD are not officially scheduled by the DEA, but GBL was classified as a List I chemical in 2000, which dictates controls and regulations for manufacturers of GBL. This was intended to limit diversion of GBL from commercial sources. There have been attempts to prosecute individuals for 1,4BD under the Federal Analog Act (as substantially similar to GHB), but these have been overturned on legal review.

Interviews with users of GHB indicate that positive experiences include increased sexual desire, decreased sexual inhibitions, and decreased anxiety; negative experiences include oversedation, loss of consciousness, motor incoordination, and mental confusion. GHB users often achieve a state similar to "light sleep," which is described as coming into and out of consciousness. This state is characteristically seen in those under the influence of GHB while driving or in drug-facilitated assault victims.[9,16,22]

GHB, GBL, and 1,4BD have been implicated in drug-assisted sexual assault cases, but the actual numbers of cases are small compared to drug-facilitated abuse using benzodiazepines.[23] The amnesia produced by GHB often makes victims unable to serve as valid witnesses. A study in 2008 looked at 189 GHB users to document the experiences they had while taking the drug.[24] Many of the studies of users of GHB indicated a high incidence of multidrug use, commonly using MDMA, ketamine, cocaine, alcohol, and methamphetamine. Similar data is not yet available for abusers of GBL and 1,4BD.

Analysis

Specimen Types and Characteristics

For antemortem specimens, the main problem with analysis for GHB is that the very short elimination half-life of 30 to 40 minutes results in many negative samples, having missed the positive "window."[25-27] This is particularly true for blood analysis, where negative results are expected after 4 hours following ingestion. Urine is slightly better, with positive results up to 12 hours. Hair has become increasingly popular, especially in the workup of potential drug-facilitated crimes.[28,29] Oral fluid is also emerging as potential specimen type.[30,31] Methods have also been reported for detection of GBL and 1,4BD in urine and whole blood.[32]

Modes of Analysis

Chromatographic methods, with or without mass spectrometry, have been the typical standard for GHB.[26] Various extraction schemes are in the literature to analyze GHB, GBL, and 1,4BD by gas chromatography-mass spectrometry (GC-MS).[33,34] Several new methods have been reported for the analysis of GHB and GBL. One of the most promising has been the use of capillary electrophoresis, where GHB can be analyzed without requiring any derivatization or extraction procedures.[35] Methods for detection of GHB in hair have steadily improved over the last decade.[28]

Known Analytical Issues

The analysis of GHB and its precursors is technically challenging due to the low concentrations of analyte in biological fluids and extensive metabolism.[3,26] Delays in specimen collection may result in concentrations below the lower limit of detection for even the most sensitive methods.

Clinical Issues

Interpretation

Interpretation of testing results for GHB may be problematic for several reasons.[3,15,26] First, the blood levels do not correlate well with symptoms. Second, the short half-life results in many patients presenting with concentrations below the limit of detection or in the range of endogenous GHB concentrations.[36] Third, there is no good screening method available for most clinical laboratories. Those laboratories that have mass spectrometry capability may not have methods for GHB since it is rarely encountered in emergency department visits for most locations. Fourth, interpretation can be difficult due to endogenous GHB levels and GHB stability in specimens.[14,37]

Interpretation of postmortem GHB concentrations has many pitfalls.[13] The concentration of GHB in non-GHB users will increase after death as a postmortem artifact even under the best of conditions. The increase is related to storage of specimens at room temperature. There is enormous variability in inter- and intraindividual GHB concentrations seen in postmortem specimens.

Overdose and Toxicity

All GHB toxicity considerations also apply to abuse of GBL and 1,4BD.[4,9,10,16] The toxicity of GHB results from its very steep dose-response curve, going from recreational use to overdose very rapidly.[4,10,13,16,38] Loss of consciousness with rapid awaking is the hallmark of a GHB overdose. Alcohol use with GHB is particularly dangerous since alcohol potentiates the CNS depressant effects of GHB.[4,10,13] Motor vehicle accidents are a common consequence of GHB ingestion.[22]

Many accidental deaths have been reported from GHB alone, combined with other illicit drugs,[4,10] and from drug-drug interactions in patients treated for narcolepsy with GHB (Xyrem).[39,40] Tragic cases of accidental GHB poisoning in young children were caused when a toy called Aqua Dots (Bindeez outside North America) contained 1,4BD, leading to a product recall in 2007 and 2008.[41] Some children mouthing the beads ingested enough 1,4BD to exhibit GHB toxicity, although fortunately with no deaths.

For GHB, GBL, and 1,4BD ingestions, no specific antidotes are available.[42,43] Flumazenil and naloxone are not effective. Withdrawal reactions can be treated with benzodiazepines. The estimated lethal dose for GHB is 5 g to 10 g, and blood concentrations in fatalities have exceeded 300 mg/L.

Dextromethorphan (DXM)

Origin

DXM was developed clinically as a less-addictive substitute for codeine and approved by the Food and Drug Administration (FDA) for over-the-counter (OTC) sale as a cough suppressant in 1958.[44] This filled the need for a cough suppressant lacking the sedative side effects, stronger potential for misuse, and physically addictive properties of codeine phosphate, the most widely used cough medication at the time. While generally safe when used as intended, consumption of large amounts of DXM can produce euphoric and intoxicating effects.[45-48] The availability of pure DXM through the internet has further fueled recreational abuse.[46]

Descriptive Chemistry[12]

DXM is a semisynthetic drug of the morphinan class with dissociative, sedative, and cough suppressant properties. DXM is found in a number of OTC products.

Synonyms: Deoxydihydrothebacodine, methorphan, (+)-3-methoxy-17-methylmorphinan, Skittles, candy, drank, robo, triple C, CCC, dex, poor man's PCP

Trade names: Romilar; ingredient of many OTC products including Benylin DM, Camydex-20, Coricidin, Delsym, Mucinex DM, Robitussin (some formulations), Vicks Dayquil

Formula: $C_{18}H_{25}NO$

Molecular mass = 271.3972 Daltons

CAS-125-71-3

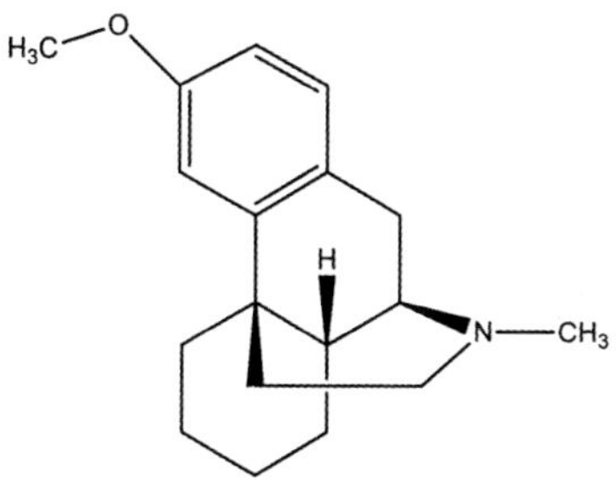

Pharmacology

Intended Uses

DXM is an OTC antitussive commonly found in cold and cough medications.[44] It is the dextro-isomer of levorphanol, an analog of codeine, but does not carry the full range of CNS effects common to opioid agonists such as morphine or codeine, nor does it produce dependence. There are currently many cough syrup preparations that contain DXM.

Mechanism of Action

DXM is a drug of the morphinan class with cough suppressant activity at typical medicinal doses and sedative, dissociative, and stimulant properties at higher doses.[44] DXM differs from codeine and morphine in having an opposite placement of the D ring, a structural feature associated with less analgesic and euphoric properties but with robust cough suppressant activity. DXM has agonist activity at the μ and σ1 opioid receptors.[44,49] At higher doses, DXM is an antagonist of the *N*-methyl-*D*-aspartate (NMDA) glutamate receptor (similar to PCP and ketamine) and inhibitor of serotonin-norepinephrine reuptake.[47,48] The latter can result in serotonin syndrome, especially when DXM abuse occurs in someone taking another drug that inhibits serotonin reuptake or metabolism.[50,51] The DXM metabolite dextrorphan also possesses pharmacologic activity and may be principally responsible for the NMDA glutamate receptor antagonism.[49]

Pharmacokinetics

DXM is rapidly absorbed from the gastrointestinal tract, with peak plasma concentrations achieved in about 2.5 hours.[52] DXM is metabolized to dextrorphan and is also demethylated to 3-methoxymorphinan and 3-hydroxymorphinan. Less than 2.5% of the DXM dose is excreted unchanged in 24 hours.

Volume of distribution and half-life information for DXM is summarized in Table 19-1.

A complicating factor in DXM use and abuse is that it is metabolized by cytochrome P450 (CYP) 2D6 and CYP3A4/5. Approximately 10% of the white population are poor metabolizers of CYP2D6 substrates like DXM.[53] CYP2D6 metabolizes DXM to dextrorphan (an active metabolite), which is conjugated (20%) with glucuronic acid or excreted as free metabolite. If inhibitors of CYP2D6 are present, the amount of DXM will increase, resulting in more toxicity.[54] Elimination half-life for DXM has been reported to be 13 hours for extensive metabolizers and 42 hours for poor metabolizers.[52]

Abuse Potential and Characteristics

DXM is often abused in high doses by adolescents and young adults to generate euphoria and visual and auditory hallucinations.[44,45,47,48,55] Illicit use of DXM is commonly referred to as *Robo-tripping* or *skittling*. These terms are derived from two of the most commonly abused products containing DXM: Robitussin and Coricidin. Novice abusers of DXM start with the OTC medications, using higher than recommended doses. This use is limited mostly by the side effects of the co-ingredients in the preparation. DXM in bulk powder form has become widely available over the internet and is often used at much higher doses than found in OTC products.[46,55]

Analysis

Specimen Types and Characteristics

DXM has been measured in urine, blood, and plasma.[12] Oral fluid is emerging as a specimen type as well.[56]

Modes of Analysis

DXM is analyzed by chromatographic methods including GC, GC-MS, and liquid chromatography-tandem mass spectrometry (LC-MS/MS).[56-59] There is no commercially available immunoassay designed for DXM testing; however, as discussed in more detail below, some of the PCP urine immunoassays have sufficient cross-reactivity to indicate a positive test result in the presence of large-dose recreational use or overdose situations.[60-62]

Known Analytical Issues

The concentrations of DXM encountered in urine in cases of abuse tend to be very high given that substantial doses are taken to achieve euphoric and intoxicating effects.[46,48,63] Thus, detection of DXM by chromatographic methods is typically straightforward.

Clinical Issues

Interpretation

Clinical laboratories who do not perform chromatographic methods for DXM instead may rely on PCP immunoassays that can cross-react with high concentrations of DXM. Cross-reactivity of DXM with PCP immunoassays varies across methods, so that DXM ingestions may be missed by PCP immunoassays with low cross-reactivity.[60,64] In addition, many laboratories no longer include PCP immunoassays in their routine drug abuse screening.

Overdose and Toxicity

DXM has a complex effect profile with markedly different effects at each dose. At smaller doses, it is also approved for very young children. There have been documented overdoses in small children as a result of parents inadvertently overmedicating their children with OTC cold/cough preparations that contain DXM.[44]

DXM users often appears "drunk" or "stoned" and may experience visual hallucinations and become ataxic.[44,45,47,48] "Recreational" doses produce a fully dissociative effect and are capable of inducing paranoia and impairing judgment, memory, language, and other mental performances. High doses may produce an irregular heartbeat, seizures, and the serotonin syndrome, the latter more common when DXM abuse occurs in someone taking another drug affecting serotonin metabolism or reuptake such as fluoxetine.[50,51] Deaths have been reported from DXM as a single agent or in combination with other drugs.[46,65]

With DXM, most patients with mild symptoms can be observed for 4 to 6 hours.[44] Naloxone has been reported effective in doses of 0.06 mg to 0.4 mg. For DXM, the estimated lethal dose is 0.5 g, and blood concentrations in fatal cases have been in the range of 3.3 mg/L to 9.2 mg/L.

3,4-Methylenedioxymethamphetamine (MDMA)

Origin

MDMA is an early designer amphetamine patented by Merck in 1914 and investigated as an appetite suppressant.[66] It did not become widely available until 1970 when it began being used as a psychotherapeutic agent. MDMA became popular on the club scene shortly thereafter.[67,68]

Descriptive Chemistry[12]

MDMA is a methylenedioxyphenethylamine within the broader family of substituted amphetamines. The most common salt is MDMA hydrochloride, which is a white or off-white powder soluble in water.

Synonyms: Ecstasy, XTC, X, ADAM, roll, M, bean, clarity, Molly, lover's speed

Formula: $C_{11}H_{15}NO_2$

Molecular mass = 193.2423 Daltons

CAS-64057-70-1

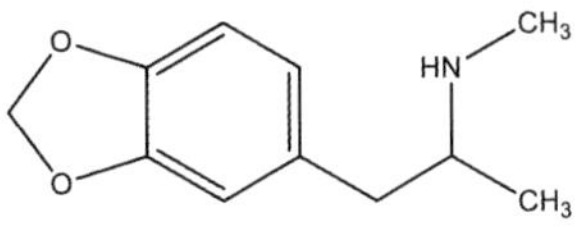

Pharmacology

Intended Uses

MDMA currently has no approved clinical applications, although it is in clinical trials for use with posttraumatic stress disorder.[69] MDMA was classified as a Schedule I controlled substance in 1985 in the US.[66] MDMA induces a sense of intimacy with others and diminished feelings of fear and anxiety, and was used in psychotherapy in the 1970s.

Mechanism of Action

MDMA is structurally related to methamphetamine and mescaline, and shares stimulant and hallucinogenic properties.[70] MDMA is an amphetamine derivative sympathomimetic, which acts as a releasing agent of serotonin, norepinephrine, and dopamine.[71] It also acts as a weak 5-HT1 and 5-HT2 receptor agonist, and its more efficacious metabolite, 3,4-methylenedioxyamphetamine (MDA), itself also a designer amphetamine drug of abuse, likely augments this action.[72] MDMA has also been shown to increase serum levels of cortisol, oxytocin, and prolactin.[73]

Pharmacokinetics

MDMA is absorbed rapidly into the bloodstream and metabolized by two separate pathways in humans.[74,75] The effects of MDMA begin 30 to 60 minutes after oral use and last up to 8 hours. Although oral use is the most common, inhalation for faster effects is also known.

Volume of distribution and half-life information for MDMA is summarized in Table 19-1.

The major metabolism pathway is demethylation by CYP2D6 to 3,4-dihydroxymethamphetamine (HHMA). HHMA is unstable and converted to 4-hydroxy-3-methoxymethamphetamine (HMMA) and further metabolized by CYP1A2 to 4-hydroxy-3-methoxyamphetamine (HMA).

In the minor metabolism pathway, MDMA is *N*-demethylated to MDA (itself also psychoactive) before ending up as HMA. 3,4-Methylenedioxy-*N*-ethylamphetamine (MDEA) is also a potential minor metabolite of MDMA. The five MDMA metabolites are excreted in urine as conjugated glucuronide and sulfate metabolites.[74] Parent drug MDMA and metabolite HMMA can be detected as early as 30 minutes. HMA is not detected until nearly 6 hours. Individual urine excretion patterns vary widely and are partially related to the urinary pH, with more acidic urine pH enhancing excretion and shortening window of detection. About 36% of the dose is excreted within the first 24 hours. Based on urine test cutoffs of 250 ng/mL for MDMA, urine specimens are not likely to be positive beyond 48 hours.[74] If metabolites other than HMMA are detected, the positive detection period could be extended to 5 days.

Abuse Potential and Characteristics

The use of MDMA spread rapidly in the 1990s and was associated with the club scene, including raves.[66-68,76] The use of MDMA then leveled off in the United States and European countries before rising again in the 2010s. MDMA typically comes in pill form, but it has increasingly been sold in the US in a powder/crystalline form known as Molly.[77] One of the challenges with studying the prevalence of MDMA use is that street preparations vary widely in purity and commonly contain adulterants such as synthetic cathinones or may even be another drug altogether. MDMA users commonly abuse other club drugs like GHB and ketamine.[78]

Analysis

Specimen Types and Characteristics

Urine is the typical specimen for MDMA screening.[79] Specimen types other than urine, blood, or oral fluid have been investigated for longer detection of MDMA use. For example, hair testing can increase the sensitivity and increase the detection time to 8 days following oral ingestion of MDMA.[80-82]

Modes of Analysis

Immunoassays have often been used to screen for the presence of MDMA in urine specimens.[79] The last decade has seen an increase in the number of marketed immunoassays specifically targeted for detection of MDMA as opposed to immunoassays marketed as targeting amphetamines, amphetamine/methamphetamine, or methamphetamine, which have widely variable cross-reactivity for MDMA. Confirmatory analysis is typically performed by GC-MS (usually with derivatization) or LC-MS/MS.[80,83-85]

Known Analytical Issues

Immunoassays marketed for MDMA detection tend to have good specificity for MDMA, although these assays may often cross-react with the structurally related MDA and MDEA (which currently have no specific immunoassays).[60,64,86] Cross-reactivity of MDMA and amphetamines immunoassays with the broad range of designer amphetamine-like drugs is complicated and has only been reported for a limited number of immunoassays.[87,88] This can present challenges because street preparations sold as MDMA may contain synthetic cathinones or other amphetamine-like stimulants that themselves may cross-react with amphetamines or MDMA immunoassays and not be targeted by standard amphetamines confirmation assays.[78,87,88]

Clinical Issues

Interpretation

Often the drugs labeled MDMA that are sold for recreational use are not what they are claimed to be. "MDMA" may really be MDA, MDEA, or one of many other amphetamine-like drugs. Positive and negative amphetamine screening results must therefore be interpreted in the light of the specific detection characteristics of the assay used. Confirmatory testing, if available, is important in providing accurate identification.

Overdose and Toxicity

MDMA can elevate body temperature, which can produce dehydration and hyperthermia, especially when exacerbated by hours of dancing or other activity.[89] Sympathetic stimulation results in tachycardia, mydriasis, diaphoresis, tremor, hyperreflexia, palpitations, and hypertension. Adverse neurologic effects include confusion, delirium, paranoia, headache, depression, insomnia, irritability, and nystagmus. Severe reactions can occur, and patients may present with seizures, cerebral edema, Parkinsonism, and the serotonin syndrome.[90-92] The combination of the musculoskeletal effects and the elevated body temperature may lead to rhabdomyolysis and renal failure.[89]

There is no antidote for MDMA intoxication, only supportive care.[67,89] Agitation and anxiety can be controlled with benzodiazepines. If hyperthermia is present, rapid cooling is a priority. For MDMA, the estimated lethal dose is 300 g, with blood concentrations of 3.1 mg/L to 4.2 mg/L blood concentrations in fatalities.

Ketamine

Origin

Ketamine was first synthesized in 1962 and gained FDA approval as a general anesthetic in 1970. Ketamine is pharmacologically related to PCP and eventually displaced PCP as an anesthetic for human clinical use due to a more favorable adverse effect profile.[93] Ketamine has short duration of action and produces dissociative anesthesia, with less respiratory depression than other general anesthetics. Reports of ketamine abuse first appeared in 1970s, with rising popularity in the club scene in the 1990s.[2,94-97]

Descriptive Chemistry[12]

Ketamine is a chiral arylcyclohexylamine derivative. Most pharmaceutical preparations of ketamine are racemic; however, the pharmaceutically more active isomer (*S*-ketamine) is being investigated for treatment-resistant depression.

Synonyms: CI-581, CL-369, K, special K, vitamin K, super K, super C, lady K, ket, Kit Kat, cat Valium

Trade Names: Ketalar

Formula: $C_{13}H_{16}ClNO$

Molecular mass = 237.7250 Daltons

CAS-6740-88-1

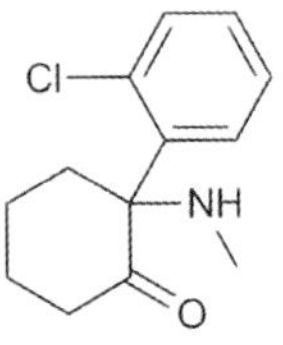

Pharmacology

Intended Uses

Ketamine is a medication mainly used for the induction and maintenance of general anesthesia.[93] Ketamine was discovered in 1962 and approved for clinical use in the US in 1970 under the trade name Ketalar. Ketamine produces dissociative anesthesia resembling a trance-like state while providing sedation, analgesia, and amnesia (memory loss). One of the main clinical advantages of ketamine is minimal effects on heart function, respiration, and airway reflexes, especially relative to other general anesthetics such as propofol or thiopental. This allows ketamine to be a good option for providing anesthesia in low-resource or remote settings. Ketamine is a core medication for intravenous anesthesia and sedation (along with propofol) in the World Health Organization Model List of Essential Medicines.[98] Nonmedical use of ketamine was first reported in the 1970s. The pharmacology of ketamine is similar to that of PCP.

Mechanism of Action

Ketamine is a dissociative anesthetic with hallucinogenic properties.[99] Ketamine is a noncompetitive antagonist of the NMDA class of glutamate receptor. Ketamine also exhibits other pharmacologic effects such as indirect activation of α-amino-3-hydroxy-5-methyl-isoxazolepropionic acid (AMPA) glutamate receptors and activation of multiple opioid receptor subtypes; however, these actions generally occur at higher concentrations than needed to inhibit NMDA receptors. Nevertheless, the pharmacodynamics of ketamine are still incompletely understood, and it is likely that mechanisms other than inhibition of NMDA glutamate receptors contribute to the effects of ketamine whether used clinically or abused.[96]

Pharmacokinetics

In clinical settings, ketamine is usually administered intravenously or intramuscularly.[93,99] Longer control of pain can be achieved by maintenance dosing of subcutaneous ketamine. Oral ketamine has low bioavailability (15-20%) due to breakdown by bile acids. Specialty pharmacies can prepare lozenges of ketamine for sublingual use that have higher bioavailability (30%) than standard oral formulations.

Volume of distribution and half-life information for ketamine is summarized in Table 19-1.

In terms of metabolism, ketamine is *N*-demethylated by CYP3A4 (major pathway), CYP2B6 (minor), and CYP2C9 to norketamine and dehydronorketamine, the two main metabolites recovered in urine.[96,100] Norketamine contributes significantly to the pharmacologic action of ketamine. Even though this metabolite is only 20% to 33% as potent as ketamine as an anesthetic, plasma levels of norketamine may reach three times that of ketamine. Duration of action of ketamine is 0.5 to 2 hours intramuscularly and 4 to 6 hours orally.

Abuse Potential and Characteristics

Ketamine emerged as a drug of abuse in the 1970s but became more popular in the 1980s.[101] The increasing abuse of ketamine, including diversion from medical and veterinary supplies, led to classification as a Schedule III controlled substance in the US in 1999.[94,96] Ketamine is abused in the club setting but also used to enhance the sexual experience. Ketamine has been implicated in drug-facilitated sexual assaults and other crimes. Ketamine abusers often aim for what is known as the "k-hole," a state characterized by physical immobility and out-of-body experience.[94] Ketamine abusers may administer the drug by intravenous, intramuscular, or intranasal routes or by smoking. Ketamine may be a preferred drug of abuse or co-abused with other substances such as DXM or GHB.[101,102]

Analysis

Specimen Types and Characteristics

Ketamine has been measured in urine, hair, oral fluid, and plasma.[96]

Modes of Analysis

Immunoassays for ketamine screening in urine have only recently become commercially available (eg, DRI Ketamine Assay, Thermo-Fisher Scientific; Ketamine Homogeneous Enzyme Immunoassay, Immunalysis). A microplate assay for urine and oral fluid is also available (OraSure Technologies). Ketamine does not show much cross-reactivity with immunoassays for screening assays for other drugs of abuse.[60] The most common analytical method for detection of ketamine is GC-MS.[82,83,96]

Known Analytical Issues

Screening immunoassays for ketamine are available but currently are not widely used by clinical laboratories. There is little published data on the performance of ketamine immunoassays except for a single report of two cases of suspected false positives on the Thermo-Fisher DRI Ketamine Assay caused by the antipsychotic drug quetiapine.[103] Ketamine may be reliably detected and quantitated by GC-MS, but this is often not routinely available in many settings.

Clinical Issues

Interpretation

The major challenge with ketamine interpretation is whether the clinical laboratory has the ability to detect the drug, whether by immunoassay or chromatographic assay. Ketamine immunoassays have only recently become commercially available and are not currently a common component of urine drugs-of-abuse testing panels. Chromatographic assays can detect ketamine but are often not available at clinical laboratories. Thus, ketamine abuse cases can be missed unless there is a high enough index of suspicion to pursue specialized testing.

Overdose and Toxicity

Acute adverse effects of ketamine include amnesia, delirium, hallucinations, hyperthermia, altered level of consciousness, tachycardia, hypertension, and impaired muscle tone.[94,104] Death is uncommon if ketamine alone is abused.[105] Chronic abuse of ketamine can lead to gastrointestinal and urinary tract toxicity including gallbladder dysfuction, hepatic toxicity, bladder injury, and hydronephrosis.[94,96] Ketamine can cause alterations to perception including out-of-body experiences, altered sense of time, and color changes.[94]

There is no specific treatment for ketamine overdose.[104] The minimum lethal dose of ketamine has not been established but is estimated to be approximately 1 g for adults given intravenously or intramuscularly in the absence of other substances. Psychotropic effects of ketamine are observed at concentrations of 0.05 mg/L to 0.3 mg/L.[106] Blood concentrations in two ketamine-associated fatalities were 1.6 mg/L and 6.9 mg/L.[105]

Phencyclidine (PCP)

Origin

PCP was first synthesized in 1926 but not utilized as an anesthetic until 1956, marketed by Parke-Davis under the trade name of Sernyl for use in humans. PCP was later abandoned for clinical use, replaced by the pharmacologically similar but safer alternative ketamine.[93] PCP became a common drug of abuse in the late 1960s through the 1980s. PCP has since faded overall as a recreational drug but still has regional popularity.[42,93]

Descriptive Chemistry[12]

PCP is an arylcyclohexylamine structurally similar to ketamine and shares many of the same pharmacologic properties. Analogs have been produced and are occasionally found in street preparations; these include cyclohexamine (PCE), phenylcyclohexylpyrrolidine (PHP), phenylcyclopentylpiperidine (PCPP), and thienylcyclohexylpiperidine (TCP).

Synonyms: PCP, angel dust, crystal, cyclone, embalming fluid, hog, killer weed, ozone, peace pills, rocket fuel, T, 1-(1-phenylcyclohexyl)-piperidine

Trade name: Sernyl

Formula: $C_{17}H_{25}N$

Molecular mass = 243.3871 Daltons

CAS-77-10-1

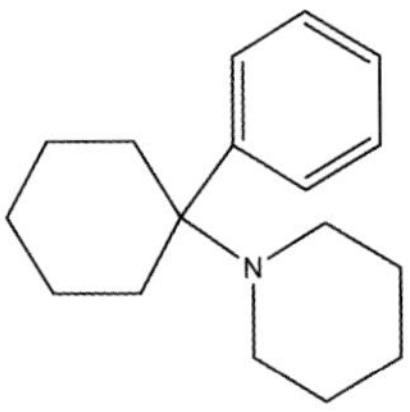

Pharmacology

Intended Uses

Clinical trials for PCP in 1957 demonstrated the short-term anesthetic properties in humans; however, psychological and physical reactions were observed, including delusions, delirium, hallucinations, muscle rigidity, and seizures.[43] It was withdrawn from human use in 1963 and is currently classified as a Schedule II controlled substance in the US. PCP currently has no clinical indications and is not produced for medical use.

Mechanism of Action

PCP is a noncompetitive antagonist of the NMDA glutamate receptor and also stimulates α-adrenergic receptors, causing sympathomimetic effects. In addition, PCP affects the actions of dopamine, which may cause the psychomotor effects seen.

Pharmacokinetics

Smoking PCP causes peak blood levels in 5 to 20 minutes and peak effect after 15 to 30 minutes, with residual effects for 4 to 6 hours.[43] Oral administration produces peak effects at 1 hour, with continued effects for 4 to 6 hours. Plasma half-life is reported to be 7 to 46 hours, with half-lives in excess of 3 days in PCP overdoses.

PCP has extensive first-pass metabolism, with 2-phenyl-4-(1-piperidinyl)-cyclohexanol (PPC) being the primary inactive metabolite. Other oxidative inactive metabolites are present as well as the glucuronide conjugates. In one study, about 20% of the dose was excreted unchanged in the urine over a 72-hour period and 80% as the polar metabolites.

Volume of distribution and half-life information for PCP is summarized in Table 19-1.

Abuse Potential and Characteristics

In the late 1960s when abuse of PCP emerged, the drug was known as the "peace pill" for its dissociative properties.[43,107] PCP has gone by many street names, including angel dust, crystal, hog, and embalming fluid. PCP may be combined with cannabis (krystal joint, supergrass, and killer weed) or cocaine (space base or tragic magic). The street-drug doses are 3 mg to 10 mg, with occasional heavy doses of >10 mg. Light doses are usually smoked, and it is common to have PCP laced in cannabis. Street preparations have variable concentrations of precursors or other unintended products, with many of them more toxic than PCP.

Analysis

Specimen Types and Characteristics

PCP is a good candidate for urinary screening, having a long excretion half-life.[79] Since plasma levels do not correlate well to symptoms, blood levels are not important except for some forensic cases. PCP has been detected in both saliva and hair as alternative specimens for analysis.[108,109]

Modes of Analysis

Screening tests for PCP are mainly immunoassays, with confirmations by GC-MS or LC-MS/MS.[79] Most immunoassays have a cutoff of 25 ng/mL, which is sufficiently sensitive to detect PCP abuse for several days if not longer. The analyte measured is the unchanged parent drug PCP, although it accounts for only 30% to 50% of the dose excreted. Few laboratories have the ability to measure any of the metabolites or glucuronide conjugates. The immunoassays utilized have mostly been standardized to a 25 ng/mL cutoff. Most screening assays will also react with some of the PCP analogs that occasionally are found as street drugs; however, their cross-reactivity varies with kit manufacturer and analytical platform.[60,64]

Known Analytical Issues

The major issue with PCP testing is cross-reactivity to structurally related compounds on the immunoassay screening test.[60] A common cross-reactive compound is DXM, especially when abused at very high doses.[61,110] Other compounds associated with false-positive PCP immunoassay results include metabolites for tramadol[111,112] and venlafaxine.[113-115] Confirmation with a reliable mass spectrometry-based confirmatory assay is important.

Clinical Issues

Interpretation

The highly variable and regionalized use of PCP makes identification of abuse challenging. When a PCP immunoassay is used in a population with low rates of PCP abuse, a high percentage (>80-90%) of the positive screens will be false positives caused by drugs such as DXM, tramadol, or venlafaxine.[60,116] Low rates of PCP abuse have prompted many laboratories to discontinue PCP screening or to use PCP immunoassays primarily for the detection of abuse of cross-reactive compounds like DXM. Confirmation by clinical history is the best interpretive method when analytical confirmation is not available. Overdoses with cocaine, amphetamines, DXM, and other hallucinogens may mimic PCP intoxication. Medical conditions including primary psychiatric disorders, head trauma, hypoglycemia, and a whole range of other conditions producing CNS symptoms need to be included in the differential diagnosis.

Overdose and Toxicity

PCP is known for its ability to induce the illusion of euphoria, omnipotence, superhuman strength, and social and sexual prowess.[42,43] Although symptoms are not directly related to dose, low doses generally produce physiological changes including increased blood pressure, perspiration, tremors, or facial grimacing. Psychological changes of agitation, euphoria, disorganization of thought, and dissociation are also seen at low doses. Moderate doses (5-10 mg) may produce nystagmus, nausea and vomiting, repetitive motor movements, muscle rigidity, fever, insomnia, loss of appetite, rage, amnesia, and hypnotic state. Acute PCP intoxication can produce a psychosis indistinguishable from acute schizophrenia.

There is no specific treatment for PCP overdose, although some have tried activated charcoal if administered 1 to 2 hours after ingestion.[42,43] Supportive care is to place the patient in quiet darkened room, and there is some data to support administering a benzodiazepine to combat anxiety or agitation. The minimum lethal dose of PCP has not been established. Blood concentrations in PCP fatalities have ranged from 0.3 mg/L to 12 mg/L.

References

1. Parks KA, Kennedy CL. Club drugs: reasons for and consequences of use. *J Psychoactive Drugs.* 2004;36(3):295-302.
2. Smith KM, Larive LL, Romanelli F. Club drugs: methylenedioxymethamphetamine, flunitrazepam, ketamine hydrochloride, and gamma-hydroxybutyrate. *Am J Health Syst Pharm.* 2002; 59(11):1067-1076.
3. Brailsford AD, Cowan DA, Kicman AT. Pharmacokinetic properties of gamma-hydroxybutyrate (GHB) in whole blood, serum, and urine. *J Anal Toxicol.* 2012;36(2):88-95.
4. Brennan R, Van Hout MC. Gamma-hydroxybutyrate (GHB): a scoping review of pharmacology, toxicology, motives for use, and user groups. *J Psychoactive Drugs.* 2014;46(3):243-251.
5. Bosch OG, Seifritz E. The behavioural profile of gamma-hydroxybutyrate, gamma-butyrolactone and 1,4-butanediol in humans. *Brain Res Bull.* 2016;126(Pt 1):47-60.
6. Klunk WE, Covey DF, Ferrendelli JA. Anticonvulsant properties of alpha, gamma, and alpha, gamma-substituted gamma-butyrolactones. *Mol Pharmacol.* 1982;22(2):438-443.
7. Wedin GP, Hornfeldt CS, Ylitalo LM. The clinical development of gamma-hydroxybutyrate (GHB). *Curr Drug Saf.* 2006;1(1):99-106.
8. Busardo FP, Kyriakou C, Napoletano S, Marinelli E, Zaami S. Clinical applications of sodium oxybate (GHB): from narcolepsy to alcohol withdrawal syndrome. *Eur Rev Med Pharmacol Sci.* 2015;19(23):4654-4663.
9. Brunt TM, van Amsterdam JG, van den Brink W. GHB, GBL and 1,4-BD addiction. *Curr Pharm Des.* 2014;20(25):4076-4085.
10. Corkery JM, Loi B, Claridge H, et al. Gamma hydroxybutyrate (GHB), gamma butyrolactone (GBL) and 1,4-butanediol (1,4-BD; BDO): a literature review with a focus on UK fatalities related to non-medical use. *Neurosci Biobehav Rev.* 2015;53:52-78.
11. van Amsterdam J, Brunt T, Pennings E, van den Brink W. Risk assessment of GBL as a substitute for the illicit drug GHB in the Netherlands: a comparison of the risks of GBL versus GHB. *Regul Toxicol Pharmacol.* 2014;70(2):507-513.
12. Moffat AC, Osselton MD, Widdop B, Watts J, eds. *Clarke's Analysis of Drugs and Poisons.* 4th ed. Chicago, IL: Pharmaceutical Press; 2011.
13. Busardo FP, Jones AW. GHB pharmacology and toxicology: acute intoxication, concentrations in blood and urine in forensic cases and treatment of the withdrawal syndrome. *Curr Neuropharmacol.* 2015;13(1):47-70.
14. LeBeau MA, Montgomery MA, Morris-Kukoski C, Schaff JE, Deakin A. Further evidence of in vitro production of gamma-hydroxybutyrate (GHB) in urine samples. *Forensic Sci Int.* 2007;169(2-3):152-156.

15. Schrock A, Hari Y, Konig S, Auwarter V, Schurch S, Weinmann W. Pharmacokinetics of GHB and detection window in serum and urine after single uptake of a low dose of GBL: an experiment with two volunteers. *Drug Test Anal.* 2014;6(4):363-366.
16. Wood DM, Brailsford AD, Dargan PI. Acute toxicity and withdrawal syndromes related to gamma-hydroxybutyrate (GHB) and its analogues gamma-butyrolactone (GBL) and 1,4-butanediol (1,4-BD). *Drug Test Anal.* 2011;3(7-8):417-425.
17. Schep LJ, Knudsen K, Slaughter RJ, Vale JA, Megarbane B. The clinical toxicology of gamma-hydroxybutyrate, gamma-butyrolactone and 1,4-butanediol. *Clin Toxicol (Phila).* 2012;50(6): 458-470.
18. Carter LP, Koek W, France CP. Behavioral analyses of GHB: receptor mechanisms. *Pharmacol Ther.* 2009;121(1):100-114.
19. Castelli MP. Multi-faceted aspects of gamma-hydroxybutyric acid: a neurotransmitter, therapeutic agent and drug of abuse. *Mini Rev Med Chem.* 2008;8(12):1188-1202.
20. Wong CG, Gibson KM, Snead OC, 3rd. From the street to the brain: neurobiology of the recreational drug gamma-hydroxybutyric acid. *Trends Pharmacol Sci.* 2004;25(1):29-34.
21. Mori T, Yoshizawa K, Shibasaki M, Suzuki T. Discriminative stimulus effects of hallucinogenic drugs: a possible relation to reinforcing and aversive effects. *J Pharmacol Sci.* 2012;120(2):70-76.
22. Centola C, Giorgetti A, Zaami S, Giorgetti R. Effects of GHB on psychomotor and driving performance. *Curr Drug Metab.* 2018.
23. Kapitany-Foveny M, Zacher G, Posta J, Demetrovics Z. GHB-involved crimes among intoxicated patients. *Forensic Sci Int.* 2017;275: 23-29.
24. Sumnall HR, Woolfall K, Edwards S, Cole JC, Beynon CM. Use, function, and subjective experiences of gamma-hydroxybutyrate (GHB). *Drug Alcohol Depend.* 2008;92(1-3):286-290.
25. Brown SD, Melton TC. Trends in bioanalytical methods for the determination and quantification of club drugs: 2000-2010. *Biomed Chromatogr.* 2011;25(1-2):300-321.
26. Ingels AS, Wille SM, Samyn N, Lambert WE, Stove CP. Screening and confirmation methods for GHB determination in biological fluids. *Anal Bioanal Chem.* 2014;406(15):3553-3577.
27. Castro AL, Dias M, Reis F, Teixeira HM. Gamma-hydroxybutyric acid endogenous production and post-mortem behaviour: the importance of different biological matrices, cut-off reference values, sample collection and storage conditions. *J Forensic Leg Med.* 2014;27:17-24.
28. Busardo FP, Pichini S, Zaami S, Pacifici R, Kintz P. Hair testing of GHB: an everlasting issue in forensic toxicology. *Clin Chem Lab Med.* 2018;56(2):198-208.
29. Xiang P, Shen M, Drummer OH. Review: drug concentrations in hair and their relevance in drug facilitated crimes. *J Forensic Leg Med.* 2015; 36:126-135.
30. De Paoli G, Bell S. A rapid GC-MS determination of gamma-hydroxybutyrate in saliva. *J Anal Toxicol.* 2008;32(4):298-302.
31. De Paoli G, Walker KM, Pounder DJ. Endogenous gamma-hydroxybutyric acid concentrations in saliva determined by gas chromatography-mass spectrometry. *J Anal Toxicol.* 2011;35(3):148-152.
32. Johansen SS, Windberg CN. Simultaneous determination of gamma-hydroxybutyrate (GHB) and its analogues (GBL, 1.4-BD, GVL) in whole blood and urine by liquid chromatography coupled to tandem mass spectrometry. *J Anal Toxicol.* 2011;35(1):8-14.
33. Brown SD, Rhodes DJ, Pritchard BJ. A validated SPME-GC-MS method for simultaneous quantification of club drugs in human urine. *Forensic Sci Int.* 2007;171(2-3):142-150.
34. Lenz D, Kroner L, Rothschild MA. Determination of gamma-hydroxybutyric acid in serum and urine by headspace solid-phase dynamic extraction combined with gas chromatography-positive chemical ionization mass spectrometry. *J Chromatogr A.* 2009;1216(18):4090-4096.
35. Gong XY, Kuban P, Scholer A, Hauser PC. Determination of gamma-hydroxybutyric acid in clinical samples using capillary electrophoresis with contactless conductivity detection. *J Chromatogr A.* 2008;1213(1):100-104.
36. Mari F, Politi L, Trignano C, Di Milia MG, Di Padua M, Bertol E. What constitutes a normal ante-mortem urine GHB concentration? *J Forensic Leg Med.* 2009;16(3):148-151.
37. Berankova K, Mutnanska K, Balikova M. Gamma-hydroxybutyric acid stability and formation in blood and urine. *Forensic Sci Int.* 2006;161(2-3):158-162.
38. Madah-Amiri D, Myrmel L, Brattebo G. Intoxication with GHB/GBL: characteristics and trends from ambulance-attended overdoses. *Scand J Trauma Resusc Emerg Med.* 2017;25(1):98.
39. Akins BE, Miranda E, Lacy JM, Logan BK. A multi-drug intoxication fatality involving Xyrem (GHB). *J Forensic Sci.* 2009;54(2):495-496.
40. Zvosec DL, Smith SW, Porrata T, Strobl AQ, Dyer JE. Case series of 226 gamma-hydroxybutyrate-associated deaths: lethal toxicity and trauma. *Am J Emerg Med.* 2011;29(3):319-332.
41. Suchard J, Nizkorodov S, Wilkinson S. 1,4-Butanediol content of aqua dots children's craft toy beads. *J Med Toxicol.* 2009;5(3):120-124.

42. Dominici P, Kopec K, Manur R, Khalid A, Damiron K, Rowden A. Phencyclidine intoxication case series study. *J Med Toxicol.* 2015;11(3):321-325.
43. Dove HW. Phencyclidine: pharmacologic and clinical review. *Psychiatr Med.* 1984;2(2):189-209.
44. Banken JA, Foster H. Dextromethorphan. *Ann N Y Acad Sci.* 2008;1139:402-411.
45. Bryner JK, Wang UK, Hui JW, Bedodo M, MacDougall C, Anderson IB. Dextromethorphan abuse in adolescence: an increasing trend: 1999-2004. *Arch Pediatr Adolesc Med.* 2006; 160(12):1217-1222.
46. Logan BK, Goldfogel G, Hamilton R, Kuhlman J. Five deaths resulting from abuse of dextromethorphan sold over the internet. *J Anal Toxicol.* 2009;33(2):99-103.
47. Martinak B, Bolis RA, Black JR, Fargason RE, Birur B. Dextromethorphan in cough syrup: the poor man's psychosis. *Psychopharmacol Bull.* 2017;47(4):59-63.
48. Schwartz RH. Adolescent abuse of dextromethorphan. *Clin Pediatr (Phila).* 2005;44(7):565-568.
49. Taylor CP, Traynelis SF, Siffert J, Pope LE, Matsumoto RR. Pharmacology of dextromethorphan: relevance to dextromethorphan/quinidine (Nuedexta) clinical use. *Pharmacol Ther.* 2016;164:170-182.
50. Ganetsky M, Babu KM, Boyer EW. Serotonin syndrome in dextromethorphan ingestion responsive to propofol therapy. *Pediatr Emerg Care.* 2007;23(11):829-831.
51. Schwartz AR, Pizon AF, Brooks DE. Dextromethorphan-induced serotonin syndrome. *Clin Toxicol (Phila).* 2008;46(8):771-773.
52. Pope LE, Khalil MH, Berg JE, Stiles M, Yakatan GJ, Sellers EM. Pharmacokinetics of dextromethorphan after single or multiple dosing in combination with quinidine in extensive and poor metabolizers. *J Clin Pharmacol.* 2004;44(10):1132-1142.
53. Takashima T, Murase S, Iwasaki K, Shimada K. Evaluation of dextromethorphan metabolism using hepatocytes from CYP2D6 poor and extensive metabolizers. *Drug Metab Pharmacokinet.* 2005;20(3):177-182.
54. Forget P, le Polain de Waroux B, Wallemacq P, Gala JL. Life-threatening dextromethorphan intoxication associated with interaction with amitriptyline in a poor CYP2D6 metabolizer: a single case re-exposure study. *J Pain Symptom Manage.* 2008;36(1):92-96.
55. Pringle G, McDonald MP, Gabriel KI. Patterns and perceptions of dextromethorphan use in adult members of an online dextromethorphan community. *J Psychoactive Drugs.* 2015;47(4):267-275.
56. Rodrigues WC, Wang G, Moore C, Agrawal A, Vincent MJ, Soares JR. Development and validation of ELISA and GC-MS procedures for the quantification of dextromethorphan and its main metabolite dextrorphan in urine and oral fluid. *J Anal Toxicol.* 2008;32(3):220-226.
57. Heneedak HM, Salama I, Mostafa S, El-Kady E, El-Sadek M. Development and validation of a sensitive UHPLC-MS/MS method for the simultaneous analysis of tramadol, dextromethorphan chlorpheniramine and their major metabolites in human plasma in forensic context: application to pharmacokinetics. *Biomed Chromatogr.* 2015;29(7):998-1007.
58. Kim EM, Lee JS, Park MJ, Choi SK, Lim MA, Chung HS. Standardization of method for the analysis of dextromethorphan in urine. *Forensic Sci Int.* 2006;161(2-3):198-201.
59. Santagati NA, Gotti R, Ronsisvalle G. Simultaneous determination of phenytoin and dextromethorphan in urine by solid-phase extraction and HPLC-DAD. *J Sep Sci.* 2005;28(11):1157-1162.
60. Krasowski MD, Pizon AF, Siam MG, Giannoutsos S, Iyer M, Ekins S. Using molecular similarity to highlight the challenges of routine immunoassay-based drug of abuse/toxicology screening in emergency medicine. *BMC Emerg Med.* 2009;9:5.
61. Marchei E, Pellegrini M, Pichini S, Martin I, Garcia-Algar O, Vall O. Are false-positive phencyclidine immunoassay instant-view multi-test results caused by overdose concentrations of Ibuprofen, metamizol, and dextromethorphan? *Ther Drug Monit.* 2007;29(5):671-673.
62. Rengarajan A, Mullins ME. How often do false-positive phencyclidine urine screens occur with use of common medications? *Clin Toxicol (Phila).* 2013;51(6):493-496.
63. Logan BK, Yeakel JK, Goldfogel G, Frost MP, Sandstrom G, Wickham DJ. Dextromethorphan abuse leading to assault, suicide, or homicide. *J Forensic Sci.* 2012;57(5):1388-1394.
64. Krasowski MD, Siam MG, Iyer M, Pizon AF, Giannoutsos S, Ekins S. Chemoinformatic methods for predicting interference in drug of abuse/toxicology immunoassays. *Clin Chem.* 2009;55(6):1203-1213.
65. Marinetti L, Lehman L, Casto B, Harshbarger K, Kubiczek P, Davis J. Over-the-counter cold medications-postmortem findings in infants and the relationship to cause of death. *J Anal Toxicol.* 2005;29(7):738-743.
66. Rosenbaum M. Ecstasy: America's new "reefer madness". *J Psychoactive Drugs.* 2002;34(2): 137-142.
67. Burgess C, O'Donohoe A, Gill M. Agony and ecstasy: a review of MDMA effects and toxicity. *Eur Psychiatry.* 2000;15(5):287-294.

68. Edland-Gryt M, Sandberg S, Pedersen W. From ecstasy to MDMA: recreational drug use, symbolic boundaries, and drug trends. *Int J Drug Policy.* 2017;50:1-8.
69. Feduccia AA, Holland J, Mithoefer MC. Progress and promise for the MDMA drug development program. *Psychopharmacology (Berl).* 2018;235(2):561-571.
70. Simantov R. Multiple molecular and neuropharmacological effects of MDMA (Ecstasy). *Life Sci.* 2004;74(7):803-814.
71. Fitzgerald JL, Reid JJ. Interactions of methylenedioxymethamphetamine with monoamine transmitter release mechanisms in rat brain slices. *Naunyn Schmiedebergs Arch Pharmacol.* 1993;347(3):313-323.
72. Lyon RA, Glennon RA, Titeler M. 3,4-Methylenedioxymethamphetamine (MDMA): stereoselective interactions at brain 5-HT1 and 5-HT2 receptors. *Psychopharmacology (Berl).* 1986;88(4):525-526.
73. Harris DS, Baggott M, Mendelson JH, Mendelson JE, Jones RT. Subjective and hormonal effects of 3,4-methylenedioxymethamphetamine (MDMA) in humans. *Psychopharmacology (Berl).* 2002;162(4):396-405.
74. Abraham TT, Barnes AJ, Lowe RH, et al. Urinary MDMA, MDA, HMMA, and HMA excretion following controlled MDMA administration to humans. *J Anal Toxicol.* 2009;33(8):439-446.
75. Barnes AJ, De Martinis BS, Gorelick DA, Goodwin RS, Kolbrich EA, Huestis MA. Disposition of MDMA and metabolites in human sweat following controlled MDMA administration. *Clin Chem.* 2009;55(3):454-462.
76. Palamar JJ, Mauro PM, Han BH, Martins SS. Shifting characteristics of ecstasy users ages 12-34 in the United States, 2007-2014. *Drug Alcohol Depend.* 2017;181:20-24.
77. Parrott AC, Downey LA, Roberts CA, Montgomery C, Bruno R, Fox HC. Recreational 3,4-methylenedioxymethamphetamine or 'ecstasy': current perspective and future research prospects. *J Psychopharmacol.* 2017;31(8):959-966.
78. Bruno R, Matthews AJ, Dunn M, et al. Emerging psychoactive substance use among regular ecstasy users in Australia. *Drug Alcohol Depend.* 2012;124(1-2):19-25.
79. Melanson SE. The utility of immunoassays for urine drug testing. *Clin Lab Med.* 2012;32(3): 429-447.
80. Cheze M, Deveaux M, Martin C, Lhermitte M, Pepin G. Simultaneous analysis of six amphetamines and analogues in hair, blood and urine by LC-ESI-MS/MS: application to the determination of MDMA after low ecstasy intake. *Forensic Sci Int.* 2007;170(2-3):100-104.
81. Johansen SS, Jornil J. Determination of amphetamine, methamphetamine, MDA and MDMA in human hair by GC-EI-MS after derivatization with perfluorooctanoyl chloride. *Scand J Clin Lab Invest.* 2009;69(1):113-120.
82. Wu YH, Lin KL, Chen SC, Chang YZ. Simultaneous quantitative determination of amphetamines, ketamine, opiates and metabolites in human hair by gas chromatography/mass spectrometry. *Rapid Commun Mass Spectrom.* 2008;22(6):887-897.
83. Lee HH, Lee JF, Lin SY, Chen PH, Chen BH. Simultaneous determination of HFBA-derivatized amphetamines and ketamines in urine by gas chromatography-mass spectrometry. *J Anal Toxicol.* 2011;35(3):162-169.
84. Middleberg RA, Homan J. Quantitation of amphetamine-type stimulants by LC-MS/MS. *Methods Mol Biol.* 2012;902:105-114.
85. Mohamed KM, Bakdash A. Comparison of 3 derivatization methods for the analysis of amphetamine-related drugs in oral fluid by gas chromatography-mass spectrometry. *Anal Chem Insights.* 2017;12:1177390117727533.
86. Melanson SE, Baskin L, Magnani B, Kwong TC, Dizon A, Wu AH. Interpretation and utility of drug of abuse immunoassays: lessons from laboratory drug testing surveys. *Arch Pathol Lab Med.* 2010;134(5):735-739.
87. Krasowski MD, Ekins S. Using cheminformatics to predict cross reactivity of "designer drugs" to their currently available immunoassays. *J Cheminform.* 2014;6:22.
88. Petrie M, Lynch KL, Ekins S, et al. Cross-reactivity studies and predictive modeling of "Bath Salts" and other amphetamine-type stimulants with amphetamine screening immunoassays. *Clin Toxicol (Phila).* 2013;51(2):83-91.
89. Graeme KA. New drugs of abuse. *Emerg Med Clin North Am.* 2000;18(4):625-636.
90. Holmes SB, Banerjee AK, Alexander WD. Hyponatraemia and seizures after ecstasy use. *Postgrad Med J.* 1999;75(879):32-33.
91. Kolbrich EA, Goodwin RS, Gorelick DA, Hayes RJ, Stein EA, Huestis MA. Physiological and subjective responses to controlled oral 3,4-methylenedioxymethamphetamine administration. *J Clin Psychopharmacol.* 2008;28(4):432-440.
92. Sprague JE, Moze P, Caden D, et al. Carvedilol reverses hyperthermia and attenuates rhabdomyolysis induced by 3,4-methylenedioxymethamphetamine (MDMA, Ecstasy) in an animal model. *Crit Care Med.* 2005;33(6):1311-1316.
93. Lodge D, Mercier MS. Ketamine and phencyclidine: the good, the bad and the unexpected. *Br J Pharmacol.* 2015;172(17):4254-4276.
94. Bokor G, Anderson PD. Ketamine: an update on its abuse. *J Pharm Pract.* 2014;27(6):582-586.

95. De Luca MT, Meringolo M, Spagnolo PA, Badiani A. The role of setting for ketamine abuse: clinical and preclinical evidence. *Rev Neurosci.* 2012; 23(5-6):769-780.
96. Han E, Kwon NJ, Feng LY, Li JH, Chung H. Illegal use patterns, side effects, and analytical methods of ketamine. *Forensic Sci Int.* 2016;268:25-34.
97. Stewart CE. Ketamine as a street drug. *Emerg Med Serv.* 2001;30(11):30, 32, 34 passim.
98. WHO Model List of Essential Medicines. 2017. http://www.who.int/medicines/publications/essentialmedicines/en/. Accessed February 14, 2019.
99. Peltoniemi MA, Hagelberg NM, Olkkola KT, Saari TI. Ketamine: a review of clinical pharmacokinetics and pharmacodynamics in anesthesia and pain therapy. *Clin Pharmacokinet.* 2016;55(9):1059-1077.
100. Xu J, Lei H. Ketamine: an update on its clinical uses and abuses. *CNS Neurosci Ther.* 2014; 20(12):1015-1020.
101. Britt GC, McCance-Katz EF. A brief overview of the clinical pharmacology of "club drugs". *Subst Use Misuse.* 2005;40(9-10):1189-1201.
102. Bobo WV, Miller SC. Ketamine as a preferred substance of abuse. *Am J Addict.* 2002;11(4):332-334.
103. Liu CH, Wang HY, Shen SH, Chiu YW. False positive ketamine urine immunoassay screen result induced by quetiapine: a case report. *J Formos Med Assoc.* 2017;116(9):720-722.
104. Gable RS. Acute toxic effects of club drugs. *J Psychoactive Drugs.* 2004;36(3):303-313.
105. Peyton SH, Couch AT, Bost RO. Tissue distribution of ketamine: two case reports. *J Anal Toxicol.* 1988;12(5):268-269.
106. Bowdle TA, Radant AD, Cowley DS, Kharasch ED, Strassman RJ, Roy-Byrne PP. Psychedelic effects of ketamine in healthy volunteers: relationship to steady-state plasma concentrations. *Anesthesiology.* 1998;88(1):82-88.
107. Thombs DL. A review of PCP abuse trends and perceptions. *Public Health Rep.* 1989;104(4):325-328.
108. Coulter C, Crompton K, Moore C. Detection of phencyclidine in human oral fluid using solid-phase extraction and liquid chromatography with tandem mass spectrometric detection. *J Chromatogr B Analyt Technol Biomed Life Sci.* 2008;863(1):123-128.
109. Paterson S, McLachlan-Troup N, Cordero R, Dohnal M, Carman S. Qualitative screening for drugs of abuse in hair using GC-MS. *J Anal Toxicol.* 2001;25(3):203-208.
110. Budai B, Iskandar H. Dextromethorphan can produce false positive phencyclidine testing with HPLC. *Am J Emerg Med.* 2002;20(1):61-62.
111. Hull MJ, Griggs D, Knoepp SM, Smogorzewska A, Nixon A, Flood JG. Postmortem urine immunoassay showing false-positive phencyclidine reactivity in a case of fatal tramadol overdose. *Am J Forensic Med Pathol.* 2006;27(4):359-362.
112. King AM, Pugh JL, Menke NB, Krasowski MD, Lynch MJ, Pizon AF. Nonfatal tramadol overdose may cause false-positive phencyclidine on Emit-II assay. *Am J Emerg Med.* 2013;31(2):444. e5-9.
113. Bond GR, Steele PE, Uges DR. Massive venlafaxine overdose resulted in a false positive Abbott AxSYM urine immunoassay for phencyclidine. *J Toxicol Clin Toxicol.* 2003;41(7):999-1002.
114. Santos PM, Lopez-Garcia P, Navarro JS, Fernandez AS, Sadaba B, Vidal JP. False positive phencyclidine results caused by venlafaxine. *Am J Psychiatry.* 2007;164(2):349.
115. Sena SF, Kazimi S, Wu AH. False-positive phencyclidine immunoassay results caused by venlafaxine and O-desmethylvenlafaxine. *Clin Chem.* 2002;48(4):676-677.
116. Johnson-Davis KL, Sadler AJ, Genzen JR. A retrospective analysis of urine drugs of abuse immunoassay true positive rates at a national reference laboratory. *J Anal Toxicol.* 2016;40(2):97-107.
117. Baselt RC, ed. *Disposition of Toxic Drugs and Chemicals in Man.* 9th ed. Forster City, CA: Biomedical Publications; 2011.

Chapter 20

Cocaine

Daniel S. Isenschmid, PhD

Introduction[1]

Origin

Cocaine is an alkaloid that is found in the plant *Erythroxylon coca,* which grows principally in the northern South American Andes. The plant favors higher elevations (up to 6000 feet) because at lower elevations (below 1500 feet) the alkaloid content is significantly diminished due to more-rapid growth. Coca leaves may first be harvested about 2 years after the time of planting. Then, depending on the altitude, the leaves may be harvested up to three times a year. The leaves are dried and converted into a coca-paste made by macerating coca leaves in an organic solvent and sulfuric acid. Further treatment of coca-paste with hydrochloric acid yields cocaine hydrochloride. The yields from 100 kg of coca leaves are about 1 kg and 800 g, respectively, for coca-paste and cocaine hydrochloride.

Descriptive Chemistry

Cocaine (methylbenzoylecgonine) is an ester of benzoic acid and the amino alcohol methylecgonine, which contains a tropine moiety and is chemically, but not pharmacologically, related to atropine. The ecgonine portion of the molecule has four asymmetric carbon atoms and can exist as four racemates (eight optically active isomers). Cocaine is structurally different from other local anesthetics by virtue of its tropine moiety. However, like other local anesthetics, cocaine consists of a hydrophobic and hydrophilic region. The hydrophobic region contains a benzene ring, while the hydrophilic region consist of a secondary or tertiary amine. Cocaine is also similar to other local anesthetics due to its ester linkages, which allow the body to hydrolyze and deactivate the drug. The ester group is also susceptible to in vitro hydrolysis.

Cocaine

Formula: $C_{17}H_{21}NO_4$

Molecular mass = 303.3529 Daltons

CAS-50-36-2

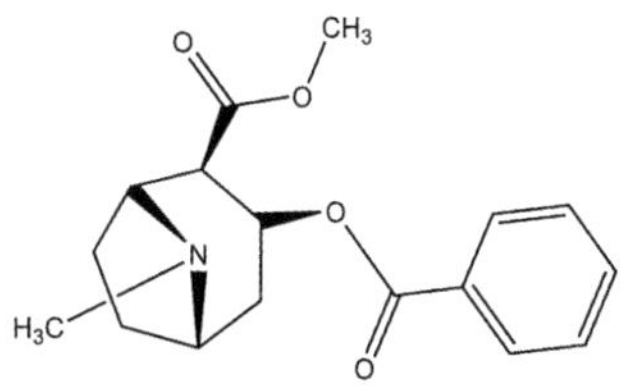

Pharmacology[1]

Intended Use

Coca (cocaine) is a psychotropic drug that has been used for over 2000 years. The Incas of Peru chewed the leaves of the coca plant in their religious ceremonies. Later, during the Spanish conquest, the Spaniards found that the Peruvian Indians could not perform heavy labor in the mines when deprived of the plant. Today, coca leaves (containing about 0.7-1.5% of total alkaloids) are still used by the indigenous populations of the high Andes, who chew them mixed with lime to cope with the rigors of life at high altitude. In the mid-19th century, Carl Wöhler, the chemist who synthesized urea, had coca leaves imported to Germany and presented them to his graduate student, Albert Niemann, to analyze. In the 1850s, Niemann was the first to successfully isolate cocaine from the coca plant. From the 1860s until the turn of the century, cocaine appeared in various elixirs and tonics purported to have "magic" properties. In 1884, Carl Koller became the first physician to use cocaine as a topical anesthetic in ophthalmologic surgery.

Popularly, it was reported to be a wonder drug that would satiate the hungry, give strength to the fatigued, and cause people to forget their misfortune. One of the more famous preparations was Vin Mariani, a mixture of wine and cocaine that received celebrity endorsements from Pope Leo XIII, US President McKinley, Thomas Edison, Auguste Rodin, and Jules Verne. For a time it was even found in Coca-Cola, which was originally introduced in 1886 as a "brain tonic." Because of the adverse effects of cocaine, appreciated even then, the Coca-Cola Company, in 1903, agreed to use (solely as a flavoring agent) only coca leaves from which the cocaine had been removed. Despite numerous early reports of cocaine toxicity, including cardiac arrhythmias and fatalities, cocaine-containing products became ever more popular.

In 1914, as cocaine abuse began to be viewed as a problem, the drug was labeled a narcotic (albeit incorrectly) under the United States Harrison Narcotic Drug Act, and over-the-counter sales were discontinued. More recently, under the Controlled Substances Act of 1970, cocaine has been scheduled as a drug with some medicinal value but a high potential for abuse (Schedule II). It continues to have some medical use but is almost exclusively limited to topical administration as a local anesthetic in ear, nose, and throat surgery (as the HCl salt in 10-20% solutions) and in ophthalmologic procedures (as a 1-4% solution). The usual maximum recommended dose for intranasal local anesthesia is 100 mg to 200 mg (1-2 mL of 10% solution). Older preparations of cocaine include tetracaine, adrenaline, and cocaine (TAC), a topical anesthetic solution used in suturing extremity wounds, in which cocaine was included because of its rapid onset of action. Topical adrenaline-and-cocaine gel is still sometimes used in pediatrics for anesthetizing children's lacerations.

Mechanism of Action

Cocaine is used medicinally as a topical local anesthetic. Therefore, it's most important clinical mechanism of action lies in its ability to block initiation and conduction of nerve impulses by decreasing axonal membrane permeability to sodium ions in fast sodium channels and thereby increase the threshold required to generate an action potential. Cocaine has additional actions that make it unique from other local anesthetics, including its ability to block reuptake of the neurotransmitters norepinephrine, dopamine, and serotonin. Norepinephrine is responsible for the classic adrenergic effects observed with cocaine use including mydriasis, vasoconstriction, hypertension, and tachycardia. The desirable effects of cocaine, mediated primarily by dopamine, include intense euphoria, psychic energy, heightened sexual excitement, and self-confidence (elevation of mood). Potential undesirable effects may include paranoia, hallucinations, and dysphoria. The central stimulatory effects ("rush") are followed by depression ("crash").[2,3] The positive reinforcement of the rush versus the negative reinforcement of the crash is the principal reason for the development of chronic cocaine abuse.

Pharmacokinetics

Cocaine is well absorbed from all routes of administration, but the time course and extent of absorption differ among them. The intravenous (IV) route of administration, sometimes called "mainlining," is the only route that consistently produces 100% drug bioavailability. Bioavailability of cocaine after nasal insufflation (IN) or smoked (SM) administration (as the free base or "crack") is quite variable, but the convenience of these two routes of administration, and the latter's rapid, intense onset of effects, makes them the most commonly used. The time course for the high in humans parallels that of the cocaine concentration in the striatum, a region in the brain implicated in control of motivation and reward. For equivalent plasma cocaine concentrations and dopamine transporter blockade, SM cocaine induced significantly greater self reports of "high" than IN cocaine and showed a trend for greater effect than IV cocaine.[4] After either IV or SM administration, the subjective euphoric response occurs in 1 to 5 minutes, with a cardiovascular response peaking in 8 to 12 minutes and lasting approximately 30 minutes. After IN administration, a euphoric effect occurs within 15 to 30 minutes, cardiovascular changes and plasma levels peak within 20 to 60 minutes, and effects last several hours, but the euphoric effects are attenuated compared to the SM route despite the extended effects.

Cocaine contains two ester moieties, rendering it susceptible to hydrolysis in vitro and in vivo. The alkyl ester of cocaine is hydrolyzed to benzoylecgonine via spontaneous hydrolysis as well as liver esterases, and the phenyl ester is hydrolyzed to ecgonine methyl ester by plasma cholinesterase and liver esterases (Figure 20-1).[5-9] Benzoylecgonine and ecgonine methyl ester are both further metabolized to ecgonine. If cocaine is used with ethanol, cocaethylene, produced by the transesterification of cocaine with ethanol, may also be observed. Unlike benzoylecgonine and ecgonine methyl ester, which are inactive metabolites, cocaethylene is an active compound that has been shown to produce even greater euphoria than cocaine itself. It is formed faster than the inactive metabolites, thereby potentially increasing the toxicity of cocaine when used with ethanol.[10,11] Other minor metabolites of cocaine include norcocaine, hydroxylated metabolites, and methylecgonidine, which has been associated primarily with smoked crack cocaine as a thermal decomposition product.[12-14] Methylecgonidine is further metabolized to ecgonidine, which may be a more useful indicator of crack smoking.[15] When smoking cocaine and using ethanol, ethylecgonidine may be produced.

Many pharmacokinetic studies have been performed with cocaine. Although considerable interindividual variation between subjects has been reported, several observations can be made. When bioequivalent doses of cocaine were administered by the IV and SM routes, similar absorption and elimination curves for cocaine were obtained with dose-related mean peak plasma concentrations.[16-18] After IN administration, the dose and mean peak plasma concentration showed a poor correlation due to dose-dependent bioavailability by that route.[19] Typical peak plasma cocaine concentrations

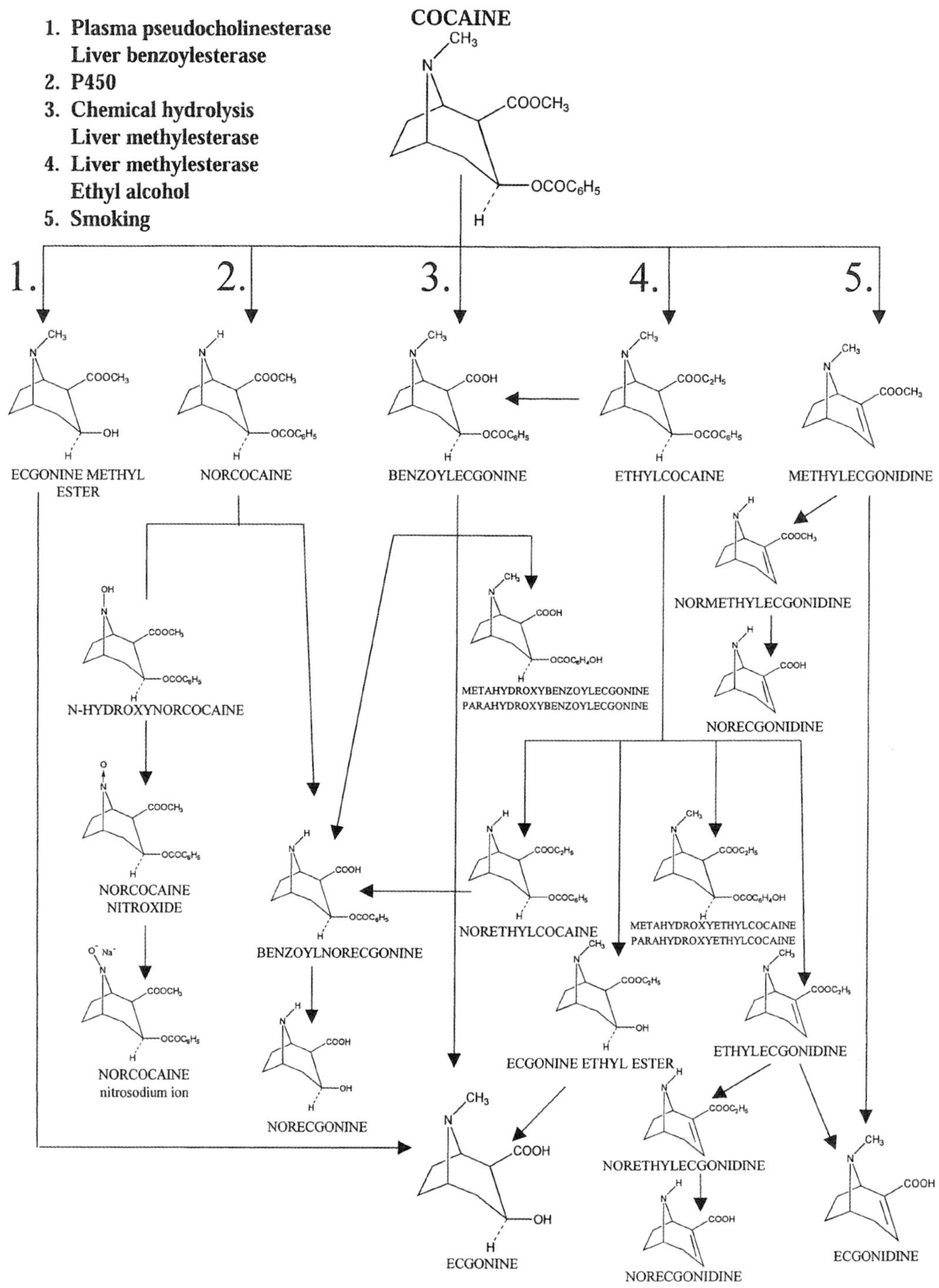

Figure 20-1. Pathways in the metabolism of cocaine.

From Isenchmid DS. Cocaine. In: Levine B, ed. *Principles of Forensic Toxicology.* Washington, DC: AACC Press; 1999:221. Reproduced with permission.

in most single-dose pharmacokinetic studies by the SM (up to 100 mg), IV (up to 64 mg), and IN (up to 100 mg) averaged between 200 and 400 ng/mL.

For IV and SM routes, the average half-life for cocaine, based on the literature, is about 60 minutes, with a somewhat longer half-life after IN administration (up to 84 minutes).[1] Benzoylecgonine appears in the plasma within 15 to 30 minutes following cocaine administration by the IV, SM, and IN routes of administration.[16,18,20] Peak plasma benzoylecgonine concentrations usually occurred within 90 minutes after SM and IV cocaine administration, and were about half the peak cocaine concentrations.[16] After IN administration of cocaine, peak benzoylecgonine concentrations were not reached until 3 hours and were about twice that of cocaine and remained elevated for the next 5 hours. The rate of benzoylecgonine elimination was slow compared to its rate of formation, accounting for its accumulation in plasma while cocaine concentrations were decreasing. The elimination half-lives for benzoylecgonine was between 5 and 6 hours after IV and SM administration and about 3.5 hours after IN administration. Ecgonine methyl ester concentrations are usually much lower than those of benzoylecgonine but are present at significant concentrations after oral cocaine administration, suggesting a possible first pass effect of liver benzoylesterase for this metabolite.[21-23] Ecgonine methyl ester may also form in vitro in blood collected without or with insufficient sodium fluoride preservative as an inhibitor of plasma cholinesterase.[24]

Cocaine and its metabolites are excreted into the urine almost exclusively by simple filtration. Thus, the urinary excretion rates and plasma concentrations of cocaine and benzoylecgonine parallel one another, indicating that the elimination rate of the drug is proportional to plasma concentration.[25] Only a small fraction of an administered dose of cocaine is excreted as parent drug, with the majority of the metabolites detected as benzoylecgonine, ecgonine methyl ester, and ecgonine.[26,27]

Abuse Potential and Characteristics[1,28]

Cocaine is one of the most popular drugs of abuse and is considered to be the most abused major stimulant in the US, exceeding methamphetamine nationally, although the predominance of one drug over the other depends on regional differences. It has acquired numerous street names including bazooka, blow, coke, crack, dust, flake, gold dust, happy dust, lady, nose, nose candy, rock, snow, speedball (when mixed with heroin and injected), stardust, tick (when smoked with phencyclidine), toot, and white. In a 2016 National Survey on Drug Use and Health, it was reported that 14.4% of the surveyed US population between the age of 12 and 17 years have used cocaine in their lifetimes, and 16.6% of those over the age of 26 used cocaine at least once.[29] The greatest mention of lifetime use was for the 55 to 59 year age group at 26.4%, reflecting the popularity of the drug back in the 1980s and 1990s. Despite this, recent reports show that cocaine-related deaths in 2015 were the highest since 2006 according to the Substance Abuse and Mental Health Services Administration, and first-time use from 2013 to 2015 increased 61%. The increase in use has been correlated to the increase in cocaine trafficking and cultivation.

Cocaine produces a drug "high" due to generalized sympathetic stimulation very similar to that of methamphetamine intoxication, including agitation, mydriasis, tachycardia, hypertension, hallucinations, hypertonia, and hyperreflexia. Subjectively, this state of euphoria may include sexual arousal, anorexia, insomnia, hyperexcitability, loquacity, grandiosity, and manic behavior. Although there is a good deal of individual variation in susceptibility to developing a dependency on cocaine, the immediate craving of the addict for more of this drug soon after use is due to the short-lived high, typically subsiding within an hour and frequently leading to a binge of multiple, repeated doses. When the binge stops, it is followed by a "crash," the onset of a severely dysphoric mood, which may include the experience of considerable anxiety, fear, depression, apathy, irritability, or suspiciousness, followed by exhaustion until sleep is achieved. Resumption of use may occur upon awakening or may not occur for several days, but psychological dependence develops from this cycle of initial euphoria followed by dysphoria, because the dysphoria may be ameliorated by repeated administration, so the user develops the need to take the drug continuously to feel relatively well. The effect, however, diminishes upon repetition, and short-term tolerance (tachyphylaxis) develops when several doses of cocaine are administered over a brief period.

Withdrawing from cocaine may produce moderate lethargy and drowsiness, hyperphagia, vivid dreams, and some mental depression—symptoms that usually abate within a few days to a few weeks. Although this does not constitute a major physical withdrawal syndrome, psychological dependence makes cocaine addiction one of the most difficult to manage, often almost impossible to overcome. Relapse rates among cocaine users range from 94% to 99%, which is the highest among all common drugs of abuse.

In a 2015 review of cocaine-related deaths from medical examiner and coroner data, the mean and median age of the decedents was 42 ($N = 3151$).[30] The common sequelae associated with chronic cocaine in patients over the age of 30 include heart disease, myocardial infarction, and exacerbation of chronic disease, strokes, and renal failure. Cocaine use is often associated with violence. This may be due to violent acts caused by the pharmacological effects of cocaine (psychopharmacological model), violent interactions resulting from involvement with an expensive but illicit commodity (systemic model), and violence as an instrumental act to obtain resources to purchase/obtain cocaine (economic-compulsive model).[31] A large percentage of homicide cases are cocaine related. From 1990 to 1991, 31.3% of homicide cases were positive for cocaine and/or benzoylecgonine in New York City.[32] Detroit reported a 28% positive rate for the parent drug in the blood of homicide victims in 2000.[33]

Cocaine is sold on the street in two forms: the hydrochloride salt or crack. The salt varies considerably in purity. It can be as low as 30%, but recently drug identification exhibits have shown the purity to be much higher, in some cases exceeding 90%, with greater than 80% typical. Historically, the salt form is typically diluted ("cut") with agents such as mannitol, lactose, and sucrose to add bulk. In addition, readily available central nervous system stimulants such as caffeine and ephedrine, and other local anesthetics such as lidocaine, procaine, and benzocaine, had been commonly used as diluents to simulate the actual drug. More recently, diphenhydramine and levamisole have been reported as cutting agents. The cocaine powder supplied by dealers is often clumpy and first needs to be chopped. This is usually done using a mirror and a razor blade. Then the cocaine is arranged into thin lines about 30 mm to 60 mm long and 2 mm wide (resulting in an average dose of 25 mg) and then snorted through a straw or "tooter." Alternatively, cocaine may be snorted from a "coke spoon" or "bullet" (a vial containing cocaine is inverted over a closed chamber and the chamber is rotated for convenient snorting). A single long fingernail may serve as a natural coke spoon.

Alkaloidal cocaine base, known as *freebase,* is made by dissolving cocaine hydrochloride salt in an aqueous alkaline solution and then extracting the free basic form with a solvent such as ether. *Crack* is a freebase form of cocaine produced by using sodium bicarbonate to create the alkaline aqueous solution, the extract of which is then dried by heating (the name coming from the "crackling" sound made by the heated extract). After heating, the mixture is cooled and filtered, and the freebase cocaine precipitates into small pellets or "rocks." A typical rock weighs about 20 mg and costs US $5.00. These rocks can then be smoked in a crack pipe. Crack pipes range from elaborate glass pipes to a soda can with a hole. The heat generated from these pipes can be very high, and chronic crack users may show stigmata of thermal injuries on the fingers.

Analysis

Specimen Types and Characteristics

Cocaine and its metabolites have been measured in whole blood, serum, plasma, urine, bile, vitreous humor, cerebral spinal fluid, postmortem tissues, hair, oral fluid, sweat, umbilical cord, meconium, and breast milk. Specimen selection depends on the availability, application, and intended purpose of the analysis.

Generally, in clinical settings urine is the most common specimen used for documenting recent exposure to cocaine, but blood is preferred for human performance testing and interpretation of potential impairment or intoxication. Increasingly, oral fluid is being used for this purpose as well. In utero exposure to cocaine can be documented through meconium or umbilical cord analysis. Hair can be particularly useful for documenting long-term cocaine use, but care needs to be taken to ensure that any environmental contamination is taken into account. For this reason, hair should be washed and the rinses analyzed. Additionally, while cocaine is the primary analyte detected in hair, some recommend that it should not be reported in the absence of benzoylecgonine or other cocaine metabolites.[34] In the case of postmortem toxicology, in addition to blood and urine, vitreous humor has been shown to be useful for the analysis of cocaine and benzoylecgonine.[35] More detailed information of testing performed on specimen matrices other than urine can be found in chapter 14 (oral fluid) and chapter 15 (hair, sweat, meconium, cord tissue, and breast milk).

Modes of Analysis[1]

Immunoassays are commonly used for screening purposes because they are readily amenable to large-batch analysis, are relatively sensitive, and require little or no sample preparation. Because immunoassays are targeted to detect benzoylecgonine, they are particularly well suited for screening urine specimens and are commonly employed for analysis of this matrix for workplace drug testing and drugs-of-abuse screening in a variety of settings, including court-ordered and hospital testing. There are several types of immunoassays on the market, and some of these, particularly enzyme-linked immunosorbent assays (ELISAs) and chemiluminescent immunoassays, have been successfully adapted to blood and tissue homogenate analysis. Although all immunoassay techniques are targeted to benzoylecgonine, cross-reactivities vary considerably by manufacturer and analytical principle. Immunoassays that possess substantial cross-reactivity to cocaine and cocaethylene are particularly useful for screening blood, where significant concentrations of parent drug might be found. Increasingly, laboratories are using liquid chromatography (LC) with accurate mass (time of flight) procedures to identify target compounds in screening procedures. These procedures are sensitive, generally highly specific (except in the case of isobaric compounds), and allow for the simultaneous analyses of metabolites along with parent compounds.

Gas chromatography (GC) is one of the most frequently used methods for the confirmatory analysis of cocaine and its metabolites. Cocaine, cocaethylene, and their *N*-desmethyl metabolites can be readily assayed without derivatization using nitrogen-phosphorous detection or mass spectrometry (MS) in both the electron impact and positive chemical ionization modes. Flame ionization detection is generally not sensitive enough for the analysis of biological samples. The main disadvantage of GC analysis is that polar metabolites, such as benzoylecgonine, must be derivatized prior to analysis. LC is very useful in confirmation procedures since cocaine and benzoylecgonine and other polar metabolites can be analyzed simultaneously without derivatization. MS or tandem mass spectrometry (MS/MS) detection procedures provide the highest degree of sensitivity and specificity of all routine detection procedures and is virtually a requirement for the forensic confirmation of cocaine and metabolites today. A particular advantage with MS detection is that isotopically labeled standards of cocaine and its major metabolites are now available and, by virtue of their nearly identical chemical characteristics, allow for optimal analytical reproducibility and accuracy when selected as internal standards. If other detectors are used, selection of internal standards should be carefully considered so that they undergo the same chemistry as the analyte. While LC-MS or MS/MS procedures have many advantages, the method must be carefully evaluated for the potential for ion suppression or enhancement.

For certain matrices, such as urine, confirmation procedures such as LC-MS/MS may be employed without any sample preparation ("dilute and shoot" injection). However, for most matrices, cocaine and its metabolites must generally be separated from the biological matrix. This is commonly accomplished by either liquid-liquid, solid-phase, or solid-phase microextraction. Solid-phase extraction procedures can be readily adapted to laboratory automation devices. Consideration must also be given to the selection of targeted analytes because the pK_a and polarity for cocaine and its metabolites varies considerably. Ecgonine, in particular, may be difficult to isolate from biological matrices.

Known Analytical Issues[1]

Cocaine contains two ester moieties that are subject to hydrolysis. Cocaine is unstable in unpreserved blood where it is hydrolyzed by plasma pseudocholinesterase to ecgonine methyl ester.[24] The addition of sodium fluoride, while inhibiting enzymatic hydrolysis of cocaine to ecgonine methyl ester, does not prevent spontaneous hydrolysis of cocaine to benzoylecgonine, but this can be minimized by storing samples in refrigerated or frozen conditions. The rate of hydrolysis of both esters has been shown to be temperature and pH dependent, with higher temperatures and pH increasing the rate of hydrolysis. Ideally, blood and plasma samples should be fluoridated and stored at refrigerated temperatures for short-term storage and frozen temperatures for longer term storage. It should be noted that standard gray top Vacutainer tubes (0.25% sodium fluoride) do not provide effective inhibition of cocaine hydrolysis in whole blood or plasma for long-term storage.[36] While cocaine hydrolysis was slower than in studies without sodium fluoride, significant hydrolysis of cocaine still occurred within 5 to 11 hours at 20°C and after 1 to 2 days at 4°C. Egonine methyl ester concentrations produced were significantly higher than benzoylecgonine concentrations, demonstrating that 0.25% sodium fluoride was not very effective at inhibiting enzymatic hydrolysis. A comprehensive stability study for cocaine and metabolites has been reported.[24] To date, there has only been a single study of the stability of cocaethylene in human blood, which confirms that the same stability issues discussed for cocaine apply to cocaethylene.[37]

The rate of cocaine hydrolysis in plasma exceeds that of whole blood. An initial plasma cocaine concentration of 100 ng/mL was no longer detectable in refrigerated (4°C) nonfluoridated plasma after 3 days.[38] In fluoridated (0.5%) plasma, it was still present after 21 days, but only at 40% to 60% of the original concentration.

The conditions to which specimens are exposed during analysis are another factor affecting stability of cocaine and metabolite concentrations. Primary specimens and aliquots should not be allowed to remain at room temperature for extended periods of time during the analytical process. Because cocaine is a basic drug, many procedures utilize basic conditions (pH 8-11) for the extraction of cocaine from the biological matrix into organic solvents. This process may be repeated during a back-extraction. The duration of exposure to these

Table 20-1. Cocaine, Cocaethylene, and Benzoylecgonine Concentrations Detected in a Population of Drivers Suspected of Impaired Driving and in Postmortem Cases[30]

	Benzoylecgonine	Cocaine	Cocaethylene
Number (DUID)	1452	644	188
Mean, ng/mL	650	84	44
Median, ng/mL	360	55	37
Range, ng/mL	50-5200	20-1000	20-210
Number (Postmortem)	3567	1927	727
Mean, ng/mL	1000	320	85
Median, ng/mL	580	90	56
Range ng/mL	50-36,000	20-39,000	20-1900

DUID, driving under the influence of drugs.

alkaline conditions, especially at room temperature, is critical and may contribute to artifactual hydrolysis of cocaine and its metabolites during analysis.

Stability of cocaine in urine is less of a concern than for blood due to a lack of esterases in that matrix. Despite this, if a urine sample contains high concentrations of cocaine, significant hydrolysis has been reported at alkaline pH, particularly at elevated temperatures.[39] Urine fortified with 1000 ng/mL of cocaine, adjusted to pH 5 and stored at 4°C, showed no appreciable cocaine loss, but urine fortified with the same amount of cocaine at pH 8 lost 40% of the original amount in 8 days, even when refrigerated.[38]

Clinical Issues

Interpretation[1]

Many factors must be considered when interpreting cocaine and metabolite concentrations in the blood. Adult (single) doses of cocaine, whether for medical or abuse purposes, are typically in the range of up to 100 mg, producing plasma or blood concentration of 200 ng/mL to 400 ng/mL. Toxic doses are highly variable, depending on the degree of individual tolerance, route of administration, presence of other drugs, and other factors. In simultaneous ethyl alcohol and cocaine users, cocaethylene concentrations should also be considered when interpreting results. Plasma cocaine concentrations >1000 ng/mL have been reported without adverse effects in some studies after chronic oral dosing and after repeated doses of smoked cocaine. Concentrations of >5000 ng/mL have generally only been reported in fatal cases, although concentrations in fatalities are usually much lower.

A search of the literature suggests that cocaine concentrations of <300 ng/mL are generally considered clinically therapeutic; however, clinical and postmortem studies have clearly shown that therapeutic, toxic, and lethal cocaine concentrations overlap. Tolerance and sensitization may play a significant role in the poor correlation observed. In a study of 130 patients who presented to an emergency department with acute cocaine toxicity, the mean plasma cocaine concentration was 340 ng/mL (range, 0.00-3920 ng/L).[40,41] The median cocaine concentration in these patients was only 70 ng/mL; however, the mean and median benzoylecgonine concentrations in these patients were 1570 ng/mL and 1060 ng/mL, respectively. There was no correlation of the cocaine and metabolite concentrations in these patients with their clinical state or outcome, but the degree of symptoms of toxicity—most notably hyperthermia, heart rate, and psychosis—was a better predictor of patient outcome. Table 20-1 provides data for cocaine, cocaethylene, and benzoylecgonine concentrations detected in a population of drivers suspected of impaired driving and postmortem cases.[30] However, the data do not take into account numerous factors such as the time of the incident versus sample collection for drivers, the site of blood sample collection or postmortem interval for postmortem cases, and the other drugs present and sample stability in both populations.

Given that cocaine is typically used in a binge of multiple doses over the course of many hours, blood concentrations of cocaine and its metabolites are usually not useful for estimating the dose or time of administration. Because the half-life of benzoylecgonine is considerably longer than that of cocaine, one would expect benzoylecgonine concentrations to increase out of proportion to the cocaine concentration during a cocaine binge. High blood benzoylecgonine concentrations with significant cocaine concentrations (>100 ng/mL) may indicate binge cocaine use, whereas similar cocaine and benzoylecgonine concentrations are more typical of a recent single dose or multiple doses within a very short period of time. As previously discussed, cocaine stability after collection and during analysis may create analytical artifacts that may alter interpretation of the results. Blood samples collected in the hospital, in particular, are usually collected in containers without preservative and may not have been stored in refrigerated conditions. Ultimately, clinical history and presentation, laboratory findings, and pathology present must be considered together because any factor taken out of context may produce an incorrect interpretation.

Most clinical tests for cocaine, whether for hospital drug testing or workplace drug testing, are performed on urine using immunoassays. These drug screens are designed to detect benzoylecgonine. Benzoylecgonine cutoffs on urine toxicology screens under the US federal drug testing program are 150 ng/mL, with a 100 ng/mL confirmation cutoff. Hospital toxicology screens may use different cutoff concentrations.

Urine is suitable only for determining an exposure to cocaine. Quantitative measurements of benzoylecgonine concentration (especially if corrected for creatinine) in serial urine samples may be useful in substance abuse treatment programs to detect a relapse during a period of abstinence, but single samples cannot be similarly interpreted because only a randomly collected urine sample is typically analyzed. Benzoylecgonine may be detected as long as 1 to 3 days after a single use; however, chronic cocaine use can increase this significantly. Therefore, these tests offer little information in terms of acute cocaine use but can be useful in documenting exposure.

Overdose and Toxicity[28]

Cocaine is among the drugs of abuse most frequently involved in emergency department visits. Symptoms of central nervous system (CNS) stimulation and sympathetic hyperactivity are very marked in overdosage with cocaine, which can result in death due to status epilepticus, hyperthermia, ventricular tachycardia, and cardiac or respiratory arrest. Signs and symptoms of acute cocaine poisoning include tachycardia, hypertension, tachypnea, and pyrexia. Patient presentations vary with the degree of toxicity. With mild poisoning, patients may show normal or nearly normal vital signs, but they exhibit anxiety, agitation, euphoria, headache, tremors, twitching, nausea, vomiting, diaphoresis, mydriasis, and pallor. With a moderate degree of poisoning, patients can present with mildly to moderately increased vital signs, confusion, hallucinations, hyperactivity, clonus, increased muscle tone, abdominal cramps, and brief tonic-clonic seizures. Rhabdomyolysis and consequent potential renal failure may be present, associated with dark urine. Patients with severe poisoning present with markedly abnormal vital signs with malignant hyperthermia, tachydysrhythmias, and status epilepticus or coma with flaccid paralysis, apnea, cyanosis, and Cheyne-Stokes respirations. Cardiovascular collapse, bradycardia, and hypotension predict a fatal outcome. Severe CNS depression with deep coma has been seen in a few cocaine abusers after prolonged binges. Laboratory abnormalities include leukocytosis, hypokalemia, and hyperglycemia.

During the cycle of euphoria and dysphoria with repeated use, cocaine abusers may present a range of physical symptoms including headache, dizziness, tremors, myoclonic jerks, and seizures. In chronic abusers, psychological deterioration may eventually occur, resulting in loss of mental function, compulsive disorders, suicidal ideation, psychopathic tendencies, and a paranoid psychosis resembling amphetamine psychosis, with stereotyped behavior, delusions, loss of impulse control, violence, and visual, olfactory, auditory, gustatory, and tactile hallucinations (including parasitosis, also called *coke bugs*). Episodes of acute dyskinesia ("crack dancing") have been seen, presenting with choreoathetoid movements of the extremities, lip-smacking, and repetitive eye-blinking. Symptoms begin minutes to hours after cocaine use and may last for several days, possibly attributable to supersensitivity to the effects of dopamine. The syndrome is usually benign and self-limited, with spontaneous resolution. The Spanish street term for this syndrome is *boca torcida,* or "twisted mouth."

The increased sympathetic activity caused by cocaine produces coronary artery vasospasm and increased platelet adhesion, decreasing the supply of blood and oxygen to myocardial tissue and at the same time elevating blood pressure and heart rate, increasing myocardial work and demand for oxygen. This combination of effects can result in angina, myocardial ischemia, or myocardial infarction. Asymptomatic myocardial ischemia manifesting as episodes of ST-segment elevation has also been reported during withdrawal of cocaine, possibly associated with coronary vasospasm, vasoconstriction, coronary thrombosis, or direct myocardiotoxicity. Vasoconstriction due to cocaine may also produce ischemia in the fingers, toes, spinal cord, kidneys, spleen, and intestines. Furthermore, with its effects on impulse conduction, the drug also can induce left ventricular dysfunction and ventricular and supraventricular arrhythmias. Chronic cocaine use accelerates the development of atherosclerosis and can also cause aortic dissection, myocarditis, or cardiomyopathy, which are frequent findings at autopsies in chronic cocaine abusers. Cardiovascular toxicity resulting from cocaine use may be related to individual sensitivity and therefore may not be predictable on the basis of dose, route of administration, or underlying heart disease. Plasma cholinesterase deficiency appears to be a marker for risk of sudden death, and, generally, other known risk factors for cardiovascular disease, such as cigarette smoking, may exacerbate cocaine's cardiotoxicity.

Chronic nasal insufflation of cocaine can result in rhinitis, epistaxis, anosmia, and septal perforation. Smoking crack cocaine can result in cough, hemoptysis, life-threatening attacks of asthma or chronic obstructive pulmonary disease, hypersensitivity pneumonitis ("crack lung"), eosinophilia with granuloma formation, noncardiogenic pulmonary edema, pulmonary hemorrhage, obliterative bronchiolitis, and abnormalities of pulmonary function. Barotrauma (eg, pneumothorax, pneumomediastinum) can be caused by crack smokers' aggressive breath-holding.

Acute renal failure can be caused by rhabdomyolysis, presenting with muscle pain, elevated creatine kinase (CK) levels, and myoglobinuria, sometimes preceded by episodes of "cocaine run amok," a syndrome of excited delirium, seizures, hypotension, and profound hyperthermia. Renal infarcts without associated rhabdomyolysis have also been reported.

Emergency department treatment of acute overdose cases may be quite involved. Basic life support is crucial, with IV access and electrocardiographic monitoring established, along with close observation. Diagnostic workup focuses on the cardiac, neurologic, and pulmonary systems through the use of continuous electrocardiographic monitoring, a chest x-ray, and frequent monitoring of vital signs, including core body temperature. Standard protocols for ruling out myocardial infarction and ischemia are followed in patients with chest pain of potential cardiac origin. Patients with a persistent or severe headache, abnormal neurologic examination, or prolonged seizures require a computed tomography scan and lumbar puncture to rule out subarachnoid hemorrhage. Cerebrovascular accidents due to ischemic or hemorrhagic stroke, subarachnoid or intracerebral hemorrhage, and cerebral vasculitis have all been seen in cocaine abusers. Patients with seizures or in a coma should be given supplemental oxygen, dextrose, and thiamine. Benzodiazepines can be used to manage seizures, and aggressive cooling may be required in instances of severe hyperthermia. Hypertension, tachycardia, and dysrhythmias may require focused intensive treatment. Gastrointestinal decontamination with activated charcoal may be appropriate for recent ingestions. Routine laboratory studies include urine drug screening, electrolytes, glucose, blood urea nitrogen, creatinine, urinalysis, urine myoglobin, complete blood count, and arterial blood gases.

References

1. Isenschmid DS. Cocaine: effects on human performance and behavior. *Forensic Sci Rev.* 2002; 14:61-100.
2. Dackis CA, Gold MS. New concepts in cocaine addiction: the dopamine depletion hypothesis. *Neurosci Biobehav Rev.* 1985;9:469-477.
3. Gawin FH, Kleber HD. Abstinence symptomatology and psychiatric diagnoses in cocaine abusers: clinical observations. *Arch Gen Psychiatry.* 1986;43:107-113.
4. Volkow ND, Wang GJ, Fischman MW, et al. Effects of route of administration on cocaine induced dopamine transporter blockade in the human brain. *Life Sci.* 2000;67:1507-1515.
5. Dean RA, Christian CD, Sample RHB, Bosron WF. Human liver cocaine esterases: ethanol-mediated formation of ethylcocaine. *FASEB J.* 1991;5:2735-2739.
6. Inaba T, Stewart DJ, Kalow W. Metabolism of cocaine in man. *Clin Pharmacol Ther.* 1978; 23:547-552.
7. Jatlow PI. Cocaine: analysis, pharmacokinetics and metabolic disposition. *Yale J Biol Med.* 1988;61:105-113.
8. Stewart DJ, Inaba T, Lucassen M, Kalow W. Cocaine metabolism: cocaine and norcocaine hydrolysis by liver and serum esterases. *Clin Pharmacol Ther.* 1979;25:464-468.
9. Stewart DJ, Inaba T, Tang BK, Kalow W. Hydrolysis of cocaine in human plasma by cholinesterase. *Life Sci.* 1977;20:1557-1563.
10. McCane-Katz EF, Kosten TR, Jatlow P. Concurrent use of cocaine and ethanol is more potent and potentially more toxic than use of either alone: a multiple dose study. *Biol Pharmacol.* 1998;44:250-259.
11. Brzezinski MR, Abraham TL, Stone CL, Dean RA, Bosron WF. Purification and characterization of a human liver cocaine carboxylesterase that catalyzes the production of benzoylecgonine and the

formation of ethylcocaine from ethanol and cocaine. *Biochem Pharm.* 1994;48:1747-1755.
12. Cone EJ, Hillsgrove M, Darwin WD. Simultaneous measurement of cocaine, ethylcocaine, their metabolites, and "crack" pyrolysis products by gas chromatography-mass spectrometry. *Clin Chem.* 1994;40:1299-1305.
13. Jacob P, Lewis ER, Elias-Baker BA, Jones RT. A pyrolysis product, anhydroecgonine methyl ester (methylecgonidine), is in the urine of cocaine smokers. *J Anal Toxicol.* 1990;14:353-357.
14. Jenkins AJ, Goldberger BA. Identification of unique cocaine metabolites and smoking by-products in postmortem blood and urine specimens. *J Forensic Sci.* 1997;42:824-827.
15. Shimomura ET, Hodge GD, Paul BD. Examination of postmortem fluids and tissues for the presence of methylecgonidine, ecgonidine, cocaine, and benzoylecgonine using sold-phase extraction and gas chromatography-mass spectrometry. *Clin Chem.* 2001;47:1040-1047.
16. Cone EJ. Pharmacokinetics and pharmacodynamics of cocaine. *J Anal Toxicol.* 1995;19:459-478.
17. Isenschmid DS, Fischman MW, Foltin RW, Caplan YH. Concentration of cocaine and metabolites in plasma of humans following intravenous administration and smoking of cocaine. *J Anal Toxicol.* 1992;16:311-314.
18. Jeffcoat AR, Perez-Reyes M, Hill JM, Sadler BM, Cook CE. Cocaine disposition in humans after intravenous injection, nasal insufflation (snorting), or smoking. *Drug Metab Disposition.* 1989;17:153-159.
19. Javaid JI, Musa MN, Fischman M, Schuster CR, Davis JM. Kinetic of cocaine in humans after intravenous and intranasal administration. *Biopharm Drug Dispos.* 1983;4:9-18.
20. Isenschmid DS, Levine BS, Caplan YH. The role of ecgonine methyl ester in the interpretation of cocaine concentrations in postmortem blood. *J Anal Toxicol.* 1992;16:319-324.
21. Jufer RA, Walsh SL, Cone EJ. Cocaine and metabolite concentrations in plasma during repeated oral administration: development of a human laboratory model of chronic cocaine use. *J Anal Toxicol.* 1998;22:435-444.
22. Jufer RA, Walsh SL, Cone EJ. Plasma concentrations of cocaine and metabolites during chronic cocaine administration in humans. Presentation at Society of Forensic Toxicologists; Snowbird, UT; October 1997.
23. Jufer RA, Wstadik A, Walsh SL, Levine BS, Cone EJ. Elimination of cocaine and metabolites in plasma, saliva, and urine following repeated oral administration to human volunteers. *J Anal Toxicol.* 2000;24:467-477.
24. Isenschmid DS, Levine BS, Caplan YH. A comprehensive study of the stability of cocaine and its metabolites. *J Anal Toxicol.* 1989;13:250-256.
25. Ambre J. The urinary excretion of cocaine and metabolites in humans: a kinetic analysis of published data. *J Anal Toxicol.* 1985;9:241-245.
26. Ambre J, Ruo T, Nelson J, Belknap B. Urinary excretion of cocaine, benzoylecgonine, and ecgonine methyl ester in humans. *J Anal Toxicol.* 1988;12:301-306.
27. Hornbeck CL, Barton KM Czarny RJ. Urine concentrations of ecgonine from specimens with low benzoylecgonine levels using a new ecgonine assay. *J Anal Toxicol.* 1995;19:133-138.
28. Bissel MG. Cocaine. In: Magnani B, Bissell MG, Kwong TC, Wu AHB, eds. *Clinical Toxicology Testing: A Guide for Laboratory Professionals.* Northfield, IL: College of American Pathologists; 2012:112-118.
29. Substance Abuse and Mental Health Services Administration. 2016 National Survey on Drug Use and Health. Methodological Resource Book Section 14: Sample Experience Report. https://www.samhsa.gov/data/sites/default/files/NSDUHmrbSampleExperience2016.pdf. Accessed February 14, 2019.
30. NMS Labs, Willow Grove, PA. Unpublished data, 2015.
31. Higgins ST. Effects of cocaine on human performance and other behavior. Workshop Presentation. Society of Forensic Toxicologists Annual Meeting; Tempe, AZ; October 1993.
32. Tardiff K, Marzuk PM, Leon AC, et al. Cocaine, opiates, and ethanol in homicides in New York City: 1990 and 1991. *J Forensic Sci.* 1995;40:387-390.
33. Isenschmid DS, Hepler BR, Kanluen S. Patterns in drugs of abuse deaths in metropolitan Detroit. Presentation. American Academy of Forensic Sciences; Seattle, WA; 2001. Updated data.
34. Cooper GA, Kronstrand R, Kintz P. Society of Hair Testing guidelines for drug testing in hair. *Forensic Sci Int.* 2012;218:20-24.
35. Mackey-Bojack S, Kloss J, Apple F. Cocaine, cocaine metabolite, and ethanol concentrations in postmortem blood and vitreous humor. *J Anal Toxicol.* 2000;24:59-65.
36. Skoop G, Klingman A, Potsch L, Mattern R. In vitro stability of cocaine in whole blood and plasma including ecgonine as a target analyte. *Ther Drug Monit.* 2001;23:174-181.
37. Taylor RW, Ramirez L. The stability of ethylcocaine in blood. Presentation. California Association of Toxicologists Quarterly Meeting; Reno, NV; February 1999.
38. Baselt RC. Stability of cocaine in biological fluids. *J Chromatogr.* 1983;268:502-505.

39. Klette KL, Poch GK, Czarny R, Lau CO. Simultaneous GC/MS analysis of meta- and para-hydroxybenzoylecgonine and norbenzoylecgonine: a secondary method to corroborate cocaine ingestion using nonhydrolytic metabolites. *J Anal Toxicol.* 2000;24:482-488.
40. Logan BK. Considerations when trying to determine the role of cocaine in death. Presentation. California Association of Toxicologists Quarterly Meeting; San Francisco, CA; February 1998.
41. Blaho K, Logan B, Winbery S, Park L, Schwilke E. Blood cocaine and metabolite concentrations, clinical findings, and outcome of patients presenting to an ED. *Am J Emerg Med.* 2000;18:593-598.

Chapter 21

Amphetamines

Matthew D. Krasowski, MD, PhD
Christine L.H. Snozek, PhD
Stacy E.F. Melanson, MD, PhD

Introduction

Origin

Amphetamine was first synthesized in the 1880s and produced as a pharmaceutical; subsequently, many illicit derivatives of amphetamine have been produced.[1] Methamphetamine, in particular, has become one of the more common illegally produced drugs. Unlike *d*-amphetamine, *d*-methamphetamine is easy to synthesize, and many laboratories producing methamphetamine have been seized by the US Drug Enforcement Administration. Preferred methods of illicit methamphetamine production have changed over time. In recent years, reduction of ephedrine or pseudoephedrine (chemicals commonly found in over-the-counter [OTC] cold medications and diet pills) has become the method of choice. Methamphetamine hydrochloride, the resulting water-soluble white crystalline powder, can then be adulterated with sugars or other cheaper stimulants for distribution. In this form, methamphetamine can be injected intravenously, ingested orally, or inhaled nasally.

Descriptive Chemistry

Amphetamines are a class of phenethylamine compounds with varying degrees of sympathomimetic activity.[2-4] They can be divided into the stimulant/illicit and sympathomimetic amines. The illicit amines include amphetamine and methamphetamine, as well as the "designer" amines 3,4-methylenedioxyamphetamine (MDA) and methylenedioxymethamphetamine (MDMA; covered in chapter 19, *Club Drugs*). Amphetamine and methamphetamine contain a chiral carbon and exist as enantiomers (ie, dextrorotatory [*d*-] and levorotatory [*l*-] forms), with the *d*-isomers possessing higher stimulant properties and the *l*-isomers possessing more pronounced vasoconstrictive properties. The sympathomimetic amines (not covered in detail in this chapter) include ephedrine, pseudoephedrine, phentermine, phenylpropanolamine, and phenylephrine.

Amphetamine

Synonyms: Amfetamine, anfetamina, racemic desoxynorephedrine

Trade names: Adderall, Benzedrine, Dexedrine, Vyvanse

Formula: $C_9H_{13}N$

Molecular mass = 135.2084/135.2062 Daltons

CAS-300-62-9

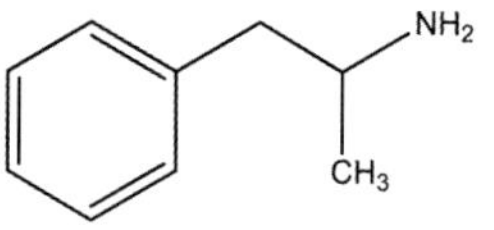

Methamphetamine

Synonyms: Metamfetamine, methylamfetamine, methylamphetamine, phenylmethylaminopropane, *d*-deoxyephedrine, desoxyephedrine

Trade names: Desoxyn, Methedrine

Formula: $C_{10}H_{15}N$

Molecular mass = 149.2328 Daltons

CAS-537-46-2

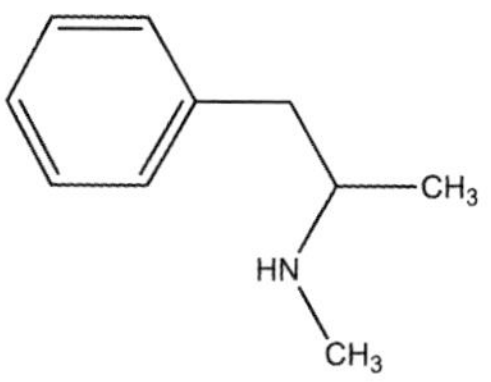

Pharmacology

Intended Uses

Historically, amphetamine has had a variety of medical uses and a legitimate place in the pharmacopeia in the treatment of depression, asthma, anxiety, barbiturate poisoning, Parkinsonism, and enuresis, as well as for appetite suppression and sleep suppression (during wartime). Use of the drug increased markedly in the 1930s when it was found to have similar effects (although with greater potency and lower production cost) to those of the widely used sympathomimetic drug ephedrine, which was extracted from plants of the genus *Ephedra*.[1] Today, the only remaining recognized therapeutic indications for *d*-amphetamines are obesity, narcolepsy, and attention deficit hyperactivity disorder. The levorotatory or *l*-forms of amphetamine and methamphetamine are not potent stimulants but are used in OTC nasal decongestants because of their vasoconstrictive properties.[2-4] The sympathomimetic amphetamines, including ephedrine, phentermine, and phenylpropanolamine, are commonly found in OTC diet pills or nonprescription cold medication.

In recent years, following the recommendations of the Combat Methamphetamine Epidemic Act of 2005, many states have limited availability of these OTC amphetamines to prevent illegal modification of these drugs to more potent illicit amphetamine derivatives, such as *d*-methamphetamine. Federal regulations classify amphetamine and methamphetamine as Schedule II drugs, indicating their high abuse potential and limited therapeutic uses. In contrast, many of the amphetamine derivatives, such as MDMA, are Schedule I (no accepted medical use in the US). See chapter 19 for more information about MDMA and other "club drugs."

Mechanism of Action

As sympathomimetics, amphetamines mimic the actions of endogenous neurotransmitters and are powerful stimulants of the sympathetic nervous system. Amphetamines increase the concentration of dopamine, norepinephrine, and epinephrine in the synaptic cleft by releasing these neurotransmitters from synaptic vesicles and have direct peripheral effects by acting at alpha- and beta-adrenergic receptors.

Pharmacokinetics

Amphetamine and methamphetamine have similar pharmacokinetic properties. Both are well absorbed orally and highly lipid soluble, with a volume of distribution (V_d) of 3 L/kg to 7 L/kg.[5,6] They possess a plasma half-life ($t_{1/2}$) of approximately 10 to 12 hours, with less than 50% of amphetamine or methamphetamine circulating bound to proteins. The bioavailability after oral ingestion ranges from 60% to 70%, whereas the bioavailability after inhalation is as high as 90%. Ingestion of 10 mg of amphetamine or methamphetamine leads to urine concentrations of 0.4 mg/L to 12.0 mg/L. Urine concentrations in abusers, who may be using up to 1500 mg/day, can reach 10 mg/L to 100 mg/L for amphetamine and 300 mg/L for methamphetamine.[5]

Amphetamine is primarily inactivated by deamination to phenylacetone followed by oxidation to benzoic acid and conjugates; however, a small amount is converted to norephedrine. Excretion is dependent on urinary pH, with higher concentrations of the parent drug seen in acidic urine. Under normal conditions, 0.9% is excreted as phenylacetone, 16% to 28% as hippuric acid, 4% as benzoylglucuronide, 2% as norephedrine, 0.3% as conjugated *p*-hydroxynorephedrine, and 2% to 4% as conjugated *p*-hydroxyamphetamine.[5] The presence of methamphetamine in urine after amphetamine ingestion cannot be explained by amphetamine use only; however, it should be noted that low concentrations of methamphetamine (<250 μg/L, or <1% of total amphetamine concentration) have been reported with very high urine amphetamine concentrations (>25 mg/L) presumably due to a manufacturing impurity.[7]

Methamphetamine is demethylated to amphetamine, its major active metabolite. At normal urine pH, up to 43% of the dose is excreted unchanged as methamphetamine, and 4% to 7% of the dose is excreted as amphetamine[5]; another 15% is excreted as free or conjugated *p*-hydroxy-methamphetamine, and the remainder of the metabolites in urine are similar to amphetamine.

Amphetamines have been shown to be very stable in urine, with recoveries ranging from 80% to 100% for specimens stored at room temperature for up to 3 months. Methamphetamine appears to be particularly stable, with near 100% recoveries for urine stored up to 6 months at room temperature or refrigerated (4°C).[8,9]

Amphetamines can be detected in urine within 3 hours of any type of administration and remain detectable for 1 to 3 days after ingestion. Some drugs, such as selegiline (a drug used to treat Parkinson disease), are metabolized to methamphetamine and further to amphetamine, while other drugs, such as fenoproporex and vyvanse, are metabolized directly to amphetamine. It should be noted that the urine of patients on these medications will have detectable levels of amphetamine or methamphetamine, or both.

Abuse Potential and Characteristics

Amphetamines, particularly methamphetamine, are frequently abused for their stimulant and euphoric properties and may be used in combination with other drugs, such as opiates or alcohol, to combat sedative effects. Ingestion of illicit amphetamines can lead to multiple effects, both desirable (wakefulness, decreased appetite, alertness, increased energy, euphoria, elevation of mood, increased ability to concentrate, and increased motor and speech activities) and undesirable (headache, palpitations, dizziness, agitation, confusion, dysphoria, delirium, aggressiveness, and hallucinations). These drugs are highly addictive, and, in extreme cases, addicts may go on "speed runs," in which they continually use the drugs for days at a time without sleeping or eating in order to maintain the "high." Tolerance to these drugs develops rapidly, particularly after intravenous use.

High doses of amphetamines can cause tachycardia, palpitations, anxiety, irritability, aggressiveness, delirium, and hallucinations. Convulsions, unconsciousness, and respiratory and/or cardiac failure may be seen with fatal doses.[5] Although signs and symptoms of the sympathomimetic toxidrome can be confused with anticholinergic ingestion, sympathomimetics do not produce urinary symptoms, dry skin, or hyperactive bowel sounds.

Sympathomimetic effects may be additive with other central nervous system stimulants. Significant interactions can occur in patients taking acidifying agents, adrenergic blockers, tricyclic antidepressants, antihistamines, chlorpromazine, meperidine, phenobarbital, phenytoin, and other medications. In addition, amphetamines should be avoided in patients in agitated states or patients with a history of drug abuse, advanced atherosclerosis, cardiovascular disease, hypertension, hyperthyroidism, or glaucoma. Amphetamines may also contribute to serotonin syndrome when ingested with other serotonergic medications. Patients with serotonin syndrome can exhibit high body temperature, hyperreflexia, sweating, dilated pupils, agitation, and diarrhea.

The minimum lethal dose of amphetamine in nonaddicted adults is estimated to be 200 mg.[5,6] The toxic range of blood concentrations has been reported as 0.2 mg/L to 3.0 mg/L, with fatalities seen at concentrations greater than 1.0 mg/L, although these are rare.[5] Measured urine concentrations in overdose situations can range from 25 mg/L to 700 mg/L. For methamphetamine, blood concentrations in fatalities range from 1.2 mg/L to 5.0 mg/L, and urine concentrations range from 28 mg/L to 320 mg/L.[5]

Analysis

Specimen Types and Characteristics

Testing for amphetamines is performed for a variety of reasons, including detection of amphetamine abuse or toxicity, screening for illicit use in the workplace, or confirmation of an amphetamine overdose for forensic or legal purposes. Several methodologies can be employed to detect amphetamines, such as gas chromatography-mass spectrometry (GC-MS), liquid chromatography-tandem mass spectrometry (LC-MS/MS), and immunoassay.[2-4,10] Urine is the specimen of choice for several reasons, including ease of collection, stability, and longer detection window. Combination chromatography-mass spectrometry techniques, as well as some immunoassays, have been modified for amphetamine testing in blood, postmortem samples, or alternative matrices (eg, hair and meconium). However, amphetamine concentrations are matrix dependent, and optimal cutoff concentrations will vary among matrices.

Oral fluid is an increasingly popular matrix for detection of amphetamine and methamphetamine use/abuse as oral fluid is less subject to adulteration than urine.[11,12] Due to their basic properties, amphetamines can concentrate in oral fluid, and studies have shown that oral fluid is a reliable matrix for the detection of amphetamines.[11,13] Additional information on the use of oral fluids in drug testing can be found in chapter 14, *Alternate Specimens for Drugs-of-Abuse Testing: Oral Fluid.*

Mode of Analysis

Although the approach to amphetamine testing is laboratory dependent, it is common to initially screen urine by an immunoassay, followed by confirmation of presumptive positives with GC-MS or LC-MS/MS. Immunoassays are frequently used to qualitatively screen for amphetamines because they are reliable, automated, relatively inexpensive, and offer a rapid turnaround time.[10] Commonly used cutoff values for screening in urine are 500 ng/mL and 1000 ng/mL. The cutoff of 1000 ng/mL was required for Federal Workplace Drug Testing Programs until May 2010, when the National Laboratory Certification Program lowered the required amphetamine/methamphetamine screening cutoff to 500 ng/mL. This lower cutoff is estimated to identify 5% to 24% more amphetamine-positive urine specimens.[14]

Amphetamines immunoassays are typically calibrated with *d*-amphetamine or *d*-methamphetamine, but the antibodies are generally designed to detect the class of compounds, rather than a specific amphetamine. This broad cross-reactivity can lead to lack of antibody specificity and variable cross-reactivity with other illicit and sympathomimetic amphetamines. Table 21-1 lists the relative cross-reactivities of various amphetamine compounds in selected amphetamine immunoassays; for example, potentially misleading positive results can be triggered by *l*-methamphetamine, one of the active compounds in nasal inhalers and a metabolite of selegiline. Patients taking these medications would be more likely to test positive by the EMIT II Plus, KIMS, and CEDIA assays than the Triage method because of the drug's higher cross-reactivity in the three assays. As another example, phentermine, a member of the amphetamine class used as an appetite suppressant, has higher potential to generate positive results by EMIT II Plus assay than the other testing methods because of its higher relative cross-reactivity in the EMIT II Plus assay (Table 21-1). Amphetamines immunoassays also have variable cross-reactivity for the designer amines, MDMA, MDA, and methylenedioxyethylamphetamine (MDEA; Table 21-1), and therefore it is important for laboratorians and clinicians to

Table 21-1. Relative Cross-Reactivity of Sympathomimetic Compounds Using Commercially Available Reagents at 1000 ng/mL Cutoff

Compound	EMIT- II Plus Amphetamines	KIMS Amphetamines II	CEDIA Amphetamine/ Ecstasy	Triage FIA Methamphetamine
d-Amphetamine	High	High	High*	N/A
d-Methamphetamine	High*	High*	High	High*
d,l-Amphetamine	High	N/A	High	N/A
d,l-Methamphetamine	High	N/A	High	N/A
l-Amphetamine	Moderate	Low	Low	N/A
l-Methamphetamine	High	Moderate	Moderate	Low
MDA	Moderate	High	High	N/A
MDMA	Low	High	High	High
MDEA	Low	High	High	Moderate
PPA	Low	Low	Low	N/A
l-Ephedrine	Low	Low	Low	N/A
Pseudoephedrine	Low	Low	Low	N/A
Phentermine	Moderate	Low	Low	N/A
Phenmetrazine	Moderate	Low	N/A	N/A
Tyramine	Low	Low	N/A	N/A

High = cross-reactivity >50%

Moderate = cross-reactivity 10-50%

Low = cross-reactivity <10%

* Indicates calibrator

EMIT, enzyme multiplied immunoassay technique; KIMS, kinetic interaction of microparticles in solution; CEDIA, cloned enzyme donor immunoassay; FIA, fluorescence immunoassay; N/A, not applicable; MDA, methylenedioxyamphetamine; MDMA, methylenedioxymethamphetamine; MDEA, methylenedioxyethylamphetamine; PPA, phenylpropanolamine.

know whether these compounds will be detected by their amphetamine assays. Some manufacturers offer assays that specifically target MDMA to improve detection of designer drugs (see chapter 19, *Club Drugs*).

Presumptive positives by immunoassay are frequently confirmed using a more specific and sensitive quantitative method, such as GC-MS or, more recently, LC-MS/MS.[2-4] Drugs measured using GC-MS or LC-MS/MS usually include amphetamine, methamphetamine, MDMA, and, less commonly, MDA, MDEA, phentermine, and amphetamine metabolites. Quantitative or qualitative results for OTC amphetamines such as phentermine, ephedrine, pseudoephedrine, and propanolamine may also be included.

In comparison with GC-MS, LC-MS/MS methods usually require little to no sample preparation, smaller sample volumes, and can provide superior selectivity and sensitivity.[15,16] Cutoffs are typically 20 to 100 times lower for LC-MS/MS compared to immunoassay. In addition, specific drugs and/or metabolites are measured (versus a qualitative result for presence of amphetamine drug[s] by immunoassay), which can be helpful to determine the drug(s) ingested. LC-MS/MS methods have also been proposed as more specific and sensitive replacements for traditional immunoassay screening methods in specialized laboratories where the high sample volume or high positivity rates make screening by LC-MS/MS a profitable alternative.

LC-MS/MS methods can be adapted to include chiral derivatization procedures or chiral columns, to distinguish the use of nonprescription nasal inhalants (*l*-methamphetamine) from illicit use (*d*-methamphetamine) or prescription *d*-amphetamine from racemic mixtures present in street amphetamine.[17,18] For example, equal concentrations of the *l*- and *d*-isomer of amphetamine are consistent with illicit amphetamine use, whereas only the *l*-isomer should be detected with selegiline use. However, chiral derivatization assays are more specialized and not routinely offered by most laboratories.

Similar to urine, both immunoassays and LC-MS/MS can be utilized to detect amphetamines in oral fluid. It has been reported that drugs are detected longer in oral fluid, which may be useful for monitoring abuse.[19] One study showed that amphetamine and methamphetamine were detected for up to 8 days in oral fluid.[19]

Known Analytical Issues

Many amphetamine immunoassays are subject to drug-related interferences due to nonspecific antibody binding, which can lead to false-positive results.[10,20-38] Parent drugs and metabolites have been reported to interfere; these include, among others, chloroquine, chlorpromazine and metabolites, bupropion and metabolites, promethazine metabolites, trazodone metabolites, ranitidine, and desipramine. Laboratorians and clinicians should be aware of potentially interfering compounds (sources of false positives) as well as compounds within the amphetamine class that may not be detected (potentially misleading negatives) by their amphetamine assays. Unexpected screening results should be followed up with more specific and/or sensitive confirmation testing when a definitive result is needed.

Despite their higher selectivity and sensitivity, confirmatory methods utilizing combination chromatography-mass spectrometry methods are not completely free from interferences. False-positive methamphetamine results by GC-MS, for example, have been reported for specimens containing high concentrations of ephedrine or pseudoephedrine.[39] In these cases, ephedrine and pseudoephedrine were converted to methamphetamine (resulting methamphetamine concentrations were always <50 ng/mL) by thermoconversion in the injection port of the GC-MS. After these reports, methods utilizing periodate sample pretreatment procedures to selectively oxidize the interfering compounds, combined with lower injection port temperatures, have been shown to effectively remove the interference from these amines. Analysis of a quality control material containing high levels of the interfering sympathomimetic amines is often included with each confirmatory batch to monitor the effectiveness of the pretreatment procedures.

False negatives may also be observed because amphetamines are volatile and can be lost during evaporation steps of extraction procedures or during GC-MS analysis. Preventative measures should be taken to prevent amphetamine losses and potential false negatives by lowering the temperature for evaporation and/or adding methanolic hydrochloride before evaporation in order to produce more stable hydrochloride salts.[14]

Because LC-MS/MS methods require minimal sample preparation and operate at lower temperatures, the potential for losses due to amphetamine volatility and false-positive interferences from thermoconversion of sympathomimetic amines to methamphetamine are minimized. However, GC-MS and LC-MS/MS methods should always be evaluated for interference from other similarly structured sympathomimetic amines, such as ephedrine, norephedrine, hydroxynorephedrine, pseudoephedrine, norpseudoephedrine, phentermine, phenylpropanolamine, and propylhexedrine. This evaluation should include the potential for co-elution with amphetamine, methamphetamine, and MDMA and similarity of their mass ions and ion ratios. Lists of selected mass ions thought to be free from interference from other sympathomimetic amines have been published.[40] Carryover should also be assessed as high concentrations of amphetamines can contaminate subsequent specimens.

Clinical Issues

Interpretation

Interpretation of amphetamine screening results by immunoassay can be challenging. The lack of uniformity among available assays and the relatively poor specificity of the assays can significantly complicate interpretation of positive and negative amphetamines results. The National Academy of Clinical Biochemistry states that for emergency department patients, the less-specific amphetamines immunoassays that will detect a broad spectrum of sympathomimetic, stimulant, and illicit amines are more useful than highly specific amphetamine immunoassays. On the other hand, assays that are more specific for either the illicit amines (such as amphetamine and/or methamphetamine) or the designer amines (such as MDMA or MDEA) are available and may be useful in addiction or chronic pain settings, or in areas with a high rate of illicit amine abuse. It is important to note that even the more-specific amphetamines assays frequently show at least moderate cross-reactivity with other compounds within the amphetamines class because of nonspecific antibody binding.[10] Amphetamines assays also suffer from false-positive results due to other, seemingly unrelated compounds.[20-38] Positive and negative amphetamine screening results must therefore be interpreted in the light of the specific detection characteristics of the assay used. Each laboratory, with the help of its clinicians, must decide which assay cross-reactivity profile and cutoffs are most appropriate for its patient population and which cases warrant confirmation testing using a more specific and/or sensitive method. A question commonly asked by providers is the negative result of the amphetamines immunoassay used in compliance testing of patients on methylphenidate. Although methylphenidate, a stimulant, has many similar clinical indications to *d*-amphetamine, it will not be detected by immunoassays designed to detect amphetamines due to structural differences.

Overdose and Toxicity

If amphetamine toxicity develops, treatment is primarily supportive. However, lowering the urine pH, thereby increasing urine acidity, can enhance the rate of amphetamine elimination. Urine acidification can be accomplished by administering ammonium chloride.[2-4]

References

1. Wills A. *Drugs of Abuse.* 2nd ed. London, England: Pharmaceutical Press; 2005:116-119.
2. Bono JP. *Criminalistics: Introduction to Controlled Substances.* Boston, MA: CRC Press; 1988:23-29.
3. Hoffman BB. *Catecholamines, Sympathomimetic Drugs, and Adrenergic Receptor Antagonists.* New York, NY: McGraw-Hill; 2001:235-241.
4. Moore KA. *Amphetamines.* Washington, DC: AACC Press; 2001:113-126.
5. Baselt RC. *Disposition of Toxic Drugs and Chemicals in Man.* 11th ed. Foster City, CA: Biomedical Publications; 2017.
6. Moffat AC, Osselton MD, Widdop B. *Clarke's Analysis of Drugs and Poisons.* 4th ed. Chicago, IL: Pharmaceutical Press; 2011.
7. Jemionek JF, Addison J, Past MR. Low concentrations of methamphetamine detectable in urine in the presence of high concentrations of amphetamine. *J Anal Toxicol.* 2009;33:170-173.
8. Hughes R, Hughes A, Levine B, Smith ML. Stability of phencyclidine and amphetamines in urine specimens. *Clin Chem.* 1991;37:2141-2142.
9. Jimenez C, de la Torre R, Ventura M, Segura J, Ventura R. Stability studies of amphetamine and ephedrine derivatives in urine. *J Chromatogr B Analyt Technol Biomed Life Sci.* 2006;843:84-93.
10. Melanson SEF. The utility of immunoassays for urine drug testing. In: Bissell MG, ed. *Toxicology Testing.* Philadelphia, PA: WB Saunders Company; 2012.
11. Choo RE, Huestis MA. Oral fluid as a diagnostic tool. *Clin Chem Lab Med.* 2004;42:1273-1287.
12. Conerman T, Gosalia AR, Kabazie AJ, et al. Utility of oral fluid in compliance monitoring of opioid medications. *Pain Physician.* 2014;17:63-70.
13. Vindenes V, Lund HM, Andresen W, et al. Detection of drugs of abuse in simultaneously collected oral fluid, urine and blood from Norwegian drug drivers. *Forsenic Sci Int.* 2012;219:165-171.
14. Broussard LA. Interpretation of amphetamines screening and confirmation testing. In: Dasgupta A, ed. *Handbook of Drug Monitoring Methods.* Totowa, NJ: Humana Press Inc; 2008.
15. Schaefer N, Peters B, Schmidt P, Ewald AH. Development and validation of two LC-MS/MS methods for detection and quantification of amphetamines, designer amphetamines, benzoylecgonine, benzodiazepines, opiates and opioids in urine using turbulent flow chromatography. *Anal Bioanal Chem.* 2013;405:247-258.
16. Comiran E, Barreto F, Meneghini LZ, et al. Method validation and determination of lisdexamfetamine and amphetamine in oral fluid, plasma and urine by LC-MS/MS. *Biomed Chromatogr.* 2017;31(3).
17. Hadener M, Bruni PS, Weinmann W, et al. Accelerated quantification of amphetamine enantiomers in human urine using chiral liquid chromatography and on-line column-switching coupled with tandem mass spectrometry. *Anal Bioanal Chem.* 2017;409:1291-1300.
18. Wang T, Shen B, Shi Y, et al. Chiral separation and determination of R/S-methamphetamine and its metabolite R/S-amphetamine in urine using LC-MS/MS. *Forensic Sci Int.* 2015;246:72-78.
19. Andas HT, Enger A, Oiestad ASL, et al. Extended detection of amphetamine and methamphetamine in oral fluid. *Ther Drug Monit.* 2016;38:114-119.
20. Colbert DL. Drug abuse screening with immunoassays: unexpected cross-reactivities and other pitfalls. *Br J Biomed Sci.* 1994;51:136-146.
21. Crane T, Badminton MN, Dawson CM, Rainbow SJ. Mefenamic acid prevents assessment of drug abuse with EMIT assays. *Clin Chem.* 1993;39:549.
22. Grinstead GF. Ranitidine and high concentrations of phenylpropanolamine cross react in the EMIT monoclonal amphetamine/methamphetamine assay. *Clin Chem.* 1989;35:1998-1999.
23. Jones R, Klette K, Kuhlman JJ, et al. Trimethobenzamide cross-reacts in immunoassays of amphetamine/methamphetamine. *Clin Chem.* 1993;39:699-700.

24. Baron JM, Griggs DA, Nixon AL. The trazodone metabolite meta-chlorophenylpiperazine can cause false-positive urine amphetamine immunoassay results. *J Anal Toxicol.* 2011;35:364-368.
25. Melanson SE, Lee-Lewandrowski E, Griggs DA, Long WH, Flood JG. Reduced interference by phenothiazines in amphetamine drug of abuse immunoassays. *Arch Pathol Lab Med.* 2006;130:1834-1838.
26. Casey ER, Scott MG, Tang S, Mullins ME. Frequency of false positive amphetamine screens due to bupropion using the Syva EMIT II immunoassay. *J Med Toxicol.* 2011; 7:105-108.
27. Merigian KS, Browning RG. Desipramine and amantadine causing false-positive urine test for amphetamine. *Ann Emerg Med.* 1993; 22:1927-1928.
28. Nixon AL, Long WH, Puopolo PR, Flood JG. Bupropion metabolites produce false-positive urine amphetamine results. *Clin Chem.* 1995;41:955-956.
29. Olsen KM, Gulliksen M, Christophersen AS. Metabolites of chlorpromazine and brompheniramine may cause false-positive urine amphetamine results with monoclonal EMIT d.a.u. immunoassay. *Clin Chem.* 1992;38:611-612.
30. Gomilia I, Quesada L, Lopez-Corominas V, et al. Cross-reactivity of chloroquine and hydroxychloroquine with DRI amphetamine immunoassay. *Ther Drug Monit.* 2017;39:192-196.
31. Liu L, Wheeler SE, Rymer JA, et al. Rantidine interference with standard amphetamine immunoassay. *Clin Chim Acta.* 2015;438:307-308.
32. Roberge RJ, Luellen JR, Reed S. False-positive amphetamine screen following a trazodone overdose. *J Toxicol Clin Toxicol.* 2001;39:181-182.
33. Schmolke M, Hallbach J, Guder WG. False-positive results for urine amphetamine and opiate immunoassays in a patient intoxicated with perazine. *Clin Chem.* 1996;42:1725-1726.
34. Smith-Kielland A, Olsen KM, Christophersen AS. False-positive results with Emit II amphetamine/methamphetamine assay in users of common psychotropic drugs. *Clin Chem.* 1995;41:951-952.
35. Johnson-Davis KL, Sadler AJ, Genzen JR. A retrospective analysis of urine drugs of abuse immunoassay true positive rates at a national reference laboratory. *J Anal Toxicol.* 2016;40:97-107.
36. Melanson SE, Baskin L, Magnani B, et al. Interpretaiton and utility of drug of abuse immunoassay: lessons from laboratory drug testing surverys. *Arch Pathol Lab Med.* 2010;134:735-739.
37. Weintraub D, Linder MW. Amphetamine positive toxicology screen secondary to bupropion. *Depress Anxiety.* 2000;12:53-54.
38. Yoo Y, Chung H, Choi H. Urinary methamphetamine concentration following famprofazone administration. *J Anal Toxicol.* 1994;18:265-268.
39. Hornbeck CL, Czarny RJ. Quantitation of methamphetamine and amphetamine in urine by capillary GC/MS, part I: advantages of trichloroacetyl derivatization. *J Anal Toxicol.* 1989;13:144-149.
40. Thurman EM, Pedersen MJ, Stout RL, Martin T. Distinguishing sympathomimetic amines from amphetamine and methamphetamine in urine by gas chromatography/mass spectrometry. *J Anal Toxicol.* 1992;16:19-27.

Chapter 22

Barbiturates

Matthew D. Krasowski, MD, PhD
Christine L.H. Snozek, PhD
Stacy E.F. Melanson, MD, PhD

Introduction

Origin

Barbituric acid was first synthesized in 1864 but was not recognized as having any medicinal value until 1903 when work at Bayer Pharmaceuticals showed that the derivative, barbital, was very effective in anesthetizing dogs. Barbital was then marketed by Bayer under the trade name Veronal. Over 2500 pharmacologically active barbituric acid derivative compounds have been synthesized, and from them a number of drugs have been marketed as anxiolytics, sedative-hypnotics, anticonvulsants, and anesthetic agents.[1] Barbiturates are still used therapeutically as anticonvulsants and anesthetics, but benzodiazepines and other drugs, such as buspirone and zolpidem, are now favored over barbiturates for sedation and anxiety.

Other barbiturates have been steadily declining in clinical usage since the 1970s.[1,2] Mephobarbital was discontinued on the United States market in 2012. Thiopental used to be a core medication in the World Health Organization Model List of Essential Medicines but has since been supplanted by propofol and ketamine for intravenous anesthesia and sedation.[3] Thiopental was discontinued on the US market in 2011 and is also now unavailable in many other countries. Amobarbital, butabarbital, and secobarbital are still available in the US but have not been among the top 400 most prescribed medications since the 1980s.[2] This is a contrast from the 1970s when six barbiturates (amobarbital, butabarbital, butalbital, pentobarbital, phenobarbital, and secobarbital) were among the most highly prescribed medications in the US.

Descriptive Chemistry

Barbiturates are a large class of central nervous system (CNS) depressants derived from barbituric acid (2,4,6-trioxohexahydropyrimidine).[4] Although barbituric acid (Figure 22-1) is inactive, substitution with an aryl or alkyl group at C-5 produces an active compound with sedative and anxiolytic properties. Substitution with a sulfur at C-2 produces the thiobarbiturates, such as thiopental, which are more lipophilic than the oxybarbiturates, which possess an oxygen at C-2. Substitutions can also occur on the nitrogen group as seen in mephobarbital.[1]

Figure 22-1. Barbituric acid.

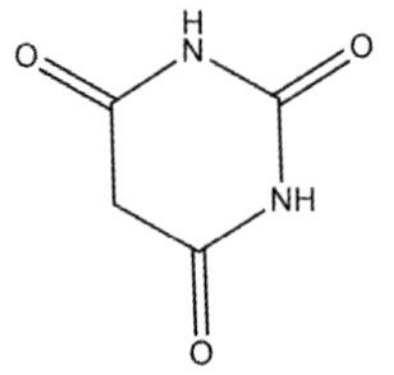

The common barbiturates include amobarbital, butalbital, butabarbital, mephobarbital, pentobarbital, phenobarbital, secobarbital, and thiopental. These drugs may be formulated alone or in combination with other drugs such as acetaminophen and caffeine (eg, Fioricet).

Amobarbital

Synonyms: Amylobarbital, amylobarbitone, pentymalum

Trade name: Amytal

Formula: $C_{11}H_{18}N_2O_3$

Molecular mass = 226.2722 Daltons

CAS-57-43-2

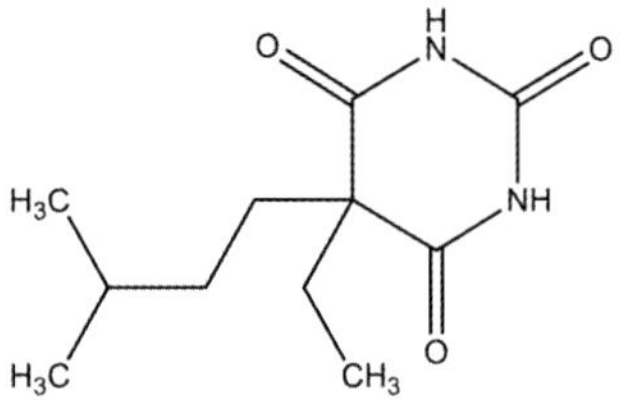

Butalbital

Synonyms: Alisobumilum, allybarbituric acid, itobarbital, tetrallobarbital

Trade names: Sandoptal, Fiorinal, Fioricet

Formula: $C_{11}H_{16}N_2O_3$

Molecular mass = 224.2563 Daltons

CAS-77-26-9

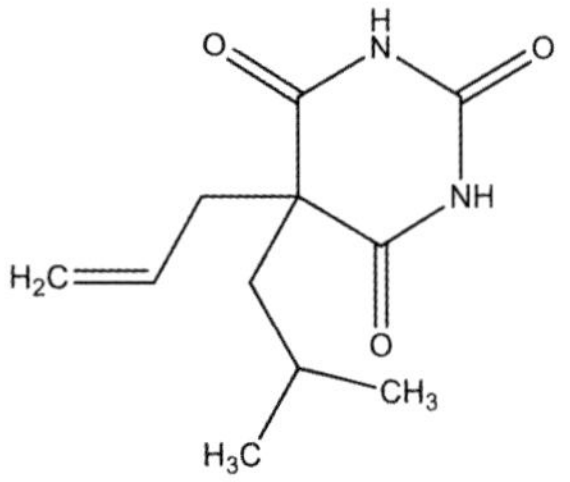

Butabarbital

Synonyms: Butethal, butobarbitalum, butobarbitone

Trade name: Butisol

Formula: $C_{10}H_{16}N_2O_3$

Molecular mass = 212.2456 Daltons

CAS-77-28-1

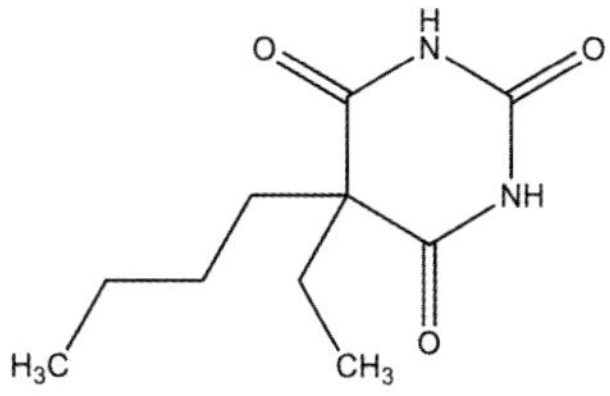

Mephobarbital

Synonyms: Methylphenylbarbital, enphenemalum, methylphenobarbitone, phemitone

Trade name: Mebaral

Formula: $C_{13}H_{14}N_2O3$

Molecular mass = 246.2619 Daltons

CAS-115-38-8

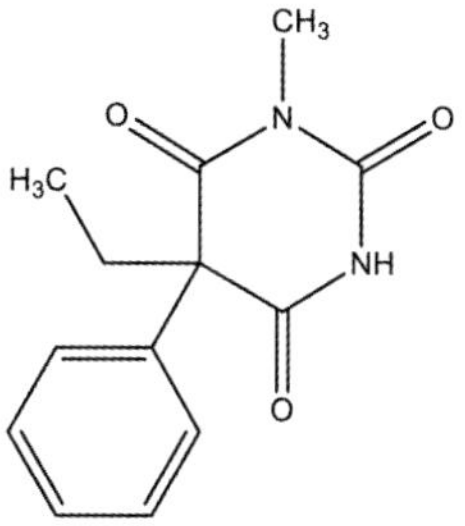

Pentobarbital

Synonyms: Aethaminalum, mebubarbital, mebumal, pentobarbitalum, pentobarbitone

Trade name: Nembutal

Formula: $C_{11}H_{18}N_2O_3$

Molecular mass = 226.2722 Daltons

CAS-76-74-4

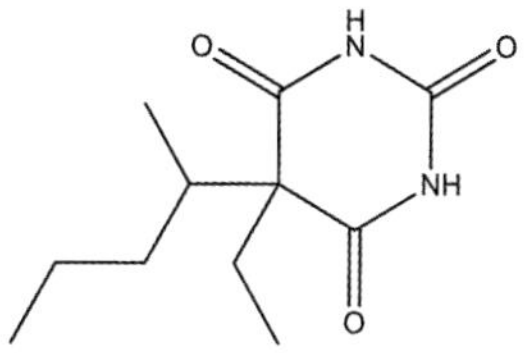

Phenobarbital

Synonyms: Fenobarbital, phenemalum, phenobarbitalum, phenobarbitone, phenylethylbarbituric acid, phenylethylmalonylurea

Trade name: Luminal

Formula: $C_{12}H_{12}N_2O_3$

Molecular mass = 232.2353

CAS-50-06-6

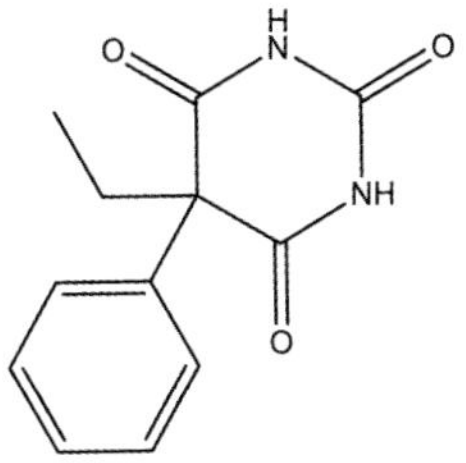

Secobarbital

Synonyms: Meballymal, quinalbarbitone, secobarbitalum, secobarbitone

Trade name: Seconal

Formula: $C_{12}H_{18}N_2O_3$

Molecular mass = 238.2829 Daltons

CAS-76-73-3

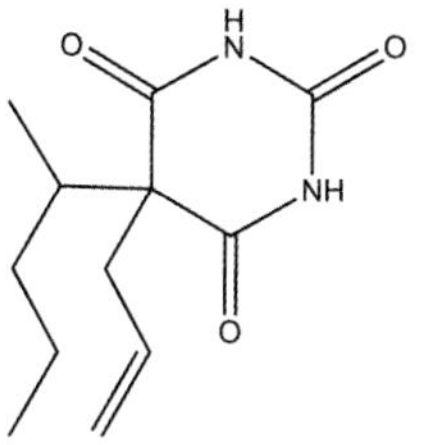

Thiopental

Synonyms: Penthiobarbital, thiomebumal, thiopentone

Trade name: Pentothal

Formula: $C_{11}H_{18}N_2O_2S$

Molecular mass = 242.3378 Daltons

CAS-76-75-5

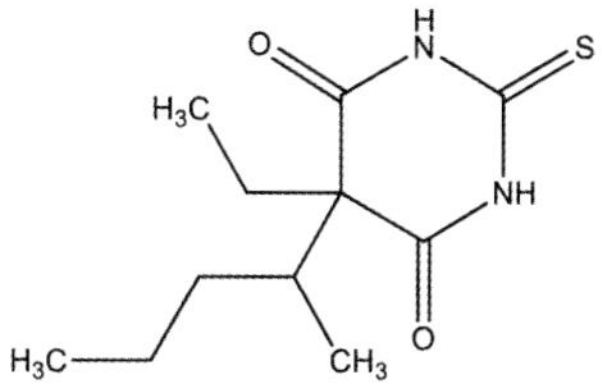

Pharmacology

Intended Uses

Barbiturates have sedative, anxiolytic, anticonvulsant, and anesthetic properties.[1] Ultra-short-acting barbiturates are more commonly used for anesthesia because they depress neuronal activity to a greater extent than longer acting barbiturates. The barbiturates were the dominant sedative-hypnotic medications for several decades starting in the 1950s and were heavily prescribed and misused

Table 22-1. Pharmacokinetic Parameters[4,9]			
Drug	**Plasma Half-Life ($t_{1/2}$, h)***	**Volume of Distribution (V_d, L/kg)***	**Plasma Clearance (mL/min/kg)***
Amobarbital	8-40	~1	~0.5
Butalbital	30-40	0.8	—
Butabarbital	34-42	—	—
Mephobarbital	48-52	2-3	—
Pentobarbital	15-50	~0.7-1.0	~0.3-0.5
Phenobarbital	48-144	~0.5-0.7	~0.06
Secobarbital	19-34	~1.5	~0.8
Thiopental	4-20	0.5-4.0	1-4

* Values are approximate.

as "sleeping pills" and tranquilizers.[1] Barbiturates then found other clinical uses such as anesthesia (pentobarbital, thiopental) and treatment of seizures (phenobarbital) and headaches (butalbital). Thiopental is an induction general anesthetic given intravenously prior to surgery. Intravenous pentobarbital or thiopental can be utilized in patients with severe head trauma or anoxic brain damage to reduce intracranial pressure and decrease cerebral oxygen demand.[5]

Currently, butalbital and phenobarbital are the most commonly utilized barbiturates in the US and the only ones to have any appreciable outpatient usage.[2] Butalbital is available only in combination with other drugs such as acetaminophen for use as a sedative-analgesic. Daily doses of butalbital in these mixtures are 30 mg to 50 mg. Phenobarbital is typically administered orally as an anticonvulsant, with daily oral doses ranging from 60 mg to 200 mg. The anticonvulsant primidone is metabolized to phenobarbital and other related compounds.

Mechanism of Action

Barbiturates produce a state of intoxication that is very similar to ethanol intoxication.[1] The effects of barbiturates range from sedation to hypnosis to coma and occur in a dose-dependent and reversible manner. The sedative stage is characterized by removal of inhibition and relief of anxiety. The hypnotic phase involves sleep induction and an increase in sleep duration. Barbiturate-induced sleep is associated with a decrease in rapid eye movement (REM). As a result, a rebound in REM sleep may be seen after barbiturate cessation.

Barbiturates decrease synaptic neurotransmission by several mechanisms, including directly decreasing release of excitatory neurotransmitters at the glutamate receptor and indirectly decreasing release at the calcium channels.[6,7] Barbiturates also enhance the binding of GABA to its receptor, $GABA_A$, and affect activity at the chloride channel, leading to anesthetic and anticonvulsant effects. However, some barbiturates may produce convulsions by directly depolarizing the neuronal membrane and increasing transmitter release. Inhibition of the reticular activating system is thought to be the reason for the sedative-hypnotic effect.[6]

Pharmacokinetics

As a class, barbiturates are largely nonionic lipid-soluble compounds. The lipid solubility of barbiturates is dependent upon the pK_a, which ranges from 7.3 to 8.0, the proportion of acid (nonionized) and base (ionized) forms in plasma, and the nature of C-5 and C-2 substituents. Nonionized forms of barbiturates, barbiturates with higher pK_a values, and thiobarbiturates, with a sulfur at C-5, in particular, are more lipophilic and will generally have faster onset of action, shorter duration of action, and greater hypnotic potency. Pharmacokinetic properties of the more common barbiturates are summarized in Table 22-1.

Based on their duration of action, barbiturates are commonly grouped into long acting, intermediate acting, short acting, and ultra short acting (Table 22-2).[8]

The *long-acting barbiturate,* phenobarbital, is primarily utilized as an anticonvulsant, hypnotic, and sedative. It is most commonly administered orally but can be given intramuscularly or intravenously. The oral bioavailability of phenobarbital is greater than 80%. The drug is approximately 50%

Table 22-2. Barbiturate Properties Based on Duration of Action[8]

Duration of Action	Barbiturates	Estimated Half-Life	Detection Window in Urine After Last Use	Clinical Use
Long acting	Phenobarbital	2-6 days	10-15 days	Anticonvulsant Sedative/hypnotic
Intermediate acting	Amobarbital Butalbital Butabarbital Mephobarbital	8-80 hours	2-7 days	Anesthetic Sedative/hypnotic
Short acting	Pentobarbital Secobarbital	15-50 hours	2-3 days	Anesthetic Sedative/hypnotic
Ultra short acting	Thiopental	4-46 hours	2-3 days	Preanesthetic

protein bound, with a volume of distribution of 0.5 L/kg to 0.7 L/kg. The usual dose of 2 mg/kg/day produces a steady-state plasma concentration of approximately 20 mg/L. Because of the long half-life of phenobarbital, ranging from 2 to 6 days, steady-state concentrations will not be achieved for several weeks. The window of detection in urine is also extended to 10 to 15 days due to the long half-life. Phenobarbital is an inducer of cytochrome P450 isoenzymes.

Intermediate-acting barbiturates, butalbital, butabarbital, amobarbital, and mephobarbital, may be used as anesthetics, hypnotics, and sedatives. Their half-lives range from 8 to 80 hours, with a detection window of 2 to 7 days. The bioavailability of oral barbiturates, utilized as sedative-hypnotics, is close to 100%, and the onset of action is 10 to 60 minutes. Peak concentrations of amobarbital are achieved after 2 hours.

Short-acting barbiturates, pentobarbital and secobarbital, possess half-lives of 15 to 50 hours and detection windows of 2 to 3 days. Pentobarbital can be administered orally, intramuscularly, rectally, and intravenously. After a single oral dose of 100 mg, peak serum concentrations of 1.2 mg/L to 3.1 mg/L can be achieved at 0.5 to 2.0 hours, whereas plasma concentrations between 25 mg/L to 40 mg/L are seen after repeated intravenous injection.

The *ultra-short-acting barbiturate,* thiopental, is utilized as an anesthetic and has a half-life of 4 to 46 hours and a detection window of 2 to 3 days. Thiopental distributes rapidly into tissues and brain due to its highly lipophilic nature. Redistribution from brain to tissues with less vascular supply, such as muscle and fat, occurs after intravenous injection. This explains why patients awaken within minutes after an anesthetic dose.

Metabolism of barbiturates occurs primarily in the liver where they are first oxidized to more polar alcohols, phenols, ketones, or carboxylic acids.[9] Oxidation of the substituents at the C-5 position is the most important for terminating pharmacological activity. Oxidation is typically followed by conjugation with glucuronic acid and renal excretion. *N*-hydroxylation, desulfuration of thiobarbiturates, and opening of the barbituric acid ring also occurs. *N*-dealkylation of *N*-alkylbarbiturates such as mephobarbital produces active metabolites such as phenobarbital.

As a specific example, phenobarbital is metabolized via *N*-glycosylation and by oxidation to *p*-hydroxyphenobarbital and subsequently conjugated with glucuronic acid. A small amount of dihydroxyphenobarbital is also produced. Approximately 25% to 33% of phenobarbital is excreted unchanged, 24% to 30% is excreted as *N*-glucosylphenobarbital, and 18% to 19% is excreted as free or conjugated *p*-hydroxyphenobarbital. However, this pattern changes with chronic use. The more lipophilic, shorter acting barbiturates undergo more extensive metabolism, and smaller fractions are excreted unchanged (eg, <5% for short acting). Urine concentrations of parent drugs range from 0.7 mg/L to 1.8 mg/L for pentobarbital and 2.5 mg/L to 3.7 mg/L for amobarbital.

Abuse Potential and Characteristics

While clinically effective, a major downside to barbiturates is their danger in overdose, which is magnified when used together with other CNS depressants such as ethanol or opioids.[1] Historically, many high-profile celebrity deaths (eg, Marilyn Monroe, Elvis Presley, Abbie Hoffman) have been attributed at least in part to barbiturate overdose.

In the 1950s, the abuse and physical dependence potential of barbiturates became recognized.[10]

When abused, barbiturates are often taken orally in combination with other sedatives such as ethanol. Chronic users have also been known to dissolve the drug and inject it intravenously. Abusers of barbiturates tend to prefer short-acting and intermediate-acting barbiturates, namely amobarbital, pentobarbital, and secobarbital. Based on the drugs' intoxicating effects, recreational abuse of barbiturates saw a sharp rise in the 1970s but has since declined due largely to the decreased therapeutic use and availability of the drugs. Depending on abuse liability, the barbiturates are found in Schedule II (amobarbital, pentobarbital), III (butalbital), or IV (phenobarbital) in the United States Controlled Substance Schedules.[11] Occasionally, barbiturates are used to offset the withdrawal effects of stimulants such as cocaine and the amphetamines.

In a study in which urine specimens from patients treated for chronic pain were screened for barbiturates, the intermediate-acting barbiturate, butalbital, was detected with the highest frequency.[12] This may be explained by the availability of headache medications that contain butalbital in combination with other medications such as acetaminophen.

Adverse effects from barbiturate use include amnesia and reflex suppression. Barbiturates may also increase the metabolism of other drugs due to their enzyme-inducing properties. In addition, precipitation of acute intermittent porphyria, systemic lupus erythematous-like effects, exfoliative dermatitis, Stevens-Johnson syndrome, and toxic epidermal necrolysis have been reported.

Analysis

Specimen Types and Characteristics

Testing for barbiturates is performed for a variety of reasons including detection of barbiturate abuse or toxicity for clinical purposes, confirmation of a barbiturate overdose for forensic or legal purposes, and screening for nonmedical use in the workplace. Urine is the specimen of choice for detecting recent or remote barbiturate use, based on its ease of collection and longer detection window. Serum testing can be used when assessing therapeutic efficacy or toxicity and can also be useful in acute overdose situations. In addition to qualitative serum barbiturate assays, quantitative drug-specific immunoassays for therapeutic monitoring of primidone and phenobarbital are available and frequently used. Immunoassays have also been used for the therapeutic monitoring of pentobarbital using laboratory-developed modifications of commercial immunoassay for barbiturates.[13,14] Barbiturates can also be analyzed in oral fluid, with stable oral fluid-to-plasma ratios over a 48-hour period.[15]

Modes of Analysis

Several methodologies can be employed to detect barbiturates. These include immunoassay, gas chromatography-mass spectrometry (GC-MS), high-performance liquid chromatography (HPLC), and liquid chromatography-tandem mass spectrometry (LC-MS/MS).[15,16] Although the approach to analysis is laboratory dependent, it is common for a qualitative urine immunoassay screen to be performed, followed by confirmation with GC-MS or LC-MS/MS. Urine immunoassays are frequently used as a front-line screen for barbiturates because they are reliable, automated, relatively inexpensive, and offer a rapid turnaround time. Cutoffs of 200 ng/mL or 300 ng/mL are typically employed, using secobarbital as the calibrator. Unlike many of the drugs-of-abuse immunoassays, the available barbiturate immunoassays are relatively specific for the barbiturate class, and false-positive results are infrequently observed.[17-19] However, barbiturates immunoassays demonstrate variable sensitivity for detecting different barbiturates within the class.[2,12,17]

Known Analytical Issues

Review of data collected from College of American Pathologists (CAP) proficiency surveys from 2011 to 2016 allows for comparison of assay performances. Performance of the urine screening assays across platforms is fairly consistent. Most immunoassays detected urine containing secobarbital, which would be expected based on the fact that secobarbital is frequently used to calibrate the assays.[17] Higher concentrations of phenobarbital and pentobarbital, above 2000 ng/mL, were generally required to produce positive results using both the 200-ng/mL and 300-ng/mL cutoffs. The majority of immunoassays using a 200-ng/mL or 300-ng/mL cutoff were also able to detect 1000 ng/mL or 1250 ng/mL butalbital; however, some immunochromatography methods resulted in less than 10% detection of butalbital at the 300-ng/mL cutoff. This may be concerning since butalbital is one of the two most commonly prescribed barbiturates in the outpatient setting. Amobarbital at 1500 ng/mL was not consistently detected across assays. It is clear from the CAP data that some barbiturates will not be detected by all urine screening assays, even at concentrations well above the assay cutoffs.

Table 22-3. Toxic Dose and Concentrations[4,9]

Drug	Minimum Lethal Dose (g)*	Toxic Plasma Concentration (mg/L)*	Fatal Plasma Concentration (mg/L)*
Amobarbital	1.5	>9	9-72
Butalbital	—	1-10	10-25
Butabarbital	—	—	30-88
Mephobarbital	—	40-60	—
Pentobarbital	2	7.5-30	12-169
Phenobarbital	1.5	4-90	4-120
Secobarbital	2.0	> 8	35-123
Thiopental	1.0	—	6-392

* Values are approximate.

Clinical Issues

Interpretation

Interpretation of qualitative urine immunoassays for barbiturates can be challenging. It is important to emphasize that a negative barbiturate screen does not necessarily mean that barbiturates and/or metabolites are absent in the tested sample. Clinicians may be unaware that immunoassay screens for barbiturates will not detect all barbiturates equally and that misleading negative results may be obtained even for a patient taking relatively high doses of some barbiturates. Negative results may also reflect barbiturate concentrations that fall below the assay cutoff. Laboratorians should review the cross-reactivity profile of their laboratory's barbiturates assays and communicate their findings with clinicians to enable proper interpretation of results. It should also be communicated to clinicians that positive results by immunoassay only indicate the presence of the drug or metabolite in urine and do not indicate or measure intoxication or efficacy of elimination. Follow-up testing using a more sensitive and specific hyphenated chromatographic-mass spectrometric techniques can provide additional information in cases of unexpected negative results or when confirmation of a positive result is required.

Overdose and Toxicity

Intoxication can result in lethargy, confusion, disorientation, and ataxia, while overdose from barbiturates leads to respiratory depression, coma, and death. Estimated minimum lethal doses for selected barbiturates along with corresponding toxic and fatal plasma concentrations are shown in Table 22-3.[4,9] Importantly, the CNS depression caused by barbiturates is additive with other sedative drugs such as ethanol and benzodiazepines, which are frequently co-ingested. Unlike opioids and benzodiazepines, there is no specific antidote to the barbiturates. Management of overdose is thus supportive and consists of supporting the respiratory and cardiac systems until the effects of the drug wear off. Furthermore, in patients with phenobarbital overdose, urine can be alkalinized to promote excretion.

References

1. Mihic SJ, Harris RA. Hypnotics and sedatives. In: Brunton L, Chabner B, Knollman B, eds. *Goodman and Gilman's The Pharmacological Basic of Therapeutics.* 12th ed. New York, NY: McGraw-Hill Co; 2011:457-480.
2. Krasowski MD, Pizon AF, Siam MG, Giannoutsos S, Iyer M, Ekins S. Using molecular similarity to highlight the challenges of routine immunoassay-based drug of abuse/toxicology screening in emergency medicine. *BMC Emerg Med.* 2009;9:5.
3. WHO Model List of Essential Medicines, 2015. http://www.who.int/medicines/publications/essentialmedicines/en/. Accessed May 21, 2019.
4. Moffat AC, Osselton MD, Widdop B. *Clarke's Analysis of Drugs and Poisons.* 3rd ed. Chicago, IL: Pharmaceutical Press; 2004.
5. Roberts I, Sydenham E. Barbiturates for acute traumatic brain injury. *Cochrane Database Syst Rev.* 2012;12:CD000033.
6. Franks NP. Molecular targets underlying general anaesthesia. *Br J Pharmacol.* 2006;147(Suppl 1):S72-81.
7. Krasowski MD, Harrison NL. General anaesthetic actions on ligand-gated ion channels. *Cell Mol Life Sci.* 1999;55:1278-1303.

8. White RM, Black ML. *Pain Management Testing Reference.* Washington, DC: AACC Press; 2007.
9. Baselt RC. *Disposition of Toxic Drugs and Chemicals in Man.* Foster City, CA: Biomedical Publications; 2011.
10. Galanter M, Kleber HD. *The American Psychiatric Publishing Textbook of Substance Abuse.* Arlington, VA: American Psychiatric Publishing, Inc; 2008:417.
11. Schedule of Controlled Substances, 2017. http://www.deadiversion.usdoj.gov/schedules. Accessed February 5, 2019.
12. Cone EJ, Caplan YH, Black DL, Robert T, Moser F. Urine drug testing of chronic pain patients: licit and illicit drug patterns. *J Anal Toxicol.* 2008; 32:530-543.
13. Earl R, Sobeski L, Timko D, Markin R. Pentobarbital quantification in the presence of phenobarbital by fluorescence polarization immunoassay. *Clin Chem.* 1991;37:1774-1777.
14. Humble RM, Ehlers A, Pakalniskis BL, et al. Therapeutic drug monitoring of pentobarbital: experience at an academic medical center. *Ther Drug Monit.* 2015;37:783-791.
15. Fritch D, Blum K, Nonnemacher S, Kardos K, Buchhalter AR, Cone EJ. Barbiturate detection in oral fluid, plasma, and urine. *Ther Drug Monit.* 2011;33:72-79.
16. Zhang X, Lin Z, Li J, et al. Rapid determination of nine barbiturates in human whole blood by liquid chromatography-tandem mass spectrometry. *Drug Test Anal.* 2017;9:588-595.
17. Krasowski MD, Siam MG, Iyer M, Pizon AF, Giannoutsos S, Ekins S. Chemoinformatic methods for predicting interference in drug of abuse/toxicology immunoassays. *Clin Chem.* 2009; 55: 1203-1213.
18. Lu NT, Taylor BG. Drug screening and confirmation by GC-MS: comparison of EMIT II and Online KIMS against 10 drugs between US and England laboratories. *Forensic Sci Int.* 2006;157:106-116.
19. Phillips JE, Bogema S, Fu P, et al. Signify ER Drug Screen Test evaluation: comparison to Triage Drug of Abuse Panel plus tricyclic antidepressants. *Clin Chim Acta.* 2003;328:31-38.

Chapter 23

Benzodiazepines

Christine L.H. Snozek, PhD
Matthew D. Krasowski, MD, PhD
Stacy E.F. Melanson, MD, PhD

Introduction

Origin

The first benzodiazepine, chlordiazepoxide, was discovered accidentally in 1955 and was later marketed as Librium in 1960 by Hoffmann–La Roche. The same company has also marketed diazepam (Valium) since 1963.[1] Diazepam was one of the most prescribed medications of the 1970s and 1980s in the United States. The '70s and '80s also saw the emergence of alprazolam (Xanax), clonazepam (Klonopin), and lorazepam (Ativan), which are now among the most prescribed benzodiazepines in US and many other countries.

Descriptive Chemistry

Benzodiazepines are composed of a benzene ring fused to a diazepine ring and a phenyl ring at the diazepine C_5 position. The chemical structure of common benzodiazepines is shown below. Five positions are available for substitutions and lead to changes in polarity, bioavailability, potency, and duration of action. For example, clonazepam and flunitrazepam contain a chloride and a fluoride, respectively, on the phenyl ring, increasing their potency. Most benzodiazepines are white or yellow crystalline powders with low solubility in water.[2] Chlordiazepoxide and clonazepam are also sensitive to sunlight.

Alprazolam

Synonym: 8-chloro-1-methyl-6-phenyl-4H-[1,2,4]-triazolo-[4,3,a][1,4]-benzodiazepine

Trade names: Niavam, Xanax

Formula: $C_{17}H_{13}ClN_4$

Molecular mass = 308.7649 Daltons

CAS-28981-97-7

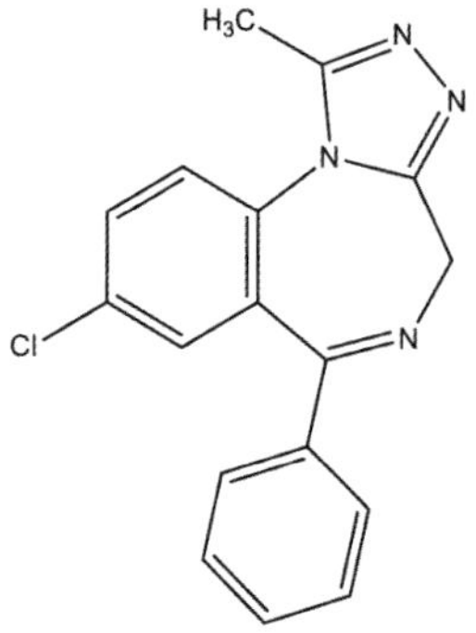

Chlordiazepoxide

Synonyms: Clopoxide, methaminodiazepoxide; 7-chloro-N-methyl-5-phenyl-3H-1,4-benzodiazepin-2-amine-4-oxide

Trade name: Librium

Formula: $C_{16}H_{14}ClN_3O$

Molecular mass = 299.7549 Daltons

CAS-58-25-3

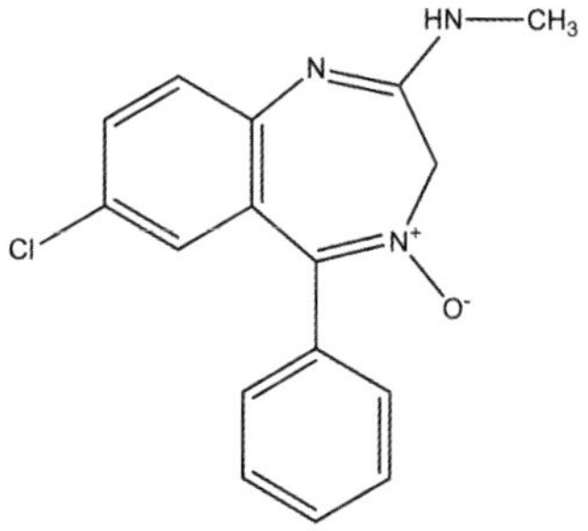

Clonazepam

Synonyms: Ro-5-4023; 5-(2-chlorophenyl)-1,3-dihydro-7-nitro-2H-1,4-benzodiazepin-2-one

Trade names: Klonopin, Rivotril

Formula: $C_{15}H_{10}ClN_3O_3$

Molecular mass = 315.713 Daltons

CAS-1622-61-3

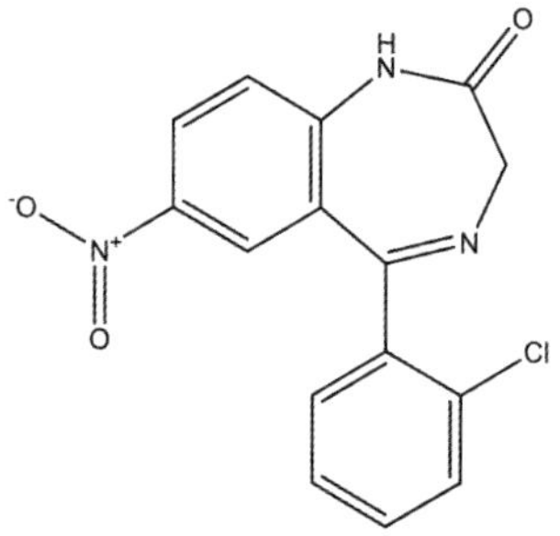

Diazepam

Synonym: 7-chloro-1,3-dihydro-1-methyl-5-phenyl-2H-1,4-benzodiazepin-2-one

Trade name: Valium

Formula: $C_{16}H_{13}ClN_2O$

Molecular mass = 284.7402 Daltons

CAS-439-14-5

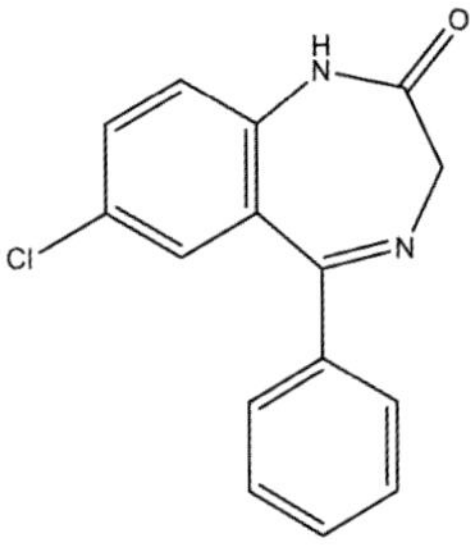

Etizolam

Synonym: 4-(2-chlorophenyl)-2-ethyl-9-methyl-6H-thieno[3,2-f][1,2,4]triazolo[4,3-a][1,4] diazepine

Trade names: Etilaam, Etizest, others

Formula: $C_{17}H_{15}ClN_4S$

Molecular mass = 342.845 Daltons

CAS-40054-69-1

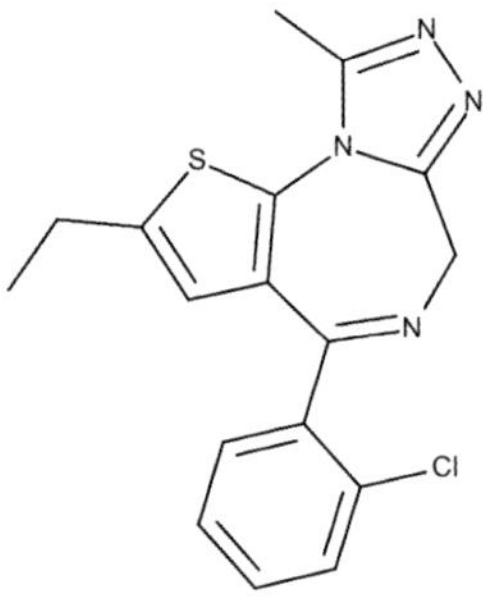

Flunitrazepam

Synonyms: Ro-5-4200; 5-(2-fluorophenyl)-1,3-dihydro-1-methyl-7-nitro-2H-1,4-benzodiazepin-2-one

Trade name: Rohypnol

Formula: $C_{16}H_{12}FN_3O_3$

Molecular mass = 313.2832 Daltons

CAS-1622-62-4

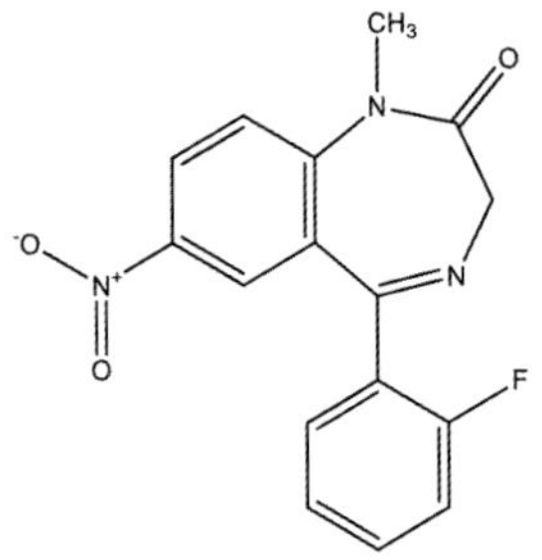

Flurazepam

Synonym: 7-chloro-1-[2-(diethylamino)ethyl]-5-(fluorophenyl)-1,3-dihydro-2H-1,4-benzodiazepin-2-one

Trade name: Dalmane

Formula: $C_{21}H_{23}ClFN_3O$

Molecular mass = 387.8782 Daltons

CAS-17617-23-1

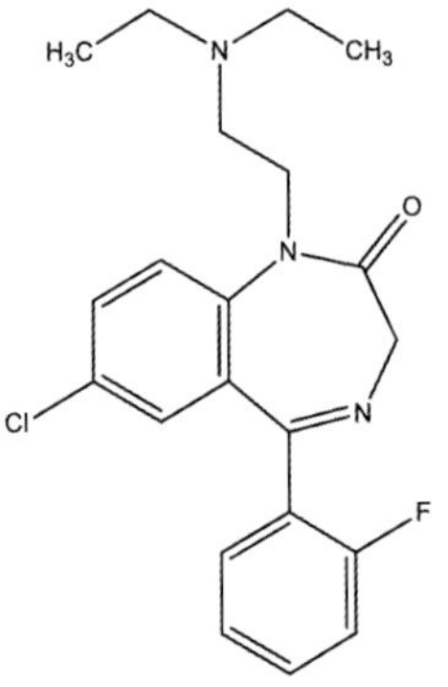

Lorazepam

Synonyms: Lorazepamum, Wy-4036; 7-chloro-5-(2chlorophenyl)-1,3-dihydro-3-hydroxy-2H-1,4-benzodiazepin-2-one

Trade name: Ativan

Formula: $C_{15}H_{10}Cl_2N_2O_2$

Molecular mass = 321.1581 Daltons

CAS-846-49-1

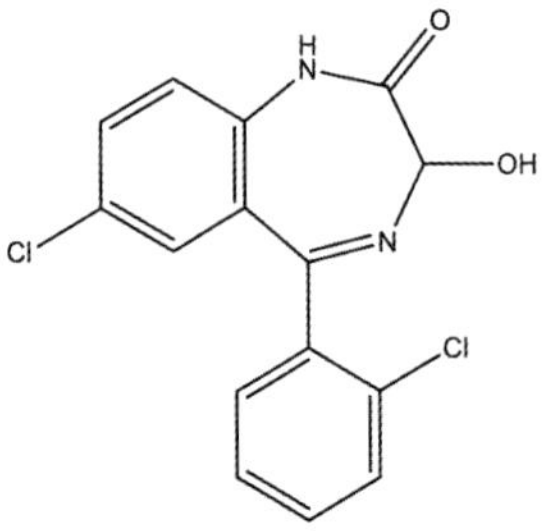

Nordiazepam

Synonyms: A-101, demethyldiazepam, desmethyldiazepam, *N*-desmethyldiazepam, Ro-5-2180

Trade names: Calmday, Madar, Nordaz

Formula: $C_{15}H_{11}ClN_2O$

Molecular mass = 270.7136 Daltons

CAS-1088-11-5

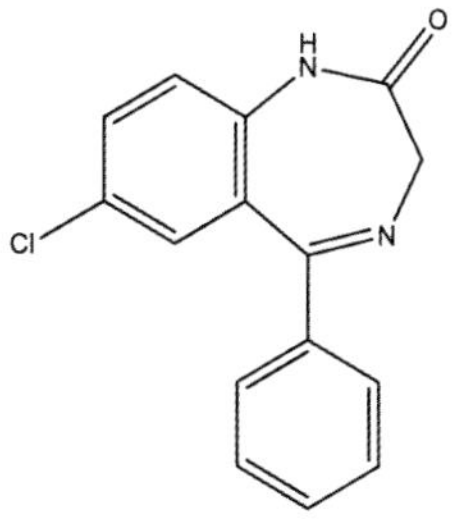

Oxazepam

Synonyms: Oxazepamum, Wy-3498; 7-chloro-1,3-dihydro-3-hydroxy-5-phenyl-2H-1,4-benzodiazepin-2-one

Trade name: Serax

Formula: $C_{15}H_{11}ClN_2O_2$

Molecular mass = 286.7130 Daltons

CAS-604-75-1

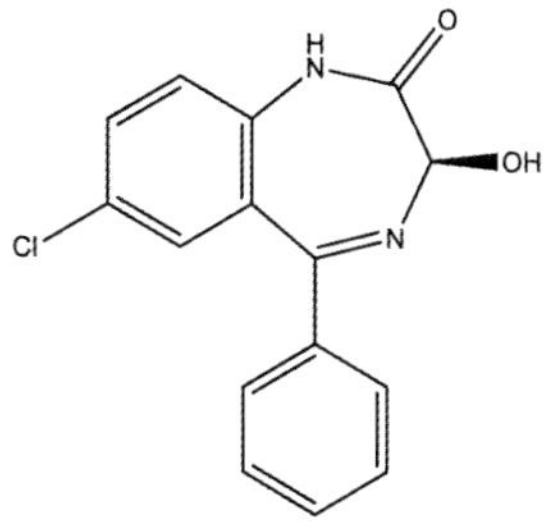

Temazepam

Synonyms: Hydroxydiazepam, methyloxazepam, oxydiazepam; 7-chloro-1,3-dihydro-3-hydroxy-1-methyl-5-phenyl-1,4-benzodiazepin-2-one

Trade name: Restoril

Formula: $C_{16}H_{13}ClN_2O_2$

Molecular mass = 300.742 Daltons

CAS-846-50-4

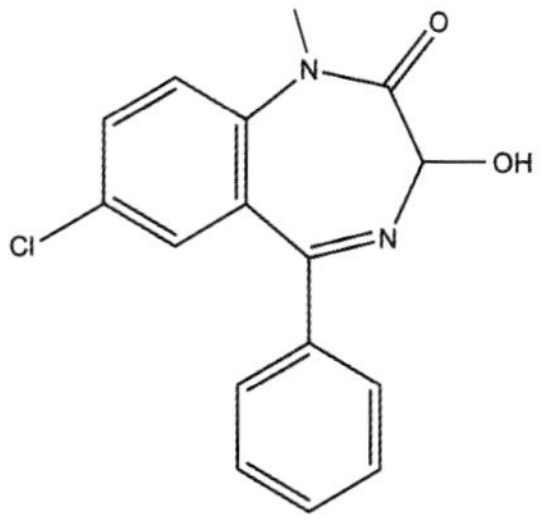

Triazolam

Synonyms: Chlorazolam, U-33030; 8-chloro-6-(-2-chlorophenyl)-1-methyl-4H-[1,2,4]-triazolo[4,3-a]-[1,4]-benzodiazepine

Trade name: Halcion

Formula: $C_{17}H_{12}Cl_2N_4$

Molecular mass = 343.2100 Daltons

CAS-28911-01-5

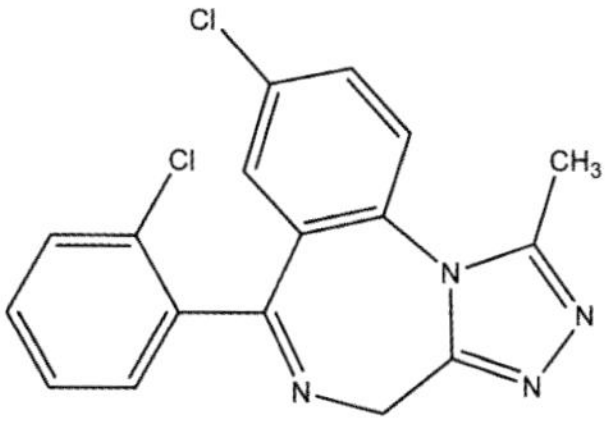

Pharmacology

Intended Uses

Due to their rapid onset of action and relatively low risk of toxicity, benzodiazepines are widely used as sedative/hypnotics, anxiolytics, anticonvulsants, and muscle relaxants. In the US, most benzodiazepines are Schedule IV, although flunitrazepam carries Schedule I penalties due to its association with drug-facilitated assault. Alprazolam, diazepam, lorazepam, and oxazepam are frequently prescribed for anxiety and other indications at typical daily oral doses of 1 mg to 10 mg.[3,4] Lorazepam and diazepam may also be administered before surgery to reduce anxiety in addition to providing anesthesia. Psychiatric disorders such as panic disorders with or without agoraphobia can be successfully managed with alprazolam and clonazepam, usually at doses higher than those prescribed for anxiety. Numerous benzodiazepines, including clonazepam, diazepam, lorazepam, and clobazam, are used to treat seizures. Chlordiazepoxide, as well as other benzodiazepines, may be used to treat delirium tremens in patients suffering from ethanol withdrawal. Based on its muscle-relaxing action, diazepam may be used to treat status epilepticus and muscle spasticity. The short-acting benzodiazepines, triazolam and flurazepam, can be used in patients with insomnia, although tolerance is a concern. Temazepam is also indicated for short-term treatment of insomnia. Etizolam is prescribed in some Asian countries for anxiety and sleep disorders, although its use in the US and Europe is primarily recreational. Flunitrazepam has no therapeutic indication, and its import is banned in the US due to its use as a "date rape" drug.

Table 23-1. Pharmacologic and Pharmacokinetic Properties of Benzodiazepines

Drug	Classification	Active Metabolite(s)	Estimated Half-Life ($t_{½}$, h)*	Detection Window in Urine After Last Use (Days)*	Volume of Distribution (V_d, L/kg)*
Alprazolam	Intermediate acting	α-Hydroxy alprazolam	11-15	2-5	<1
Chlordiazepoxide	Intermediate acting	Nordiazepam Oxazepam	5-30	2-5	<1
Clonazepam	Intermediate acting	7-Amino clonazepam	20-40	2-5	>1
Diazepam	Long acting	Nordiazepam Oxazepam Temazepam	20-40	7-10	0.5-2.5
Etizolam	Short acting	α-Hydroxy etizolam	3-17	2-5	<1
Flunitrazepam	Intermediate acting	7-amino flunitrazepam	6-24	2-5	>1
Flurazepam	Short acting	Hydroxyethyl-flurazepam	2-3	1-2	>1
Lorazepam	Intermediate acting	None	9-24	2-5	>1
Nordiazepam	Long acting	Oxazepam	Variable, but typically >24	7-10	0.5-2.5
Oxazepam	Intermediate acting	None	4-15	2-5	0.5-2.5
Temazepam	Intermediate acting	Oxazepam	8-20	2-5	>1
Triazolam	Short acting	α-Hydroxy triazolam	1.5-3	1-2	>1

* Values are approximate.

Mechanism of Action

Benzodiazepines have anxiolytic, sedative-hypnotic, muscle relaxant, and anticonvulsant properties.[3,4] Sedation occurs at lower doses, whereas hypnosis occurs at higher doses. Notably, benzodiazepines lack autonomic nervous system, antipsychotic, and extrapyramidal effects. The binding of benzodiazepines to a single benzodiazepine binding site on the $GABA_A$ receptor induces a conformational change in the receptor, which increases receptor binding to GABA, leading to higher chloride influx, hyperpolarization, and inhibition of neuronal firing. Central nervous system (CNS) receptors in the thalamus, limbic system, and cerebral cortex have high affinity for benzodiazepines, while peripheral receptors have a lower affinity.[3] The pharmacologic activity and potency of benzodiazepines vary widely depending upon the affinity of each benzodiazepine for the benzodiazepine receptor.

Pharmacokinetics

Table 23-1 provides a summary of the pharmacokinetic properties of benzodiazepines.[2] All benzodiazepines are well absorbed from the gastrointestinal tract, with bioavailabilities >90% in most cases. Peak plasma concentrations are observed within 30 to 90 minutes after oral administration.[2] Approximately 70% to 90% of benzodiazepines in the plasma are protein bound. Volumes of distribution vary between the benzodiazepines, with alprazolam, chlordiazepoxide, and etizolam having the smallest volume of distribution of <1.0 L/kg, while clonazepam, flunitrazepam, lorazepam, temazepam, and triazolam have larger volumes of distribution of >1.0 L/kg. Diazepam, nordiazepam, and oxazepam have volumes of distributions ranging between 0.5 L/kg to 2.5 L/kg. Most benzodiazepines, with the exception of oxazepam, are lipid soluble and readily cross the blood-brain barrier.[2,5] Due to their lipid solubility, they also pass into breast milk and cross the placenta.

Benzodiazepines undergo extensive hepatic metabolism by dealkylation, demethylation, hydroxylation, and conjugation, often forming metabolites with pharmacologic activity. For example, many of the benzodiazepines are metabolized to oxazepam (Table 23-1), a pharmacologically active benzodiazepine, which is then inactivated and excreted as a glucuronide conjugate.[6] Most benzodiazepines are inactivated via glucuronidation as the only or most important metabolic transformation. The urine primarily contains free and conjugated metabolites, and parent compounds are typically not detected unless a test incorporates preanalytical hydrolysis.

Abuse Potential and Characteristics

Benzodiazepines are frequently abused for their euphoric properties, particularly those with short half-lives (eg, alprazolam, etizolam) and high lipophilicity (eg, diazepam). It is common for the benzodiazepines to be abused in combination with other addictive substances such as ethanol. Benzodiazepines are also frequently diverted to street use and as such have been utilized to sedate others for so-called drug-facilitated sexual assault or date rape. Recently, newer benzodiazepines (eg, clonazolam, deschloroetizolam, flubromazepam, pyrazolam) have emerged as designer drugs and are often high potency; designer drugs are discussed in chapter 26, *Novel Psychoactive Substances*. Many of these compounds are neither approved nor scheduled in the US, although some, like etizolam, are used medically in other countries.[7,8]

Analysis

Specimen Types and Characteristics

Urine has historically been the specimen of choice to detect benzodiazepine use and abuse, based on its ease of collection and longer detection window, but serum, oral fluid, and other specimen types can also be used. Screening for benzodiazepines by immunoassay can be a valuable aid in evaluating an unknown cause of CNS depression. Benzodiazepines may be quantified by gas chromatography or liquid chromatography coupled to mass spectrometry, but quantification is generally unwarranted in overdose situations because neither serum nor urine concentrations are predictive of dose exposure or severity of intoxication.

Modes of Analysis

Testing for benzodiazepines is typically performed in the clinical setting to detect benzodiazepine toxicity, compliance with therapy, and potential abuse. Benzodiazepine testing is also performed in forensic and occupational toxicology. Several methodologies can be employed to detect benzodiazepines including immunoassay, gas chromatography-mass spectrometry (GC-MS), high-performance liquid chromatography (HPLC), and liquid chromatography-tandem mass spectrometry (LC-MS/MS).[9] Although the approach to analysis is laboratory dependent, front-line testing commonly includes a benzodiazepine immunoassay screen, after which presumptive positives may or may not be confirmed by a more specific method such as GC-MS or LC-MS/MS, depending on the clinical scenario.[4]

Urine confirmation cutoffs are typically ≤100 ng/mL, with recommended cutoffs in the setting of drug-facilitated assault at 5 ng/mL to 10 ng/mL.[10] An enzymatic hydrolysis pretreatment with β-glucuronidase can be performed prior to confirmatory testing to improve sensitivity for benzodiazepines that are excreted primarily as glucuronide conjugates; alternatively, conjugated metabolites can be reported in addition to parent drugs in confirmation assays. Acid hydrolysis is not recommended because this process leads to the formation of benzophenones, some of which are common between various benzodiazepines, making interpretation more difficult. Due to the polar nature of benzodiazepines, GC-MS methods require a derivatization step prior to analysis, usually to trimethylsilyl derivatives, while LC-MS/MS offers the advantage that derivatization is unnecessary.

Urine confirmation testing panels generally include, at a minimum, oxazepam, nordiazepam, diazepam, temazepam, lorazepam, α-hydroxyalprazolam, and 7-aminoclonazepam. Other benzodiazepines and their metabolites, eg, glucuronide conjugates for assays that do not involve a pre-extraction hydrolysis, may also be included. Some, like etizolam and flunitrazepam, are more commonly included in designer drug and/or drug-facilitated assault panels. Several benzodiazepines have shared metabolites, so that detection of a single metabolite alone, such as oxazepam, will not allow determination of the specific benzodiazepine ingested.

Known Analytical Issues

Immunoassays are frequently employed to qualitatively screen for benzodiazepines because they are reliable, automated, relatively inexpensive, and offer a rapid turnaround time. While currently available immunoassays can reliably detect longer acting benzodiazepines and some of the designer benzodiazepines,[11,12] they suffer from variable and often poor sensitivity for newer, shorter acting benzodiazepines. Common cutoff concentrations of 200 ng/mL or 300 ng/mL were established years ago when less potent and longer acting benzodiazepines, such as diazepam, were primarily prescribed. These same cutoffs may not be low enough to detect the shorter acting and more potent benzodiazepines, such as lorazepam, alprazolam, and flunitrazepam. It should also be noted that even confirmatory methods may fail to detect the more potent and rapidly metabolized benzodiazepines such as clonazepam, triazolam, and flunitrazepam.

Sensitivity of the immunoassays for the various benzodiazepines and their metabolites also varies within and across assays.[13-16] Most urine benzodiazepine assays have antibodies that are designed to detect either parent compounds or unconjugated metabolites, such as oxazepam. However, many commonly prescribed benzodiazepines, such as lorazepam and clonazepam, and the illicitly used flunitrazepam are excreted primarily as metabolites (lorazepam-glucuronide, 7-aminoclonazepam, and 7-aminoflunitrazepam, respectively), which generally have substantially lower cross-reactivities in the assays. Including a β-glucuronidase pretreatment step can improve assay sensitivity for highly glucuronidated benzodiazepines such as lorazepam. However, pretreatment is time consuming and not practical if results are needed emergently; in addition, pretreatment may not increase sensitivity of immunoassays sufficiently to meet clinical needs.[16] Enzyme-linked immunosorbent assay (ELISA) methods for sensitive and specific detection of the primary flunitrazepam metabolite, 7-aminoflunitrazepam, have also been developed. It is important for laboratorians and clinicians to know which compounds will be detected by their benzodiazepine assays and be aware that false-negative results can be observed even in patients with high urine concentrations of benzodiazepines, particularly flunitrazepam, alprazolam, clonazepam, and lorazepam. On-line hydrolysis or a redesign of the assays such that the antibody will detect conjugated metabolites in urine is necessary to improve performance. In the absence of a sufficiently sensitive immunoassay, direct analysis by a more sensitive method such as GC-MS or LC-MS/MS may be indicated.[17,18]

Sensitivity is also a concern for benzodiazepine testing in oral fluid. Oral fluid is an increasingly common matrix for testing, particularly in setting such as roadside collections for suspected drugged driving and when urine adulteration is a concern.[19] Many benzodiazepines are only present in low (<1 ng/mL) concentrations in oral fluid, which likely contributes to the poor sensitivity for these drugs that has been published in some studies.[20] However, oral fluid does have the benefit that most benzodiazepines are present as parent rather than metabolite,[19] which addresses some of the concerns with urine testing described above.

False-positive results can be obtained when immunoassay screening for benzodiazepines is performed due to nonspecific antibody binding. Commonly prescribed drugs, including the arthritis medication oxaprozin (Daypro),[21] the antiviral efavirenez,[22] and the antidepressant sertraline,[23] can cross-react with some benzodiazepine assays, producing a false-positive response. Due to the limitations of current urine benzodiazepine assays, clinicians should be aware that screen results are presumptive and that confirmatory testing may be necessary. However, especially with the emergence of several newer benzodiazepines onto the illicit drug market, clinicians and laboratorians should be aware that apparently false-positive results by immunoassay might reflect use of a benzodiazepine not included in a given confirmatory panel, consistent with a false-negative result by the confirmation method.

Clinical Issues

Interpretation

Clinicians are frequently unaware that benzodiazepine immunoassay screening methods do not detect all drugs within the class equally[24] and that false-negative and false-positive results may be observed. For these reasons, the National Academy of Clinical Biochemistry (now the AACC Academy) cautions against the use of immunoassay screens for benzodiazepines.[17,18] If benzodiazepines screens are utilized, the laboratory should assist with result interpretation. The cross-reactivity profile for the laboratory's benzodiazepine assays, as well as a list of possible interferences, should be available to clinicians. Results should also be reported as presumptive positive or presumptive negative according to a defined cutoff value to assist with interpretation. It is important to emphasize that negative results may reflect concentrations that are below the sensitivity limits of the assay and do not necessarily exclude the presence of the drug or metabolite. It should also be clarified that presumptive positive results only indicate the presence of a cross-reacting drug or metabolite and do not indicate or measure intoxication or efficacy of elimination. A positive benzodiazepines screening

Table 23-2. Toxic Dose and Concentrations[2,6,25]

Drug	Lethal Dose (g)*	Toxic Plasma Concentration (mg/L)*	Blood Concentration in Fatalities (mg/L)*
Alprazolam	—	0.1-0.4	0.12-2.1
Chlordiazepoxide	>2	>3	20-26
Clonazepam	>1	>0.1	>1
Diazepam	>2	3-5	>5
Etizolam	—	>0.03	—
Flunitrazepam	—	>0.1	0.45
Flurazepam	>2	>0.2	>0.5
Lorazepam	—	0.3-0.6	0.5
Nordiazepam	—	1.5-2	—
Oxazepam	—	>2	> 3
Temazepam	—	>1	>8
Triazolam	>0.002	>0.04	>0.12

* Values are approximate.

result also cannot be used to establish which benzodiazepine is ingested or differentiate recent versus long-term use or compliance versus abuse. In the emergency department setting, lorazepam and other benzodiazepines may be used for sedation and agitation control before specimen collection, making positive results even more difficult to interpret. More sensitive and specific confirmatory testing should be performed when it is important to know which benzodiazepines are present, when testing results do not match the clinical picture, or when definitive results are necessary. It should also be noted that some benzodiazepines (eg, diazepam, nordiazepam) can be detected for an extended period after the last dose due to long half-lives of both the parent drug and metabolites.

Overdose and Toxicity

Benzodiazepines possess a very high therapeutic index, and the adverse effects are generally minor.[3,4] However, hypotension, tachycardia, palpitations, amnesia, ataxia, and behavioral disturbances can be seen. Due to the central disinhibition, a paradoxical rage or psychosis may be induced by benzodiazepines. Respiratory depression may also occur from high doses, especially in children or the elderly, or when used in conjunction with other CNS depressants such as ethanol.

One of the more frequent and important side effects of benzodiazepines is the occurrence of tolerance and dependence. Tolerance to the hypnotic effects develops more rapidly than tolerance to the anxiolytic effects. If a dependent patient stops medicating, convulsions, muscle cramps, abdominal cramps, and sweating can result. In 1993, the United Kingdom removed triazolam (Halcion), which was primarily prescribed for insomnia, from the market due to its adverse effects, rapid development of tolerance, and rebound insomnia (when treatment stopped), particularly in the elderly. The US Food and Drug Administration did not ban triazolam but revised the labeling to ensure the drug was used for short-term (7-10 days) treatment of insomnia and to recommend lower doses in the elderly. Estimated toxic dose and concentration information is summarized in Table 23-2.[2,6,25]

Benzodiazepine overdose and toxicity may be treated with the receptor antagonist, flumazenil. Multiple treatments are needed for the longer acting benzodiazepines, and care should be taken to avoid precipitation of withdrawal symptoms and seizure.

References

1. Shorter E. Benzodiazepines. In: Shorter E. *A Historical Dictionary of Psychiatry*. London, UK: Oxford University Press; 2005:41-42.
2. Moffat AC, Osselton MD, Widdop B. *Clarke's Analysis of Drugs and Poisons*. 3rd ed. Chicago, IL: Pharmaceutical Press; 2004.

3. Theoharides TC. *Essentials of Pharmacology.* 2nd ed. Boston, MA: Little, Brown and Company; 1992:479.
4. Fraser AD. *Psychotropic Agents: The Benzodiazepines.* Washington, DC: AACC Press; 2001:211-221.
5. Etizolam. https://pubchem.ncbi.nlm.nih.gov/compound/3307. Accessed May 21, 2019.
6. Baselt RC. *Disposition of Toxic Drugs and Chemicals in Man.* 8th ed. Foster City, CA: Biomedical Publications; 2008.
7. Etizolam. Drug Enforcement Agency. https://www.deadiversion.usdoj.gov/drug_chem_info/etizolam.pdf. Accessed May 21, 2019.
8. Moosmann B, King LA, Auwärter V. Designer benzodiazepines: a new challenge. *World Psychiatry.* 2015;14(2): 248.
9. Bono JP. *Criminalistics: Introduction to Controlled Substances.* Boca Raton, FL: CRC Press; 1988: 23-29.
10. Recommended Minimum Performance Limits for Common DFC Drugs and Metabolites in Urine Samples. Society of Forensic Toxicologists. http://www.soft-tox.org/files/MinPerfLimits_DFC2017.pdf. Accessed May 21, 2019
11. O'Connor LC, Torrance HJ, McKeown DA. ELISA detection of phenazepam, etizolam, pyrazolam, flubromazepam, diclazepam and delorazepam in blood using Immunalysis® Benzodiazepine Kit. *J Anal Toxicol.* 2016;40(2):159-161.
12. Bertol E, Vaiano F, Furlanetto S, Mari F. Cross-reactivities and structure-reactivity relationships of six benzodiazepines to EMIT® immunoassay. *J Pharm Biomed Anal.* 2013;84:168-172.
13. Fraser AD, Meatherall R. Comparative evaluation of five immunoassays for the analysis of alprazolam and triazolam metabolites in urine: effect of lowering the screening and GC-MS cut-off values. *J Anal Toxicol.* 1996;20:217-223.
14. Way BA, Walton KG, Koenig JW, Eveland BJ, Scott MG. Comparison between the CEDIA and EMIT II immunoassays for the determination of benzodiazepines. *Clin Chim Acta.* 1998;271:1-9.
15. DeRienz RT, Holler JM, Manos ME, Jemionek J, Past MR. Evaluation of four immunoassay screening kits for the detection of benzodiazepines in urine. *J Anal Toxicol.* 2008;32:433-437.
16. Darragh A, Snyder ML, Ptolemy AS, Melanson S. KIMS, CEDIA, and HS-CEDIA immunoassays are inadequately sensitive for detection of benzodiazepines in urine from patients treated for chronic pain. *Pain Physician.* 2014;17(4):359-366.
17. Wu AH, McKay C, Broussard LA, et al. National Academy of Clinical Biochemistry laboratory medicine practice guidelines: recommendations for the use of laboratory tests to support poisoned patients who present to the emergency department. *Clin Chem.* 2003;49:357-379.
18. Langman LJ, Jannetto PJ, eds. AACC Academy Laboratory Medicine Practice Guidelines: Using clinical laboratory tests to monitor drug therapy in pain management patients. https://www.aacc.org/science-and-practice/practice-guidelines/using-clinical-laboratory-tests-to-monitor-drug-therapy-in-pain-management-patients. Accessed May 21, 2019.
19. Allen KR. Screening for drugs of abuse: which matrix, oral fluid or urine? *Ann Clin Biochem.* 2011;48:531-541.
20. Verstraete AG. Oral fluid testing for driving under the influence of drugs: history, recent progress and remaining challenges. *Forensic Sci Int.* 2005;150:143-150.
21. Fraser AD, Howell P. Oxaprozin cross-reactivity in three commercial immunoassays for benzodiazepines in urine. *J Anal Toxicol.* 1998;22:50-54.
22. Blank A, Hellstern V, Schuster D, et al. Efavirenz treatment and false-positive results in benzodiazepine screening tests. *Clin Infect Dis.* 2009; 48:1787-1789.
23. Nasky KM, Cowan GL, Knittel DR. False-positive urine screening for benzodiazepines: an association with Sertraline?: a two-year retrospective chart analysis. *Psychiatry (Edgmont).* 2009;6:36-39.
24. Durback LF, Scharman EJ, Brown BS. Emergency physicians' perceptions of drug screens at their own hospitals. *Vet Hum Toxicol.* 1998;40:234-237.
25. Schulz M, Iwersen-Bergmann S, Andresen H, Schmoldt A. Therapeutic and toxic blood concentrations of nearly 1,000 drugs and other xenobiotics. *Crit Care.* 2012;16(4):R136.

Chapter 24

Opioids I: Opiates and Semisynthetic Opioids

Matthew D. Krasowski, MD, PhD
Gwendolyn A. McMillin, PhD

Introduction

Opioids are a diverse group of substances that bind to one or more opioid receptors, which are primarily located in the central nervous system (CNS) and gastrointestinal (GI) tract.[1] The opioids in general are classified as narcotic analgesics and CNS depressants. Medically, opioids are primarily used for pain control but also exhibit antitussive and other therapeutic actions. Of major concern is the widespread use of opioid drugs for nonmedical or recreational purposes, which has contributed to escalating rates of addiction, drug overdoses, and drug-related deaths.[2-5] Opioids are often described based on origin: endogenous (eg, endorphins), natural opiates (ie, derived from the opium poppy), semisynthetic (ie, derived from natural opiates), synthetic (ie, prescription drugs exhibiting activity at the opioid receptors but not of endogenous or natural origin), and designer (ie, nonprescription drugs exhibiting activity at the opioid receptors but not of endogenous or natural origin). Although endogenous opioids may become commercialized drugs someday, a detailed discussion of endogenous opioids is beyond the scope of this book.[6,7] This chapter will cover the common opiates as well as semisynthetic opioids including heroin, hydrocodone, hydromorphone, oxycodone, and oxymorphone. Natural opiates other than morphine and codeine are not emphasized.

Origin

The term *opium* comes from the Greek word for juice, *opos*. Opium is the viscous fluid within the unripe capsule of the flowering head of the opium poppy and is the source of the natural opiates. The history of opium extends at least as far as 300 BCE wherein Theophrastus describes opium distributed by Helen, the daughter of Zeus, to help alleviate grief and suffering. As early as the 8th century, opium was being traded throughout Asia, Europe, India, and other parts of the world. Abuse of and tolerance to opium is described in the 16th century. In 1806, the active ingredient of opium was isolated and named "morphine" after the god of dreams.[8] Morphine accounts for approximately 10% of the weight of dried opium and is responsible for most of the characteristic analgesic and psychotropic effects. During the American Civil War, opiates were widely utilized and many soldiers developed an addiction to morphine.[9] In addition to morphine and codeine, the opium poppy produces many compounds, among which are a variety of alkaloids including thebaine, papaverine, and noscapine. In 1898, diacetylmorphine (heroin) was produced as the first commercial semisynthetic opioid. Heroin was derived from morphine and is metabolized to morphine but was originally marketed as a cough remedy that exhibited less abuse potential than morphine. Other semisynthetic opioids emerged on the market including hydrocodone, oxycodone, and the more potent analogs hydromorphone and oxymorphone. The semisynthetic opioids are simple chemical modifications of natural opiates. Thus, hydrocodone and hydromorphone are morphine derivatives, while oxycodone and oxymorphone are thebaine derivatives. The codeine derivative dihydrocodeine (hydrocodol) is a semisynthetic opioid that is also a metabolite of hydrocodone. Dihydrocodeine is co-formulated for antitussive properties with acetaminophen and caffeine (eg, Panlor) or with aspirin and caffeine for moderate to severe pain (eg, Synalgos), but dihydrocodeine is not routinely targeted in clinical drug testing and is not discussed further in this chapter.

Descriptive Chemistry[10-13]

Opiates and semisynthetic opioids are commonly prescribed in combination with other drugs such as acetaminophen, ibuprofen, aspirin, caffeine, and many other therapeutic drugs. Most are available in generic formulations. Diverse formulations to support various routes of administration and controlled or extended versus immediate release products are available as well. The example trade names listed here do not identify co-formulated medications or product types, and the lists are not comprehensive. Understanding the results of drug testing that is designed to detect use of or exposure to opiates and semisynthetic opioids requires familiarity with the relationships between parent drug use, recognized metabolites, and pharmaceutical impurities. See Figure 24-1 for a simplified schematic illustrating the known relationships between these compounds.

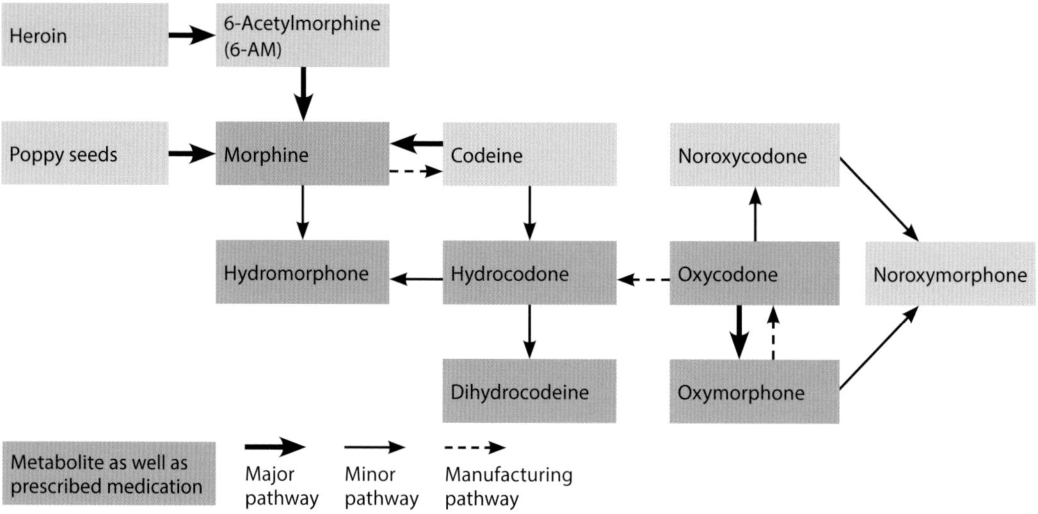

Figure 24-1. Simplified metabolic relationships between opiates and common semisynthetic opioids. Note that many other metabolites exist and that the predominance of one pathway over another may vary based on drug-drug interactions and genetics associated with metabolism. Additional pharmaceutical impurities may also exist but were omitted from this figure for clarity.

Morphine

Synonyms: Morphia; (5α,6α)-7,8-didehydro-4,5-epoxy-17-methylmorphinan-3,6-diol monohydrate; dreamer, emsel, God's drug, MS, Mister Blue, Morpho

Trade names: Astramorph, DepoDur, Duramorph, Kadian, Morphabond, MS Contin, Oramorph SR, Roxanol

Formula: $C_{17}H_{19}NO_3$

Molecular mass = 285.3377 Daltons

CAS-57-27-2 (anhydrous);
6008-81-0 (monohydrate)

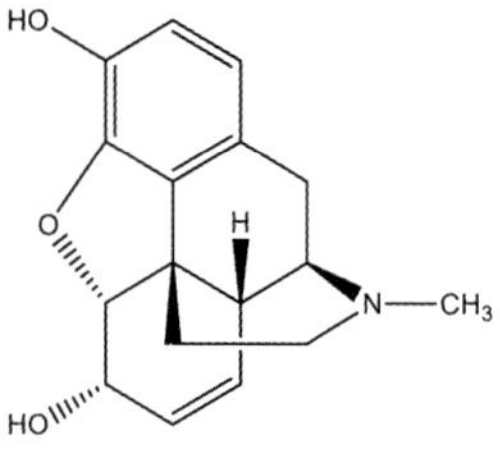

Detection of morphine in a biological specimen is most consistent with use of or exposure to a drug containing morphine. Morphine is the most common metabolite of heroin and may also be the only metabolite detected after heroin use. Proportionately low concentrations of morphine may reflect metabolism of codeine, poppy seed ingestion, or pharmaceutical impurity of hydromorphone.

Codeine

Synonyms: Codeinum, methylmorphine, metilmorfina, morphine methyl ether; (5α,6α)-7,8-didehydro-4,5-epoxy-3-methoxy-17-methylmorphinan-6-ol monohydrate

Trade names: Tylenol 3 or 4 with codeine, Contin, Fioricet with codeine, Soma Compound with codeine, Triacin-C, Tuzistra-XR

Formula: $C_{18}H_{21}NO_3$

Molecular mass = 299.3642 Daltons

CAS-76-57-3 (anhydrous);
6059-47-8 (monohydrate)

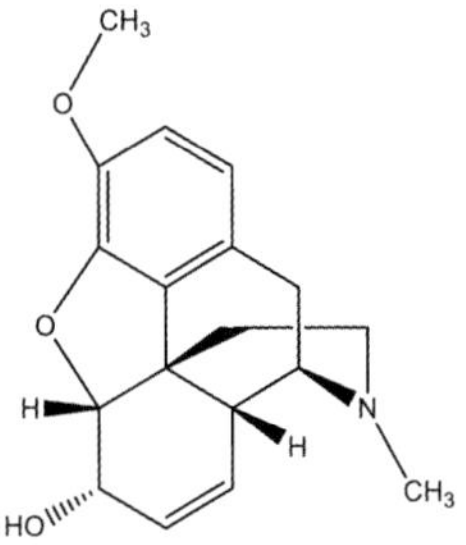

Detection of codeine in a biological specimen is most consistent with use of or exposure to a drug containing codeine. Proportionately low concentrations of codeine may reflect poppy seed ingestion, contamination of heroin, or pharmaceutical impurity of either hydrocodone or morphine.

Heroin

Synonyms: Acetomorphine, diacetylmorphine, diamorphine; (5α,6α)-7,8-didehydro-4,5-epoxy-

17-methylmorphinan-3,6-d diacetate (ester); big H, black tar, Chiva, Hell dust, smack, thunder

Trade names: Heroin is not currently marketed in the US as an independent drug but is marketed for palliative care in some other countries.

Formula: $C_{21}H_{23}NO_5$

Molecular mass = 369.4110 Daltons

CAS-561-27-3

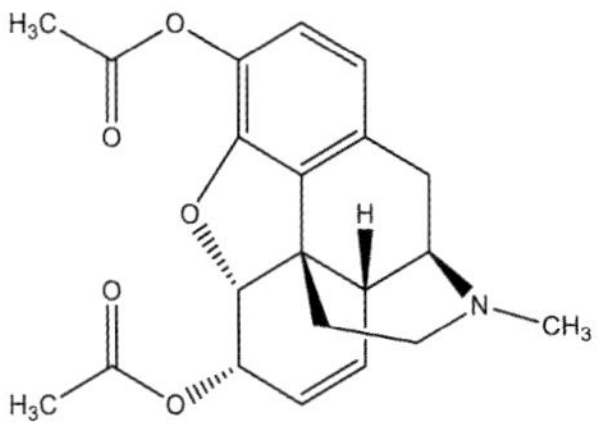

Detection of heroin or the metabolite 6-monoacetylmorphine (6-AM) in a biological specimen is considered definitive evidence for use of or exposure to a drug containing heroin. Due to the relatively rapid metabolism and elimination of heroin and 6-AM, morphine may be the only evidence of heroin use that is detected. It is common that codeine is a detectable contaminant in heroin, which may be detected with its metabolite hydrocodone. The morphine metabolite hydromorphone may also be observed. Codeine, hydrocodone, and hydromorphone would be expected in very low concentrations compared to morphine. Although rare, cases of little to no morphine after heroin use have been reported.[14,15] Further, heroin products may not be pure and may thereby include other opioids such as fentanyl analogs.[16]

Hydrocodone

Synonyms: Dihydrocodeinone; 4,5-epoxy-3-methoxy-17-methylmorphinan-6-one; hydro, narco, vickies, vike

Trade names: Anexsia, Hycet, Hysingla, Hycodan, Lorcet, Lortab, Norco, Tussionex, Tussigon, Vicodin, Xodol, Zamicet, Zohydro, Zydone

Formula: $C_{18}H_{21}NO_3$

Molecular mass = 299.3642 Daltons

CAS-125-29-1

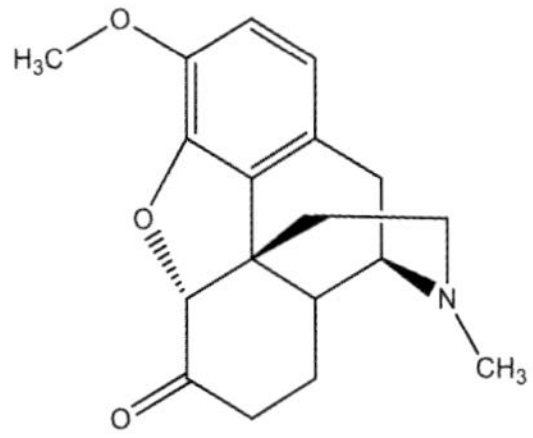

Detection of hydrocodone in a biological specimen is most consistent with use of or exposure to a drug containing hydrocodone. Proportionately low concentrations of hydrocodone may reflect metabolism of codeine or pharmaceutical impurity of oxycodone. The presence of hydrocodone in some oxycodone preparations is the most common of the opioid pharmaceutical impurities recognized to date that is detected by laboratory testing, which is why it was included in Figure 24-1. Note that oxycodone is not described as an impurity of hydrocodone.[13]

Hydromorphone

Synonyms: Dihydromorphinone, dimorphone; 4,5-epoxy-3-hydroxy-17-methylmorphinan-6-one; D, dillies, dust, footballs, juice, smack

Trade names: Dilaudid, Exalgo, Palladone

Formula: $C_{17}H_{19}NO_3$

Molecular mass = 285.3377 Daltons

CAS-466-99-9

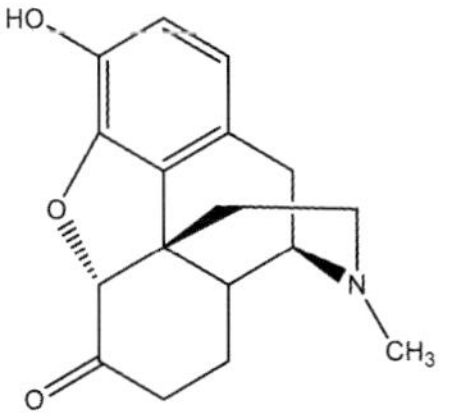

Detection of hydromorphone in a biological specimen is most consistent with use of or exposure to a drug containing hydromorphone. Proportionately low concentrations of hydromorphone may reflect metabolism of hydrocodone, metabolism of morphine, or pharmaceutical impurity of oxymorphone.

Oxycodone

Synonyms: 7,8-Dihydro-14-hydroxycodeinone; dihydrone, oxycone; (5α)-4,5-epoxy-14-hydroxy-3-methoxy-17-methylmorphinan-6-one; hillbilly heroin, kicker OC, ox, roxy, perc, oxy

Trade names: Dazidox, Endodan, Oxaydo, Oxecta, Oxycontin, Percocet, Percodan, Roxicet, Roxicodone, Xartemis, Xolox, Xtampza

Formula: $C_{18}H_{21}NO_4$

Molecular mass = 315.3636

CAS-76-42-6

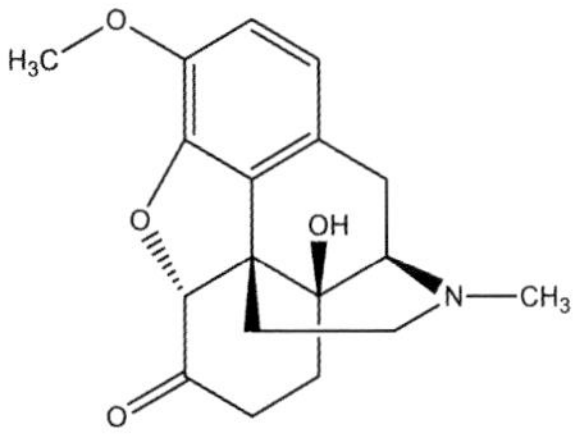

Detection of oxycodone in a biological specimen is most consistent with use of or exposure to a drug containing oxycodone. Proportionately low concentrations of oxycodone may reflect pharmaceutical impurity of oxymorphone.

Oxymorphone

Synonyms: 7,8-Dihydro-14-hydroxymorphinone; oximorphone, oxydimorphone; (5α)-4,5-epoxy-3,14-dihydroxy-17-methylmorphinan-6-one; blue heaven, blues, Mrs O, new blues, octagons, pink, pink heaven, stop signs

Trade name: Opana

Formula: $C_{17}H_{19}NO_4$

Molecular mass = 301.3371 Daltons

CAS-76-41-5

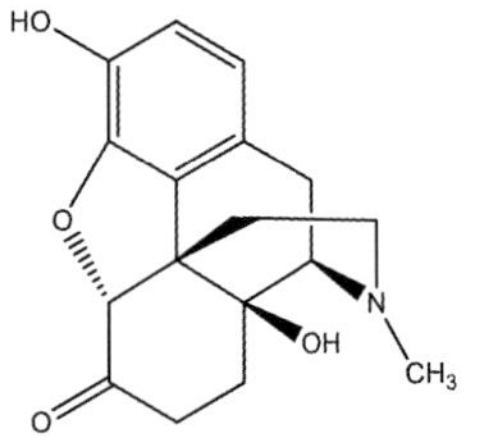

Detection of oxymorphone in a biological specimen is most consistent with use of or exposure to a drug containing oxymorphone. Proportionately low concentrations of oxymorphone may reflect metabolism of oxycodone.

Pharmacology

Pharmacology of opiates and semisynthetic opioids is very similar and is therefore discussed all together in this chapter.

Intended Uses

Opiates and semisynthetic opioid drugs remain among the most widely utilized prescription analgesics, indicated for moderate to severe pain.[1] Opiates and semisynthetic opioids may also be used for antitussive effects, nausea and vomiting, and diarrhea. The depressant effects of opioids on both the respiratory system and CNS can be fatal. Either unintentional or intentional overdose with these drugs, particularly when used in combination with other depressant drugs (eg, benzodiazepines, ethanol), has become an epidemic in the US and is associated with escalating rates of drug-related deaths.[4,5] Opioids are among the most common drugs used and abused for nonmedical purposes. Effective prescribing and dispensing guidelines for the opioids are available and have been adopted widely to guide opioid utilization and minimize the risk of misuse and overdose.[2,17-19]

Mechanisms of Action

Opioids are classified based on their affinity and effect at the classes of opioid receptors as agonists, partial agonists, mixed agonists/antagonists, and antagonists.[1,20] Opioid receptors are G-coupled ligand-gated receptors. When an agonist binds to an opioid receptor, the alpha subunit of the G-protein initiates a cell signaling cascade that results in a reduction of intracellular cyclic adenosine monophosphate (cAMP) concentrations, activation of potassium conductance, and inhibition of calcium conductance. As a consequence, release of neurotransmitters associated with pain, such as glutamate, substance P, and calcitonin-related peptide, is reduced, leading to decreased synaptic transmission. There are four classes of opioid receptors described. Most clinically useful opioids act with relative agonist selectivity for the mu (μ) opioid receptor, named for the prototype ligand morphine. Likewise, the kappa (κ) receptor is named for the prototype ligand ketocyclazocine. The delta (δ) receptor is named for vas deferens, the tissue from which it was first isolated. Each of the opioid receptor classes is associated with subclasses, which work in combination to influence the pharmacodynamics of opioids. The classification of opioid receptors is also defined by variation in the genes that code for the receptors. Selective ligands used in research have helped to elucidate the specific roles played by each receptor subtype as well as the affinities of the receptor subtypes for specific drugs. Further, the competitive antagonists naloxone and naltrexone have been used to study opioid receptors, as they block all three major receptor classes.

Opioid receptors are widely distributed in most tissues but are best recognized for their effects in the CNS and GI tract. Drugs such as methynaltrexone that do not penetrate the blood-brain barrier have proven effective in reversing opioid-related GI side effects such as constipation.[21] The myriad responses and individual sensitivity to opioids reflect the landscape of specific opioid receptor subtypes expressed in both the CNS and GI tract of an individual patient, coupled with the affinity of the specific opioid(s) utilized to each receptor, dose, route of administration, co-medications, and other pharmacologically relevant factors. Tolerance and hyperalgesia are recognized as well, further complicating the selection of an appropriate and safe dose.[22]

Pharmacokinetics

Route of administration will influence opioid bioavailability. While intravenous administration should represent near complete bioavailability, orally administered formulations vary tremendously. For example, bioavailability of an orally administered dose of morphine ranged from approximately 12% to 46% among participants in a controlled pharmacokinetic study, due in large part to variation in first-pass metabolism.[23] Opioids are extensively metabolized through both phase I oxidation/reduction reactions and through phase II conjugation reactions. The most prominent metabolites in urine are typically normetabolites and glucuronide conjugates. As such, detection of opioid exposure in urine is improved by targeted detection of normetabolites and glucuronide conjugates and/or by implementing preanalytical hydrolysis. Common routes of phase I metabolism are summarized in Figure 24-1 along with annotations for pharmaceutical impurities that can complicate interpretation.

For many opiates and semisynthetic opioids, both active and inactive metabolites that exhibit unique elimination profiles may contribute to the efficacy and toxicity profiles of these drugs. For example, codeine is a prodrug that is metabolized to morphine by a reaction mediated primarily by cytochrome P450 isozyme 2D6 (CYP2D6). Genetic variation and drug-drug interactions can impact the proportion of codeine that is activated to morphine, wherein poor metabolizers may fail to produce the active drug, and ultrarapid metabolizers may produce excess proportions of morphine. Variation in patterns of drugs detected in biological samples may complicate the interpretation. A similar phenomenon is recognized for hydrocodone and oxycodone.[24] Estimates for volume of distribution (V_d) and plasma half-life ($t_{1/2}$) of the opiates and semisynthetic opioids discussed here are listed in Table 24-1, considering immediate release formulations. Actual $t_{1/2}$ will vary with the specific opioid used, formulation, dose, and the pharmacokinetics exhibited by the associated person at the time of use. Likewise, lethal doses and fatal plasma concentrations are relative and must be evaluated in context of a specific case. Due to the relatively large V_d of the opiates and semisynthetic opioids, postmortem redistribution is likely to occur.

Table 24-1. Volume of Distribution (V_d) and Half-Life ($t_{1/2}$) Estimates for Immediate-Release Drug Formulation[12]

Drug	V_d (L/kg)	$t_{1/2}$
Codeine	2.5-3.5	1.2-3.9 h
Heroin	25	2-6 min
6-Monoacetyl-morphine (6-AM)	—	6-25 min
Hydrocodone	3.3-4.7	3.4-8.8 h
Hydromorphone	2-4	3-9 h
Morphine	2-5	1.3-6.7 h
Oxycodone	1.8-3.7	3-6 h
Oxymorphone	2-4	4-12 h

Table 24-2. Estimated Morphine Equivalents of Opiates and Semisynthetic Opioids[11]

Drug	Morphine Equivalent Conversion Factor (mg)
Codeine	0.15
Hydrocodone	1
Hydromorphone	4
Morphine	1
Opium	1
Oxycodone	1.5
Oxymorphone	3

Abuse Potential and Characteristics

Abuse potential of the opiates and semisynthetic opioids is substantial, leading to development of many programs to minimize prescribing opioids, reduce quantities and limit morphine equivalents, and widely distribute naloxone to paramedics and family members.[2,25,26] Estimated morphine equivalents for the drugs discussed in this chapter are shown in Table 24-2.[11] Actual morphine equivalents will vary with the specific opioid used, formulation, dose, and the pharmacokinetics and pharmacodynamics exhibited by the associated person at the time of use. While efforts to manage prescription opioids have shown promise, opioid-related deaths continue to increase. The wide availability of illegal and designer opioids on the street and by mail (eg, ordered on the internet), as well as increased demand from addicted individuals, is contributing significantly to this concern. For example, "heroin" is supplied in varying degrees of purity on the street and is nearly always "cut" with other substances as it works its way through the chain of distribution, being commonly adulterated with other depressant drugs like benzodiazepines or other opioids and/or diluted with neutral powders like sugar.[27] In the last decade, street heroin has been more commonly mixed with fentanyl and fentanyl analogs, in some cases resulting in very potent products associated with waves of overdose deaths.[28] The chemical form of the heroin itself depends to some extent on where the opium was originally harvested and processed, the two main opium-growing regions being in central Asia (Afghanistan, Pakistan, Iran), known as the "Golden Crescent," and in southeast Asia (Laos, Myanmar, Thailand), known as the "Golden Triangle." Heroin is among the most widely abused opioids because of its combination of being lipophilic and water soluble, making it bioavailable and potent, facilitating rapid achievement of psychoactive concentrations in the brain. See chapter 25 for additional discussion of abuse potential with synthetic and designer opioids.

Analysis

Recently published laboratory practice and consensus guidelines provide detailed discussion and references regarding aspects of analysis including specimens, analytical approaches, assay content, and reporting.[29-31] These topics are discussed briefly below.

Specimen Types and Characteristics

Opiates and semisynthetic opioids are most commonly measured in urine.[29-32] Common reasons for opiate testing include detection of undisclosed drug use, to support treatment in acute care or emergency settings, and for evaluating adherence/abstinence in chronic pain and addiction management clinics. Due to concerns about adulteration or substitution of urine and for monitoring patients that cannot (or will not) provide urine, other specimens with observed collections are also utilized such as oral fluid and blood. The detection windows for these specimens are not as long as for urine, and metabolites may be limited. Not all drugs deposit in oral fluid due to protein binding and chemical properties of the drug analytes (eg, pK_a). Blood is the preferred specimen for correlating symptoms of response, impairment, and toxicity with drug concentrations, although interpretation of concentrations of opiate and semisynthetic opioids is limited due to factors such as specific drug product used, tolerance, and individual response characteristics. Specimens that may reflect the longest period of detection include hair, which is surrounded by its own limitations and controversies. The specific drug analytes targeted by testing laboratories will vary based on the sensitivity and specificity of the sample processing and analytical methods. Consult with the laboratory to learn what analytes may be detected in specimens that are available for testing. For detection of drug-exposed newborns, meconium and umbilical cord tissue are preferred.[33]

Modes of Analysis

The primary modes of analysis utilized in clinical drug testing include immunoassays and targeted testing, generally performed by chromatography coupled to mass spectrometric detection.[29,30] To some extent, the analysis of opioids is dependent on the specimen to be tested, the drug to be detected, and the circumstances surrounding the analysis. There are a number of commercial immunoassays available, including enzyme immunoassays (automated and ELISA format), fluorescence immunoassays, lateral flow (point of collection), and microparticle immunoassays. It is common for automated urine immunoassays to offer at least two different positive cutoffs, including 300 ng/mL and 2000 ng/mL. The lower cutoff is common in the medical setting and can be easily exceeded by recent ingestion of poppy seed-containing products.[34] The higher 2000 ng/mL cutoff is standard for workplace testing and is much less likely to be exceeded by dietary poppy seed ingestion alone, although foods with high poppy seed content (eg, ethnic dishes using concentrated poppy seed paste) might do so. There exists variable specificity of opiate immunoassays for natural and semisynthetic opiates.[35-37] Standard opiates urine immunoassays commonly used clinically have high cross-reactivity with morphine and codeine, usually using morphine as the target compound (calibrator). The specificity of opiates immunoassays for the semisynthetic opiates is variable, although many cross-react reasonably well with morphine-6-glucuronide, codeine, hydrocodone, hydromorphone, and other opioids of similar chemical structure.[35,38] Standard opiates immunoassays often cross-react poorly with oxycodone and oxymorphone, leading to the development of oxycodone-specific immunoassays and, to a more limited extent, specific immunoassays for other semisynthetic opiates such as 6-AM.

Confirmation procedures are usually based on either gas chromatography (GC) or liquid chromatography (LC) coupled to mass spectrometric detection. Single stage techniques (eg, GC-MS) and triple quadrupole configurations, known as tandem mass spectrometry (eg, LC-MS/MS) are common. Accurate mass technologies, such as Orbitrap and time-of-flight (TOF) mass spectrometry, and direct injection (ie, no chromatography) methods are also available. These laboratory-developed methods are not standardized and should be scrutinized based on assay design, sample clean-up, preanalytical processing (eg hydrolysis), cutoff concentrations, cutoffs, and approaches to data qualification and analysis. Methods may be designed to be qualitative or quantitative and may be targeted to detect only specific compounds or designed to detect unknown compounds.[29,30,39]

Known Analytical Issues

There are a large number of opioids that will not cross-react with commercially available opiate immunoassays.[34,35] Further, confirmation testing must align with cutoffs and cross-reactivity profiles of immunoassays to increase the likelihood of detecting an expected drug(s). Specimen quality (eg, dilution of urine, timing of blood collection) will influence detection as well. False positives and false negatives are possible with all methods due to, for example, cross-reactivity of a specific immunoassay or isobaric interferences in a mass spectrometric assay. Failure to efficiently extract and recover the drug(s) of interest and/or matrix effects are also potential analytical problems with chromatographic and mass spectrometric assays.[39]

Clinical Issues

Interpretation

The interpretation of opiate testing in blood, urine, and other specimens should be approached with caution.[32,33,40] There are a number of patient factors that need to be considered, including consumption of poppy seeds in food, drug tolerance, the pharmacodynamics in seriously ill and geriatric patients, co-medications, pharmaceutical impurities, and pharmacogenetics. The metabolism pathways summarized in Figure 24-1 can be helpful in interpretation of targeted opiate and semisynthetic opioid testing, which may reveal multiple compounds, some of which can be both parent drugs and metabolites or manufacturing impurities of other opiates. Pharmaceutical impurities may only be resolved with targeted quantitative test methods.

The presence of morphine and codeine in poppy seeds complicates interpretation of opiate testing because dietary consumption of poppy seeds may produce positive drug screens.[34] For example, detection of morphine in body fluids can result from the use of heroin, codeine, or morphine, or the ingestion of poppy seeds. Heroin use may be missed unless 6-AM or, less commonly, heroin itself is detected.

If immunoassays are utilized for opiate and semisynthetic opioid detection, the laboratory should assist with result interpretation. The cross-reactivity profile for the laboratory's opiates assays, as well as a list of possible interferences, should be available to clinicians. It is important to emphasize that negative results do not necessarily exclude the presence of the drug or metabolite. A positive opiates screening result also cannot be used to establish which opiate is ingested or differentiate recent versus long-term use or compliance versus abuse. In the emergency department setting, opiates are widely used for analgesia, making positive screening results even more difficult to interpret if specimens are collected after medications are administered. Specific confirmatory testing (qualitative or quantitative) should be performed when it is important to know which opiates are present, when testing results do not match the clinical picture, or when definitive results are necessary.

When evaluating quantitative results, it is tempting to correlate concentration with dose, but many studies have demonstrated overlap in the distributions of opioid drugs and metabolites relative to dose. Proportional relationships may be of value, particularly when looking at pharmaceutical impurities.[13]

Overdose and Toxicity[1,41]

Opiate overdose classically manifests as pinpoint pupils accompanied by respiratory and CNS depression and loss of consciousness from which patients awaken after naloxone injection. Needle track marks and other signs of intravenous drug abuse may be evident. Specific drug concentrations are usually not utilized in the acute overdose situation, but qualitative urine screening may confirm recent opiate use. Since many of the opiate products are mixed with acetaminophen, it is important to also obtain serum acetaminophen levels if overdose of opiates is suspected.

In the emergency situation, airway management and assisted ventilation may be necessary, along with supplemental oxygen. As an antidote, naloxone, an opioid antagonist without any agonist properties, may usually be given safely in doses up to 10 mg to 20 mg, but with the relatively short 1- to 2-hour duration of naloxone effects, it is generally recommended that, after awakening, opiate coma patients should be held and/or admitted for observation for at least 6 to 12 hours.[42]

References

1. Yaksh TL, Wallace MS. Opioids, analgesia, and pain management. In: Brunton LL, Chabner BA, Knollman BC, eds. *Goodman and Gilman's The Pharmacological Basis of Therapeutics*. 12th ed. New York City, NY: McGraw-Hill Co; 2011:481-526.

2. Centers For Disease Control and Prevention Public Health Service. US Department of Health and Human Services. Guideline for prescribing opioids for chronic pain. *J Pain Palliat Care Pharmacother.* 2016;30(2):138-140.
3. Han B, Compton WM, Jones CM, Cai R. Nonmedical prescription opioid use and use disorders among adults aged 18 through 64 years in the United States, 2003-2013. *JAMA.* 2015;314(14):1468-1478.
4. Huang X, Keyes KM, Li G. Increasing prescription opioid and heroin overdose mortality in the United States, 1999-2014: an age-period-cohort analysis. *Am J Public Health.* 2018;108(1):131-136.
5. Ruhm CJ. Corrected US opioid-involved drug poisoning deaths and mortality rates, 1999-2015. *Addiction.* 2018;113(7):1339-1344.
6. Aldrich JV, McLaughlin JP. Opioid peptides: potential for drug development. *Drug Discov Today Technol.* 2012;9(1):e23-e31.
7. Spetea M, Asim MF, Wolber G, Schmidhammer H. The micro opioid receptor and ligands acting at the micro opioid receptor, as therapeutics and potential therapeutics. *Curr Pharm Des.* 2013;19(42):7415-7434.
8. Brownstein MJ. A brief history of opiates, opioid peptides, and opioid receptors. *Proc Nat Acad Sci U S A.* 1993;90(12):5391-5393.
9. Courtwright DT. Opiate addiction as a consequence of the Civil War. *Civ War Hist.* 1978; 24(2):101-111.
10. Moffat AC, Osselton MD, Widdop B. *Clarke's Analysis of Drugs and Poisons.* 3rd ed. Chicago, IL: Pharmaceutical Press; 2004.
11. Association AP. *Lexicomp Drug Information Handbook.* 27th ed. Wolters Kluwer; 2018.
12. Baselt RC, ed. *Disposition of Toxic Drugs and Chemicals in Man.* 9th ed. Forster City, CA: Biomedical Publications; 2011.
13. Officers AAoMR. *MRO Advisory: Interpreting Test Results for Prescription Opiates.* Research Triangle Park, NC: Quadrangle Research, LLC; 2010:1-2.
14. Crews B, Mikel C, Latyshev S, et al. 6-Acetylmorphine detected in the absence of morphine in pain management patients. *Ther Drug Monit.* 2009;31(6):749-752.
15. Glass LR, Ingalls ST, Schilling CL, Hoppel CL. Atypical urinary opiate excretion pattern. *J Anal Toxicol.* 1997;21(6):509-514.
16. Tiscione NB, Alford I. Carfentanil in impaired driving cases and the importance of drug seizure data. *J Anal Toxicol.* 2018;42(7):476-484.
17. Bohnert ASB, Guy GP Jr, Losby JL. Opioid prescribing in the United States before and after the Centers for Disease Control and Prevention's 2016 Opioid Guideline. *Ann Intern Med.* 2018; 169(6):367-375.
18. Carlson CL. Effectiveness of the World Health Organization cancer pain relief guidelines: an integrative review. *J Pain Res.* 2016;9:515-534.
19. Forbes K. Pain in patients with cancer: the World Health Organization analgesic ladder and beyond. *Clin Oncol.* 2011;23(6):379-380.
20. Ghelardini C, Di Cesare Mannelli L, Bianchi E. The pharmacological basis of opioids. *Clin Cases Miner Bone Metab.* 2015;12(3):219-221.
21. Sobczak M, Salaga M, Storr MA, Fichna J. Physiology, signaling, and pharmacology of opioid receptors and their ligands in the gastrointestinal tract: current concepts and future perspectives. *J Gastroenterol.* 2014;49(1):24-45.
22. Varrassi G, Fusco M, Skaper SD, et al. A pharmacological rationale to reduce the incidence of opioid induced tolerance and hyperalgesia: a review. *Pain Ther.* 2018;7(1):59-75.
23. Hoskin PJ, Hanks GW, Aherne GW, Chapman D, Littleton P, Filshie J. The bioavailability and pharmacokinetics of morphine after intravenous, oral and buccal administration in healthy volunteers. *Br J Clin Pharmacol.* 1989;27(4):499-505.
24. Caudle KE, Klein TE, Hoffman JM, et al. Incorporation of pharmacogenomics into routine clinical practice: the Clinical Pharmacogenetics Implementation Consortium (CPIC) guideline development process. *Curr Drug Metab.* 2014;15(2):209-217.
25. Peglow SL, Binswanger IA. Preventing opioid overdose in the clinic and hospital: analgesia and opioid antagonists. *Med Clin North Am.* 2018;102(4):621-634.
26. Vashishtha D, Mittal ML, Werb D. The North American opioid epidemic: current challenges and a call for treatment as prevention. *Harm Reduct J.* 2017;14(1):7.
27. Cole C, Jones L, McVeigh J, Kicman A, Syed Q, Bellis M. Adulterants in illicit drugs: a review of empirical evidence. *Drug Test Anal.* 2011;3(2):89-96.
28. Pergolizzi JV, Jr., LeQuang JA, Taylor R Jr, Raffa RB, Group NR. Going beyond prescription pain relievers to understand the opioid epidemic: the role of illicit fentanyl, new psychoactive substances, and street heroin. *Postgrad Med.* 2018;130(1):1-8.
29. Langman LJ, Jannetto PJ, eds. *Laboratory Medicine Practice Guidelines. Using Clinical Laboratory Tests to Monitor Drug Therapy in Pain Management Patients.* Washington, DC: AACC Academy; 2018.
30. *Laboratory Support for Pain Management Programs.* 1st ed. Wayne, PA; Clinical and Laboratory Standards Institute; 2018. CLSI guideline C63.
31. Jarvis M, Williams J, Hurford M, et al. Appropriate use of drug testing in clinical addiction medicine. *J Addict Med.* 2017;11(3):163-173.

32. Mahajan G. Role of urine drug testing in the current opioid epidemic. *Anesth Analg.* 2017;125(6):2094-2104.
33. Wabuyele SL, Colby JM, McMillin GA. Detection of drug-exposed newborns. *Ther Drug Monit.* 2018;40(2):166-185.
34. Tenore PL. Advanced urine toxicology testing. *J Addict Dis.* 2010;29(4):436-448.
35. Krasowski MD, Pizon AF, Siam MG, Giannoutsos S, Iyer M, Ekins S. Using molecular similarity to highlight the challenges of routine immunoassay-based drug of abuse/toxicology screening in emergency medicine. *BMC Emerg Med.* 2009;9:5.
36. Magnani B, Kwong T. Urine drug testing for pain management. *Clin Lab Med.* 2012;32(3):379-390.
37. Melanson SE. The utility of immunoassays for urine drug testing. *Clin Lab Med.* 2012;32(3):429-447.
38. Melanson SE, Baskin L, Magnani B, Kwong TC, Dizon A, Wu AH. Interpretation and utility of drug of abuse immunoassays: lessons from laboratory drug testing surveys. *Arch Pathol Lab Med.* 2010;134(5):735-739.
39. McMillin GA, Slawson MH, Marin SJ, Johnson-Davis KL. Demystifying analytical approaches for urine drug testing to evaluate medication adherence in chronic pain management. *J Pain Palliat Care Pharmacother.* 2013;27(4):322-339.
40. Kwong TC, Magnani B, Moore C. Urine and oral fluid drug testing in support of pain management. *Crit Rev Clin Lab Sci.* 2017;54(6):433-445.
41. Ciejka M, Nguyen K, Bluth MH, Dubey E. Drug toxicities of common analgesic medications in the emergency department. *Clin Lab Med.* 2016;36(4):761-776.
42. Goldfrank L, Weisman RS, Errick JK, Lo MW. A dosing nomogram for continuous infusion intravenous naloxone. *Ann Emerg Med.* 1986;15(5):566-570.

Chapter 25

Opioids II: Synthetic Opioids

Hoi-Ying Elsie Yu, PhD
Nicholas Heger, PhD

Introduction

Opioids are a diverse group of substances that bind to one or more opioid receptors, which are primarily located in the central nervous system (CNS) and gastrointestinal (GI) tract.[1] The opioids in general are classified as narcotic analgesics and CNS depressants. Medically, opioids are primarily used for pain control but also exhibit antitussive and other therapeutic actions. Of major concern is the widespread use of opioid drugs for nonmedical or recreational purposes, which has contributed to escalating rates of addiction, drug overdose, and drug-related deaths.[2-5] Opioids are often described based on origin: endogenous (eg, endorphins), natural opiates (ie, derived from the opium poppy), semisynthetic (ie, derived from natural opiates), synthetic (ie, prescription drugs exhibiting activity at the opioid receptors but not of endogenous or natural origin), and designer (ie, nonprescription drugs exhibiting activity at the opioid receptors but not of endogenous or natural origin). Although endogenous opioids may become commercialized drugs someday, a detailed discussion of endogenous opioids is beyond the scope of this book.[6,7] This chapter will cover the common synthetic opioids including buprenorphine, fentanyl, meperidine, methadone, propoxyphene, tramadol, and tapentadol.

Origin

Of the synthetic opioids, meperidine is the oldest commercially produced drug, developed in 1939.[8] Propoxyphene entered the US market in 1957[8] but was removed from the US market in 2010. Fentanyl was developed by Janssen in 1960[9] and introduced in the US in 1968.[10] Tramadol (Ultram) was developed by Grünenthal in Germany in 1962 and entered the West German market in 1977.[11] It was introduced in the US in 1995. A structurally similar drug, tapentadol (Nucynta), became available in the US in 2008.[12] Methadone was developed in Germany and became available for use in the US in 1947.[13] The first two high-dose sublingual formulations of buprenorphine, Subutex (buprenorphine) and Suboxone (buprenorphine and naloxone combination), were approved in the US for treating opioid addiction in 2002 but were soon also used for chronic pain management.[14] In 2010, a transdermal form of buprenorphine (Butrans) was approved for use in the US. In 2016, a subdermal implant form (Probuphine) was introduced in the US.

Descriptive Chemistry

The synthetic opioids are man-made chemical agents designed to bind to opioid receptors. Buprenorphine is a thebaine derivative, fentanyl and meperidine are phenylpiperidine derivatives, methadone is a diphenylheptane derivative, propoxyphene is a phenylheptylamine derivative, and tramadol and tapentadol are aminocyclohexanol derivatives. Diverse formulations to support various routes of administration and controlled or extended versus immediate release products are available as well. The example trade names listed here do not identify co-formulated medications or product types, and the lists are not comprehensive.

Buprenorphine

Synonyms: Buprenorphinum, RX-6029-M; 2-(N-cyclopropylmethyl-4,5alpha-epoxy-3-hydroxy-6-methoxy-6,14-endo-ethanomorphinan-7alpha-yl)-3,3-dimethyl-2-butanol

Trade names: Buprenex, Butrans, Buprex, Subutex, Probuphine, Transtec, ingredient of Suboxone

Formula: $C_{29}H_{41}NO_4$

Molecular mass = 467.64 Daltons

CAS-52485-79-7

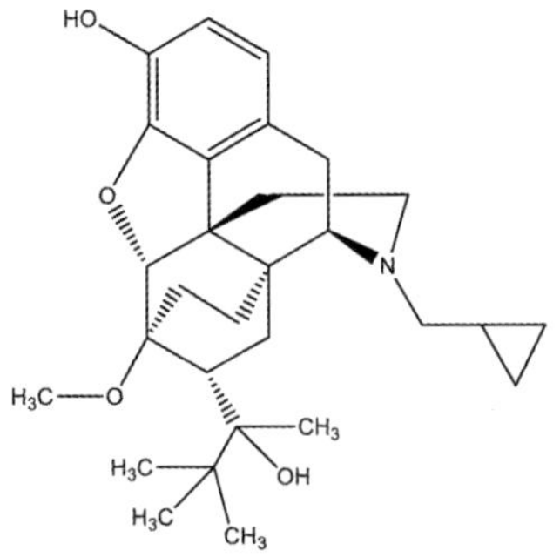

Pharmaceutical preparations of buprenorphine typically contain buprenorphine hydrochloride. It is chemically identified as 17-cyclopropylmethyl-4,5alpha-epoxy-7alpha-((S)-1-hydroxy-1,2,2-trimethylpropyl-6-methoxy-6,14-endo-ethanomorphinan-3-ol (formula $C_{29}H_{42}ClNO_4$; nominal formula weight 504.108 g/mol; CAS 53152-21-9).

Fentanyl

Synonyms: Fentanalum, phentanyl, N-phenyl-N-[1-(2-phenylethyl)-piperidin-4-yl]-propanamide

Trade names: Duragesic, Durogesic, Matrifen, Fentora, Ionsys, Actiq, Onsolis

Formula: $C_{22}H_{28}N_2O$

Molecular mass = 336.4705 Daltons

CAS-437-38-7

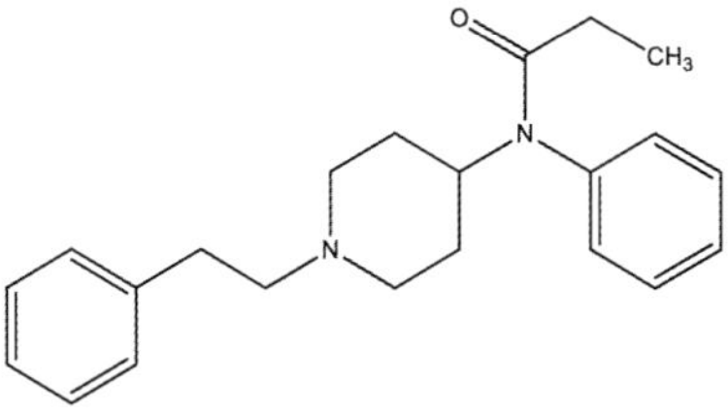

Pharmaceutical preparations of fentanyl typically contain fentanyl citrate. It is chemically identified as N-(1-phenethyl-4-piperidyl)propionanilide citrate (1:1) (formula: $C_{22}H_{28}N_2O \cdot C_6H_8O_7$; nominal formula weight: 528.59 g/mol; CAS 990-73-8).

Methadone

Synonyms: Amidine, amidone; 6-dimethylamino-4,4-diphenyl-3-heptanone

Trade names: Dolophine, Methadose

Formula: $C_{21}H_{27}NO$

Molecular mass = 309.445 Daltons

CAS-76-99-3; 297-88-1 (racemic)

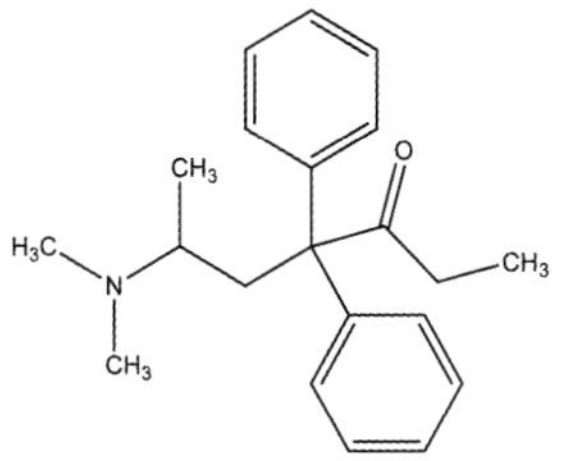

Methadone is currently available as a racemic mixture of the hydrochloride salt (*S*- and *R*- isomers) in medications. It is chemically identified as 6-(dimethylamino)-4,4-diphenylheptan-3-one hydrochloride (formula $C_{21}H_{28}ClNO$; nominal formula weight 345.911 g/mol; CAS 1095-90-5, 125-56-4).

Meperidine

Synonyms: Pethidine, isonipecaine, ethyl-1-methyl-4-phenylpiperidine-4-carboxylate

Trade name: Demerol

Formula: $C_{15}H_{21}NO_2$

Molecular mass = 247.3327 Daltons

CAS-57-42-1

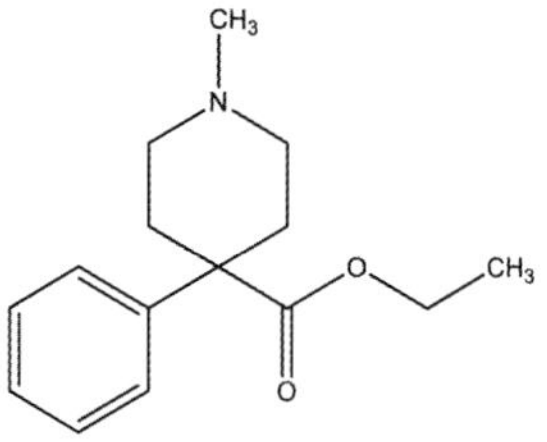

Meperidine hydrochloride is the meperidine salt that is frequently used in medications. It is chemically identified as ethyl-1-methyl-4-phenylpiperidine-4-carboxylate hydrochloride (formula: $C_{15}H_{22}ClNO_2$; nominal formula weight: 283.8 g/mol; CAS 50-13-5).

Propoxyphene

Synonyms: Dextropropoxyphene; [(2S,3R)-4-(dimethylamino)-3-methyl-1,2-di(phenyl)butan-2-yl] propanoate

Trade names: Darvon, Wygesic

Formula: $C_{22}H_{29}NO_2$

Molecular mass = 339.4712 Daltons

CAS-469-62-5

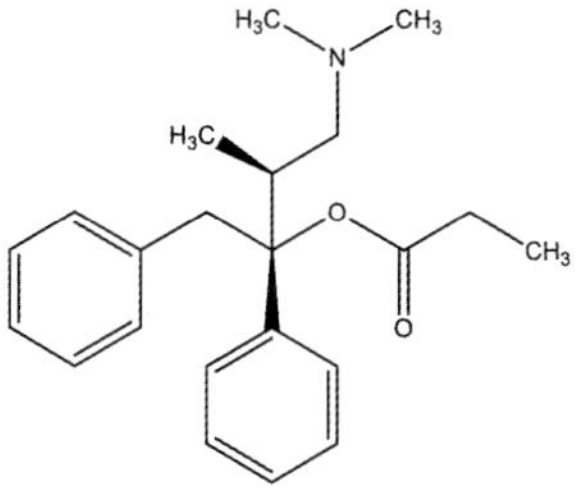

Propoxyphene hydrochloride and napsylate are the two salts that were frequently used in medication. Propoxyphene hydrochloride is chemically identified as [(2S,3R)-4-(dimethylamino)-3-methyl-1,2-diphenylbutan-2-yl] propanoate hydrochloride (formula: $C_{22}H_{30}ClNO_2$; nominal formula weight: 379.5 g/mol; CAS-6585-54-2). Propoxyphene napsylate is chemically identified as [(2S,3R)-4-(dimethylamino)-3-methyl-1,2-diphenylbutan-2-yl] propanoate; naphthalene-2-sulfonic acid; hydrate (formula: $C_{32}H_{39}NO_6S$; nominal formula weight: 565.7 g/mol; CAS 66943-72-4).

Tapentadol

Synonyms: 3-((1R,2R)-3-(dimethylamino)-1-ethyl-2-methylpropyl)phenol

Trade names: Nucynta, Palexia

Formula: $C_{14}H_{23}NO$

Molecular mass = 221.339 Daltons

CAS-175591-23-8

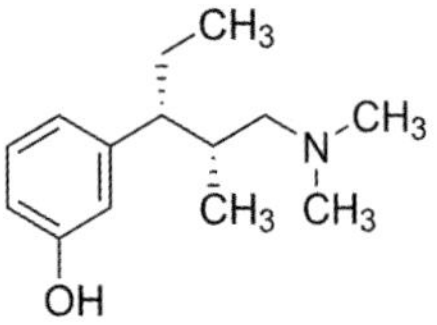

Tapentadol hydrochloride is the salt that is frequently used in medication. It is chemically identified as 3-[(2R,3R)-1-(dimethylamino)-2-methylpentan-3-yl]phenol hydrochloride (formula: $C_{14}H_{24}ClNO$; nominal formula weight: 257.802 g/mol; CAS 175591-09-0).

Tramadol

Synonyms: It consists of two enantiomers, (1RS,2RS)-2-(dimethylaminomethyl)-1-(3-methoxyphenyl)cyclohexan-1-ol

Trade names: Ultram, ConZip, Dromodol, Zydol, etc

Formula: $C_{16}H_{25}NO_2$

Molecular mass = 263.3752 Daltons

CAS-53611-16-8

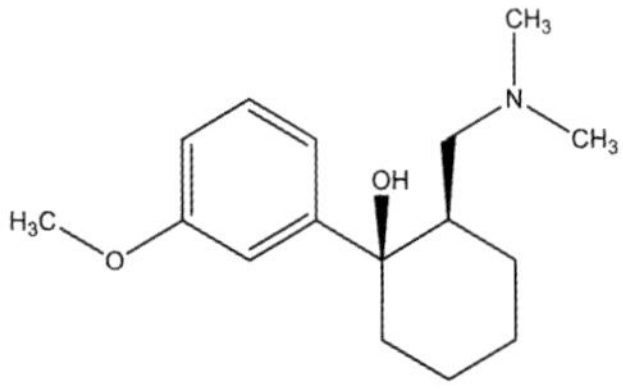

Pharmaceutical preparations of tramadol often contain tramadol hydrochloride. It is chemically identified as (1RS,2RS)-2-(dimethylaminomethyl)-1-(3-methoxyphenyl)cyclohexan-1-ol hydrochloride (formula: $C_{16}H_{26}ClNO_2$; nominal formula weight: 299.8 g/mol; CAS 36282-47-0).

Pharmacology

See chapter 24, *Opioids 1: Opiates and Semisynthetic Opioids,* for introductory remarks on pharmacology.

Intended Use

The synthetic opioids are largely prescribed for pain management or for opioid substitution when treating addiction. Buprenorphine is a controlled Schedule III analgesic prescribed for moderate to severe chronic pain. Similar to methadone, buprenorphine is also approved for treatment of opioid addiction although can only be prescribed in the outpatient setting by specially trained and certified physicians, nurse practitioners, and physician assistants. Clinically, buprenorphine has fewer undesirable opioid CNS and GI side effects than other opioids used in pain management and treatment of opioid addiction.[15] Buprenorphine may also be combined with the opioid receptor antagonist naloxone (eg, Suboxone), which serves as an abuse deterrent. Studies comparing methadone and buprenorphine for opioid substitution treatment have shown similar efficacy at suppressing illicit opioid use and retention in treatment programs when prescribed at fixed medium to high doses.[16,17] European studies have shown enhanced therapeutic benefits for chronic pain management with the use of new transdermal buprenorphine delivery systems because of its higher safety profile, better patient compliance, and fewer undesirable side effects compared to other opioid medications.[15,18]

Fentanyl is a controlled Schedule II analgesic available in a variety of routes of administration. A transdermal patch (Durogesic/Duragesic/Matrifen) is most commonly used for chronic pain management. In 2006, the US Food and Drug Administration (FDA) approved the fentanyl iontophoretic transdermal system (Ionsys) for the management of acute, moderate to severe postoperative pain in the inpatient setting. Iontophoresis uses a weak electrical current to deliver fentanyl across the skin into the systemic circulation, thereby allowing for rapid rate of drug absorption and eliminating the fat depot effect that is commonly seen in the passive transdermal patch system. The needleless Ionsys may therefore be more convenient than intravenous infusion for acute pain treatment. For breakthrough pain management, intranasal formulations are thought to be better than transmucosal applications, as intranasal fentanyl provides more rapid relief.[19,20]

Meperidine is a controlled Schedule II analgesic prescribed for moderate to severe pain. It has been used to manage postoperative pain, labor pain, dental pain, and migraines.[21] Meperidine has not been shown to provide better pain relief than other opioids.[22] In fact, many nonopioids have been shown to be superior.[22] Compared to other opioids, use of meperidine has declined.[23]

Methadone is a controlled Schedule II analgesic and is prescribed for management of moderate to severe chronic pain. Methadone is also approved by the FDA for drug detoxification treatment and maintenance treatment of opioid addiction. Methadone may only be dispensed for detoxification or maintenance purposes in the oral formulation by opioid treatment programs certified by the Substance Abuse and Mental Health Services Administration (SAMHSA).[24]

Propoxyphene was a controlled Schedule IV analgesic prescribed for mild to moderate pain, with lower abuse potential than fentanyl or meperidine.

However, due to its cardiotoxicity (prolongation of the QRS interval and resultant dysrhythmias), propoxyphene was withdrawn from the European and US markets in 2009 and 2010, respectively.[25,26]

Tapentadol is a controlled Schedule II analgesic. It is generally used to treat nociceptive pain. In addition, tapentadol can also be used to treat moderate to severe diabetic neuropathic pain. It provides similar analgesic efficacy as oxycodone but with fewer adverse GI side effects.[12] Also, the development of tolerance appears to be delayed compared to other opiates like morphine.[12]

Tramadol is an analgesic prescribed for moderate to moderately severe pain, with lower abuse potential than other opioids.[27] In 2014, the US Drug Enforcement Administration (DEA) officially classified it as a Schedule IV substance. Tramadol has also been used to treat both chronic and acute pain including postoperative pain, trauma pain, labor pain, cancer pain, and neuropathic pain.[28] Its analgesic effect is enhanced when used with nonopioid analgesia. Tramadol can also be used in the patient-controlled analgesia setting, where the patient can dispense a preprogrammed amount of tramadol as needed.[28] Although it has similar potency to meperidine, tramadol may be superior because it is well tolerated, with fewer side effects.[28] Unlike other opioids, tramadol produces less constipation[27] and respiratory depression.[11]

Mechanism of Action

The synthetic opioids are analgesic μ opioid receptor agonists with varying degrees of potency. Buprenorphine is estimated to be 30 to 40 times more potent than morphine by the intravenous route—and potentially higher with chronic administration or other routes of delivery.[29,30] Fentanyl is about 80 times more potent than morphine. Methadone is estimated to be three to four times more potent than morphine and is also an *N*-methyl-*D*-aspartate (NMDA) receptor antagonist.[31,32] Meperidine is much weaker, with potency only about 10% that of morphine.[21] Propoxyphene is weaker yet (~100 times weaker than morphine[11]) and, similar to methadone, is a weak NMDA receptor antagonist, with analgesic potency similar to that of codeine or acetaminophen.[21] Tapentadol is a weak μ receptor agonist (~50 times lower affinity than morphine). However, because it also exerts its analgesic effect by inhibiting norepinephrine reuptake, it is only two to three times less potent than morphine.[12] Tramadol, as a parent drug, has similar potency as meperidine (~10% of morphine). Its metabolite, *O*-desmethyltramadol, however, has about six times higher affinity for the μ receptor than the parent drug.[21] Tramadol's ability to inhibit norepinephrine and serotonin reuptake for pain relief is also well documented.[33]

Unlike morphine and the other opiates discussed in chapter 24, *Opioids 1: Opiates and Semisynthetic Opioids,* the synthetic opioids discussed in this chapter, with the exception of buprenorphine and tapentadol,[34] have all been shown to be, or have been implicated as, weak serotonin reuptake inhibitors.[35] Therefore, they can enhance the descending pain inhibitory tracts in the spinal cord, providing another mechanism of pain relief in addition to being opioid receptor agonists. In addition, meperidine appears to have unique properties to treat shivers and rigors as compared to other opioids.[36] The mechanism of action is not fully understood. However, the interaction of the thermoregulatory center in the hypothalamus and opioid and muscarinic CNS receptors is thought to be involved.[36]

Both methadone and buprenorphine are utilized in the treatment of opioid abuse. Methadone's analgesic potency, long duration of action, and availability of oral preparations make this drug useful in chronic pain management and opioid abuse/withdrawal treatment applications.[37] Buprenorphine is a partial agonist at μ opioid receptors, with high affinity, low intrinsic activity, and slow receptor dissociation rate. These characteristics explain the reduced incidence of abstinence syndrome observed with this drug and make buprenorphine particularly suitable for substitution therapy for opioid dependency.[38] Buprenorphine also acts at other opioid receptors including δ, κ, and a newly described opioid-receptor–like (ORL-1) receptor as an agonist/antagonist, which explains its unique and complex pharmacology.[39] Though buprenorphine is more potent than morphine at lower doses, it reaches a ceiling where higher doses do not result in increasing opioid effects, contributing to an improved safety profile as it is less likely than full agonists to produce respiratory depression in overdose situations.[13,15,38,40]

Pharmacokinetics

Buprenorphine

Buprenorphine has poor oral bioavailability due to extensive first-pass metabolism. The development of sublingual dosage forms significantly improved drug absorption (oral bioavailability ~30-50%[41]), though oral fluid pH and length of time the dose is held under the tongue play a role. Buprenorphine is highly lipid soluble with a large volume of distribution (V_d) of 1.4 L/kg to 6.2 L/kg[13] and reaches peak serum/plasma concentration (t_{max}) in 1 hour.[41] It is highly protein bound (up to 96%), especially to alpha and beta globulins.[42]

Buprenorphine is extensively metabolized in the liver by *N*-dealkylation to pharmacologically active norbuprenorphine, which has 50 times less analgesic potency than buprenorphine. Metabolism is primarily mediated by CYP3A4, and its metabolism is therefore influenced with concomitant administration of medications that inhibit or induce CYP3A4 activity.[13,42] Both buprenorphine and norbuprenorphine undergo glucuronidation, which makes them inactive. The mean elimination half-life ($t_{½}$) for buprenorphine is 2 to 4 hours if given by parenteral route and 18 to 49 hours if given by sublingual route.[13] Most of the dose is eliminated in feces, with only 10% to 30% being excreted in urine.[13,42]

Fentanyl

Fentanyl is highly lipophilic (V_d ~3-8 L/kg[13]), with a rapid onset of action. Its dissociation with the receptor is rapid ($t_{½}$ 2.5 min), explaining its short-acting property.[43] After transdermal patch application, t_{max} is achieved in 12 to 48 hours.[44] It takes about 3 days to reach steady state, which can be maintained with replacement of patches.[43] Patch dosage should be prescribed in micrograms per hour, not by patch size, even though fentanyl concentration is uniform on the patch. Duragesic comes in different patch sizes, ranging from 12.5 mcg/hour to 100 mcg/hour. Since fentanyl is lipophilic, the cutaneous depot will continue to release fentanyl into systemic circulation after removal of the patch. For iontophoretic administration, Ionsys is preprogrammed to deliver 40 mcg of fentanyl in 10 minutes, and patients can self-administer as many as 6 doses per hour. Ionsys t_{max} is achieved in 39 minutes, and terminal $t_{½}$ is about 11 hours, similar to that of intravenous infusion (t_{max} ~35 min, $t_{½}$ ~13 h).[44] For breakthrough pain management, intranasal formulations have a t_{max} as short as 5 minutes as compared to 20 to 60 minutes with transmucosal routes.[43] Different transmucosal formulations are currently available, including buccal tablets (Fentora), lozenges (Actiq), and films (Onsolis).

Two commonly used fentanyl derivatives, alfentanil and sufentanil, have similar properties.[46] Remifentanil, a unique fentanyl derivative, may be superior because it is metabolized to inactive metabolites by plasma and tissue esterases, thereby making it more short acting than fentanyl.[45,47] Like fentanyl, it is a potent μ opioid receptor agonist. Because of its rapid onset of action (~1 min)[47] and elimination ($t_{½}$ ~3 min),[47] it is becoming a popular analgesic in the intensive care unit[45] and in labor pain management.[47] Fentanyl is primarily metabolized to norfentanyl by CYP3A4.[48]

Meperidine

Meperidine can be administered orally (t_{max} ~2 h), intravenously (t_{max} ~1.2 min), intramuscularly (t_{max} ~15-60 min), and epidurally.[22] The duration of analgesic effect lasts 2 to 4 hours.[11] Depending on the clinical situation, it is administered 50 mg to 150 mg every 3 to 4 hours, with a daily maximum of 600 mg and a maximum administration duration of 48 hours due to potential toxicity.

Only approximately 50% to 60% of meperidine parent compound reaches the systemic circulation when taken orally due to extensive first-pass metabolism.[22] The $t_{½}$ is 2 to 5 hours, with a V_d of 3.7 L/kg to 4.2 L/kg.[13] Meperidine is mainly *N*-demethylated by CYP3A4 and 2B6 to a neurotoxic metabolite, normeperidine ($t_{½}$ ~15-30 h).[8,21] Oral intake of meperidine may result in higher concentrations of normeperidine as a result of first-pass metabolism.[22] In addition, patients with kidney dysfunction may have increased risk of normeperidine toxicity, as renal clearance is compromised.[36]

Methadone

The pharmacokinetics of methadone is characterized by high interindividual variability, especially in absorption and metabolism, making it difficult to predict its effects (both clinical and toxic) and blood concentrations based upon the dose administered.[48] The *R*-enantiomer is 10 times more effective at the μ receptor and has 50 times more analgesic activity compared to *S*-enantiomer,[49] though it is sold as a racemic mixture in pharmaceutical preparations. Methadone undergoes first-pass metabolism (oral bioavailability ~41-99%[50]) and has a prolonged $t_{½}$ (15-55 h[13]). The t_{max} is also variable, ranging from 1 to 6 hours when administered orally. Due to high lipid solubility, 98% of the drug is distributed to the tissues with a large volume of distribution (V_d 4-7 L/kg).[13] The proportion of free methadone present in blood is low (1-2%), with 60% to 70% of the drug being bound to the plasma proteins.[50,51]

Methadone is metabolized in the liver (major: CYP3A4 and 2B6; minor: 2C9 and 2C19[37,51]) to inactive *N*-demethylated derivatives, 2-ethylidene-1,5-dimethyl-3,3diphenylpyrrolidine (EDDP) and 2-ethyl-5-methyl-3,3-diphenylpyrrolidine (EMDP).[13] A minor component is reduced to methadol and then to normethadol, although neither has any apparent pharmacological activity. Recent studies have shown that the metabolism is stereoselective especially with 2B6 enzyme, which along with the genetic polymorphisms and variable expression of these enzymes may explain the interindividual variability in its pharmacokinetics.[52] The rate of metabolism is higher when the drug is administered by the oral route compared to intramuscular route.[53] Methadone, EDDP, and EMDP are the primary excretory products identified in the urine.[13]

Propoxyphene

Prior to its removal from the market, propoxyphene was available as oral tablets, with or without acetaminophen (Darvocet or Darvon, respectively). The V_d for propoxyphene is 12 L/kg to 26 L/kg,[13] $t_{1/2}$ is 8 to 24 hours, and t_{max} is ~2 hours.[13] Propoxyphene exhibits an analgesic effect for 3 to 5 hours.[21] It is metabolized to norpropoxyphene ($t_{1/2}$ ~30-60 h) by CYP3A4 and excreted into the urine.[8,21]

Tapentadol

Tapentadol (Nucynta) is available as oral tablets (t_{max} ~1.5 h), with $t_{1/2}$ of 3 to 5 hours.[12,13] The V_d for tapentadol is 6 L/kg to 9 L/kg.[13] The bioavailability is about 32% due to extensive first pass metabolism.[12] Tapentadol is mainly metabolized by UGT1A9 and UGT2B7 via glucuronidation and excreted into the urine.[12] All tapentadol metabolites are inactive.

Tramadol

Tramadol can be administered orally (t_{max} ~2 h), intravenously (t_{max} ~0.5 h), intramuscularly (t_{max} ~0.75 h), or rectally (t_{max} ~3.3 h).[28,54] Sustained-release tablets contain 100 mg to 200 mg tramadol and are taken only twice daily.[28] The bioavailability of oral formulations is about 70%.[28] Tramadol is also available in combination with acetaminophen (Ultracet) or aspirin.

The V_d for tramadol is 2.6 L/kg to 2.9 L/kg,[13] and the $t_{1/2}$ is 4.3 to 8.3 hours.[13] Tramadol is *N*-demethylated by CYP2B6 and 3A4 and *O*-demethylated by CYP2D6. These metabolites are then conjugated to glucuronide and sulfates.[28] Tramadol and its metabolites are excreted in the urine.[28]

See Table 25-1 for V_d and $t_{1/2}$ estimates for the synthetic opioids.

Table 25-1. Volume of Distribution (V_d) and Half-Life ($t_{1/2}$) Estimates[13]

Drug	V_d (L/kg)	$t_{1/2}$ (h)
Buprenorphine	1.4-6.2	2-4 (parenteral); 18-49 (sublingual)
Fentanyl	3-8	3-12
Meperidine	3.7-4.2	2-5
Methadone	4-7	15-55
Propoxyphene	12-26	8-24
Tapentadol	6-9	3-5
Tramadol	2.6-2.9	4.3-8.3
O-desmethyl-tramadol		6.3-9.5

Abuse Potential and Characteristics

Opioids are attractive recreational drugs because they produce a feeling of euphoria. In addition, many perceive the use of prescription opioids as safer and less illegal when compared to other illicit drugs. Unfortunately, as one becomes tolerant with the drug, a higher dose is needed to maintain the euphoric feeling and mitigate withdrawal symptoms. Dependency and diversion of these drugs from legitimate medical use has therefore become a problem of epidemic proportions as the total number of opioid prescriptions increases. From 1991 to 2010, the total number of prescriptions tripled as a result of changes in health care practice, where opioids were beginning to be used for chronic pain.[55] As a result of increased effort to address the opioid epidemic issue, the average dosage of opioid prescriptions in the US has steadily decreased since 2010.[56] However, the dosage prescribed in 2015 was still three times higher compared to that in 1999.[56] With the increased use of prescription opioids, nonmedical use continues to be an issue and is the second most prevalent illicit drug use compared to cannabis.[57] Expectedly, the estimated number of opioid-related emergency department visits increased from ~300,000 to 855,000 cases in the US between 2004 and 2011.[58] More specifically, buprenorphine-related cases increased by 34 times, methadone-related and fentanyl-related cases both almost doubled, and tramadol-related cases tripled. There was, however, a significant decrease in cases related to meperidine and propoxyphene[58] as they were not commonly used or sold in the US anymore. Overall, opioid-related deaths continued to rise in the US, with the latest statistic from the Centers for Disease Control and Prevention showing an alarming increase of 27.7% from 2015 to 2016.[59]

Abuse of fentanyl transdermal patches can take the form of ingestion, inhalation, and excessive application.[48,60] The matrix design used in many of the transdermal systems is thought to be less suitable for transmucosal abuse because the fentanyl matrix maintains its basic delivery system even if cut into pieces. On the other hand, the reservoir design allows for direct access of fentanyl. Intravenous administration of residual fentanyl from the reservoir after use is common among drug abusers. However, it is unlikely that either design can prevent abuse from ingestion.[48] In addition, abuse of illicit fentanyl analogs (eg, acetylfentanyl, furanylfentanyl, carfentanil) has become an issue in the US in recent years.[61]

To reduce potential illicit use, especially intravenous use of sublingual medication, buprenorphine may be sold as a combination sublingual tablet containing buprenorphine and the opioid antagonist naloxone at a ratio of 4:1 (Suboxone). When this combination is taken as intended (sublingually), very little naloxone is absorbed or available systemically because it has low sublingual bioavailability and short elimination half-life. However, if the sublingual combination tablet is crushed and injected intravenously, the naloxone is rapidly distributed and will precipitate withdrawal symptoms, making this formulation less likely to be abused by this route.[38,42] The transdermal patch formulation of buprenorphine (Butrans) may also present a risk for illicit use (or accidental exposure), as discarded patches may still contain significant amounts of drug.

Although tramadol has low abuse potential, deaths have been reported as a result of suicide or abuse.[60] In 2010, the FDA added a new warning label to emphasize the risk of suicide and abuse.

Analysis

Specimen Types, Requirements, and Characteristics

Urine and blood are the most commonly used specimen types for detection of opioids. Oral fluid has also grown in popularity in recent years. Medication compliance is usually monitored by analyzing urine as it offers a longer detection window compared to blood or oral fluid. Both the parent drug and metabolite(s) should be measured because patients who attempt to cheat a urine drug test by dissolving their medication in the urine sample will not have metabolites present.

Modes of Analysis

Mass spectrometry (MS)-based methods (gas chromatography-mass spectrometry [GC-MS], liquid chromatography-tandem mass spectrometry [LC-MS/MS], time-of-flight mass spectrometry [TOF-MS]) are considered the "gold standard." These methods are more sensitive and specific than immunoassays and can be designed to provide quantitative measurement of parent drug and metabolites. These characteristics make MS-based methods ideal for use in monitoring medication compliance status for pain management and addiction programs.[62] (See also chapter 3, *Laboratory Support of Chronic Opioid Therapy.*)

Immunoassay-based methods are available for automated instruments and, in some cases, point-of-care testing urine cups. Advantages include minimal sample preparation and rapid analysis. As such, immunoassay methods are most appropriate for use by the emergency department in cases of drug overdose. However, immunoassays may have variable sensitivity and specificity, and variation in cutoffs, which may result in false positives and false negatives, depending upon the product used.

Known Analytical Issues

As is generally true with any preliminary screening immunoassay, review of the assay's sensitivity, specificity, and cross-reactivity information is recommended. Further, when indicated, confirmation of presumptive positives or unexpected negatives should be performed with a more sensitive and specific method such as MS.

Buprenorphine immunoassays are primarily targeted to cross-react with the parent drug. Some immunoassays have significant cross-reactivity with the major metabolite norbuprenorphine, as well as glucuronidated forms of parent drug and metabolite. Depending upon the method and generation of the assay, there may be considerable cross-reactivity with other opiates/opioids, including codeine, dihydrocodeine, hydrocodone, nalorphine, naltrexone, norpropoxyphene, methadone, morphine, and tramadol, as well as nonopiates such as chloroquine and hydroxychloroquine.[63-66]

Urine immunoassays for fentanyl are primarily designed to cross-react with fentanyl, but not the metabolite norfentanyl. Some immunoassays will also detect fentanyl analogs such as acetylfentanyl, butyrylfentanyl, and sufentanil. False positives have been noted in patients taking labetalol, trazodone, or risperidone with some immunoassays.[67,68] According to the manufacturers, immunoassays for propoxyphene detect mainly propoxyphene, but with about 70% cross-reactivity with norpropoxyphene. However, Pesce et al[69] discovered a false-negative rate of 23.4% in one of the immunoassays, likely attributable to poor cross-reactivity with norpropoxyphene.

Immunoassays for methadone are targeted to the parent drug and do not cross-react significantly with methadone metabolites or other opioid drugs. There have been occasional reports of

Table 25-2. Toxic Dose

Drug	Estimated Minimum Lethal Dose	Toxic Plasma Concentration (mg/L)	Fatal Plasma Concentration
Buprenorphine	Not reported	Not reported	0.3-7.7 ng/mL (blood)
Fentanyl	2 mg	Not reported	1.89-139 mcg/L
Meperidine	1 g	>2	Not reported
Methadone	40-50 mg	Overlaps therapeutic range	0.06-3.1 mg/L
Propoxyphene	0.5 g	>1	>2 mg/L
Tapentadol	Not reported	Not reported	0.3-5.2 mg/L
Tramadol	Not reported	>1	>2.0 mg/L

cross-reactivity with structurally and pharmacologically unrelated drugs with some of the immunoassays, including tramadol,[70] tapentadol,[71] quetiapine, and verapamil.[63] Immunoassays for the methadone metabolite EDDP appear to be more specific.[70]

Rapid drug-screening test cups/cards are immunoassays in nature. Therefore, specificity and sensitivity are variable, depending upon the product used.[72] They should not be used for pain management or preemployment drug screen purposes without definitive testing by MS-based methods.[62]

Clinical Issues

Interpretation

Most of the commercially available "opiates/opioids" immunoassays are designed to detect morphine and codeine and may have variable cross-reactivity with semisynthetic opioids. These assays will not, however, detect the synthetic opioids described in this chapter. It is imperative that ordering clinicians do not interpret a negative "opiates" result as the absence of all opioids. Although there is no "cocktailed" immunoassay that can detect all the commonly used synthetic opioids, targeted screening immunoassays are becoming increasingly available for automated chemistry instruments. Laboratorians should be familiar with the cross-reactivity of these immunoassays used at their institution. Immunoassays from different manufacturers may have variable cross-reactivity with metabolites. Depending on the accuracy of the screening assay, such implementation may offer a faster turnaround time than MS-based quantitative assays, particularly in the emergency setting. In the event that an initial immunoassay screen is unexpectedly negative, definitive testing by MS-based methods may identify the presence of metabolites that are not detected by the immunoassay. If clinical suspicion is high for diversion/abuse, definitive testing for the presence of metabolite should be performed. This is particularly true in addiction treatment programs as patients who have diverted the drug for sale may attempt to add a small amount of the parent drug into their urine sample to produce a positive result.

Overdose and Toxicity

As with the opiates (as described in chapter 24), confusion, dizziness, miosis, hallucinations, hypotension, respiratory depression, seizures, and coma are features of toxicity. Additive effects may occur if ethanol, other opioids, or CNS depressants (eg, benzodiazepines) are taken concomitantly with opioids. In 2016, the FDA issued a drug safety communication warning about the serious risks of combining opioid pain medications with benzodiazepines due to potentially lethal suppression of the CNS.[74] The known toxic doses and plasma concentrations are summarized in Table 25-2.

Naloxone is commonly used to reverse respiratory depression caused by an opioid overdose. However, it is important to note that naloxone has a much shorter duration of action than the respiratory depressant effects of opioids. Consequently, the patient's respiratory status should be continuously monitored, and multiple administrations of naloxone may be required.[74] With propoxyphene/norpropoxyphene/methadone toxicity, naloxone is not effective in treating cardiotoxicity, and additional therapeutic interventions are needed.

In the case of meperidine overdose, the side effects are mainly attributed to the neurotoxic metabolite normeperidine. As such, naloxone cannot reverse the toxicity.[22] Paradoxically, naloxone may induce convulsions as a result of meperidine removal from opioid receptors.[22] Signs of normeperidine toxicity include irritability, agitation, tremors, tachycardia, muscle twitches, hypertension, disorientation, and seizures.[36] Unfortunately, these signs can be suggestive of inadequate pain relief, which in turn leads to further administration of meperidine.[36] Due to this neurotoxic side effect, meperidine is not recommended as a first-line agent for pain treatment[22] and should not be used in elderly patients.[36] Expectedly, sales of meperidine dropped 32% from 1997 to 2007.[23] Similarly, both propoxyphene and its metabolite, norpropoxyphene, are neurotoxic (in addition to being cardiotoxic). Propoxyphene was withdrawn from the US market in 2010.

Deaths and life-threatening side effects have been reported due to inappropriate prescriptions and illicit use of fentanyl. Fentanyl overdose has resulted from improper use such as replacing patches more frequently than instructed, using more patches than prescribed, or applying heat to the patch and inhaling the vapors. As a result, the FDA issued a second warning on the fentanyl patch in December 2007 to highlight some of this safety information. There were also several product recalls as a result of potential leakage of fentanyl from the reservoir of the transdermal design.[48]

The range of blood concentrations observed in patients with methadone toxicity significantly overlap with those in patients on methadone maintenance treatment, making it difficult to distinguish these two situations based upon blood concentrations alone. High interindividual variability in methadone pharmacokinetics necessitates caution when initiating, switching, or titrating the dose of methadone, especially if other CYP450 inducers or inhibitors are used. On January 1, 2008, as part of an effort to reduce the number of adverse events related to methadone use, an advisory was issued by the DEA to restrict the distribution and availability of high-strength (40-mg) methadone tablets only to facilities authorized for detoxification and maintenance treatment of opioid addiction and to hospitals; the lower strength formulations, which are FDA approved for pain management use, continue to be available to all authorized registrants and retail pharmacies.[75]

Buprenorphine toxicity is clinically indistinguishable from overdoses with other opioids. However, life-threatening respiratory depression is attenuated due to the partial agonist effect. Similar to other opioid-related deaths, most buprenorphine fatalities have been attributed to co-administration with other CNS depressants such as alcohol or benzodiazepines.[76]

Many of the opioids (meperidine, tramadol, methadone, propoxyphene, fentanyl) discussed in this chapter have been shown or implicated to inhibit serotonin reuptake, so they must not be taken with monoamine oxidase inhibitors or other serotonin reuptake inhibitors, otherwise patients may suffer from serotonin toxicity.[35] Symptoms of serotonin toxicity include agitation, mental confusion, myoclonus, hyperreflexia, tachycardia, and diaphoresis. Fatalities from serotonin toxicity involving fentanyl, meperidine, propoxyphene, and tramadol have been reported.[35] All of the synthetic opioids (except for tapentadol) described here are metabolized by CYP3A4. Therefore, administration of CYP3A4 inducers like phenobarbital or phenytoin[8] will increase the production of metabolites and shorten the half-life of the parent compounds. In the cases of meperidine and propoxyphene, intake of inducers may result in toxicity because their CYP3A4 metabolites are toxic. CYP2D6 also plays a role in the metabolism of tramadol, tapentadol, and methadone. Genetic variations in CYP2D6 would therefore affect their effectiveness.

As with many other drugs, metabolism of the opioids discussed in this chapter relies heavily on the function of the liver. Therefore, liver dysfunction as a result of illness or acetaminophen overdose may alter pharmacokinetics. Similarly, renal impairment can affect the clearance of these drugs. Therefore, dose adjustment may be required in patients who have liver or renal dysfunction to prevent life-threatening issues.

References

1. Yaksh TL, Wallace MS. Opioids, analgesia, and pain management. In: Brunton LL, Chabner BA, Knollman BC, eds. *Goodman and Gilman's The Pharmacological Basic of Therapeutics.* 12th ed. New York, NY: McGraw-Hill Co; 2011:481-526.
2. Centers For Disease Control and Prevention Public Health Service. US Department of Health and Human Services. Guideline for prescribing opioids for chronic pain. *J Pain Palliat Care Pharmacother.* 2016;30(2):138-140.
3. Han B, Compton WM, Jones CM, Cai R. Nonmedical prescription opioid use and use disorders among adults aged 18 through 64 years in the United States, 2003-2013. *JAMA.* 2015;314(14):1468-1478.
4. Huang X, Keyes KM, Li G. Increasing prescription opioid and heroin overdose mortality in the United States, 1999-2014: an age-period-cohort analysis. *Am J Public Health.* 2018;108(1):131-136.
5. Ruhm CJ. Corrected US opioid-involved drug poisoning deaths and mortality rates, 1999-2015. *Addiction.* 2018;113(7):1339-1344.

6. Aldrich JV, McLaughlin JP. Opioid peptides: potential for drug development. *Drug Discov Today Technol.* 2012;9(1):e23-e31.
7. Spetea M, Asim MF, Wolber G, Schmidhammer H. The micro opioid receptor and ligands acting at the micro opioid receptor, as therapeutics and potential therapeutics. *Curr Pharm Des.* 2013;19(42):7415-7434.
8. Armstrong SC, Wynn GH, Sandson NB. Pharmacokinetic drug interactions of synthetic opiate analgesics. *Psychosomatics.* 2009;50: 169-176.
9. Stanley TH. The history and development of the fentanyl series. *J Pain Symptom Manage.* 1992;7: S3-S7.
10. Ropero-Miller JD, Goldberger BA. Opioids. In: Shaw LM, Kwong TC, eds. *The Clinical Toxicology Laboratory: Contemporary Practice of Poisoning Evaluation.* Washington DC: AACC Press; 2001.
11. Leppert W, Luczak J. The role of tramadol in cancer pain treatment: a review. *Support Care Cancer.* 2005;13:5-17.
12. Vadivelu N, Chang D, Helander EM, et al. Ketorolac, oxymorphone, tapentadol, and tramadol: a comprehensive review. *Anesthesiol Clin.* 2017;35(2):e1-e20.
13. Baselt RC. *Disposition of Toxic Drugs and Chemicals in Man.* 11th ed. Seal Beach, CA: Biomedical Publications; 2017.
14. Campbell ND, Lovell AM. The history of the development of buprenorphine as an addiction therapeutic. *Ann N Y Acad Sci.* 2012;1248:124-139.
15. Likar R. Transdermal buprenorphine in the management of persistent pain: safety aspects. *Ther Clin Risk Manag.* 2006;2:115-125.
16. Wills S. *Drugs of Abuse.* 2nd ed. London, UK: Pharmaceutical Press; 2005:46-53.
17. Mattick RP, Breen C, Kimber J, Davoli M. Buprenorphine maintenance versus placebo or methadone maintenance for opioid dependence. *Cochrane Database Syst Rev.* 2014;(2):CD002207.
18. James IG, O'Brien CM, McDonald CJ. A randomized, double-blind, double-dummy comparison of the efficacy and tolerability of low-dose transdermal buprenorphine (BuTrans seven-day patches) with buprenorphine sublingual tablets (Temgesic) in patients with osteoarthritis pain. *J Pain Symptom Manage.* 2010;40(2):266-278.
19. Hagelberg NM, Olkkola KT. Fentanyl for breakthrough cancer pain: what's new? *Pain.* 2010;151:565-566.
20. Plante GE, VanItallie TB. Opioids for cancer pain: the challenge of optimizing treatment. *Metabolism.* 2010;59(Suppl 1):S47-S52.
21. Trescot AM, Datta S, Lee M, Hansen H. Opioid pharmacology. *Pain Physician.* 2008;11:S133-S153.
22. Clark RF, Wei EM, Anderson PO. Meperidine: therapeutic use and toxicity. *J Emerg Med.* 1995;13:797-802.
23. Manchikanti L, Fellows B, Ailinani H, Pampati V. Therapeutic use, abuse, and nonmedical use of opioids: a ten-year perspective. *Pain Physician.* 2010;13:401-435.
24. US Federal Register. 42 CFR 8.12 Federal opioid treatment standards.
25. Barkin RL, Barkin SJ, Barkin DS. Propoxyphene (dextropropoxyphene): a critical review of a weak opioid analgesic that should remain in antiquity. *Am J Ther.* 2006;13:534-542.
26. *Prescription Drugs and the Elderly: Many Still Receive Potentially Harmful Drugs Despite Recent Improvements.* Washington, DC: US General Accounting Office; July 1995. GAO/HEHS-95-152. http://www.gao.gov/archive/1995/he95152.pdf. Accessed May 7, 2019.
27. Inciardi JA, Cicero TJ, Munoz A, et al. The diversion of Ultram, Ultracet, and generic tramadol HCL. *J Addict Dis.* 2006;25:53-58.
28. Grond S, Sablotzki A. Clinical pharmacology of tramadol. *Clin Pharmacokinet.* 2004;43:879-923.
29. Cuschieri RJ, Morran CG, McArdle CS. Comparison of morphine and sublingual buprenorphine following abdominal surgery. *Br J Anaesth.* 1984;56:855-859.
30. Foster B, Twycross R, Mihalyo M, Wilcock A. Buprenorphine. *J Pain Symptom Manage.* 2013;45(5):939-949.
31. Ayonrinde OT, Bridge DT. The rediscovery of methadone for cancer pain management. *Med J Aust.* 2000;173(10):536-540.
32. Mercadante S, Casuccio A, Fulfaro F, et al. Switching from morphine to methadone to improve analgesia and tolerability in cancer patients: a prospective study. *J Clin Oncol.* 2001;19(11):2898-2904.
33. Codd EE, Shank RP, Schupsky JJ, Raffa RB. Serotonin and norepinephrine uptake inhibiting activity of centrally acting analgesics: structural determinants and role in antinociception. *J Pharmacol Exp Ther.* 1995;274:1263-1270.
34. Langford RM, Knaggs R, Farquhar-Smith P, Dickenson AH. Is tapentadol different from classical opioids? A review of the evidence. *Br J Pain.* 2016;10(4):217-221.
35. Gillman PK. Monoamine oxidase inhibitors, opioid analgesics and serotonin toxicity. *Br J Anaesth.* 2005;95:434-441.
36. Koczmara C, Perri D, Hyland S, Rousseaux L. Meperidine (Demerol) safety issues. *Dynamics.* 2005;16:8-12.
37. Methadone hydrochloride. In: Budavari S, O'Neil M, Smith A, Heckelman P, Obenchain J. *The Merck Index.* 12th ed. Boca Raton, FL: CRC Press; 1996:1015-1016.

38. Center for Substance Abuse Treatment. *Clinical Guidelines for the Use of Buprenorphine in the Treatment of Opioid Addiction.* Treatment Improvement Protocol (TIP) Series 40. DHHS Publication No. (SMA) 04-3939. Rockville, MD: Substance Abuse and Mental Health Services Administration; 2004.
39. Lutfy K, Cowan A. Buprenorphine: a unique drug with complex pharmacology. *Curr Neuropharmacol.* 2004; 2:395-402.
40. Heit HA, Gourlay DL. Buprenorphine: new tricks with an old molecule for pain management. *Clin J Pain.* 2008;24:93-97.
41. Kuhlman JJ, Lalani S, Magluillo J, et al. Human pharmacokinetics of intravenous, sublingual, and buccal buprenorphine. *J Clin Pharmacol.* 1997;37:31-37.
42. Elkader A, Sproule B. Buprenorphine: clinical pharmacokinetics in the treatment of opioid dependence. *Clin Pharmacokinet.* 2005;44:661-680.
43. Prommer E. The role of fentanyl in cancer-related pain. *J Palliat Med.* 2009;12:947-954.
44. Power I. Fentanyl HCl iontophoretic transdermal system (ITS): clinical application of iontophoretic technology in the management of acute postoperative pain. *Br J Anaesth.* 2007;98:4-11.
45. Gommers D, Bakker J. Medications for analgesia and sedation in the intensive care unit: an overview. *Crit Care.* 2008;12(Suppl 3):S4.
46. Wilhelm W, Kreuer S. The place for short-acting opioids: special emphasis on remifentanil. *Crit Care.* 2008;12(Suppl 3):S5.
47. Evron S, Ezri T. Options for systemic labor analgesia. *Curr Opin Anaesthesiol.* 2007;20:181-185.
48. Nelson L, Schwaner R. Transdermal fentanyl: pharmacology and toxicology. *J Med Toxicol.* 2009; 5:230-41.
49. Eap CB, Buclin T, Baumann P. Interindividual variability of clinical pharmacokinetics of methadone: implications for the treatment of opioid dependence. *Clin Pharmacokinet.* 2002;41:1153-1193.
50. Fredheim OMS, Moksnes K, Borchgrevink PC, Kaasa S, Dale O. Clinical pharmacology of methadone for pain. *Acta Anaesthesiol Scand.* 2008;52:879-889.
51. Ferrari A, Coccia CP, Bertolini A, Sternieri E. Methadone: metabolism, pharmacokinetics and interactions. *Pharmacol Res.* 2004;50:551-559.
52. Totah RA, Allen KE, Sheffels P, Whittington D, Kharasch ED. Enantiomeric metabolic interactions and stereoselective human methadone metabolism. *J Pharm Exp Ther.* 2007;321:389-399.
53. Methadone. DRUGDEX® System [internet database]. Version 5.1. Greenwood Village, CO: Thomson Micromedex.
54. Lintz W, Beier H, Gerloff J. Bioavailability of tramadol after i.m. injection in comparison to i.v. infusion. *Int J Clin Pharmacol Ther.* 1999;37:175-183.
55. Yu HY. The prescription drug abuse epidemic. *Clin Lab Med.* 2012; 32: 361-377.
56. Guy GP, Zhang K, Bohm MK, et al. Vital signs: changes in opioid prescription in the United States, 2006-2015. *MMWR Morb Mortal Wkly Rep.* 2017;66:697-704.
57. Lipari RN, Van Horn SL, Hughes A, Williams M. *State and Substrate Estimates of Nonmedical Use of Prescription Pain Relievers: The CBHSQ Report.* Rockville, MD: Substance Abuse and Mental Health Services Administration; 2013-2017.
58. *Drug Abuse Warning Network, 2011: Selected Tables of National Estimates of Drug-Related Emergency Department Visits.* Rockville, MD: Center for Behavioral Health Statistics and Quality, SAMHSA; 2013.
59. Vivolo-Kantor AM, Seth P, Gladden RM, et al. Vital signs: trend in emergency department visits for suspected opioids overdose – United States, July 2016 – September 2017. *MMWR Morb Mortal Wkly Rep.* 2018;67:279-285.
60. Bronstein AC, Spyker DA, Cantilena LR Jr, et al. 2008 Annual Report of the American Association of Poison Control Centers' National Poison Data System (NPDS): 26th Annual Report. *Clin Toxicol (Phila).* 2009;47:911-1084.
61. O'Donnell JK, Halpin J, Mattson CL, Goldberger BA, Gladden RM. Deaths involving fentanyl, fentanyl analogs and U-47700: 10 States, July-December 2016. *MMWR Morb Mortal Wkly Rep.* 2017; 66:1197-1202.
62. Yu H-Y. Pitfalls of Point-of-Care Urinary Drug Screening for Pain Management. *AACC CLN.* Ask the Expert. July 2015:48.
63. Saitman A, Park HD, Fitzgerald RL. False-positive interferences of common urine drug screen immunoassays: a review. *J Anal Toxicol.* 2014;38(7):387-396.
64. Berg JA, Schjøtt J, Fossan KO, Riedel B. Cross-reactivity of the CEDIA buprenorphine assay in drugs-of-abuse screening: influence of dose and metabolites of opioids. *Subst Abuse Rehabil.* 2015;6:131-139.
65. Melanson SE, Snyder ML, Jarolim P, Flood JG. A new highly specific buprenorphine immunoassay for monitoring buprenorphine compliance and abuse. *J Anal Toxicol.* 2012;36(3):201-206.
66. Shaikh S, Hull MJ, Bishop KA, et al. Effect of tramadol use on three point-of-care and one instrument-based immunoassays for urine buprenorphine. *J Anal Toxicol.* 2008;32:339-343.

67. Snyder ML, Jarolim P, Melanson SE. A new automated urine fentanyl immunoassay: technical performance and clinical utility for monitoring fentanyl compliance. *Clin Chim Acta.* 2011;412(11-12):946-951.
68. Wang BT, Colby JM, Wu AH, Lynch KL. Cross-reactivity of acetylfentanyl and risperidone with a fentanyl immunoassay. *J Anal Toxicol.* 2014; 38(9):672-675.
69. Pesce A, Rosenthal M, West R, et al. An evaluation of the diagnostic accuracy of liquid chromatography-tandem mass spectrometry versus immunoassay drug testing in pain patients. *Pain Physician.* 2010;13:273-281.
70. Sneidman MR, Yu HE. Comparison of Roche methadone screening assay with DRI methadone metabolite (EDDP) screening assay. *Clin Chem.* 2014;60:S245 (B390).
71. Collins AA, Merritt AP, Bourland JA. Cross-reactivity of tapentadol specimens with DRI methadone enzyme immunoassay. *J Anal Toxicol.* 2012;36(8):582-587.
72. Sneidman MR, Yu HE. Performance comparison of six different rapid screening drug test cards/cups. *Clin Chem.* 2015;61:S220 (B319).
73. FDA Drug Safety Communication: FDA warns about serious risks and death when combining opioid pain or cough medicines with benzodiazepines; requires its strongest warning. https://www.fda.gov/Drugs/DrugSafety/ucm518473.htm. Accessed May 7, 2019.
74. van Dorp E, Yassen A, Sarton E, et al. Naloxone reversal of buprenorphine-induced respiratory depression. *Anesthesiology.* 2006;105(1):51-57.
75. US Department of Justice, Drug Enforcement Administration, Office of Diversion Control. Methadone Hydrochloride Tablets USP 40 mg (Dispersable). January 1, 2008. https://www.deadiversion.usdoj.gov/pubs/advisories/methadone_advisory.htm. Accessed May 7, 2019.
76. Kintz P. A new series of 13 buprenorphine-related deaths. *Clin Biochem.* 2002;35(7):513-516.

Chapter 26

Novel Psychoactive Substances

Donna Papsun, MS

Introduction

Novel psychoactive substances (NPS) is a designation used to refer to substances that have emerged onto the recreational drug scene that may have either been chemically modified from existing drugs of abuse or repurposed from pharmaceutical and/or academic research chemicals for abuse with the intent to skirt legal controls. NPS are very diverse in terms of their effects and chemistries, with the majority of those identified to date mimicking the effects of the six main groups of substances controlled under international drug conventions, including opioids, synthetic cannabinoid receptor agonists, stimulants, classic hallucinogens, dissociatives, and sedatives/hypnotics. The appeal of NPS lies in accessibility, which has been aided by the internet and e-commerce, circumventing drug laws and evading detection through traditional toxicology testing. The emergence of this group with little to no understanding of human interactions while evading regulatory controls has led to their increased abuse, hospital emergency admissions, and fatalities.

The European Monitoring Centre for Drugs and Drug Addiction (EMCDDA) has reported a steady increase in the number of NPS every year since 2008; 66 new substances were notified for the first time in 2016, bringing the total number of substances being monitored to 628.[1] Although more substances are reported each year, many NPS are transient in nature and remain on illicit drug markets for a few years until they become regulated, in which case their popularity tends to drop off and a new substance takes its place.

Novel psychoactive substances represent a major challenge in relation to their chemistry, pharmacology, and toxicity. Though the general pharmacological classes of NPS are known, information regarding specific associated effects and toxicity is still limited and typically obtained from case reports and series, with very few, if any, controlled dosage studies. Pharmacokinetic parameters are largely unknown for all NPS due to the lack of human studies. The small amount of information that is known for certain compounds is typically gleaned from animal studies or may only involve studies of analytes that are no longer relevant in the current landscape of NPS.

Synthetic Cannabinoids

Origin

Synthetic cannabinoids are a class of NPS derived from a body of research involving a large number of substances synthesized to investigate the cannabinoid receptor system as potential therapeutic agents. The diversity of chemical structures seen in the synthetic cannabinoid class includes modifications, substitutions, halogenation, and alkyl homolog variations that retain receptor binding activity. In general, synthetic cannabinoids are chemically classified based on a structure consisting of core, ring, link, and a tail, as described in an EMCDDA report; the newest generations of synthetic cannabinoids may no longer feature a ring.[2]

The first incidence of synthetic cannabinoids detected in the United States occurred in 2008 when US Customs and Border Patrol verified the presence of HU-210 and JWH-018 in packets of herbal incense products called "Spice"; since then, the formulation of synthetic cannabinoids found in these products has changed quickly over time. UR-144 and its fluorinated counterpart XLR-11 emerged sometime around 2012 following a decline in JWH-018 positivity, and AB-CHMINACA emerged circa 2014, following a decline in prevalence and scheduling by the Drug Enforcement Administration (DEA) in 2013 of XLR-11. Example compounds are described below.

Descriptive Chemistry

JWH-018

Synonyms: AM-678, 1-pentyl-3-(1-naphthoyl) indole

Formula: $C_{24}H_{23}NO$

Molecular mass = 341.45 g/mol

CAS-209414-07-3

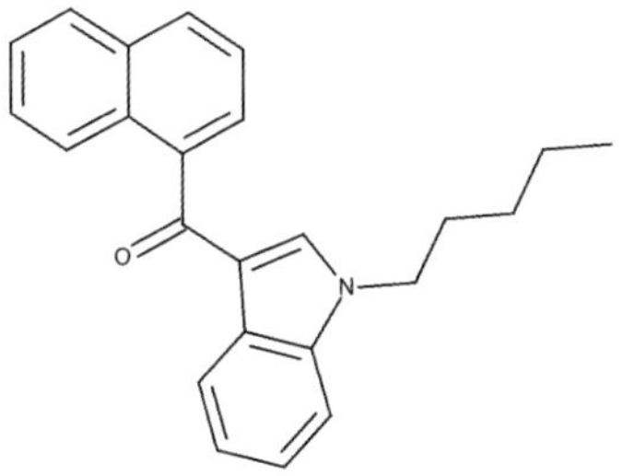

XLR-11

Synonym: 5"-fluoro-UR-144

Formula: $C_{21}H_{28}FNO$

Molecular mass = 329.46 g/mol

CAS-1364933-54-9

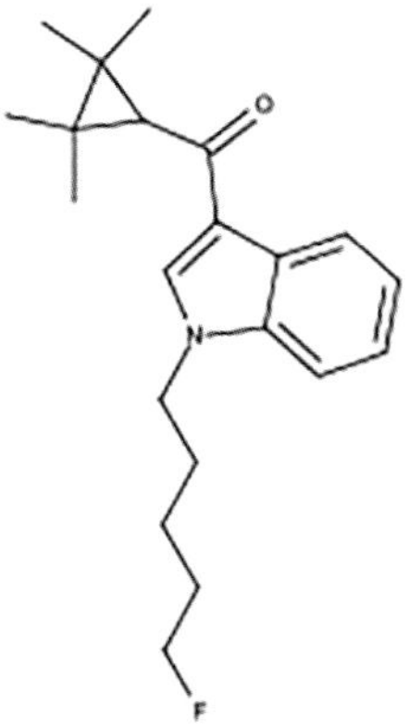

AB-CHMINACA

Synonyms: Not applicable

Formula: $C_{20}H_{28}N_4O_2$

Molecular mass = 356.46 g/mol

CAS-1185887-21-1

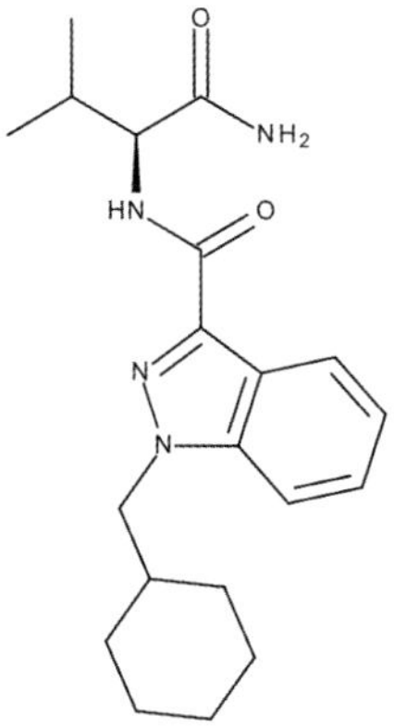

Pharmacology

Studies of synthetic cannabinoids indicate higher cannabinoid receptor binding affinities, with effects two to 100 times more potent than delta-9-tetrahydrocannabinol (Δ^9-THC), the primary psychoactive compound in the cannabis plant; in addition, many of these substances also have noncannabinoid receptor binding, which has led to additional adverse side effects not consistent with the side effect profile of traditional cannabinoids. The potency for the three synthetic cannabinoids listed above compared to Δ^9-THC is listed in Table 26-1; these synthetic cannabinoids are provided as examples of the different types of structures seen in this group of NPS.

Synthetic cannabinoids refer to the class of drugs targeting the endogenous cannabinoid receptors,

Table 26-1. Potency Compared to Delta-9-THC as Determined by Mouse-Tetrad Studies

Compound	Potency
JWH-018[86]	2.9
XLR-11[87]	6.3
AB-CHMINACA[88]	26

THC, tetrahydrocannabinol.

CB_1 and CB_2, with CB_1 receptor activation producing desired euphoria and relaxation effects, while CB_2 receptors are involved in immune functions and are typically the targets for therapeutic agents. Certain substitutions will change the affinity and potency; for example, a single atom substitution of fluorine on the terminal position of the pentyl chain increases the compound's ability to bind at the CB_1 receptor.

Intended Use and Mechanism of Action

Synthetic cannabinoids are recreational substances repurposed from pharmaceutical research that are intended to mimic the effects of Δ^9-THC. Synthetic cannabinoids are psychoactive chemicals dissolved in solvent, which are then applied to plant material. This plant material is then packaged and sold online or in head shops in colorful branded packaging, with common product names of "K2," "Spice," and herbal incense; these packages feature a disclaimer "Not for Human Consumption" to circumvent regulatory control. Traditionally, synthetic cannabinoids are smoked, but the active substances themselves have also been detected in electronic cigarette solutions and powder products.

Pharmacokinetics

During one study, blood specimens were obtained from an individual smoking an herbal incense product containing JWH-018 and JWH-073; peak concentrations of both compounds were observed after 19 minutes and then decreased to less than half after 53 minutes, with further decrease by 199 minutes. This initial data suggests that the half-life of JWH-018 is very short.[3] This was corroborated by a later study, where maximum concentrations of JWH-018 reached 2.9 ng/mL to 9.9 ng/mL minutes after smoking 2 mg to 3 mg, with a half-life estimated to be between 1.3 and 5.7 hours.[4]

In general, metabolic pathways for synthetic cannabinoids include hydroxylation along the tail, terminal carboxylation of the tail, and hydroxylation of the ring. Some, but not all, of the halogenated compounds also undergo dehalogenation. Newer synthetic cannabinoids, which do not have a ring structure, undergo hydroxylation of the terminal amide.[5]

Detection of the parent compound in urine is rare for synthetic cannabinoids. Urine analysis inclusive of metabolites helps to broaden the detection interval for drug abuse. JWH-018 metabolites include JWH-018 *N*-pentanoic acid and JWH-018 *N*-(5-hydroxypentyl).[6] The major exclusive metabolite of XLR-11, not shared with UR-144, is 2'carboxy-XLR-11.[7] Major metabolites of AB-CHMINACA were identified to be products of monohydroxylation and amide hydrolysis producing the carboxylated metabolite, AB-CHMINACA-COOH.[8]

Many of the hydroxylated and carboxylic acid metabolites undergo phase II metabolism, including conjugation with glucuronic acid facilitated by UGT enzymes.[9] Many of the hydroxylated metabolites have also been demonstrated to be pharmacologically active.

Peak concentrations of JWH-018 and JWH-073 in urine were detected between 3 and 16.5 hours after smoking a blend of the two compounds, with a detection window of 2 to 3 days inclusive of metabolites.[10]

Abuse Potential and Characteristics

Synthetic cannabinoids produce physiological and psychoactive effects similar to Δ^9-THC, but with greater intensity, resulting in medical and psychiatric emergencies.[11] Case reports have indicated that use of synthetic cannabinoids can produce effects beyond acute intoxication, with tolerance and withdrawal symptoms described following prolonged use, which suggests dependence may be associated with chronic use.[12,13]

Overdose and Toxicity

Acute synthetic cannabinoid exposure causes a range of mild to severe neuropsychiatric, cardiovascular, and renal symptoms in addition to other effects. General adverse effects associated with synthetic cannabinoid use include nausea, vomiting, anxiety, agitation, paranoia, tachycardia, hypertension, hallucinations, tremors, seizures, and chest pain. Additional serious medical complications include acute renal failure/acute kidney injury (AKI), myocardial infarction, ischemic strokes, psychosis, suicidal ideation, and cognitive impairment. The type and degree of effect depends on the dose and compound used; in addition, multiple synthetic cannabinoids have been found in the same product, which poses additional risks to the end user.

Between 2010 and 2015, physicians in the Toxicology Investigators Consortium (ToxIC) treated 456 patients with synthetic cannabinoid intoxications; 277 of the 456 reported synthetic cannabinoids as the sole toxicologic agent. Among these 277 patients, the most common clinical signs of intoxication were neurological (agitation, central nervous system [CNS] depression/coma, and delirium/toxic psychosis).[14]

Synthetic cannabinoids have been linked to fatalities. No deaths have been reported with JWH-018; however, several intoxications have been reported, with serum concentrations ranging from <0.10 ng/mL to 13 ng/mL.[15] Postmortem blood concentrations of JWH-018 have ranged from 0.1 ng/mL to 199 ng/mL.[16] Blood concentrations in two deaths associated with XLR-11 use were reported as 0.61 ng/mL and 1.4 ng/mL.[17] In a case where a young man died after ingesting an herb product containing synthetic cannabinoids, toxicological analyses of blood samples revealed AB-CHMINACA of 7.61 ng/mL and trace amounts of 5-fluoro-AMB, FUB-PB-22, and AB-FUBINACA; autopsy revealed pulmonary edema resulting in hypoxic encephalopathy.[18]

In addition to XLR-11 and AB-CHMINACA, deaths have been attributed to 5-fluoro-PB-22, 5-fluoro-AMB, 5-fluoro-ADB, ADB-CHMINACA, and MDMB-CHMICA, while severe adverse effects have been linked to several other compounds, such as AKI associated with XLR-11 and agitated delirium associated with ADB-PINACA.[19] Adulterants may also cause toxicity and contribute to severe adverse effects. Severe bleeding was experienced by a series of individuals (including a few fatalities) who used synthetic cannabinoids laced with the anticoagulant brodifacoum; FUB-AMB was the primary psychoactive synthetic cannabinoid found in the contaminated product.[20]

Patients admitted to the emergency department (ED) for synthetic cannabinoid overdose generally receive supportive care, benzodiazepines, and fluids, except in cases with serious complications such as seizures, which often also require intubation. Acute adverse effects generally subside within 24 to 38 hours.

Serious medical complications have developed after subacute exposures, including myocardial infarction, ischemic strokes, seizures, and AKI, which required hemodialysis and corticosteroid treatment.

Synthetic Stimulants

Origin

Synthetic stimulants are a chemically diverse groups of substances (including phenethylamines, cathinones, aminoindanes, and piperazines), the effects of which include those considered stimulant, entactogenic, and hallucinogenic in nature. Substances in this group mimic the effects of traditional drugs such as cocaine, methamphetamine, and 3,4-methylenedioxymethamphetamine (MDMA). One of the more popular groups of synthetic stimulants are synthetic cathinones, structural derivatives of cathinone, the active compound in the khat plant and alkaloid structurally similar to amphetamine. These substances first appeared in the US illicit drug market around 2009, although first references on internet drug forums were in 2007. Synthetic structural modifications of cathinone have led to a number of cathinone derivatives, such as adding substituents on the aromatic ring and/or the *alpha*-carbon, *N*-alkylation, and incorporation of the nitrogen atom in a ring structure.

Methylone, along with mephedrone and methylenedioxypyrovalerone (MDPV), was part of the first wave of synthetic stimulants to achieve popularity in the US, with methylone frequently being seen as an alternative to MDMA. Methylone was a popular entactogen amongst attendees at electronic music festivals but over time was replaced by ethylone followed by butylone and subsequently dibutylone. *Alpha*-PVP emerged as an alternative to MDPV in 2013 after it was federally scheduled. *N*-ethylpentylone emerged on the recreational drug scene in 2016, following a decline in *alpha*-PVP popularity, which was potentially caused by a Chinese export ban that was levied in October 2015. Example compounds are described below.

Descriptive Chemistry

Methylone

Synonyms: βk-MDMA, MDMC; 3,4-methylenedioxy-*N*-methylcathinone

Formula: $C_{11}H_{13}NO_3$

Molecular mass = 207.23 g/mol

CAS-186028-80-8

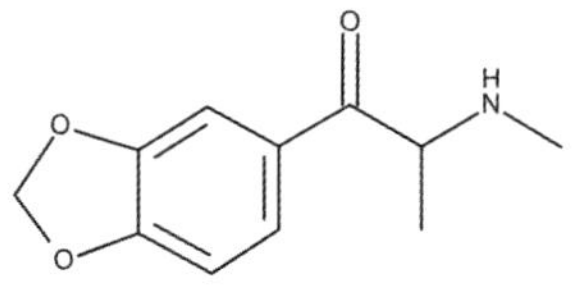

Alpha-PVP

Synonyms: α-PVP, *alpha*-pyrrolidinovalerophenone, *alpha*-pyrrolidinopentiophenone

Formula: $C_{15}H_{21}NO$

Molecular mass = 231.34 g/mol

CAS-5485-65-4

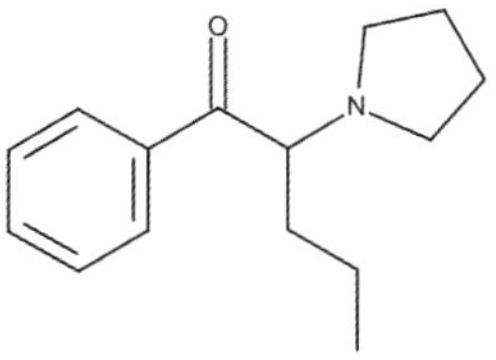

N-Ethylpentylone

Synonyms: Ephylone, βk-ethyl-K, βk-EBDP, β-keto-ethylbenzodioxolylpentanamine

Formula: $C_{14}H_{19}NO_3$

Molecular mass = 249.31 g/mol

CAS-17763-02-9

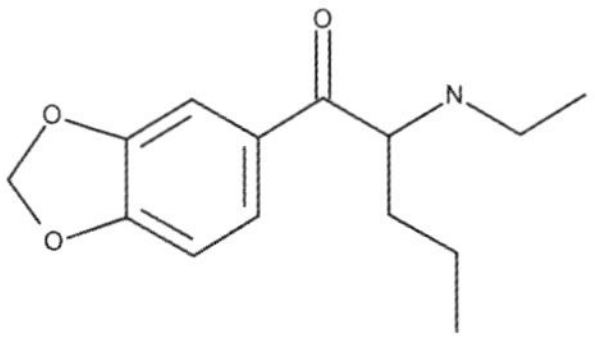

Pharmacology

Intended Use and Mechanism of Action

The synthetic stimulants, similar to synthetic cannabinoids, are packaged and sold online or in head shops in colorful branded packaging, with common product names of "bath salts," "legal highs," and "party powders"; these packages also typically feature a disclaimer "Not for Human Consumption." The true contents of the products may be obscured as advertising, and packaging of the products is often misleading, both in terms of number and identity of active substance as well as legality. The products are sold as tablets, capsules, and powders; modes of abuse include ingestion, inhalation, injection, and insufflation.

Synthetic stimulants act as CNS stimulants by increasing monoamine neurotransmitter concentrations; this involves interactions with dopamine, serotonin, and norepinephrine transporters to varying degrees of affinity and selectivity. More stimulant activity is associated with higher potency at the dopamine transporter, while more emphathogenic activity is associated with higher potencies at the serotonin transporter or those with similar potencies at dopamine and serotonin transporters. Ring substituted cathinones, such as methylone and *N*-ethylpentylone, typically act as transporter substrates that increase the release of dopamine, serotonin, and norepinephrine in addition to blocking reuptake from the synaptic cleft.[21] The presence of a pyrrolidine ring, as in *alpha*-PVP, acts as a transport blocker (reuptake inhibitors) at the dopamine transporter. Increasing the length of the *alpha*-carbon chain increases affinity and potency at the dopamine transporter in addition to stimulating the release of dopamine and norepinephrine.[22]

Pharmacokinetics

Generally, the presence of a β-keto group increases the polarity of cathinone derivatives, resulting in a decrease of their ability to cross lipid membranes, which may lead to higher doses or binge consumption of cathinones to attain effects.[23] Methylone exhibits rapid kinetics with peak blood concentrations occurring 30 minutes after oral administration in rats and readily crosses the blood-brain barrier, but not as readily as *alpha*-PVP.[24] Pyrovalerone cathinones are highly lipophilic, thus having a high blood-brain barrier penetration and a high volume of distribution, which results in longer plasma and tissue half-lives due to the presence of the pyrrolidine ring. In a study of one patient, the half-life of *alpha*-PVP was predicted to be approximately 4 hours.[25]

Metabolic pathways for cathinones include reduction of the keto group, desalkylation, hydroxylation, and desmethyleneation in cathinones containing a methylenedioxy moiety. When a methylenedioxy group is present, it undergoes ring opening to afford a dihydroxy intermediate that is eventually converted to its corresponding 3-hydroxy-4-methoxy and/or 4-hydroxy-3-methoxy counterparts; with pyrrolidine-containing compounds, the pyrrolidine ring can either be oxidized to a lactam or converted to an iminium salt that is hydrolyzed to a corresponding ketone.[26] Methylone is metabolized by *N*-demethylation, reduction of the keto group, and oxidation of the tolyl moiety.[27] The main metabolites targeted for *alpha*-PVP analysis are β-hydroxy-α-PVP and α-PVP lactam.[28,29] Reduction of the beta-ketone to an alcohol resulted in the most prominent and unique metabolite for *N*-ethylpentylone.[30] Some cathinones metabolize to other cathinones, which also have activity and may obscure the true identity of parent substance.

Both methylone and 4'-hydroxy-3'-methoxymethcathinone urine concentrations peaked 4 hours after administration.[31] Methylone was undetectable 36 hours after exposure, while its metabolite persisted for 48 hours after.[31]

The urinary half-life of *alpha*-PVP was estimated to be 22 hours based on the first 5 days of urinary analysis.[32]

Abuse Potential and Characteristics

The desired effects of synthetic cathinones include increased energy, empathy, euphoria, mental alertness, concentration, talkativeness, sexual arousal, a focused mind, and overall positive feelings, similar to those of cocaine and amphetamine; the effects generally occur within 15 to 45 minutes following administration and last from 2 to 7 hours.[33] Small chemical changes to the structure of cathinone and/or amphetamine result in several new drugs that pharmacologically behave very similarly, producing the same spectrum of stimulant effects while potentially evading toxicological detection and the law.

Overdose and Toxicity

Cardiac, psychiatric, and neurological signs and symptoms are the most common adverse effects in synthetic cathinone users who require medical care. The most frequently reported clinical signs with synthetic cathinone toxicity include agitation, paranoia, hallucinations, psychosis, myoclonus, and headaches. Other common symptoms of synthetic cathinone toxicity include bruxism, hyperthermia, hypertension, tachycardia, vasoconstriction, hyponatremia, nausea, vomiting, and chest pains. Synthetic cathinone hallucinations are frequently auditory and tactile in nature and paired with psychoses that can be severe and long lasting; patients may be admitted days after cessation of drug use, with psychotic symptoms persisting for several days thereafter, even while receiving treatment. More serious symptoms of synthetic cathinone toxicity that require substantial and prolonged medical treatment—and in some cases lead to death—include cardiac arrest, liver failure, kidney failure, rhabdomyolysis, and the development of compartment syndrome, which can lead to muscle and nerve damage and problems with blood flow. The abuse of synthetic cathinones has also led to violent behaviors including self-harm and suicide.

Symptoms fall on a scale of serotonin syndrome as a consequence of excess serotonin in the CNS and excited delirium. Excited delirium syndrome may include clinical features of psychomotor agitation, delirium, tachycardia and hyperthermia, cardiac arrest, rhabdomyolysis, renal failure, hepatic injury, anoxic brain injury, and death. This syndrome has been debated in medical literature; its mechanism is postulated to be excessive overstimulation of the heart by catecholamines brought on by drug exposure, leading to increased contractility, blood pressure, and heart rate, resulting in increased oxygen demand, followed by myocardial ischemia, fatal cardiac arrhythmias, and sudden death.[34] Excited delirium syndrome has been cited as a contributing factor in fatal cases involving highly agitated persons physically restrained in police custody.[35]

Methylone peripheral blood concentrations in excess of 500 ng/mL may result in lethal toxicity, including hyperthermia and other sympathomimetic-like symptoms.[36] In three fatal intoxications of methylone, the deceased exhibited seizure-like activity and elevated body temperature, with two cases exhibiting metabolic acidosis; peripheral blood concentrations were determined to be 840 ng/mL, 3300 ng/mL, and 560 ng/mL. Three other deaths attributed to methylone were reported in blood at 100 ng/mL, 4310 ng/mL, and 11,000 ng/mL.[37]

It has been suggested that serum or blood concentrations exceeding 100 ng/mL to 200 ng/mL of *alpha*-PVP are considered high and may be associated with adverse effects.[38] A man in his mid-20s died as a result of sudden heart failure following restraint after exhibiting sudden violent behavior; his *alpha*-PVP serum concentration was 411 ng/mL.[39] A 32-year-old male who died of sudden cardiac arrest had an *alpha*-PVP plasma concentration of 1500 ng/mL; a second individual who experienced visual hallucinations, psychotic symptoms, bilateral mydriasis, sinus tachycardia, and rhabdomyolysis had a plasma level of 235 ng/mL.[40] Another case was a 28-year-old male who arrived at the ED in asystole and had a blood *alpha*-PVP concentration of 901 ng/mL; pulmonary edema, atherosclerotic lesions, and heart failure cells were noted on autopsy.[41] The most recent reported fatality involved a 28-year-old male admitted to the ED due to cardiac arrest. His *alpha*-PVP blood concentration was 174 ng/mL after 5 hours of treatment in the ED, and his cause of death was ruled cardiac arrest secondary to intoxication with *alpha*-PVP.[42]

N-ethylpentylone was qualitatively confirmed in a case where an individual died after presenting to the ED displaying agitation and unusual behavior; clinical laboratory analysis revealed elevated troponins, rhabdomyolysis, hypoglycemia, hepatic and renal injury, respiratory failure, and disseminated intravascular coagulation.[43] *N*-ethylpentylone concentrations ranged from 12 ng/mL to 50,000 ng/mL in 26 cases submitted as part of toxicological death investigations and drugged driving casework.[44] In one case where cause of death was ruled complications of acute *N*-ethylpentylone intoxication, the blood concentration was 953 ng/mL; three other deaths in the same case series reported concentrations of 31 ng/mL, 45 ng/mL, and 121 ng/mL, with the two lower concentrations associated with deaths by gunshot wounds.[45]

Patients showing signs of the sympathomimetic toxidrome after exposure to synthetic cathinones, including agitation, psychosis, significant tachycardia, hypertension, and seizures, should be treated with benzodiazepines to counteract excessive epinephrine and norepinephrine release and reuptake inhibition, and to control agitation, anxiety, and seizures.[46] Treatment is primarily supportive, as there is no specific antidote. Hyperthermia should be treated with aggressive cooling. Anxiolytic and antipsychotic drugs such as lorazepam, haloperidol, diazepam, and risperidone have been used alone or in combination to successfully treat cathinone-induced neurologic disorders.[47-49] However, haloperidol should be used with caution since it may exacerbate hyperthermia and trigger the development of neuroleptic malignant syndrome.

Physical restraints may be warranted but are contraindicated, especially for patients exhibiting signs of excited delirium; persistent hyperthermia and excessive muscle activity induced by restraint can exacerbate rhabdomyolysis and facilitate life-threatening kidney failure, leading to death. Preferred therapy includes sedation and adrenergic blockade.[50]

Novel Illicit Opioids

Origin

Illicit fentanyl use started to rise as a profitable alternative to heroin. In 2013, the first fentanyl derivative, acetylfentanyl, appeared, and other nontraditional opioid agonists gleaned from pharmaceutical research into morphine alternatives such as AH-7921 and MT-45 emerged soon after. In 2014 and 2015, additional fentanyl derivatives and other novel illicit opioids emerged, with a large increase in use and breadth of substances between 2016 and 2017. Some of the more prevalent compounds include furanylfentanyl, U-47700, carfentanil, para-fluoroisobutyrylfentanyl (FIBF), 3-methylfentanyl, cyclopropylfentanyl, and methoxyacetylfentanyl. Example compounds are described below.

Descriptive Chemistry

Acetylfentanyl

Synonym: Desmethylfentanyl

Formula: $C_{21}H_{26}N_2O$

Molecular mass = 322.44 g/mol

CAS-3258-84-2

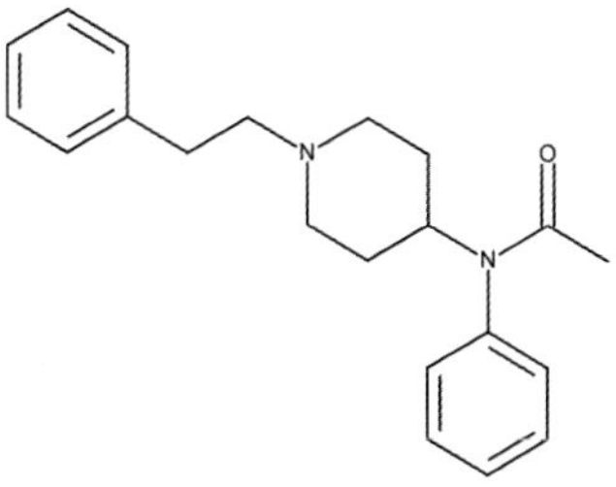

Furanylfentanyl

Synonym: Fu-F

Formula: $C_{24}H_{26}N_2O_2$

Molecular mass = 374.48 g/mol

CAS-101365-56-4

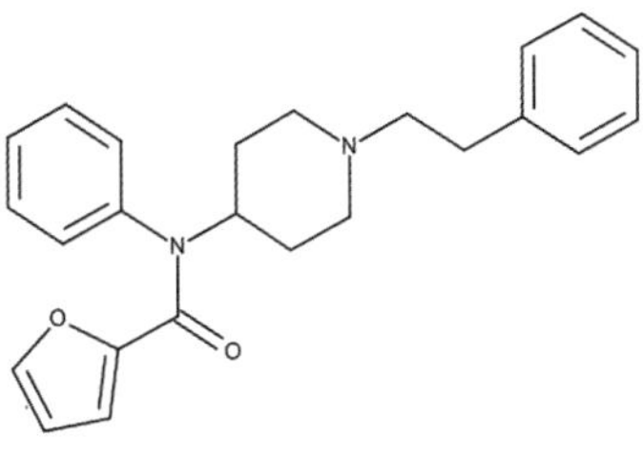

U-47700

Synonym: U-47

Formula: $C_{16}H_{22}Cl_2N_2O$

Molecular mass = 329.27 g/mol

CAS-82657-23-6

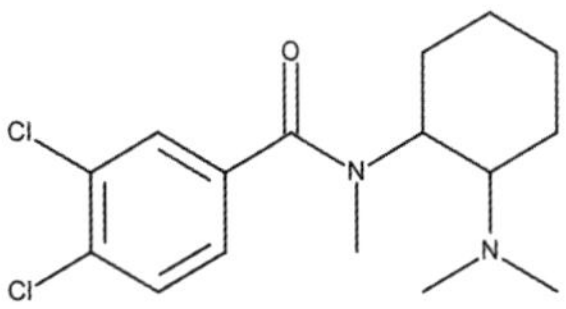

Pharmacology

Intended Use and Mechanism of Action

The pharmacological activity of fentanyl, its analogs, and other structurally dissimilar novel opioids is due to their activation of opioid receptors, with primary activity resulting from activation of the μ opioid receptor. See chapter 24, *Opioids 1: Opiates and Semisynthetic Opioids,* for a discussion of opioid pharmacology.

Due to the multiple positions at which substitutions can be made to the fentanyl core structure, such as replacement of or substitution on the phenyl or piperidinyl rings, alteration of chain length or substitution on the alkyl chain, and halogenation on multiple sites, a very large number of permutations and consequently fentanyl analogs are possible. These structural changes can dramatically affect the analgesic activity and potency of such compounds, in addition to altering their legal status. Table 26-2 summarizes the analgesic activity and potency relative to morphine for fentanyl and selected analogs derived from animal models in preclinical studies.

Commonly, novel illicit opioids are sold as powders, nasal sprays, liquids, or in tablet forms. These substances can be purchased online and shipped from countries such as China under the pretense of "research chemicals." In addition, these substances have been distributed into the street heroin supply where they are often mixed with or substituted for heroin and/or illicit fentanyl, which may lead to life-threatening respiratory depression and death to the unsuspecting end user. Counterfeit pharmaceuticals sold on the street have also been chemically confirmed to contain novel illicit opioids.

Table 26-2. Analgesic Activity and Potency Relative to Morphine for Specified Novel Illicit Opioids

Compound	Analgesic Activity ED50 (mg/kg)	Analgesic Potency Relative to Morphine
Morphine[89]	13.9	1
Fentanyl[89]	0.062	224
Acetylfentanyl[90]	0.021	16
Furanylfentanyl[91]	0.02	7
U-47700[92,93]	0.21	7.5 -12

Pharmacokinetics

Data regarding pharmacokinetic and pharmacodynamic properties of fentanyl analogs and/or novel synthetic opioids in humans is scarce, and most data is only derived from animal models. Fentanyl analogs are known for their high potency, low cardiovascular toxicity, rapid onset, and short duration of action, which made the group attractive to initial clinical investigation. High lipophilicity, ease of crossing the blood-brain barrier, and high receptor affinity are reasons for increased potency, in addition to high selectivity and specificity for the μ opioid receptor subtype, all of which contribute to clinical effects.[51]

The major route of metabolism for fentanyl is *N*-dealkylation on the piperidine nitrogen to norfentanyl, its primary inactive metabolite, with minor pathways involving amide hydrolysis to despropionylfentanyl and alkyl hydroxylation to hydroxyl fentanyl.[52] Fentanyl has a phenethylpiperidine core in its structure, and since many of the analogs typically incorporate variations on this core, they follow the established metabolic pathways of fentanyl.

Acetylnorfentanyl is the metabolite of acetylfentanyl. The major metabolites of furanylfentanyl were generated by amide hydrolysis and dihydrodiol formation; this is attributed to its aromatic, heterocyclic furan ring, which undergoes characteristic reactions.[53] Based on the above considerations, it is likely that other fentanyl analogs that have not been studied are similarly metabolized through the same phase I reactions to their respective

Table 26-3. Dose and Duration of Action of Synthetic Opioids Compared to Heroin and Fentanyl

Drug/Route of Administration	Dose			Action		
	Light	Common	Strong	Onset	Duration	After-Effects
Heroin						
Insufflation	7.5-20 mg	20-35 mg	35-50 mg	10-15 min	3-6 h	1-24 h
Smoked	5-15 mg	15-25 mg		5-10 min	3-5 h	1-24 h
Intravenous		5-10 mg	8-15 mg	0-5 min	4-5 h	1-24 h
Fentanyl						
Intranasal	10-25 μg	25-50 μg	50-75 μg			
Transdermal	12.5 μg/h	25-50 μg/h	50-100 μg/h	2-4 h	48-72 h	
Buccal				15-30 min	1-4 h	
Insufflated				15-30 min	1-4 h	
Acetylfentanyl						
Oral	1-3 mg	3-5 mg	5-7 mg	Minutes	Hours	1-8 h
Furanylfentanyl						
Oral	0.3-0.5 mg	0.5-0.9 mg	0.9-1.6 mg			
Insufflation	0.2-0.4 mg	0.4-0.8 mg	0.8-1.6 mg	1-10 min	1-3 h	1-3 h
U-47700	5-7.5 mg	7.5-15 mg	15-25 mg			
Oral				15 min	5-7 h	1-4 h
Insufflation				15 min	3-4 h	1-4 h
Intravenous				0-1 min	1-2 h	1-4 h

Adapted with permission from Zawilska JB.[94]

nor-metabolites via *N*-dealkylation on the piperidine ring and via other common metabolic pathways, including hydroxylation, dihydroxylation, and carboxylation, often in combination with *N*-dealkylation. Although not a fentanyl variant, *N*-desmethyl-U-47700 was determined to be the primary metabolite of U-47700 after undergoing *N*-dealkylation.[54]

Due to similar structures and shared metabolic pathways, the metabolism of many fentanyl variants can result in shared metabolites, which may complicate interpretation of toxicological data as well as obscure the true identity of parent substance.

Abuse Potential and Characteristics

Novel synthetic opioids are appealing due to the desired opioid-type effects of analgesia, sedation, and euphoria; ease of availability; profitability; and increasing restrictions on prescription opioids with a large opioid-abusing population.[55] Opioids, in general, are known for their high abuse potential; regular use leads to habituation and dependence that is dose and frequency related. Tolerance to the analgesic and euphoric effects of opioids develops quickly, with doses frequently requiring adjustment for effective pain management. Doses and durations of action for listed substances are compared to heroin and fentanyl in Table 26-3. Cessation of opioid agonist use leads to a withdrawal syndrome characterized by drug craving, dysphoria, anxiety, insomnia, irregular heart rate, loss of appetite, diarrhea, sweating, nausea, vomiting, abdominal cramps, and shivers.

Overdose and Toxicity

Because fentanyl analogs and novel synthetic opioids share the same mechanism of action as fentanyl and/or morphine, clinical features after their use are indistinguishable. Many patients who present to the ED after novel synthetic opioid use report decreased consciousness, respiratory depression, and miosis. Common adverse effects may include dizziness, nausea, vomiting, anxiety, sweating, and disorientation. Other effects that have been reported include hypoxic respiratory failure and diffuse alveolar hemorrhage after butyrylfentanyl use[56] and folliculitis/dermatitis with hair loss and ototoxicity after MT-45 use.[57]

Due to the high potencies of these compounds causing profound respiratory and CNS depression, unsuspecting end users are particularly at risk for death, especially if expecting heroin and/or pharmaceutical opioids. Fentanyl and fentanyl analogs are highly potent and fast-acting synthetic compounds that can trigger rapid progression to loss of consciousness and death. No regulation of dose, poly-drug use, and patterns of repeated use are most likely contributors to the high rates of overdose, respiratory depression, and death associated with these drugs. Serious interactions can occur when these substances are mixed with heroin, cocaine, and other CNS depressants, particularly benzodiazepines.

The main mechanism of fatal opioid overdose is respiratory depression, which can result in cerebral and pulmonary edema. Novel illicit opioids have been implicated in thousands of deaths in recent years, although often seen with other substances. Acetylfentanyl concentrations were reported to be 31 ng/mL to 600 ng/mL in four deaths attributed to only acetylfentanyl.[58] Three deaths in which furanylfentanyl was the only substance reported had blood concentrations of 0.43 ng/mL, 1.16 ng/mL, and 7.66 ng/mL.[59] A 27-year-old male was found deceased after snorting an unknown powder; his serum concentration was 1460 ng/mL of U-47700, along with quetiapine, amphetamine, and naproxen.[60] U-47700 was confirmed in 16 fatalities across the US between 2015 and 2016, with blood concentrations ranging from 17 ng/mL to 490 ng/mL, often with other drugs, including five cases with furanylfentanyl.[61]

As with other intoxication with all opioids, treatment is focused on protecting the airway and maintaining breathing and circulation; naloxone has proven useful in reversing the central and peripheral opioid effects rapidly. Potent synthetic opioids may require large and often repeated doses of naloxone, likely due to the higher affinities and potentially longer durations of action of novel synthetic opioids.

Designer Hallucinogen

Origin

25I-NBOMe, the best-characterized designer hallucinogen, is the *N*-benzoyl-methoxy derivative of the substituted phenethylamine 2C-I. It was originally investigated as a radiotracer for positron emission tomography (PET) as a highly potent serotonin agonist but subsequently emerged as a recreational drug of abuse due to its psychedelic and hallucinogenic effects in 2010. 25B-NBOMe and 25C-NBOMe are two other analogs, with the iodine substituted with a bromine and chlorine, respectively.

Descriptive Chemistry

25I-NBOMe

Synonyms: 25I, 2C-I-NBOMe, Cimbi-5

Formula: $C_{18}H_{22}INO_3$

Molecular mass = 427.28 g/mol

CAS-1043868-97-8

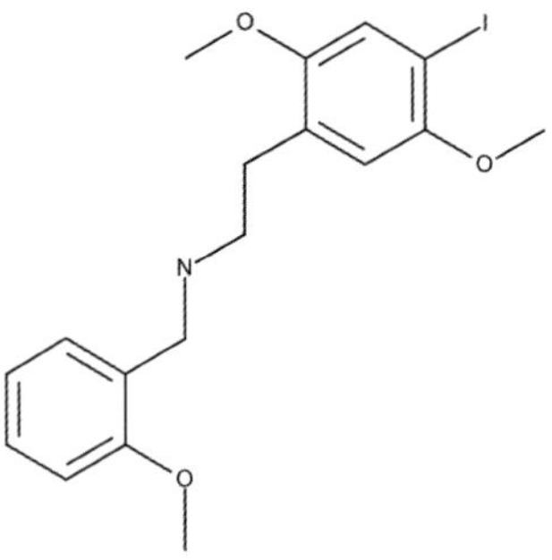

Pharmacology

Intended Use and Mechanism of Action

NBOMes, like the classical hallucinogen lysergic acid diethylamine (LSD), are agonists of the serotonergic system, binding to the serotonin 5-HT_{2A} receptor. 25I-NBOMe is a full agonist with a dissociation constant (K_i) of 0.044 ± 0.006 nM, making it 16 times the potency of 2C-I itself at the receptor and an effective concentration observed in 50% of subjects tested (EC50) of 0.44 ± 0.07 nM.[63] As a hallucinogenic compound with a mechanism of action as an agonist of the 5-HT_{2A} receptor, effects range from mild to profound alterations in cognition and affect, powerful sensory and somatic effects, and mystical experiences.

Common routes of administration include sublingual, buccal, and nasal/intranasal. 25I-NBOMe has been routinely reported as being ingested by blotter tabs, often being mistakenly sold as LSD. It has also been encountered in liquid formulations to be dropped into the nasal cavity. Sublingual doses as low as 50 μg may produce psychoactive effects; typical doses are reported to range from 500 μg to 800 μg.

Pharmacokinetics

The pharmacokinetics of NBOMe compounds have not been studied in man or whole animals. However, demethylated metabolites and 2C-I were identified after a 25I-NBOMe ingestion.[64] Urine collected 13 hours post admission did not reveal presence of parent compound, in which case testing for metabolites is likely recommended.[65]

Abuse Potential and Characteristics

NBOMes are typically used for their sympathomimetic and serotonergic effects. Hallucinogenic effects include vivid auditory and visual hallucinations and a change in time perception. Onset of action for 25I-NBOMe varies from 15 to 120 minutes, with duration of effects lasting 6 to 10 hours depending on route of administration.

Overdose and Toxicity

NBOMe ingestion often presents as a serotonin toxidrome that begins shortly after ingestion, characterized by prominent neuropsychiatric effects (agitation, delirium, perceptual disturbances, and seizures) and autonomic instability (tachycardia, hypertension, diaphoresis, and dilated pupils).

Adverse effects from analytically confirmed human NBOMe ingestion has been reported; in one review looking at 20 individual patients, fatalities were reported in three cases (15%). Seven individuals (35%) were discharged after a period of observation, while eight (40%) required intensive care unit admission; common adverse effects were agitation (85%), tachycardia (85%), hypertension (65%), and seizures (40%), with laboratory abnormalities including elevated creatinine kinase (45%), leukocytosis (25%), and hyperglycemia (20%).[66]

Case reports of seven males who were presented to an emergency department due to analytically confirmed 25I-NBOMe intoxication reported the following adverse effects: tachycardia (n=7), hypertension (4), agitation and aggression (6), visual and auditory hallucinations (6), seizures (3), hyperpyrexia (3), clonus (2), elevated white cell count (2), elevated creatinine kinase (7), metabolic acidosis (3), and AKI (1).[67] Cardiac ischemia is considered to be a concern as well, due to 25I-NBOMe's ability to cause vasoconstriction in addition to blood platelet aggregation due to the release of thromboxane A2.

A number of deaths associated with 25I-NBOMe have also been reported, attributable either to pharmacologic toxicity, such as status epilepticus producing anoxic brain injury, or behavioral effects resulting in severe traumatic injuries. Concentrations have varied from as little as 0.034 ng/mL in serum in an individual who stabbed himself in the neck to as high as 28 ng/mL in the blood of a female who collapsed and become unresponsive after exhibiting aggressive behavior, seizures, and vomiting.[68,69]

Most users who seek medical attention recover, but a number have required extended stays in intensive care with ventilator support. Management of NBOMe ingestion should include aggressive fluid repletion using intravenous fluids and benzodiazepines for sedation.

Designer Dissociative

Origin

3-MeO-PCP (3-methoxy-phencyclidine), the best-characterized designer dissociative, is a methoxy-substituted derivative of the drug of abuse PCP (phencyclidine). Dissociative drugs, such as PCP, ketamine, and dextromethorphan, have been used nonmedically for mind-altering effects for decades. Many of these compounds have also been used clinically and in legitimate research. Derivatives based on the arylcyclohexylamine backbone have formed the basis of conventional drug discovery and drug development for conditions such as neuropathic pain and a variety of neurodegenerative disorders, and subsequently have been repurposed for recreational abuse; one of the first compounds of this class to reach the NPS market was methoxetamine. 4-MeO-PCP, a positional isomer of 3-MeO-PCP, first appeared on internet drug markets in 2008.

Descriptive Chemistry

3-MeO-PCP

Synonym: 3-Methoxy-phencyclidine

Formula: $C_{18}H_{27}NO$

Molecular mass = 273.42 g/mol

CAS-91164-58-8

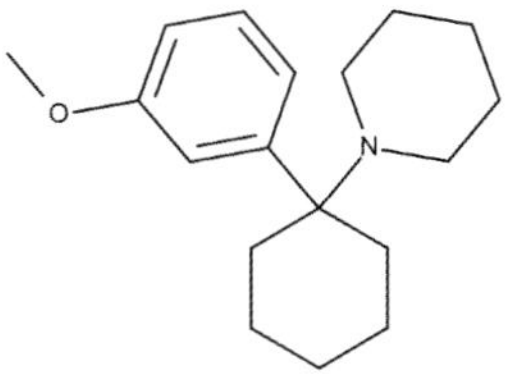

Pharmacology

Intended Use and Mechanism of Action

Arylcyclohexylamines is a miscellaneous group of dissociative anesthetic-type substances, acting by antagonism on *N*-methyl-*D*-aspartate (NMDA) receptors.[70] The binding affinity (K_i) of 3-MeO-PCP to the NMDA receptor is one of the highest known, with a K_i of 20 nM, roughly three times that of PCP.[71] It is an NMDA antagonist. In lower concentrations, effects of NMDA antagonism are amnesia and analgesia; in higher concentrations, side effects include hallucinations, paranoid delusions, ataxia, hyperreflexia, clonus, confusion, and agitation.[72] Drugs of the arylcyclohexylamine class are also dopamine reuptake inhibitors, which can produce stimulant and euphoric effects as well as tachycardia, hypertension, psychosis, and aggression.

Pharmacokinetics

3-MeO-PCP is active via oral, insufflation, inhalation, and injection routes in the single milligram range. 3-MeO-PCP's activity threshold is reported at 3- to 5-mg doses and generally strong dissociative effects are attained after 10- to 20-mg doses.[70] The duration of the effects has been reported to be ~4.5 hours, with onset within 30 minutes of an oral intake and a peak of approximately 2 hours; the half-life was estimated to be 11 hours.[70]

3-MeO-PCP metabolism was studied in rats; metabolic pathways included aliphatic and aromatic hydroxylation, carboxylation after ring opening, *O*-demethylation, and glucuronidation.[73] No other pharmacokinetic parameters have been studied for 3-MeO-PCP.

Abuse Potential and Characteristics

The main desired effects for dissociative drugs include euphoria, empathy, dissociation, and hallucinations, although side effects can include psychomotor agitation, cognitive impairment, and confusion. Dissociative intoxication shows a high degree of dose-dependent variation; stimulation may occur at low doses, while sedation, amnesia, and anesthesia generally occur at high doses. Perceptual alterations include proprioceptive disorders, ataxia, tingling, floating sensations, numbness, depersonalization, and derealization; visual effects may include impaired depth perception and synesthesia. Effects on cognition include altered thought patterns in addition to paranoia and grandiose ideology or full-blown delusions.[70]

Overdose and Toxicity

During a 21-month period in Sweden between July 2013 and March 2015, 59 patients presented to the ED after exposure to either 3-MeO-PCP or 4-MeO-PCP. Only seven cases were single-substance intoxications of 3-MeO-PCP; prominent clinical signs were hypertension, tachycardia, and altered mental status including confusion, disorientation, dissociation, and hallucinations. Patients testing positive for 3-/4-MeO-PCP were typically under medical care for 1 to 2 days, and 37% graded as severe intoxications; besides supportive care, 49% of patients were treated with benzodiazepines and propofol.[74] Serum concentrations ranged from 1 ng/mL to 242 ng/mL, with a mean and median of 29 ng/mL and 16 ng/mL, respectively.

It was reported that two men who consumed a powdered drug along with alcohol at a party started to experience disorientation, hallucinations, spastic leg postures, and facial grimacing after 15 minutes. Emergency medical services transported the men to the hospital. Upon admission, the first male remained hypertensive and tachycardic, and displayed prominent signs of psychosis, altered neurological status, and increased muscle tone with spastic leg postures. The second individual was also hypertensive and tachycardic, and displayed altered state of consciousness, isochoric and miotic pupils, and elevated arterial levels of lactate (3.2 mmol/L) with a pH of 7.289. Preliminary immunochemical screening of urine indicated presence of PCP in both patients; 3-MeO-PCP serum levels 2 hours post drug ingestion were 49 ng/mL and 66 ng/mL in these patients. Methamphetamine and metabolite amphetamine were also detected in the first male at 121 ng/mL and 10 ng/mL, respectively, while blood alcohol concentration was 0.102% in the second male.[75]

In a death attributed to intoxication of 3-MeO-PCP, the femoral blood concentration was 0.39 mcg/g.[76] A second case where death was determined to be combined 3-MeO-PCP, diphenhydramine, and amphetamine involved a concentration of 139 ng/mL in blood.[77]

Treatment of 3-MeO-PCP poisoning is symptomatic as there is no specific antidote. Management follows supportive measures similar to those of ketamine toxicity, such as use of intravenous fluids to prevent and manage rhabdomyolysis and promote renal excretion of the drug, and benzodiazepines for agitation and seizure. The mainstay is securing the airway, stabilizing hemodynamics, anticonvulsive therapy when indicated, total gastrointestinal washout, managing hyperpyrexia, and preventative measures in rhabdomyolysis/crush syndrome. Antipsychotics (haloperidol/olanzapine) are recommended to control neuropsychiatric status.

Designer Benzodiazepines

Origin

Many designer benzodiazepines were originally synthesized by pharmaceutical companies as therapeutic drug candidates; most were not developed, forwarded to clinical trials, or approved for medicinal use on the basis of safety and/or efficacy, although some are prescribed in a few countries. Such substances are potentially more harmful than pharmaceutical benzodiazepines with unknown pharmacological/toxicological profiles and have added to the complexity and dangers of the illicit market for benzodiazepines. Etizolam, the best-characterized designer benzodiazepine, was introduced to Japan in 1983 as a prescription benzodiazepine for treatment of anxiety and muscle relaxant properties. It is also approved in Korea and Italy, but not currently approved for medicinal use in the US. Etizolam appeared in the illicit US market in 2012, with a total of 2445 reports between its first appearance and June 2018, according to the DEA.[78] Other compounds that have been reported from this class include phenazepam, flubromazepam, flubromazolam, delorazepam, diclazepam, and clonazolam.

Descriptive Chemistry

Etizolam

Synonyms: Etilaam, Etizest, Depas

Formula: $C_{17}H_{15}ClN_4S$

Molecular mass: 342.07 g/mol

CAS-40054-69-1

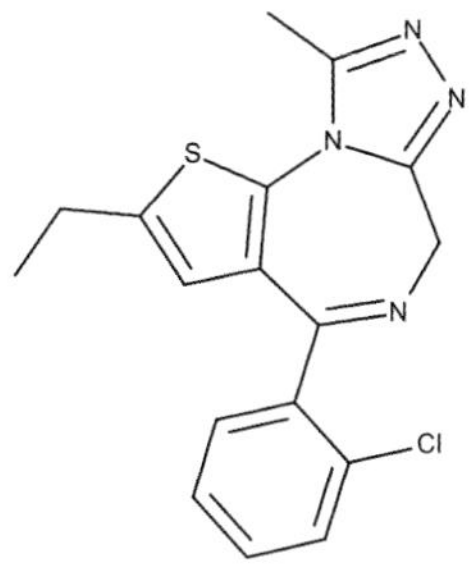

Pharmacology

Intended Use and Mechanism of Action

Designer benzodiazepines are agonists at the $GABA_A$ receptor and potentiate the inhibitory action of gamma-amino butyric acid (GABA). Benzodiazepines, as a class of CNS depressants, have anxiolytic, sedative-hypnotic, muscle relaxant, and anticonvulsant properties, and are often prescribed as anxiolytics, anesthetic adjuncts, and treatment for obsessive-compulsive disorders. The phenyl group appears to be a requirement for benzodiazepine activity; modifications of the benzodiazepine structure affect both the potency and duration of action.

Pharmacokinetics

Since etizolam is therapeutically prescribed in certain countries, pharmacokinetic studies have been performed. The single-dose kinetic profile of etizolam suggests absorption after oral dosage as reasonably rapid, with maximum plasma concentrations being achieved within 0.5 to 2 hours. The mean elimination half-life averaged 3.4 hours.[79]

Highly lipophilic compounds typically exhibit greater plasma protein binding and can generally cross the blood-brain barrier with greater ease; etizolam's lipophilicity was experimentally determined to be similar to clonazepam, a commonly prescribed benzodiazepine.[80]

Etizolam is metabolized by hydroxylation of the methyl and ethyl groups to form alpha-hydroxyetizolam and 8-hydroxyetizolam. These metabolites show longer half-lives than unchanged etizolam. Both metabolites have activity, with 8-hydroxyetizolam demonstrating higher activity than etizolam itself in mouse studies, which suggests that the metabolites may contribute significantly to the clinical effects of the parent compound.[81]

Additional designer benzodiazepines may metabolize to active substances and/or other known benzodiazepines, such as diclazepam to delorazepam, which is also subsequently metabolized to lorazepam, a common prescription benzodiazepine with its own activity. Therefore, detection of lorazepam could indicate exposure to diclazepam and/or delorazepam, in addition to the use of lorazepam itself.

Based on the kinetic characteristics of the parent drug and metabolites, etizolam can be regarded as a short-acting benzodiazepine, with elimination kinetics between those of short-intermediate derivatives and ultra-rapidly eliminated benzodiazepines.[81]

Abuse Potential and Characteristics

All benzodiazepines have sedating effects, which make them a target for abuse. Desired effects of benzodiazepines include relief of tension, mental stress, and anxiety; positive feelings of calmness; relaxation and well-being in anxious individuals; improved coping with situational pressures or psychological problems; and relief of side effects associated with overstimulation or withdrawal of other drugs. Etizolam is chemically and pharmacologically similar to diazepam, but six to 10 times more potent based on preclinical data.[79] Benzodiazepines may be administered orally, intravenously, or intramuscularly. Designer benzodiazepines are most often encountered in tablet forms but are also seen as powder, pellets, blotters, and capsules.

Overdose and Toxicity

Some signs and symptoms of benzodiazepine overdose include anxiety, agitation, dizziness, confusion, nystagmus, slurred speech, altered mental state, amnesia, hypotension, and impaired cognition. Respiratory depression may occur with benzodiazepine use, which will be significantly increased if used in combination with other CNS depressants such as alcohol or opioids. Chronic use of benzodiazepines may result in the development of tolerance and dependence. Abrupt cessation may lead to withdrawal syndrome, which can include insomnia, anxiety, perceptual hypersensitivity, tremors, irritability, nausea and vomiting, mental confusion, and life-threatening convulsions.

Etizolam is considered relatively safe, with the possibility of poisoning by etizolam alone being low; however, it can contribute to muscle-relaxing properties that may contribute to other mechanisms of death such as drowning or a drugged driving traffic fatality. Etizolam in 14 impaired driving cases ranged in concentrations from 19 ng/mL to 170 ng/mL, with a median of 50 ng/mL.[82]

A 59-year-old female with chronic kidney disorder was found deceased by drowning in a bathtub in her house; etizolam was confirmed at 263 ng/mL in blood, which is higher than typical therapeutic levels of 25 ng/mL.[81]

Flumazenil is a specific antidote for benzodiazepine overdose, but the risk of flumazenil may outweigh potential benefits, so it is ideally only used to treat acute overdose in the benzodiazepine-naïve individual.

Analysis

Specimen Types, Requirements, and Characteristics

For the detection of NPS in antemortem specimens, challenges include potential stability issues, the requirement for specialized toxicology testing due to unknown but often low concentrations of drug analytes, target analytes detectable in biological matrices after exposure, and unknown detection windows for drug analytes.

Concentrations in biological matrices are influenced not only by sampling time after drug intake and intake amount, but also postcollection variables. In addition to the lack of established pharmacokinetic parameters for most NPS, data regarding chemical stability properties in biological matrices is also scarce. Mechanisms involved in chemical conversion of compounds that occur both during enzymatic metabolism and degradation due to instability may include reduction, oxidation, and hydrolysis; instability of compounds is affected by external environmental factors such as temperature, pH, light exposure, type of matrix, and duration of storage.[83] In one example, a stability test carried out for the analysis of cathinones reported approximately 20% to 80% degradation in 5 days at 20 ± 2°C and approximately 15% to 20% loss in 6 days at 5 ± 2°C in human whole blood at physiological pH, even in the presence of fluoride-oxalate preservative.[84]

In general, storage of specimens with parameters of time, temperature, specimen type, and preservative have not been examined for the majority of NPS or related metabolites. Although preferred specimen collection tubes and stability data are largely unknown for many substances, parent drugs and/or metabolites of NPS substances have been reported in the literature in blood, serum, and urine, in addition to postmortem specimens such as tissues and fluids. The extent of the effect stability has on concentrations may be unknown but does not invalidate the identification of NPS in biological specimens. In general, gray and lavender top tubes are suggested, while serum separator tubes are generally not recommended for toxicological detection. Best practices include specimen retention, maintaining biological specimens either refrigerated or frozen, and submitting for expedited analysis.

Modes of Analysis

The analysis of NPS poses several issues, including limited analytical methods for detecting and monitoring these substances based on the need for sensitive, specialized instrumentation. In addition, the appearance of new substances typically outpaces availability of standardized reference material, which is required for development of a toxicological assay, all before a time-consuming validation of that assay can be performed. Most screening methodology for NPS employs some type of mass spectrometry (MS)-based technique such as liquid chromatography time of flight (LC-TOF) and other accurate mass technologies. Traditional screening techniques such as immunoassay or gas chromatography-mass spectrometry (GC-MS) can be used but lack specificity and sensitivity for the detection of most NPS analytes. Extensive extraction techniques, such as liquid-liquid extraction or solid-phase extraction, are also required to isolate the analytes of interest from biological matrix components, which may be resource prohibitive.

Although immunoassays are typically not designed for the detection of NPS, certain compounds may cross-react and therefore trigger positive immunoassay results. However, unless confirmatory tests include the specific NPS, the causal agent may go undetected and the confirmatory test will be negative. Since the structures of novel benzodiazepines such as etizolam and fentanyl analogs such as furanylfentanyl are similar to those of which the immunoassay screens are targeted towards, many compounds cross-react. Table 26-4 provides cross-reactivity information for specific compounds of these two classes. There are some synthetic cannabinoid-targeted immunoassays, but these were originally developed for the original JWH-type compounds; the quick turnover of NPS as well as the large variation in chemical structures does not lend itself to the development and implantation of routine immunoassay tests for use in clinical laboratories. Methoxylated PCP analogs also cross-react with PCP immunoassays, although the responses are lower than that of the parent substance (~7-fold lower for 3-MeO-PCP and ~40-fold for 4-MeO-PCP); it is postulated that metabolites may contribute to the degree of cross-reactivity.

Table 26-4. Percent Cross-Reactivity of Fentanyl Analogs and Benzodiazepines Derivatives to Commercial Immunoassays[95,96]

Fentanyl Analog	% Cross-Reactivity	Benzodiazepine Derivative	% Cross-Reactivity
Acetylfentanyl	111	Phenazepam	90
Butyrylfentanyl	77	Etizolam	107
Para-fluorofentanyl	87	Flubromazepam	84
Cis-3-methylfentanyl	3	Diclazepam	79
Trans-3-methylfentanyl	50	Delorazepam	80

The rapid expansion of substances, in addition to the rapid-turnover and potential short lifespan of NPS, has resulted in the limited capacity of the laboratory to detect all of the substances with contemporaneous standards. In addition to the need to acquire reference material, which may or may not be commercially available, testing for these substances requires very sensitive instrumentation to detect very low concentrations of NPS in biological specimens, which may not be available in most clinical settings.

Purity, dosage, and composition of products containing NPS are often not known, ranging from one to multiple active substances in addition to potentially harmful adulterants such as anticoagulants. The products may lack homogeneity, so two individuals using the same product may get differing doses of the active components. These limitations coupled with the lack of human metabolism studies, receptor efficacy, and binding affinity profiles subsequently means that false-negative and false-positive results are possible. Further, the toxicologist cannot say much in a case other than confirming its presence or absence, effectively making a quantitative result almost as useful as a qualitative result.

References

1. *EMCDDA-Europol 2016 Annual Report on the Implementation of Council Decision 2005/387/JHA*. Luxembourg: European Monitoring Centre for Drugs and Drug Addiction, Publications Office of the European Union; 2017. Implementation reports.
2. Perspective on drugs. Synthetic cannabinoids in Europe. European Monitoring Centre for Drugs and Drug Addiction. http://www.emcdda.europa.eu/topics/pods/synthetic-cannabinoids. Accessed August 1, 2019.
3. Kacinko S, Xu A, Homan JW, et al. Development and validation of a liquid chromatography-tandem mass spectrometry method for the identification and quantification of JWH-018, JWH-073, JWH-019, and JWH-250 in human whole blood. *J Anal Toxicol.* 2011; 35(7):386-393.
4. Toennes SW, Geraths A, Pogoda W, et al. Pharmacokinetic properties of the synthetic cannabinoid JWH-018 and of its metabolites in serum after inhalation. *J Pharm Biomed Anal.* 2017;140:215-222.
5. Logan BK, Mohr ALA, Friscia M et al. Reports of adverse events associated with use of novel psychoactive substances, 2013-2016: a review. *J Anal Toxicol.* 2017;41(7):573-610.
6. Erol Ozturk Y, Yeter O, Alpertunga B. Validation of JWH-018 and its metabolites in blood and urine by UPLC-MS/MS: monitoring in forensic cases. *Forensic Sci Int.* 2015;248:88-93.
7. Wohlfarth A, Pang S, Zhu M, et al. First metabolic profile of XLR-11, a novel synthetic cannabinoid, obtained by using human hepatocytes and high-resolution mass spectrometry. *Clin Chem.* 2013;59(11):1638-1648.
8. Erratico C, Negreira N, Norouzizadeh H, et al. In vitro and in vivo human metabolism of the synthetic cannabinoid AB-CHMINACA. *Drug Test Anal.* 2015;7(10):866-876.
9. Presley BC, Gurney SM, Scott KS, Kacinko SL, Logan BK. Metabolism and toxicological analysis of synthetic cannabinoids in biological fluids and tissues. *Forensic Sci Rev.* 2016;28(2):103-169.
10. de Jager AD, Warner JV, Henman M, Ferguson W, Hall A. LC-MS/MS method for the quantitation of metabolites of eight commonly-used synthetic cannabinoids in human urine: an Australian perspective. *J Chromatography B Analyt Technol Biomed Life Sci.* 2012;897:22-31.
11. Castaneto MS, Gorelick DA, Desrosiers NA, et al. Synthetic cannabinoids: epidemiology, pharmacodynamics, and clinical implications. *Drug Alcohol Depend.* 2014;144:12-41.

12. Every-Palmer S. Synthetic cannabinoid JWH-018 and psychosis: an explorative study. *Drug Alcohol Depend.* 2011;117:152-157.
13. Zimmerman US, Winkelmann PR, Pilhatsch M, et al. Withdrawal phenomena and dependence syndrome after the consumption of "spice gold". *Dtsch Arztebl Int.* 2009;106(27):464-467.
14. Riederer AM, Campleman SL, Carlson RG, et al. Acute poisonings from synthetic cannabinoids - 50 U.S. Toxicology Investigators Consortium Registry Sites, 2010-2015. *MMWR Morb Mortal Wkly Rep.* 2016;65(27):692-695.
15. Hermanns-Clausen M, Kneisel S, Szabo B, Auwärter V. Acute toxicity due to the confirmed consumption of synthetic cannabinoids: clinical and laboratory findings. *Addiction.* 2013;108(3):534-544.
16. Shanks KG, Dahn T, Terrell AR. Detection of JWH-018 and JWH-073 by UPLC-MS-MS in postmortem whole blood casework. *J Anal Toxicol.* 2012;36(3):145-152.
17. Shanks KG, Winston D, Heidingsfelder J, Behonick G. Case reports of synthetic cannabinoid XLR-11 associated fatalities. *Forensic Sci Int.* 2015;252:e6-e9.
18. Maeda H, Kikura-Hanajira R, Kawamura M, Nagashima E, Yoshida KI. AB-CHMINACA-induced sudden death from non-cardiogenic pulmonary edema. *Clin Toxicol (Phila).* 2018;56(2):143-145.
19. Trecki J, Gerona RR, Schwartz MD. Synthetic cannabinoid-related illnesses and deaths. *N Engl J Med.* 2015;373(2):103-107.
20. Hacker C. 3 arrested after synthetic pot linked to severe bleeding, 2 deaths. *Daily Herald.* http://www.dailyherald.com/news/20180402/3-arrested-after-synthetic-pot-linked-to-severe-bleeding-2-deaths. Accessed April 23, 2018.
21. German CL, Fleckenstein AE, Hanson GR. Bath salts and synthetic cathinones: an emerging designer drug phenomenon. *Life Sci.* 2014;97(1):2-8.
22. Marusich JA, Antonazzo KR, Wiley JL, Blough BE, Partilla JS, Baumann MH. Pharmacology of novel synthetic stimulants structurally related to the "bath salts" constituent 3,4-methylenedioxypyvovalerone (MDPV). *Neuropharmacology.* 2014;87:206-213.
23. Prosser JM, Nelson LS. The toxicology of bath salts: a review of synthetic cathinones. *J Med Toxicol.* 2012;8(1):33-42.
24. López-Arnau R, Martinez-Clemente J, Carbó MI, Pubill D, Escubedo E, Camarasa J. An integrated pharmacokinetic and pharmacodynamic study of a new drug of abuse, methylone, a synthetic cathinone sold as "bath salts". *Prog Neuropsychopharmacol Biol Psychiatry.* 2012;45: 64-72.
25. Quesada L, Gomila I, Yates C, Barcelo C, Puiqurique J, Barcelo B. Elimination half-life of alpha-pyrrolidinovalerophenone in an acute non-fatal intoxication. *Clin Toxicol (Phila).* 2016; 54(6):531-532.
26. Glennon RA. Bath salts, mephedrone, and methylenedioxypyrovalerone as emerging illicit drugs that will need targeted therapeutic intervention. *Adv Pharmacol.* 2014;69:581-620.
27. Meyer MR, Wilhelm J, Peters FT, Maurer HH. Beta-keto amphetamines: studies on the metabolism of the designer drug mephedrone and toxicological detection of mephedrone, butylone, and methylone in urine using gas chromatography-mass spectrometry. *Anal Bioanal Chem.* 2010;397(3):1225-1233.
28. Shima N, Katagi M, Kamata H, et al. Metabolism of the newly encountered designer drug α-pyrrolidinovalerophenone in humans: identification and quantitation of urinary metabolites. *Forensic Toxicol.* 2014;32(1):59-67.
29. Grapp M, Sauer C, Vidal C, Muller D. GC-MS analysis of the designer drug α-pyrrolidinovalerophenone and its metabolites in urine and blood in an acute poisoning case. *Forensic Sci Int.* 2016;259:e14-e19.
30. Krotulski AJ, Papsun DM, De Martinis BS, Mohr ALA, Logan BK. N-ethyl pentylone (ephylone) intoxications: quantitative confirmation and metabolite identification in authentic human biological specimens. *J Anal Toxicol.* 2018;42(7);467-475.
31. Kamata HT, Shima N, Zaitsu K, et al. Metabolism of the recently encountered designer drug, methylone, in humans and rats. *Xenobiotica.* 2006;36(8):709-723.
32. Namera A, Konuma K, Kawamura M, et al. Time-course profile of urinary excretion of intravenously administered α-pyrrolinovalerophenone and α-pyrrolidinobutiophenone in a human. *Forensic Toxicol.* 2014;32(1):68-74.
33. Rosenbaum CD, Carreiro SP, Babu KM. Here today, gone tomorrow... and back again? A review of herbal marijuana alternatives (K2, Spice), synthetic cathinones (bath salts), kratom, Salvia divinorium, methoxetamine, and piperazines. *J Med Toxicol.* 2012;8(1):15-32.
34. Sellors K, Jones A, Chan B. Death due to intravenous use of α-pyrrolidinopentiophenone. *Med J Aust.* 2014;201(10):601-603.
35. Mash DC. Excited delirium and sudden death: a syndromal disorder at the extreme end of the neuropsychatric continuum. *Front Physiol.* 2016;7(435):1-9.
36. Pearson JM, Hargraves TL, Hair LS, et al. Three fatal intoxications due to methylone. *J Anal Toxicol.* 2012;36(6):444-451.

37. Elliott S, Evans J. A 3-year review of new psychoactive substances in casework. *Forensic Sci Int.* 2014;243:55-60.
38. Beck O, Franzén L, Bäckberg M, Signell P, Helander A. Toxicity evaluation of α-pyrrolidinovalerophenone (α-PVP): results from intoxication cases within the STRIDA project. *Clin Toxicol (Phila).* 2016;54(7):568-575.
39. Nagai H, Saka K, Nakajima M, et al. Sudden death after sustained restraint following self-administration of the designer drug α-pyrrolidinovalerophenone. *Int J Cardiol.* 2014;172(1):263-265.
40. Eiden C, Mathieu O, Cathala P, et al. Toxicity and death following recreational use of 2-pyrrolidino valerophenone. *Clin Toxicol.* 2013;51(9):899-903.
41. Sykutera M, Cychowska M, Bloch-Boguslawska E. A fatal case of pentedrone and α-pyrrolidinovalerophenone poisoning. *J Anal Toxicol.* 2015; 39(4):324-329.
42. Potocka-Banaś B, Janus T, Majdanik S, Banaś T, Dembrińska T, Borowiak K. Fatal intoxication with α-PVP, a synthetic cathinone derivative. *J Forensic Sci.* 2017;62(2):553-556.
43. Thirakul P, Hair SL, Bergen LK, Pearson MJ. Clinical presentation, autopsy results and toxicology findings in an acute N-ethylpentylone fatality. *J Anal Toxicol.* 2017;41(4):342-346.
44. Krotulski AJ, Papsun DM, De Martinis BS, Mohr ALA, Logan BK. N-ethyl pentylone (ephylone) intoxications: quantitative confirmation and metabolite identification in authentic human biological specimens. *J Anal Toxicol.* 2018;42(7):467-475.
45. Atherton D, Dye D, Robinson CA, Beck R. N-ethyl pentylone-related deaths in Alabama. *J Forensic Sci.* 2018;e1-e4.
46. Prosser JM, Nelson LS. The toxicology of bath salts: a review of synthetic cathinones. *J Med Toxicol.* 2012;8(1):33-42.
47. Kasick DP, McKnight CA, Klisovic E. "Bath salt" ingestion leading to severe intoxication delirium: two cases and a brief review of the emergence of mephedrone use. *Am J Drug Alcohol Abuse.* 2012;38(2):176-180.
48. Mas-Morey P, Visser MH, Winkelmolen L, Touw DJ. Clinical toxicology and management of intoxications with synthetic cathinones ("bath salts"). *J Pharm Pract.* 2013;26(4): 353-357.
49. Stoica MV, Felthous AR. Acute psychosis induced by bath salts: a case report with clinical and forensic implications. *J Forensic Sci.* 2013;58(2):530-533.
50. Karila L, Lafaye G, Scocard A, Cottencin O, Benyamina A. MDPV and α-PVP use in humans: the twisted sisters. *Neurophamacology.* 2018;134(Pt A):65-72.
51. Maguire P, Tsai N, Kamal J, Cometta-Morini C, Upton C, Loew G. Pharmacological profiles of fentanyl analogs at mu, delta and kappa opiate receptors. *Eur J Pharmacol.* 1992;213(2):219-225.
52. Schneider E, Brune K. Opioid activity and distribution of fentanyl metabolites. *Naunyn Schmiedebergs Arch Pharmacol.* 1986;334: 267-274.
53. Goggin MM, Nguyen A, Janis GC. Identification of unique metabolites of the designer opioid furanylfentanyl. *J Anal Toxicol.* 2017;41:367-375.
54. Krotulski AJ, Mohr ALA, Papsun DM, Logan BK. Metabolism of novel opioid agonists U-47700 and U-49900 using human liver microsomes with confirmation in authentic urine specimens from drug users. *Drug Test Anal.* 2018;10(1):127-136.
55. Armenian P, Vo KT, Barr-Walker J, Lynch KL. Fentanyl, fentanyl analogs, and novel synthetic opioids: a comprehensive review. *Neuropharmacology.* 2018;134(Pt A):121-132.
56. Cole JB, Dunbar JF, McIntire SA, Regelmann WE, Slusher TM. Butyrfentanyl overdose resulting in diffuse alveolar hemorrhage. *Pediatrics.* 2015;135(3);740-743.
57. Helander A, Bäckberg M, Beck O. MT-45, a new psychoactive substance associated with hearing loss and unconsciousness. *Clin Toxicol (Phila).* 2014;52(8); 901-904.
58. Poklis J, Poklis A, Wolf C, et al. Postmortem tissue distribution of acetylfentanyl, fentanyl, and their respective nor-metabolites analyzed by ultrahigh performance liquid chromatography with tandem mass spectrometry. *Forensic Sci Int.* 2016;257:435-441.
59. Guerrieri D, Rapp E, Roman M, Druid H, Kronstrand R. Postmortem and toxicological findings in a series of furanylfentanyl-related deaths. *J Anal Toxicol.* 2017;41(3):242-249.
60. Elliott SP, Brandt SD, Smith C. The first reported fatality associated with the synthetic opioid 3,4-dichloro-N-[2-(dimethylamino)cyclohexyl]-N-methylbenzamide (U-47700) and implications for forensic analysis. *Drug Test Anal.* 2016;8: 875-879.
61. Mohr AL, Friscia M, Papsun D, Kacinko SL, Buzby D, Logan BK. Analysis of novel synthetic opioids U-47700, U-50488, and furanylfentanyl by LC-MS/MS in postmortem casework. *J Anal Toxicol.* 2016;40(9):709-717.
62. Nichols DE, Frescas SP, Chemel BR, Rehder KS, Zhong D, Lewin AH. High specific activity tritium-labeled N-(2-methoxybenzyl)-2,5-dimethoxy-4-iodophenethylamine (INBMeO): a high affinity 5-HT2A receptor – selective agonist radioligand. *Bioorg Med Chem.* 2008;16(11): 6116-6123.
63. 25I-NBOMe: Critical Review Report. Geneva: 36th Meeting, Expert Committee on Drug Dependence, World Health Organization. 2014.

64. Wohlfarth A, Roman M, Anderson M, et al. 25C-NBOMe and 25I-NBOMe metabolite studies in human hepatocytes, in vivo mouse and human urine with high resolution mass spectrometry: metabolism of 25C- and 25I-NBOMe. *Drug Test Anal.* 2017;9(5):680-698.
65. Poklis JL, Dempsey SK, Liu K, et al. Identification of metabolite biomarkers of the designer hallucinogen 25I-NBOMe in mouse hepatic microsomal preparations and human urine samples associated with clinical intoxication. *J Anal Toxicol.* 2015;39(8):607-616.
66. Suzuki J, Dekker MA, Valenti ES, et al. Toxicities associated with NBOMe ingestion, a novel class of potent hallucinogens: a review of the literature. *Psychosomatics.* 2015;56(2):129-139.
67. Hill SL, Doris T, Gurung S, et al. Severe clinical toxicity associated with analytically confirmed recreational use of 25I-NBOMe: case series. *Clin Toxicol (Phila).* 2013;51(6):487-492.
68. Suzuki J, Poklis JL, Poklis A. "My friend said it was good LSD": a suicide attempt following analytically confirmed 25I-NBOMe ingestion. *J Psychoactive Drugs.* 2014;46(5):379-382.
69. Kueppers VB, Cooke CT. 25I-NBOMe related death in Australia: a case report. *Forensic Sci Int.* 2015;249:e15-e18.
70. Morris H, Wallach J. From PCP to MXE: a comprehensive review of the non-medical use of dissociative drugs. *Drug Test Anal.* 2014;6(7-8):614-632.
71. Roth BI, Gibbons S, Arunotayanun W, et al. The ketamine analogue methoxetamine and 3- and 4-methoxy analogues of phencyclidine are high affinity and selective ligands for the glutamate NMDA receptor. *PLoS One.* 2013:8(3):e59334.
72. Misselbrook GP, Hamilton EJ. Out with the old, in with the new? Case reports of the clinical features and acute management of two novel designer drugs. *Acute Med.* 2012;11(3):157-160.
73. Michely JA, Manier SK, Caspar AT, Brandt SD, Wallach J, Maurer HH. New psychoactive substances 3-methoxyphencyclidine (3-MeO-PCP) and 3-methoxyrolicyclidine (3-MeO-PCPy): metabolic fate elucidated with rat urine and human liver preparations and their detectability in urine by GCMS, "LC-(High Resolution)-MSn, and "LC-(High Resolution)-MS/MS". *Curr Neuropharmacol.* 2017;25(5):692-712.
74. Bäckberg M, Beck O, Helander A. Phencyclidine analog use in Sweden: intoxication cases involving 3-MeO-PCP and 4-MeO-PCP from the STRIDA project. *Clin Toxicol (Phila).* 2015;53(9):856-864.
75. Zidkova M, Hlozek T, Balik M, et al. Two cases of non-fatal intoxication with a novel street hallucinogen: 3-methoxy-phencylidine. *J Anal Toxicol.* 2017;41(4):350-354.
76. Johansson A, Lindstedt D, Roman M, et al. A non-fatal intoxication and seven deaths involving the dissociative drug 3-MeO-PCP. *Forensic Sci Int.* 2017;275:76-82.
77. Bakota E, Arndt C, Romoser AA, Wilson SK. Fatal intoxication involving 3-MeO-PCP: a case report and validated method. *J Anal Toxicol.* 2016;40(7):504-510.
78. Etizolam. Drug Enforcement Agency, Diversion Control Division, Drug and Chemical Identification Section; October 2018.
79. Fracasso C, Confalonieri S, Garattini S, Caccia S. Single and multiple dose pharmacokinetics of etizolam in healthy subjects. *Eur J Clin Pharmacol.* 1991:40(2):181-185.
80. Manchester KR, Maskell PD, Waters L. Experimental versus theoretical log D7.4, pKa, and plasma protein binding values for benzodiazepines appearing as new psychoactive substances. *Drug Test Anal.* 2018 March 26. Epub ahead of print.
81. Nakamae T, Shinozuka T, Sasaki C, et al. Case report: etizolam and its major metabolites in two unnatural death cases. *Forensic Sci Int.* 2008;182(1-3):e1-e6.
82. Høiseth G, Tuv SS, Karinen R. Blood concentrations of new designer benzodiazepines in forensic cases. *Forensic Sci Int.* 2016;268:35-38.
83. Soh YN, Elliott S. An investigation of the stability of emerging new psychoactive substances. *Drug Test Anal.* 2014;6(7-8):696-704.
84. Sørenson LK. Determination of cathinones and related ephedrines in forensic whole-blood samples by liquid chromatography-electrospray tandem mass spectrometry. *J Chromatogr B Analyt Technol Biomed Life Sci.* 2011;879(11-12):727-736.
85. Gerostamoulos D, Elliott S, Walls HC, Peters FT, Lynch M, Drummer OH. To measure or not to measure? That is the NPS question. *J Anal Toxicol.* 2016;40(4):318-320.
86. Gurney SM, Scott KS, Kacinko SL, Presley BC, Logan BK. Pharmacology, toxicology, and adverse effects of synthetic cannabinoid drugs. *Forensic Sci Rev.* 2014;26(1):53-78.
87. Wiley JL, Marusich JA, Lefever TW, Grabenauer M, Moore KN, Thomas BF. Cannabinoids in disguise: Δ9-tetrahydrocannabinol-like effects of tetramethylcyclopropyl ketone indoles. *Neuropharmacology.* 2013;75:145–154.
88. Wiley JL, Marusich JA, Lefever TW, et al. AB-CHMINACA, AB-PINACA, and FUBIMINA: Affinity and potency of novel synthetic cannabinoids in producing Δ9-tetrahydrocannabinol-like effects in mice. *J Pharmacol Exp Ther.* 2015; 35(3):328–339.

89. Ujváry I, Jorge R, Christie R, et al. Acryloylfentanyl, a recently emerged new psychoactive substance: a comprehensive review. *Forensic Toxicol.* 2017;35(2):232-243.
90. Higashikawa Y, Suzuki S. Studies on 1-(2-phenethyl)-4-(N-propionylanilino) piperidine (fentanyl) and its related compounds, VI: structure-analgesic activity relationship for fentanyl, methyl-substituted fentanyls and other analogues. *Forensic Toxicol.* 2008;26(1):1-5
91. Huang BS, Terrell RC, Deutsche KH, et al. N-aryl-N-(4-piperidinyl)amides and pharmaceutical compositions and method employing such compounds. US4584303A, 1986.
92. Harper NJ, Veitch GB, Wibberley DG. 1-(3,4-dichlorobenzamidomethyl) cyclohexyldimethylamine and related compounds as potential analgesics. *J Med Chem.* 1974;17(11):1188-1193.
93. Baumann MH, Majumdar S, Le Rouzic V. Pharmacological characterization of novel synthetic opioids (NSO) found in the recreational drug marketplace. *Neurophamacology.* 2018;134(Pt A):101-107.
94. Zawilska JB. An expanding world of novel psychoactive substances: opioids. *Front Psychiatry.* 2017;8(110):1-14.
95. Ruangyuttikarn W, Law MY, Rollins DE, Moody DE. Detection of fentanyl and its analogs by enzyme-linked immunosorbent assay. *J Anal Toxicol.* 1990;14(3):160-164.
96. O'Connor LC, Torrance HJ, McKeown DA. ELISA detection of phenazepam, etizolam, pyrazolam, flubromazepam, diclazepam, and delorazepam in blood using Immunalysis® benzodiazepine kit. *J Anal Toxicol.* 2016;40(2):159-161.

Acknowledgment

The author would like to express her appreciation to Melissa Fogarty for her assistance with this manuscript.

Chapter 27

Over-the-Counter Analgesics

Hoi-Ying Elsie Yu, PhD
Gary L. Horowitz, MD

Introduction

A wide array of nonprescription analgesics is used in over-the-counter (OTC) painkillers and cold medications. Aspirin, Tylenol, Advil, and Aleve represent common trade names for salicylate, acetaminophen, ibuprofen, and naproxen, respectively. This chapter will address the first two of these compounds, salicylate and acetaminophen, which are highly associated with risk of acute overdose and poisoning.

The ready availability of these OTC analgesics probably contributes to the large number of toxic exposures each year. In 2016, the American Association of Poison Control Centers (AAPCC) reported ~74,000 exposures related to acetaminophen, with 93 fatalities, and ~19,000 cases related to salicylate exposures, with 22 fatalities.[1] In the United Kingdom and Hong Kong, blister packaging has been demonstrated to reduce overdose exposures, probably as a result of the inconvenience in opening many individual packages to obtain large numbers of tablets.[2,3] In the United States, the Food and Drug Administration (FDA) has mandated warning labels on OTC analgesics to state the potential danger of liver damage on acetaminophen-containing medications and stomach bleeding on other nonsteroidal anti-inflammatory drugs in an attempt to heighten the awareness of their toxicity.

Salicylate

Origin

Use of the inner bark of the white willow tree (*Salix alba*) for pain relief goes back to ancient times. Hippocrates in the 5th century BCE described a bitter powder extracted from willow bark that could ease aches and pains and reduce fevers. It was also mentioned in texts from the ancient Near East. The Cherokee and other Native Americans used an infusion of the bark for fever and other medicinal purposes for centuries.[4] The first formal medical description of this effect was in England in 1763 when Edward Stone noted willow bark's effectiveness in reducing a fever.[5] The active extract of the bark, called *salicin,* was first isolated in Germany in 1826 and in 1828 was converted into a sugar and a second component, which on oxidation becomes salicylic acid.[6] Salicylic acid was also isolated from the herb meadowsweet (*Filipendula ulmaria,* formerly classified as *Spiraea ulmaria*) by German researchers in 1839. This extract was somewhat effective but when consumed in high doses was also noted to cause digestive problems, such as gastric irritation, bleeding, and diarrhea, and even to cause death. The salicylates are a group of compounds derived from salicylic acid in which an ester or salt is added.

Descriptive Chemistry[7]

Synonym: 2-Hydroxybenzoate

Trade names: Aspirin, Excedrine

Formula: $C_7H_5O_3$-

Molecular mass = 137.1128 Daltons

CAS-69-72-7

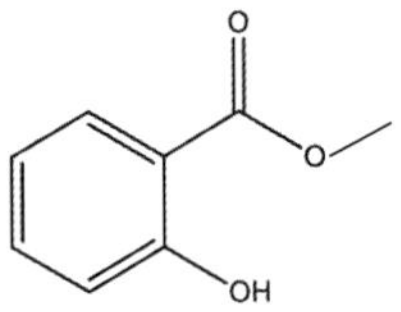

Pharmacology

Intended Use

Acetylsalicylic acid (ASA) has become one of the most commonly used therapeutic salicylates, both in pure form and in combination with other drugs. Today, this compound can be found in a variety of OTC drugs under different brand names, including Aspirin and Excedrin. In addition to aspirin, salicylate can be found in fragrance. In particular, methyl salicylate (oil of wintergreen) is available as OTC lotions, liniments, and ointments, and is usually used to treat musculoskeletal discomfort. Salicylic acid is also an active ingredient in many skin care products owning to its antifungal and bacteriostatic properties.

Mechanism of Action

Salicylate has antiplatelet, antipyretic, analgesic, and anti-inflammatory properties, many of which are attributed to its ability to inhibit prostaglandins and thromboxane via inactivation of cyclooxygenase (COX) enzymes.

Pharmacokinetics

Each "aspirin" tablet contains 325 mg to 650 mg of acetylsalicylic acid. The volume of distribution for

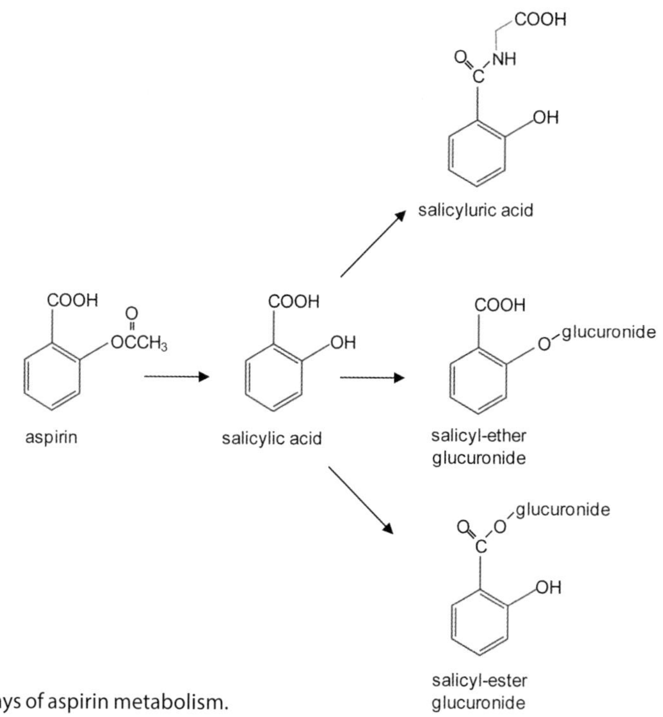

Figure 27-1. Pathways of aspirin metabolism.

salicylate is about 0.1 L/kg to 0.2 L/kg. Therapeutic concentrations of aspirin are usually 2 mg/dL to 10 mg/dL for analgesia and 10 mg/dL to 25 mg/dL for use as an anti-inflammatory agent.[8] Lower doses, such as the 81-mg baby aspirin, are available and are used for its antiplatelet effect, primarily for prevention of myocardial infarction. Aspirin is rapidly absorbed after oral administration. Nearly the entire dose of acetylsalicylic acid is hydrolyzed to salicylic acid (Figure 27-1), the bioactive form of the drug.

Peak plasma concentrations of salicylates are reached approximately 2 hours after ingestion of a therapeutic dose. However, ingestion of large amounts of aspirin inhibits gastric emptying, which may cause the tablets to form a bezoar or a concretion of the ingested pills in the stomach. Both bezoars and enteric-coated aspirin products delay absorption, and therefore peak concentrations are reached later than the expected 2 hours after ingestion.

Aspirin is metabolized to salicylic acid rapidly, with a half-life between 13 and 20 minutes. The half-life of salicylic acid, however, is dose dependent. If the dose is less than 3 g, the half-life is about 2 to 4 hours; in larger doses, the half-life may be extended up to 19 hours. Nearly all of a single dose is eliminated in the urine as salicylic acid (5%), salicyluric acid (80%), salicyl phenolic glucuronide (10%), and salicyl acyl glucuronide (5%; Figure 27-1). Trace amounts of other metabolites have also been noted.

Abuse Potential and Characteristics

Salicylate toxicity ranges from the hypersensitive asthmatic who may have sudden death with ingestion of as little as a single tablet to the overdose patient who may ingest over 50 tablets. Oil of wintergreen is particularly toxic because it is often found in a liquid form. One Chinese preparation of methyl salicylate, Koong Yick Hung Far Oil, is 67% methyl salicylate and equivalent to the ingestion of about 184 300-mg aspirin tablets.[9] Reye syndrome, an acute encephalopathy, is associated with sporadic cases of mortality in children from ingestion of aspirin for flu-like illness. Laboratory findings for Reye syndrome include rapid extreme elevation in ammonia, aspartate aminotransferase (AST), and prothrombin time (PT). Due to enhanced public awareness against the use of aspirin in children with fever, the incidence of Reye syndrome has been greatly reduced.[10]

Salicylates exert their antiplatelet effects at very low concentrations, explaining why a dose of 81 mg/day is sufficient for prevention of myocardial infarction. For its antipyretic and analgesic effect, serum salicylate concentrations of 5 mg/dL to 10 mg/dL (50-100 mg/L) are adequate. To achieve anti-inflammatory effects, salicylate concentrations of 15 mg/dL to 30 mg/dL are usually required. As shown in Table 27-1, serum salicylate

Table 27-1. Toxic Dose and Concentrations of Over-the-Counter Analgesics[1,20]

Drug	Estimated Lethal Dose (g)	Toxic Plasma Concentration Range (mg/L)	Blood Concentrations in Fatalities (mg/L)
Salicylate	15	>300	660 (average)
Acetaminophen	~10	120-300	160-390

Table 27-2. Common Symptoms Associated With Acute and Chronic Salicylate Exposure

Acute	Nausea Vomiting Abdominal pain Tinnitus (at concentrations >20 mg/dL) Respiratory alkalosis Metabolic acidosis Hypokalemia Confusion and agitation Coma Hyperthermia with a potential for rhabdomyolysis
Chronic	Altered mental status Lethargy Irritability Tinnitus Confusion Metabolic acidosis Pulmonary edema

concentrations above 30 mg/dL (300 mg/L) are associated with toxicity; concentrations in reported fatalities have averaged higher than 60 mg/dL (600 mg/L). However, concentrations associated with toxicity may vary depending on whether the intoxication is acute or chronic. As shown in Table 27-2, acute and chronic salicylate intoxication present differently. Toxicity is at the cellular and organelle level as a result of the uncoupling of oxidative phosphorylation (Krebs cycle) and impaired production of adenosine triphosphate (ATP).

Patients with acute toxicity may exhibit gastric pain, vomiting, hematemesis, agitation, seizures, and central nervous system (CNS) depression. In addition, there may be two findings particularly characteristic of salicylate toxicity: patients may complain of tinnitus or they may manifest tachypnea or hyperpnea. As a result of hyperventilation, patients typically present with a respiratory alkalosis, which is later followed by development of an increased anion gap metabolic acidosis (distinct from renal compensation for the respiratory alkalosis). It is worth noting that the increase in the anion gap represents more than simply the salicylate concentration, which, even at 50 mg/dL, is just 3.6 mmol/L. Rather, it represents in addition the accumulation of other organic acids related to the uncoupling of oxidative phosphorylation. In cases of salicylate-induced hyperthermia, rhabdomyolysis may occur with markedly increased serum creatine kinase concentrations.

Chronic intoxication is often seen in the elderly, who may be taking aspirin or aspirin products for either inflammatory conditions or chronic pain. The presentation is usually nonspecific and may not be recognized without a thorough history and a clinical suspicion, which prompts obtaining a salicylate concentration. Patients present with symptoms of confusion, dehydration, and increased anion gap metabolic acidosis. Chronic salicylism has also presented as noncardiogenic pulmonary edema.[11]

Analysis

Specimen Types and Characteristics

Serum/plasma is the preferred specimen for salicylate measurement.

Modes of Analysis

Traditional colorimetric assays are based on the degree of purple color development when salicylate combines with ferric ion. This is the principle underlying spot tests, which have been used to determine whether specific tablets, creams, lotions, and solutions contain salicylate.[12] An adaptation of the method uses Trinder's reagent, which consists of mercuric chloride, hydrochloric acid, and ferric nitrate. This method is used on many automated chemistry instruments.

More recently, an enzymatic reaction has been introduced. It uses the enzyme salicylate hydroxylase, which catalyzes the conversion of salicylate in the presence of NADH to catechol and NAD+ (Figure 27-2). The conversion of NADH to NAD+ is monitored photometrically at a wavelength of 340 nm. In some adaptations, catechol, the converted product of salicylate, is monitored. Immunoassays (eg, enzyme-multiplied immunoassay technique [EMIT]) are also available to measure salicylate.

Chromatographic assays (gas chromatography or liquid chromatography) are capable of

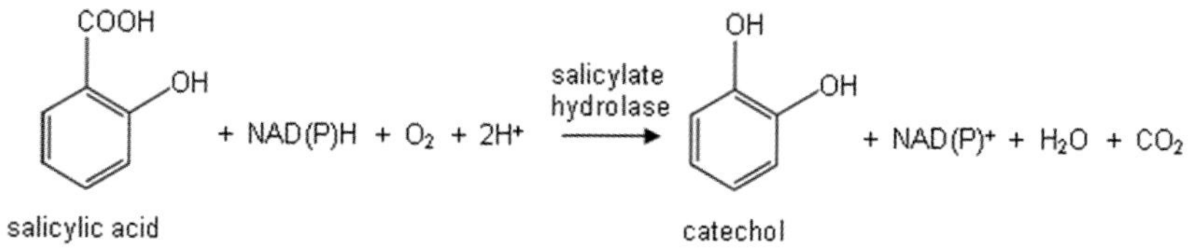

Figure 27-2. Enzymatic assay for salicylate measurement.

measuring salicylate and will eliminate many interferences that can affect the assays mentioned below. However, these assays are typically not available around the clock and take much longer to perform, so they are not effective in the emergency setting; measurements on automated chemistry analyzers provide better turnaround time and are therefore more suitable for hospital settings.

Known Analytical Issues

With the automated Trinder method, many common endogenous substances, such as bilirubin, ketone bodies, and catecholamines, may interfere with the assay.[30] Interference by bilirubin is assay and concentration dependent. In contrast, salicylate concentrations measured by enzymatic reactions tend to show minimal interference from bilirubin (up to ~20 mg/dL bilirubin). Enzymatic assays show minimal interference with ketones, benzoate, and p-OH-benzoate but may be affected by high concentrations of lactate dehydrogenase with sufficient substrate. However, monitoring the formation of the end product catechol instead of NAD+ will minimize the problems.[13] Diflunisal, which is structurally similar to salicylate, has been shown to seriously interfere with several different assays, with cross-reactivities as high as 200%.[14,15]

In short, because of the large number of potential interferences, laboratories should check their specific manufacturer's package insert to be sure they know the limitations of the assay they use, and they should be aware that chromatographic methods may overcome potential interferences and can be used when questions arise.

Clinical Issues

Interpretation

Ideally, a salicylate concentration should be obtained at about 2 hours post ingestion in order to determine the peak concentration. However, in a suspected overdose, a salicylate concentration should be obtained as soon as the patient presents. This should be followed with serial measurements approximately every 2 hours until a peak is identified, and then every 4 to 6 hours thereafter until there is evidence that the serum concentration has decreased below toxic concentrations (typically <30 mg/dL).[16] If both the number and concentration of pills are known, the clinician can estimate the amount ingested and predict toxicity based on the patient's weight. Ingestions between 150 mg/kg and 200 mg/kg will cause mild intoxication, while higher doses (ie, >300 mg/kg) are likely to produce severe intoxication. Chronic intoxication usually occurs with doses in the range of 100 mg/kg over several days. Of particular importance, laboratories report results in either mg/dL or mg/L. This may present some confusion to clinicians if they work with more than one laboratory or have had prior experience at a hospital that reports in different units. The clinical laboratory should clearly communicate to the medical staff the units used, such that a concentration of "200" is 200 mg/L and not 200 mg/dL.

Additional laboratory tests that are helpful in assessing the severity of the intoxication, as well as following the efficacy of treatment, include blood gas measurements (to monitor acid-base status), electrolytes (to assess anion gap and to monitor for hypokalemia), glucose (to monitor for hypoglycemia), creatinine, liver function tests (including PT), and potentially creatine kinase (CK; if rhabdomyolysis is a concern).

Overdose and Toxicity

Treatment includes respiratory and cardiovascular support, as needed. If the overdose is recent on presentation to the emergency department, gastric decontamination with activated charcoal is warranted. With suspicion of bezoar formation or ingestion of enteric-coated aspirin, whole bowel irrigation with polyethylene glycol can be helpful. In general, patients are usually dehydrated, and intravenous fluids are necessary for hydration and correction of electrolyte imbalances, including hypokalemia or hypoglycemia.

The mainstay of treatment is to alkalinize the urine, which facilitates excretion of salicylate. Administration of intravenous sodium bicarbonate is used to produce a urine with a pH ≥7.5.[17] Complications such as hypokalemia can be corrected by giving potassium supplements.[17] In cases where urinary alkalinization is not sufficient, hemodialysis may be required. Both acetylsalicylic acid and salicylic acid have a low volume of distribution, making hemodialysis ideal in reducing toxicity. In acute toxicity, indications for hemodialysis include a serum concentration >100 mg/dL (1000 mg/L), acute respiratory distress syndrome requiring supplemental oxygen, severe acidosis (pH <7.20) refractory to standard therapy, or altered mental status.[18] Patients with chronic intoxication, or if they present with pulmonary edema, may need dialysis at lower concentrations (>60 mg/dL).

Acetaminophen

Origin

Acetanilide, the first aniline derivative discovered to have analgesic/antipyretic properties, was introduced under the name of Antifebrin in 1886,[19] but unacceptable toxic effects, especially cyanosis due to methemoglobinemia, prompted the search for less toxic aniline derivatives.[20] Acetaminophen had been synthesized via reduction of *p*-nitrophenol with tin in glacial acetic acid in 1877,[21,22] but it was not until 1887 that it was administered to patients.[20] In 1893, clinical results of acetaminophen were compared in the literature with phenacetin, another aniline derivative,[23] and it was claimed that acetaminophen was slightly more likely to produce methemoglobinemia. This led to acetaminophen being discarded in favor of phenacetin, the sales of which established Bayer as a leading pharmaceutical company.[24] In 1947, researchers in the US analyzed the metabolism of acetanilide and acetaminophen,[24] showing that acetaminophen was a major metabolite of acetanilide in human blood and did not cause methemoglobinemia,[25] which instead is produced in humans mainly by another metabolite, phenylhydroxylamine. This led to a "rediscovery" of acetaminophen,[20] which has been marketed in the US since 1953.

Descriptive Chemistry[7]

Synonyms: Paracetamol, *N*-acetyl-*p*-aminophenol, APAP

Trade names: Tylenol, Panadol

Formula: $C_8H_9NO_2$

Molecular mass = 151.1626 Daltons

CAS-103-90-2

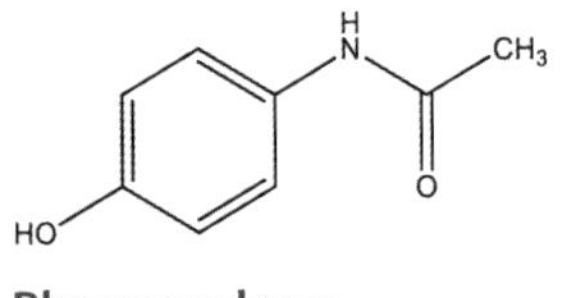

Pharmacology

Intended Use

Acetaminophen is a widely used painkiller in the US. When used properly, it is safe and free from the side effects to the heart and stomach that many other OTC painkillers have. It can be found in Tylenol, Excedrin, NyQuil, and many other OTC headache and cold medications. Some prescription medications, such as Percocet, Lortab, Vicodin, and Norco, also contain acetaminophen.

Mechanism of Action

Acetaminophen is an analgesic/antipyretic agent, but its mechanism of action has not been completely clear. An active metabolite of acetaminophen, *N*-arachidonoylphenolamine (AM404; Figure 27-3), has been shown to induce analgesic/antipyretic activities via the production of endogenous cannabinoids and possibly also the inhibition of COX enzymes and prostaglandin E2.[20] AM404 is thought to be present only in the nervous system and is of minimal abundance in the overall metabolism of acetaminophen.[26]

Pharmacokinetics

Oral doses for pain or fever relief are about 650 mg to 1000 mg acetaminophen in adults and 10 mg/kg to 15 mg/kg in children, taken every 4 hours if needed. Depending on the formulations (immediate release tablets, extended release tablets, liquid acetaminophen), peak plasma concentrations of acetaminophen may be reached 30 to 120 minutes after ingestion. The volume of distribution for acetaminophen is about 1 L/kg. This results in a therapeutic serum concentration of approximately 10 mcg/mL to 20 mcg/mL.

At therapeutic dosage, acetaminophen is metabolized in the liver where ~90% of it is transformed into nontoxic glucuronide or sulfate conjugates (Figure 27-3), which are subsequently eliminated via renal excretion. However, the remaining ~10% of acetaminophen is metabolized by the P450 enzymes (CYP2E1) to highly reactive toxic *N*-acetylbenzoquinoneimine (NAPQI), which binds to hepatic macromolecules and leads to oxidative hepatocellular necrosis.[27] Fortunately, hepatic glutathione rapidly complexes with NAPQI to form nontoxic cysteine or mercapturic acid conjugates (Figure 27-3), which are then excreted in urine.[28] Normally, the elimination half-life is 1 to 3 hours.

Abuse Potential and Characteristics

Acetaminophen overdose results in excessive buildup of the hepatotoxic metabolite NAPQI because of (1) increased production of NAPQI as a result of saturation of the glucuronidation and sulfation pathways and (2) reduced elimination of NAPQI as a result of depletion of glutathione stores. In general, a single ingestion of >250 mg/kg or multiple ingestions of >12 g/day will induce toxicity. The clinical manifestations are typically

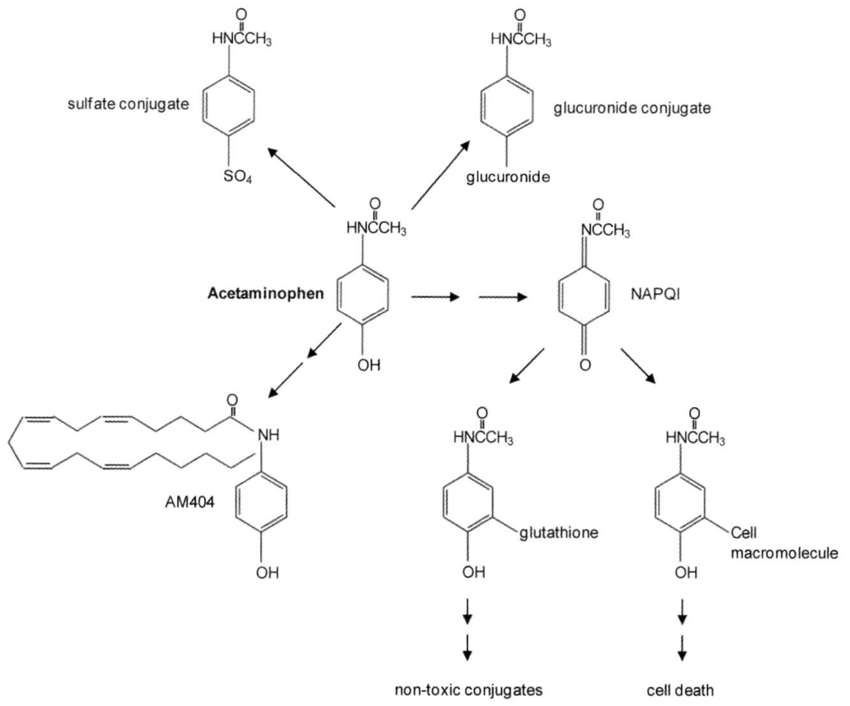

Figure 27-3. Pathways of acetaminophen metabolism.

categorized into four stages.[29] Stage I occurs within the first 24 hours post toxic ingestion and is considered the "preclinical toxic phase" where patients present with nonspecific symptoms, such as nausea, vomiting, pallor, and lethargy, with normal liver function laboratory results. Stage II occurs about 24 to 72 hours post ingestion where patients usually show improvement of stage I symptoms. However, acetaminophen-induced hepatic injury starts to become evident. Patients usually present with liver enlargement and tenderness, where the first laboratory evidence of liver toxicity is increased PT, followed by elevated alanine aminotransferase (ALT) and AST (typically 100 times above the upper limit of the normal reference interval). Stage III occurs about 72 to 96 hours post ingestion where patients return to the nonspecific stage I symptoms. If left untreated, patients will progress to hepatic encephalopathy, lactic acidosis, renal failure, and eventually death. Stage IV occurs about 96 hours to 2 weeks post ingestion and is the "recovery phase" for those who survive. Some patients may take longer to recover depending on severity of toxicity. Clinical improvement should be evident during this phase. Laboratory results, however, may take longer to return to normal.

Toxic acetaminophen exposure could be intentional (eg, suicide) or accidental (eg, unaware of taking multiple acetaminophen-containing medications). In children, most toxicity is a result of inappropriate dosing. In July 2009, advisers to the FDA recommended a reduction of a single adult acetaminophen dose from the current 1000 mg to 650 mg and more specific and accurate dosing instructions for children. In March 2014, products with more than 325 mg acetaminophen were withdrawn from the US market. Estimated lethal doses and concentrations are shown in Table 27-1.

Analysis

Specimen Types and Characteristics

Although urine can be used to screen for acetaminophen poisoning,[30] plasma and serum are the preferred specimens in determining the extent of acetaminophen intoxication. Serial measurement of plasma acetaminophen concentrations can also be used to calculate half-life or elimination of acetaminophen and monitor treatment progress.

Modes of Analysis

Most commercially available assays for clinical acetaminophen analysis measure only the unconjugated drug. This is important because only the unconjugated acetaminophen induces hepatotoxicity, and the level of unconjugated acetaminophen corresponds to that on the Rumack-Matthew nomogram for prediction of hepatotoxicity.[31] Most clinical laboratories use either enzymatic assays or immunoassays on automated chemistry instruments because they are rapid (~10 minutes) and accurate. These assays have higher specificity than

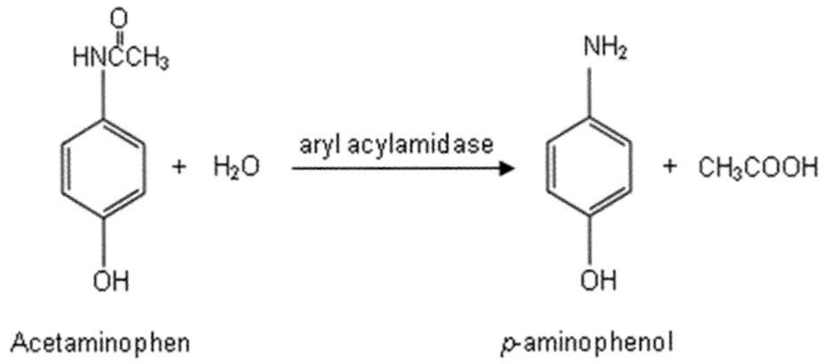

Figure 27-4. Enzymatic assay for acetaminophen measurement.

the Glynn and Kendal nitration-based colorimetric method[32] that was once widely used. Enzymatic assays use aryl acylamidase to hydrolyze acetaminophen to *p*-aminophenol (Figure 27-4). The production of *p*-aminophenol is hence directly proportional to acetaminophen concentration in plasma/serum. Measurement of *p*-aminophenol is followed colorimetrically at ~600 nm as it oxidizes or reacts with a dye. Various kinds of immunoassays to measure acetaminophen are currently available, including immunoturbidimetric assay and EMIT.

Known Analytical Issues

Icterus,[33] hemolysis, and lipemia interfere with enzymatic (aryl acylamidase) assays since the end points are commonly measured colorimetrically at ~600 nm. High bilirubin concentrations (>10 mg/dL) in patients with liver failure have been shown to cause falsely high acetaminophen concentrations when enzymatic assays are used.[33-35] Since acetaminophen is a common cause of drug-induced hepatotoxicity, a falsely high acetaminophen concentration may lead to incorrect diagnoses in patients with liver failure. Similarly, a falsely high acetaminophen result might result in unnecessary alarm in liver transplant patients. In addition to bilirubin, an IgM paraprotein can cause falsely low acetaminophen result in enzymatic assays.[36] *N*-acetylcysteine (NAC), the drug commonly used to treat acetaminophen overdose, has also been shown to cause falsely low acetaminophen results in enzymatic assays.[37] On the other hand, immunoassays appear to have minimal interference by icterus and hemolysis.[34] Therefore, perhaps it is not surprising that at least one commercial vendor is moving from the enzymatic assay to the immunoassay methodology.

Clinical Issues

Interpretation

In acute acetaminophen overdose, plasma acetaminophen concentration and time of ingestion can help predict risk of toxicity based on the Rumack-Matthew nomogram.[38] To use this nomogram, several criteria must be followed. First, this nomogram only applies to acute acetaminophen overdose. In chronic acetaminophen overdose patients, toxicity typically occurs at lower concentrations that do not correlate with the nomogram. Second, ingestion time is required to predict hepatotoxicity using the nomogram. Third, plasma acetaminophen concentration must be obtained after 4 hours of ingestion to ensure absorption is complete.[39] Fourth, the nomogram applies to immediate-release formulations of acetaminophen only and does not take into consideration the co-ingestion of other substances that may affect absorption of acetaminophen. Fifth, patients with reduced glutathione or induced P450 systems are more susceptible to acetaminophen-induced toxicity. This includes patients with liver diseases, cystic fibrosis,[40] and alcoholism, as well as the use of microsomal enzyme-inducing drugs (anticonvulsants, antituberculosis drugs, OTC herbs like St John's wort),[29] and patients who are malnourished.

In addition to the Rumack-Matthew nomogram, other prediction tools may also be useful to predict hepatotoxicity in acetaminophen overdose.[41] These include the "paracetamol-aminotransferase (ALT) multiplication product" where a product above the 10,000 mg/L × 1 U/L cutoff is strongly associated with hepatotoxicity and a product below 1500 mg/L × 1 U/L is considered having very low risk of hepatotoxicity.

While there is no standard practice in situations where risk stratification may not be possible, initiation of NAC treatment can likely improve outcome in a patient who has overdosed and has detectable serum acetaminophen levels even if hepatic injury is not evident,[42] particularly since NAC treatment is relatively safe. NAC treatments are also recommended in patients who have increased risk of hepatic failure.[40,42]

Overdose and Toxicity

NAC administration is often used as the antidote for acetaminophen overdose. NAC acts by increasing production of glutathione and possibly also sulfate, thereby preventing the formation of toxic

NAPQI.[29] It has been shown to be most effective when administered to patients who have not yet developed hepatic injury.[42] Once hepatic injury becomes evident, treatment with NAC is less effective but can improve hemodynamics and oxygen delivery.[43] NAC can be administered orally or intravenously, depending on the clinical situation. There does not appear to be an advantage of one over the other. However, some patients cannot withstand the unpleasant smell or taste of NAC, thereby requiring intravenous administration. Once treatment starts, the patient's acetaminophen concentration, liver function (AST, ALT, PT), and kidney function (creatinine concentration) should be evaluated every 12 hours.[42] Treatment can be discontinued if the acetaminophen concentration is no longer detectable and liver/kidney function tests show signs of improvement.[42] Complete normalization of laboratory results may take several weeks during recovery. In summary, acetaminophen overdose is common and deadly if left untreated. However, timely administration of NAC could prevent hepatotoxicity.

References

1. Gummin DD, Mowry JB, Spyker DA, Brooks DE, Fraser MO, Banner W. 2016 Annual Report of the American Association of Poison Control Centers' National Poison Data System (NPDS): 34th Annual Report. *Clin Toxicol (Phila).* 2017; 55:1072-1254.
2. Chan TY. Improvements in the packaging of drugs and chemicals may reduce the likelihood of severe intentional poisonings in adults. *Hum Exp Toxicol.* 2000;19:387-391.
3. Hawton K, Townsend E, Deeks J, et al. Effects of legislation restricting pack sizes of paracetamol and salicylate on self poisoning in the United Kingdom: before and after study. *BMJ.* 2001;322:1203-1207.
4. Hemel PB, Chiltoskey MU. *Cherokee Plants and Their Uses: A 400 Year History.* Sylva, NC: Herald Publishing Co; 1975.
5. Stone E. An account of the success of the bark of the willow in the cure of agues. *Philosophical Transactions.* 1763;53:195–200.
6. Jeffreys D. Aspirin. *The Remarkable Story of a Wonder Drug.* New York, NY: Bloomsbury; 2005:38-40.
7. Moffat AC, Osselton MD, Widdop B, eds. *Clarke's Analysis of Drugs and Poisons.* 3rd ed. London, UK: Pharmaceutical Press; 2004.
8. Warner A, Annesley T, eds. *Guideline for Therapeutic Drug Monitoring Services.* Washington, DC: National Academy of Clinical Biochemistry; 1999:83.
9. Chan TY, Chan AY. Use of a plasma salicylate assay service in a medical unit in Hong Kong: a follow-up study. *Vet Hum Toxicol.* 1996;38:278-279.
10. Belay ED, Bresee JS, Holman RC, Khan AS, Shahriari A, Schonberger LB. Reye's syndrome in the United States from 1981 through 1997. *N Engl J Med.* 1999;340(18):1377-1382.
11. Cohen DL, Post J, Ferroggiaro AA, Perrone J, Foster MH. Chronic salicylism resulting in noncardiogenic pulmonary edema requiring hemodialysis. *Am J Kidney Dis.* 2000;36:E20
12. Hoffman RJ, Nelson LS, Hoffman RS. Use of ferric chloride to identify salicylate-containing poisons. *J Toxicol Clin Toxicol.* 2002;40:547-549.
13. Kwong TC. Methods for salicylate and acetaminophen measurement. In: Shaw LM, Kwong TC, eds *The Clinical Toxicology Laboratory Contemporary Practice of Poisoning Evaluation.* Washington, DC: AACC Press; 2001:499-502.
14. Sarma L, Wong SH, DellaFera S. Diflunisal significantly interferes with salicylate measurements by FPIA-TDx and UV-VIS aca methods. *Clin Chem.* 1985;31:1922-1923.
15. Dalrymple RW, Stearns FM. Diflunisal interference with determination of salicylate by the Trinder, Abbott TDx, and Du Pont aca methods. *Clin Chem.* 1986;32:230.
16. White S, Wong SH. Standards of laboratory practice: analgesic drug monitoring. National Academy of Clinical Biochemistry. *Clin Chem.* 1998;44:1110-11123.
17. Proudfoot AT, Krenzelok EP, Vale JA. Position paper on urine alkalinization. *J Toxicol Clin Toxicol.* 2004;42:1-26.
18. Juurlink DN, Gosselin S, Kielstein JT, et al. Extracorporeal treatment for salicylate poisoning: systematic review and recommendations from the EXTRIP workgroup. *Ann Emerg Med.* 2015;66:165-181.
19. Cahn A, Hepp P. Das Antifebrin, ein neues Fiebermittel. *Centralbl Klin Med.* 1886;7:561-564.
20. Bertolini A, Ferrari A, Ottani A, Guerzoni S, Tacchi R, Leone S. Paracetamol: new vistas of an old drug. *CNS Drug Rev.* 2006;12:250-275.
21. Morse HN. Ueber eine neue Darstellungsmethode der Acetylamidophenole. *Berichte der Deutschen Chemischen Gesellschaft.* 1878;11:232-233.
22. Silverman M, Lydecker M, Lee PR. Bad Medicine. *The Prescription Drug Industry in the Third World.* Stanford, CA: Stanford University Press; 1992:88-90.
23. Von Mering J. Beitrage zur Kenntniss der Antipyretica. *Ther Monatsch.* 1893;7: 577–587.
24. Sneader W. *Drug Discovery: A History.* Hoboken, NJ: Wiley; 2005:439.

25. Lester D, Greenberg LA, Carroll RP. The metabolic fate of acetanilid and other aniline derivatives, II: major metabolites of acetanilid appearing in the blood. *J Pharmacol Exp Ther.* 1947;90: 68-75.
26. Hogestatt ED, Jonsson BA, Ermund A, et al. Conversion of acetaminophen to the bioactive N-acylphenolamine AM404 via fatty acid amide hydrolase-dependent arachidonic acid conjugation in the nervous system. *J Biol Chem.* 2005;280(36):31405-31412.
27. Jollow DJ, Mitchell JR, Potter WZ, Davis DC, Gillette JR, Brodie BB. Acetaminophen-induced hepatic necrosis, II: role of covalent binding in vivo. *J Pharmacol Exp Ther.* 1973;187:195-202.
28. Mitchell JR, Jollow DJ, Potter WZ, Gillette JR, Brodie BB. Acetaminophen-induced hepatic necrosis, IV: protective role of glutathione. *J Pharmacol Exp Ther.* 1973;187:211-217.
29. Yoon E, Babar A, Choudhary M, Kutner M, Pyrsopoulos N. Acetaminophen-induced hepatotoxicity: a comprehensive update. *J Clin Transl Hepatol.* 2016;4:131-142.
30. Perrone J, Hollander JE, Shaw L, De Roos F. Predictive properties of a qualitative urine acetaminophen screen in patients with self-poisoning. *J Toxicol Clin Toxicol.* 1999;37:769-772.
31. Porter WH. In acetaminophen assay, only unconjugated drug should be measured. *Clin Chem.* 1984;30:1884-1885.
32. Glynn JP, Kendal SE. Letter: paracetamol measurement. *Lancet.* 1975;1:1147-1148.
33. Bertholf RL, Johannsen LM, Bazooband A, Mansouri V. False-positive acetaminophen results in a hyperbilirubinemic patient. *Clin Chem.* 2003;49:695-698.
34. Liang S, Bae H, Horowitz GL. Falsely-elevated acetaminophen results in icteric and hemolyzed specimens. *Clin Chem.* 2008;54(6 Suppl):A223.
35. Fong BM, Siu TS, Tam A. Persistently increased acetaminophen concentrations in patient with acute liver failure. *Clin Chem.* 2011;57:9-13.
36. Hullin DA. An IgM paraprotein causing a falsely low result in an enzymatic assay for acetaminophen. *Clin Chem.* 1999;45:155-157.
37. Mayer M, Salpeter L. More on interference of N-acetylcysteine in measurement of acetaminophen. *Clin Chem.* 1998;44:892-893.
38. Rumack BH, Peterson RC, Koch GG, Amara IA. Acetaminophen overdose: 662 cases with evaluation of oral acetylcysteine treatment. *Arch Intern Med.* 1981;141:380-385.
39. Rumack BH. Acetaminophen hepatotoxicity: the first 35 years. *J Toxicol Clin Toxicol.* 2002;40:3-20
40. Wong A, Cheung B, Nejad C, Gantier M, Graudins A. Hepatotoxicity after paracetamol overdose in a patient with cystic fibrosis despite early acetylcysteine and utility of microRNA to predict hepatotoxicity. *Clin Toxicol.* 2018;56:904-906.
41. Wong A, Graudins A. Risk prediction of hepatotoxicity in paracetamol poisoning. *Clin Toxicol.* 2017;55:879-892.
42. Heard KJ. Acetylcysteine for acetaminophen poisoning. *N Engl J Med.* 2008;359:285-292.
43. Harrison PM, Wendon JA, Gimson AE, Alexander GJ, Williams R. Improvement by acetylcysteine of hemodynamics and oxygen transport in fulminant hepatic failure. *N Engl J Med.* 1991;324:1852-1857.

Chapter 28

Lead and Other Toxic Metals

Robert A. Middleberg, PhD

Introduction

Metals and metalloids (substances having properties of a metal and a nonmetal) comprise the majority of the periodic chart. Not all metals and metalloids have been well characterized in respect to toxicity. While the term *heavy metals* is used, this term is without consensus definition in chemistry and toxicology.[1] Unfortunately, there is some fictional association of the term heavy metals with toxicity. Often, even toxicologists refer to "heavy metals" as those composed of lead, arsenic, mercury, cadmium, and thallium, as well as others that fit the day. More properly, the term heavy metals should be disregarded, with the relevant term being *metals*.

The use of, and exposure to, metals by man is well documented in history. Metals most likely represent the oldest characterized toxins known to man. Some of the earliest writings in toxicology revolve around metals, especially concerning those who were occupationally exposed. Hippocrates, in 370 BCE, documented abdominal colic in a man who extracted metals. Many other physician-historians have documented exposure of man to metals.[2]

Metals, as elements, are neither created nor destroyed by humans. In this respect, metals are both toxins (found in the earth's crust or in ores) and toxicants (anthropogenic uses). The toxicokinetics and toxicodynamics of metals are quite variable, not only between different metals, but also within different chemical species of the same metal, eg, inorganic arsenic versus organic arsenicals. The term given to this latter principle is *speciation*. The toxic effects of metals are significantly affected by the species present. Half-lives of metals can vary from hours to months to years depending on the metal and species. Many metals are essential for normal physiological and biochemical functions and are termed *essential trace elements*. For example, glucose regulation requires the presence of chromium in the +3 oxidation state, while chromium in the +6 oxidation state is highly toxic. Other significant essential trace elements include cobalt, copper, iron, manganese, molybdenum, selenium, and zinc. Other metals are also thought to be essential trace elements.[3,4]

Humans are exposed to metals through numerous sources including the environment, food, water, and lifestyle choices, eg, smoking cigarettes, and one's occupation. Once exposed, humans have several metal-binding proteins to assist in the transport, storage, and elimination of metals. Included in these specific proteins are metallothioneins (Cd, Cu, Hg, Ag, Zn), transferrin (Fe, Al, Mn), ferritin (Fe, Cd, Zn, Be, Al), and ceruloplasmin (Cu). Since a particular protein can bind several metals, the presence of competing metals may cause deficiencies in essential trace elements.[5,6]

Biological monitoring for metals is usually performed in whole blood, serum/plasma, red blood cells, and urine. Additional issue-critical specimens include organ biopsies (eg, liver biopsies for copper determination in the diagnosis of Wilson disease), hair and nails (for chronic exposure), and autopsy specimens (for disease and cause-of-death determination). It is imperative that caution be taken when collecting biosamples for metals analysis due to the omnipresence of metals in the environment and the potential for inadvertent contamination of a given specimen.

In addition to measuring the metal itself, biomarkers are also sometimes useful. A biomarker is the product of an interaction between a xenobiotic agent and some target molecule or cell that is measurable (biomarker of exposure) or a biochemical, physiological, behavioral, or other alteration within the individual (biomarker of effect).[7] For example, blood can be used to measure cadmium as a biomarker of exposure, while β-2 microglobulin in urine can be measured as a biomarker of effect.

The monitoring of individuals in respect to correlating broad-based metal concentrations to general health status must be viewed skeptically. Many factors, including environmental contamination, diet, hobbies, etc, will influence the interpretation of such assessments. This testing should not be confused with testing for potential significant toxic exposures to any particular metal.

In general, numerous treatment protocols exist after significant human exposure to metals. Such treatment is often guided by biomonitoring of blood, urine, and other specimens in relation to clinical manifestations and can range from symptomatic treatments to specific metal-based options. Many metals have antidotes in the form of chelating agents. These substances are generally not specific

Table 28-1. Selected Physico-Chemical Properties of Metals[6,8-14]

Element	Lead	Arsenic	Cadmium	Mercury	Thallium
Symbol	Pb	As	Cd	Hg	Tl
Synonym	Plumbum	[none]	[none]	Quicksilver; Hydrargyrum	[none]
Isotopes	^{208}Pb (~52%) ^{206}Pb (~25%) ^{207}Pb (~22%) ^{204}Pb (~1%)	^{75}As	^{106}Cd (1.22%) ^{108}Cd (0.88%) ^{110}Cd (12.9%) ^{111}Cd (12.75%) ^{112}Cd (24.07%) ^{113}Cd (12.6%) ^{114}Cd (28.86%) ^{116}Cd (7.5%)	^{196}Hg (0.15%) ^{198}Hg (9.97%) ^{199}Hg (16.87%) ^{200}Hg (23.10%) ^{201}Hg (13.18%) ^{202}Hg (29.86%) ^{204}Hg (6.87%)	^{203}Tl (29.524%) ^{205}Tl (70.476%)
Atomic mass	207.2000	74.9216	112.4110	200.5900	204.3833

for a particular metal and thus can lead to deficiencies in trace elements when used. The effectiveness of chelation therapy can be variable based, in part, on the time of administration versus time of exposure (for example, the efficacy of chelation therapy for lead once the compound is incorporated into bone is low) as well as other factors. In addition, many chelators have their own toxicity profiles.

While most metals have established toxicity profiles, this chapter is meant to highlight a few of the classically recognized metal poisons, including lead, arsenic, cadmium, mercury, and thallium. See Table 28-1 for basic physico-chemical properties of the discussed metals.

Lead

Origin and Uses

Lead is found in ore deposits throughout the world, with the predominant ore being galena (PbS). Man has used lead in its various forms, eg, salts, alloys, and organic forms, for probably thousands of years. With that, lead has long been recognized as a toxin (natural forms) and toxicant (man-made forms). Its toxic effects were noted approximately 3000 years ago and can be found in the earliest of biomedical scientific writings, including those of Nikander and Hippocrates. Despite its recognized toxicities, and due to some of its properties, including resistance to corrosion, malleability, acid resistance, and low melting point, lead has played a significant role in man's history in respect to utility. Some significant uses or applications of lead and related compounds have included plumbing, batteries, paint, and gasoline.[2,6] In the United States, there has been significant curtailing of the use of lead in products that ordinarily present widespread exposure of the population. The basis for the legislated decrease in lead use was based on its known toxicities, especially in children with a developing central nervous system (CNS). Two major initiatives have been credited with the decreased exposure to lead:

- House paints used prior to 1940 generally contained lead, which imparted pigment as well as durability and moisture resistance. In the 1930s, it was recognized that childhood lead poisoning was an issue in the US. The American Public Health Association recommended not using lead-based paint on items such as baby toys and carriages. By 1940, little lead-based paint was being used for interior painting, and by 1950, it was recognized that peeling and chipping paint in older homes presented hazards to children.[15] It wasn't until 1971, however, that the first lead-based paint legislation was passed in the US. This legislation, the Lead-Based Paint Poisoning Prevention Act (LBPPPA), was amended in 1973 and generally dealt with lead-based paint in federally funded housing. In 1978, the Consumer Product Safety Commission banned the residential use of lead-based paint.[16] Today, however, lead-based paint is still used in certain industrial applications, especially outside the US.[17,18]
- In 1921, at a General Motors Research Corporation laboratory, tetraethyl lead (TEL) was found to reduce internal combustion engine pinging or knocking. By the mid-1920s, the toxicity associated with TEL was well established with deaths in some individuals working with the compound. Nonetheless, TEL became the domestic and international antiknock agent. Continued reports of toxicity were prevalent, but in the US, it wasn't

until 1970, with the passage of the Clean Air Act, that there were initiatives to squelch lead emissions from gasoline with phase-outs beginning in 1972 and ending in 1986. Finally, amendments to the Clean Air Act in 1990 banned the presence of lead in gasoline.[19]

Based on the abatement initiatives in paint and gasoline in the US, an 80% drop in blood lead levels in children was observed between 1976 and 1999.[18] Even so, it is estimated that approximately one million children remain at risk for lead poisoning based on living conditions and parental occupations.[19,20]

Toxicology

Mechanism of Action

Lead exerts adverse effects on various cellular and subcellular entities essential for normal physiological and biochemical functionality. Several essential enzymes are impaired by lead, leading to various pathophysiological states. Like many other metals, lead has an affinity for sulfhydryl groups, which are essential for many enzymes to function properly. For example, lead interferes with a number of enzymes important in the synthesis of steroids and vitamin D as well as in maintaining the integrity of cell membranes. Specific enzyme interactions of note include aminolevulinic acid dehydratase (ALA-D) and ferrochelatase. These two enzymes are essential for proper heme synthesis. ALA-D is a cytoplasmic enzyme, whereas ferrochelatase is a mitochondrial enzyme. Accumulation of ALA occurs with inhibition of ALA-D, while there is a build-up of protoporphyrin in red cells after ferrochelatase impairment. Both ALA and protoporphyrin (and related entities) are measurable biomarkers of lead exposure.

Other mechanisms of action of lead toxicity include effects on DNA transcription factors and interference with calcium-related activity.[6,12,20,21]

Toxicokinetics

Absorption of lead after oral ingestion in adults ranges between 5% and 15%, whereas in children, it can be as high as approximately 40%, thus further facilitating its toxicity in the latter age group. Organic lead compounds may be readily absorbed through the skin. Once absorbed, lead in the bloodstream is almost entirely bound to hemoglobin. Once distributed, the majority of lead resides in long bones, whereas the target organ for toxicity is soft tissue (liver, kidney, brain, etc). Lead crosses the placenta and therefore has effects on the developing fetus. The half-life for distribution/elimination of lead from blood is 1 to 2 months, whereas for bone it is greater than 20 years.[6,20]

Acute Exposure

Acute poisoning with lead is rare and is generally manifested as gastrointestinal (GI) disturbances (nausea, vomiting, abdominal pain), CNS effects (paresthesias, pain, muscle weakness), and renal damage. Death can occur in 1 to 2 days. If one survives, effects associated with chronic exposure may be expected, potentially with permanent neurologic and/or behavioral problems.[12,16,22-24]

Chronic Exposure

The effects of chronic exposure to lead are dependent upon the organ system involved as well as the age of the individual (child vs adult [see Figure 28-1]), amount of exposure, and other factors. Chronic lead poisoning is known as *plumbism.*

CNS: Lead encephalopathy is more common in children than adults.[25] Early signs include ataxia, falling, headache, clumsiness, restlessness, and irritability. As the condition progresses, excitement and confusion, visual disturbances, delirium with convulsions, and coma become evident. The death rate amongst those with cerebral involvement was as high as 65% prior to the use of chelation therapy but is now approximately 5%.[26] Long-term sequelae in children include impaired mental capacity, electroencephalogram (EEG) changes, seizures, and cerebral palsy.

In young children with significant lead exposure, normal development may be noted up to 18 months or longer. This "normal period" may be followed by a steady loss of motor and speech skills. Hyperkinetic behavior and aggressive behavior may be evident, thus being confused for attention deficit/hyperactivity disorders.[27,28] Learning disabilities, decrements in IQ, and behavioral problems may be seen even in children that are exposed to low levels of lead. All of these effects are exacerbated as the blood lead level increases. It is estimated that there is an IQ deficit of 1 to 5 points with a 10 mcg/dL increase in blood lead.[29] At blood lead concentrations less than 10 mcg/dL, quantitative estimates of IQ loss have also been defined.[30]

Neuromuscular: Muscle weakness and fatigue progressing to *lead palsy* can occur. Foot and wrist drop are most noteworthy.[27]

Hematologic: Basophilic stippling in erythrocytes is identifiable when blood lead concentrations approach 80 mcg/dL. The more commonly observed hematologic effect of lead, however, is a hypochromic microcytic anemia. This results from a decreased life span of the erythrocytes as well as inhibition of heme synthesis.[27]

Other known effects of lead include renal tubular disorder and irreversible interstitial nephropathy,

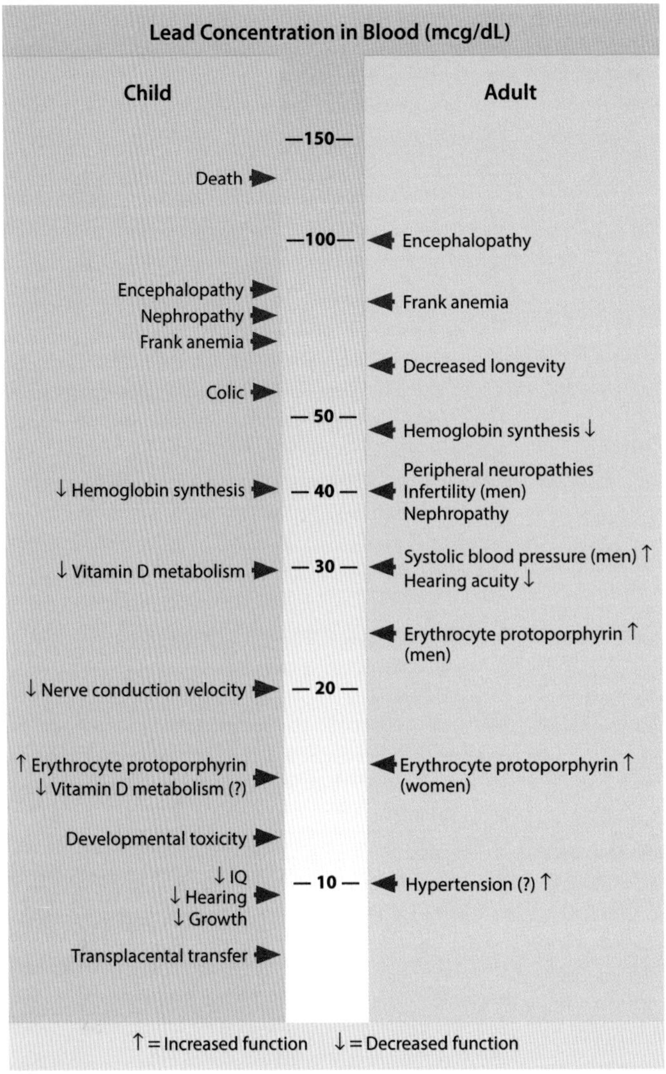

Figure 27-1. Toxic effects of lead.

From Ellenhorn MJ. *Ellenhorn's Medical Toxicology: Diagnosis and Treatment of Human Poisoning.* 2nd ed. Baltimore, MD: Williams & Wilkins; 1997. Modified with permission.

ashen color of the face, retinal stippling, lead-lines along the gums (blue-black, black, or grayish lines known as Burton's lines) due to lead sulfide deposition, and potential cancers.[31] Lead is also a significant reproductive toxicant. It can cause diminished or aberrant sperm in males and can act as an abortifacient in women.[16,24,32]

Analysis

Specimen Types and Characteristics

Whole blood lead is the best measure of inorganic lead in the body. Bone densitometry and x-ray may also be useful. Urine lead concentration is the specimen of choice for organic lead exposure, with concentrations generally exceeding 200 mcg/L in poisoning. Fatalities from organic lead may have urinary concentrations exceeding 1000 mcg/L. In organic lead exposure, there is a disproportionally high ratio of urine lead to blood lead compared to that observed with inorganic lead exposure.[12]

Modes of Analysis

Common methods of analysis include inductively-coupled plasma mass spectrometry (ICP-MS), graphite furnace atomic absorption spectroscopy (GFAAS), and anodic stripping voltammetry (ASV). Modern laboratory-based methods can easily achieve limits of quantitation of at least 1 mcg/dL. Point-of-care screening devices facilitate rapid blood lead concentration determinations; however, when elevated concentrations are detected, retesting of a new blood sample utilizing laboratory-based methods must occur. Also, such devices can be adversely affected by a number of factors, including tube type.[34]

Clinical Issues

Unexpected positive or highly elevated results should be confirmed with a newly collected specimen with an appropriate collection method to mitigate the risk of contamination. Treatment is generally supportive, and if the blood lead concentration is high enough, chelation with $CaNa_2EDTA$ may be useful.[35] Chelation is not effective for organic lead exposure.[7] See Table 28-2 for management recommendations in pediatric exposures.

Arsenic

Origin and Uses

Arsenic is classified as a metalloid. It is often isolated as a byproduct of the smelting of other metals, eg, copper and gold ores. In respect to biology and toxicology, arsenicals can be categorized three ways: (1) inorganic arsenicals, (2) organic arsenicals, and (3) arsine gas. When compounded, arsenic generally exists in the –3, +3 and +5 oxidation states. The form of arsenic together with its oxidation state are important determinants of toxicity.[36] The focus of the content in this chapter is inorganic arsenicals.

Table 28-2. Blood Lead Concentrations and Indicated Treatment in Children[33]	
<5 mcg/dL*	No treatment; nutritional and developmental milestones assessment; lead education; follow-up testing at recommended age-based intervals
5-9 mcg/dL	Nutritional and developmental milestones assessment; environmental assessment for potential sources of lead; nutritional counseling related to calcium and iron intake; follow-up testing at recommended age-based intervals
10-19 mcg/dL	Nutritional and developmental milestones assessment; environmental assessment for potential sources of lead, including a home visit; nutritional counseling related to calcium and iron intake; potential laboratory testing for iron status; follow-up testing at recommended age-based intervals
20-44 mcg/dL	Complete history and physical; neurodevelopmental assessment; environmental investigation of home to include hazard reduction; iron status and hemoglobin or hematocrit determinations; abdominal x-ray with gut decontamination if warranted; follow-up testing at recommended age-based intervals
45-69 mcg/dL	Complete history and physical; complete neurological exam, including neurodevelopmental assessment; environmental investigation of home to include hazard reduction; iron status and hemoglobin or hematocrit determinations; abdominal x-ray with gut decontamination if warranted; oral chelation therapy with hospitalization if not lead safe at home; follow-up testing at recommended age-based intervals
≥70 mcg/dL	Hospitalize and begin chelation therapy with consultation of a medical toxicologist or pediatric environmental health specialty unit; other actions under the 45-69 mcg/dL category

*5 mcg/dL is termed the "reference value" for blood lead concentration in children and represents the 97.5th percentile of blood lead concentrations based on 2007-2008 and 2008-2009 National Health and Nutrition Examination Survey (NHANES) data. This statistical figure is not meant to mean that concentrations below 5 mcg/dL are without consequence.

Arsenicals were used as medicinal agents as early as 400 BCE for such ailments as protozoal and spirochetal (including syphilis) diseases, psoriasis, and leukemia. While Western medicine abandoned the use of arsenicals by the 1980s, there has been a recurrence of use in conditions such as promyelocytic leukemia (ie, arsenic trioxide). Additionally, an organic arsenical is used in the treatment of African tryppanosomiasis.[37] Besides medicinal uses, arsenic has had widespread use as a pesticide, as a wood preservative, and in livestock feed (as an antibiotic and to promote growth). Arsine and arsenic trioxide are used in the manufacture of computer chips.[13]

While intentional exposures to arsenic, both homicidal and suicidal, still occur, most people are exposed to arsenic through soil, water (ground and well), food, and air. Certain fish and seafood are known to contain significant concentrations of arsenosugars (organic arsenic forms) and other arsenic-containing compounds, primarily in the form of arsenobetaine and arsenocholine, with the latter compound found mainly in shrimp. These compounds generally present little risk of toxicity; however, they can contribute significantly to one's body burden of arsenic. Therefore, care must be taken in the interpretation of arsenic findings in blood and urine in respect to risk for toxicity, especially if samples were taken within 1 to 2 days of consumption of these foods. For this reason, speciation of arsenic is recommended as a confirmation test for elevated arsenic concentrations in blood or urine.[38]

In general, risk of toxicities from the different species of arsenic can be summarized as follows:

$$\text{organic arsenicals} < As^{+5} \text{ (arsenate)} < As^{+3} \text{ (arsenite)} < \text{arsine gas } (AsH_3)$$

Arsenic is a recognized human carcinogen causing lung, skin, and bladder cancers.[12]

Toxicology

Mechanism of Action

The mechanism of action of arsenic is form dependent. Pentavalent arsenicals uncouple mitochondrial oxidative phosphorylation with associated sequelae. Trivalent arsenicals bind with sulfhydryl groups, thus inhibiting many enzymes, including those involved in glycolysis and the citric acid cycle.[39] Arsine gas interacts with hemoglobin by unknown specific mechanisms to cause hemolysis.[40]

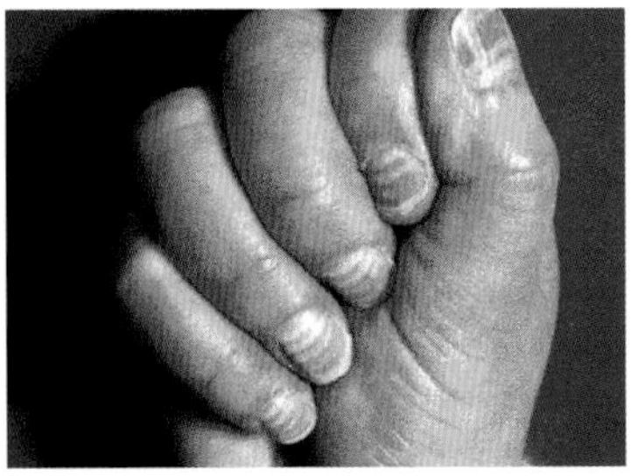

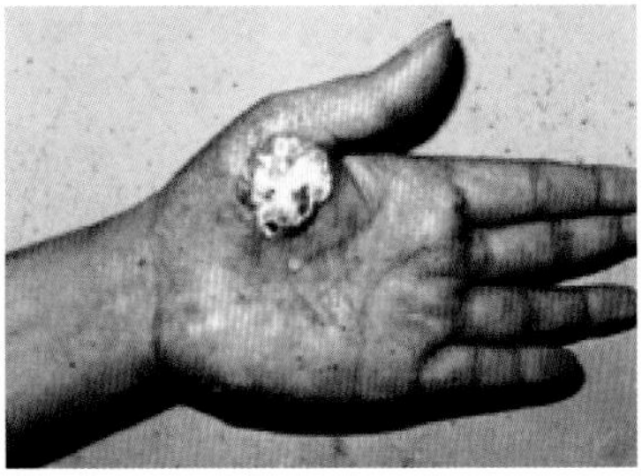

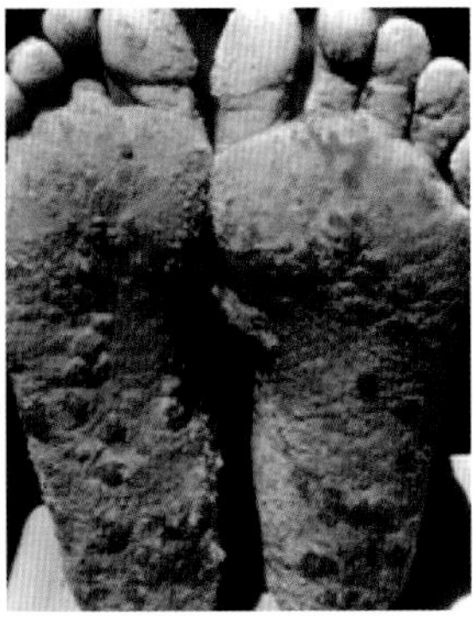

Figure 28-2. (Left) Mees' lines.[43]
Figure 28-3. (Center) Cancerous lesion on palm of hand.[44]
Figure 28-4. (Right) Cancerous lesions on soles of feet.[45]

Toxicokinetics

Arsenic is readily absorbed following inhalation or ingestion and through parenteral and dermal routes (excluding inorganic arsenicals). Exposure to arsenate or arsenite leads to initial accumulation in the liver, kidneys, and lungs. As arsenic exists in different forms and oxidation states, its biotransformation is somewhat complex. Basically, for inorganic arsenicals, reduction/oxidation reactions that interconvert As (III) and As (V) occur as well as methylations that convert As (III) to monomethylarsonic acid (MMA) and dimethylarsinic acid (DMA). Typically, the biotransformation process is as follows:

$$\text{inorganic arsenate} \xrightarrow[\textit{reduction}]{} \text{arsenite} \xrightarrow[\textit{methylation}]{} \text{MMA (V)}$$

$$\xrightarrow[\textit{reduction}]{} \text{MMA (III)} \xrightarrow[\textit{methylation}]{} \text{DMA (V)}$$

After exposure to inorganic arsenic, a mixture of arsenic, MMA, and DMA is found in urine. Arsenobetaine does not appear to be biotransformed and is found intact in urine, while arsenocholine is oxidized to arsenobetaine. Whole body clearance of arsenic generally takes place with half-lives of 40 to 60 hours. Seafood containing arsenic is generally cleared with a half-life of less than 20 hours. Ingested MMA and DMA are mostly eliminated within 1 day.[13,41]

Acute Exposure

After oral ingestion of inorganic arsenicals, gastrointestinal disturbances are usually noted within 1 hour (can be delayed). Projectile vomiting and diarrhea are common. Rice water stools (clear feces with a whitish flocculent material that is the sloughing of gastrointestinal cellular material) are also noted. Burning of the lips, constriction of the throat, and difficulty swallowing are also noted. Muscle cramps and thirst are common. Acute renal tubular necrosis can be observed with or without other renal effects, eg, oliguria, proteinuria, hematuria. Nervous system effects may include confusion, muscle weakness, and peripheral neuropathy, which can have a latency period of days to weeks. Hypoxic convulsions may be terminally present.[13,42]

Chronic Exposure

Common signs and symptoms of chronic exposure to inorganic arsenicals include weight loss, anorexia, muscle weakness and aching, skin pigmentation, and hyperkeratosis and peripheral neuritis. Like many metals, arsenic can induce a metallic, or "garlic," odor to breath and sweat. Numbness and tingling of extremities is not uncommon. Alopecia can also be noted, but again, several metals can cause this sign. Mees' lines (transverse white deposits of arsenic on the nails; see Figure 28-2) can appear approximately 6 weeks after exposure. Hepatic and renal dysfunction can be observed along with peripheral neuropathies. In respect to cancers, skin lesions include intraepidermal, basal cell, and squamous cell carcinomas, while carcinomas of the lung and bladder may occur (see Figures 28-3 and 28-4).[13,27,42]

Analysis

Specimen Types and Characteristics

For suspect exposures, blood and urine arsenic concentrations (both total and speciated) should be determined. For chronic exposures, hair and/or nail analysis may be informative as well. Additionally, in postmortem cases, arsenic determination in visceral organs, especially kidney and liver, can be valuable.

Mode of Analysis

For unspeciated, total arsenic determination, typical analytical methods of analysis include AAS and ICP-MS. Speciation is generally performed using ion chromatography (IC), high-performance liquid chromatography (HPLC), or IC-ICP/MS or HPLC-ICP/MS.

Clinical Issues

Unexpected positive or highly elevated results should be confirmed with a newly collected specimen with an appropriate collection method to mitigate the risk of contamination. Supportive care should be commenced as needed. In severe cases, chelation with dimercaprol (BAL) for acute symptoms (3 mg/kg IM every 4 h) followed by oral penicillamine may be used. Succimer may be used in place of dimercaprol due to its higher therapeutic index.[46] Exchange transfusion and hemodialysis may be effective in arsine poisoning.[40]

Cadmium

Origin and Uses

Cadmium is a relatively modern metal, not having been discovered until 1817. It is a widely but sparsely distributed element in the earth's crust typically mined as sulfide minerals in association with other metal ores. This element has chemical similarity to zinc. It gained substantial use over the last 50 or so years due mainly to its noncorrosive properties. Based on this latter property, it has, and continues to be, used in the electroplating and galvanizing industries. It is also a pigment in paints and plastics, including those found in laboratories (eg, yellow pipette tips) and is used in the manufacturing of batteries.[9,14]

Man is mainly exposed to cadmium through food, smoking, or the workplace. Shellfish and fish may contain high amounts of cadmium due to polluted water. *Itai-itai* ("ouch-ouch" in Japanese) disease was coined when a Japanese population was exposed to a cadmium-contaminated rice field beginning in 1912. The contamination resulted from a lead-zinc processing plant effluent. The known painful effects of cadmium exposure, however, were recognized in the early 1900s. Livestock and fruit accumulate cadmium from soil, food, and water sources, adding to the human body burden of cadmium. Smoking a pack of cigarettes per day can double one's body burden of cadmium.[47,48]

Cadmium toxicity is of significant concern to workers. Fumes and airborne concentrations can cause significant effects in workers. It is one of only a few compounds where the US Occupational Safety and Health Administration (OSHA) mandates monitoring of exposed workers. Cadmium exposure has been correlated with lung and prostate cancers.[49]

Toxicology

Mechanism of Action

Cadmium appears to exert its effects through oxidative stress, epigenetic changes in DNA expression, competitive interference with the actions of zinc or magnesium, and a host of other means.[50]

Toxicokinetics

The toxicokinetics of cadmium are affected by the route of administration. While exposure to cadmium can take place through dermal absorption, data is limited; thus, this route of administration will not be discussed.

Inhalation: Since cadmium metal and salts have low volatility, they generally exist in air as suspensions of particulate matter. In this respect, inhalation results in deposition into alveoli, a major site of absorption. It is estimated that approximately 25% of inhaled cadmium gets absorbed. Once absorbed, the majority of cadmium deposits in kidney and liver. Cadmium that makes its way into the gastrointestinal tract via the mucocilliary escalator generally gets excreted unabsorbed in the feces. Once absorbed, cadmium is excreted mainly through urinary and fecal routes. Urinary excretion of cadmium increases with developing kidney damage.[9,14]

Oral: Only approximately 1% to 10% of orally ingested cadmium gets absorbed. As most people are exposed to cadmium through diet, practically all organs and tissues have measurable cadmium concentrations, with the majority in kidney and liver. Since absorption is low via the oral route, most cadmium ends up in the feces. That which is absorbed is eliminated mainly through the kidneys and feces.[9,14]

Once absorbed, cadmium is found mainly in the blood cells bound to a metallothionein-like protein. In plasma, cadmium is transported by metallothionein. The cadmium-metallothionein complex facilitates entrance of cadmium into the kidneys. Cadmium exposure also induces the synthesis of metallothionein. Estimates of the biological half-lives of cadmium in the various organs and tissues of the body are 10 to 30 years.[5,9,14]

Acute Exposure

Local irritation is usually present at the site of exposure. If swallowed, irritation of the GI tract, with associated nausea, vomiting, diarrhea, and cramping, is observed. If inhaled (a more toxic situation), pneumonitis progressing to potentially fatal pulmonary edema or other long-term pulmonary sequelae may occur; GI disturbances are also common.[27]

Chronic Exposure

Renal problems (tubular or glomerular insufficiency) are significant with chronic cadmium exposure. If inhaled, chronic pulmonary dysfunction and disease are often noted. Osteopenia-osteomalacia (causing musculoskeletal pain) is progressive and is the progenitor of the name of the *itai-itai* disease (see Figure 28-5). Yellow teeth lines may also be present.[51]

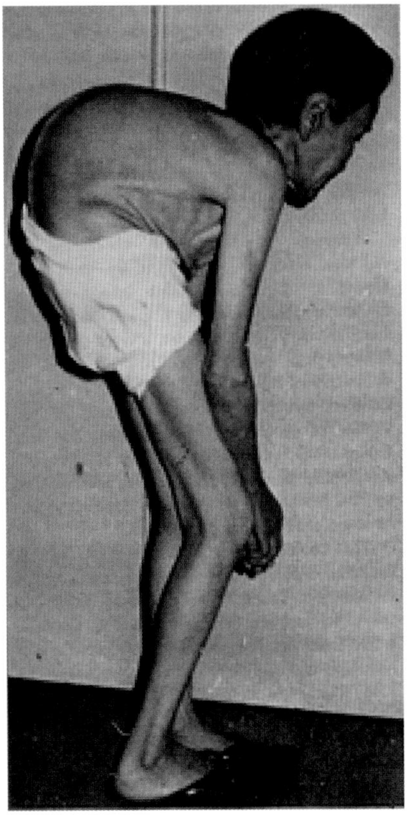

Figure 28-5. Sequelae of itai-itai disease.[52]

Analysis

Specimen Types and Characteristics

Blood is usually used to identify recent exposure to cadmium, while urine can give a better indication of body burden. However, even urine is subject to change with recent exposure to cadmium. Other useful tissues and biomaterials include hair, nail, feces, liver, and kidney. Often, urine concentrations are creatinine corrected.

In addition to measuring cadmium itself, common biomarkers of renal function are often measured, including urinary β-2 microglobulin, urinary retinol-binding protein (RBP), and N-acetyl-β-D-glucosaminidase (NAG) as well as others. These markers, however, are not specific for cadmium toxicity.[53]

Modes of Analysis

For cadmium determination in biomaterials, typical methods of analysis include AAS and ICP-MS.

Clinical Issues

Unexpected positive or highly elevated results should be confirmed with a newly collected specimen with an appropriate collection method to mitigate the risk of contamination. Initial treatment is supportive and symptomatic, especially with respiratory-induced sequelae. Attempts to reduce the body burden of cadmium must be undertaken with care and, in fact, are not recommended by many sources since some chelating agents may increase the mobilization of cadmium, thus facilitating kidney and liver damage.[54]

Mercury

Origin and Uses

Mercury is the only metal that is liquid at room temperature. It is mainly found in mercury-rich ores as the red sulfide known as cinnabar. Through degassing of the earth's crust and oceans, 30,000 to 50,000 tons of mercury are released naturally into the atmosphere. It has been used for centuries for therapeutic treatment of many conditions, including as a diuretic, antibacterial (eg, syphilis), antiseptic, and laxative. While no longer a traditional therapeutic agent, it may be found in nontraditional therapeutic treatments (eg, folk medicine). Mercury also has been used in dental amalgams and has many industrial uses, including the manufacture of electrical equipment, thermometers, and paints. In general, however, the body burden of mercury found in most people is due to consumption of contaminated food, most commonly fish.

Mercury exists in three toxicologically relevant forms: elemental, inorganic, and organic mercurials. Each form has distinct toxicokinetics and toxicodynamic properties. In our environment, due to bioconversion and redox chemistry, humans are exposed to the various forms of mercury. For example, methylmercury is produced by microbial activity on inorganic mercurials; in vivo, man demethylates methylmercury to produce inorganic mercury.[10,55]

Mercury is present in sea and fresh water either through environmental contamination or natural processes. It generally exists as methylmercury in water and becomes part of our food chain. Fish have been shown to contain differing amounts of methylmercury, primarily based on what they eat and how long they live. Consuming fish high in mercury content is a concern for humans, especially pregnant and nursing women and those with particular vulnerabilities. Guidelines on safe consumption of fish have been published.[56,57,58] Aryl- and alkoxyalkyl mercurials were once used as diuretics and produce effects similar to mercuric salts. Alkyl mercury has been used in fungicides.

Toxicology

Mechanism of Action

The primary mechanism of action of mercurials is based on the covalent bond between mercury and sulfur, as found in sulfhydryl groups, which can significantly disrupt many enzymatic and biological processes. Other less-significant pathophysiological mechanisms of action are known.[55]

Toxicokinetics

Liquid (elemental) mercury is poorly absorbed from the GI tract and through skin. As such, ingested elemental mercury is usually not a medical emergency. Once absorbed from the GI tract, elemental mercury is transported mainly by erythrocytes. The danger of ingested elemental mercury lies in its volatility should it get caught in pathophysiological sites such as fistulas and diverticula or should it be aspirated into lungs. Mercury vapor can readily pass through the blood-brain barrier, resulting in significant amounts of mercury in brain. Due to redox reactions, most elemental mercury is eliminated as mercuric mercury, while some may be eliminated in breath. Most elemental mercury accumulated in the body is eliminated with a half-life of approximately 60 days, while that in brain could be years.[10,55]

While inorganic mercury can be divided into mercurous (Hg+1) and mercuric (Hg+2) entities, in vivo, the predominant species is in the mercuric form. In fact, mercurous mercury may only serve as an intermediary in the redox conversion of elemental mercury to the mercuric form. In an intact GI tract, approximately 2% of mercuric chloride is absorbed, although due to its corrosive action, absorption characteristics may change. Interestingly, there is some skin absorption of mercuric mercury. Once absorbed, mercuric mercury is distributed between erythrocytes and plasma, and may accumulate in kidney and liver; very little crosses the blood-brain barrier. Excretion is mainly by the kidney, in feces, and through sweat. The estimated half-life is about 60 days.[10,55]

Toxicokinetics of organic mecurials can vary with the specific compound(s). The following represents generalities. Organic mercurials can be absorbed through oral means, inhalation, and the skin. Absorption from the GI tract is predicted to be greater than inorganic mercurials (up to 90%) due to increased lipid solubility. It is distributed mainly by erythrocytes and its interaction with sulfhydryl-containing proteins in plasma. Organic mercurials are found mainly in the liver, kidney, brain, hair, and epidermis. Aryl and long-chain compounds are biotransformed to inorganic mercury. Half-life is approximately 70 days. Elimination is mainly via the bile/feces and kidneys. These compounds are subject to enterohepatic recirculation, thus prolonging their residence time in the body.[10,55]

Acute Exposure

Acute exposure to elemental mercury can cause GI disturbances, a metallic taste in the mouth, cough, chest tightness, and pulmonary toxicity (potential residual fibrosis). These latter effects are especially noteworthy in mercury vapor inhalation.[59]

Chronic Exposure

Chronic exposure to elemental mercury produces CNS effects. One such condition, known as *asthenic vegetative syndrome (micromercurialism),* is characterized by neurasthenia, gingivitis, and thyroid disturbances (eg, goiter). Continued exposure leads to tremors and psychological changes (eg, depression, confusion, irritability). Vasomotor sequelae consisting of excessive perspiration and blushing called *erethism* is also common. The classic triad of effects from mercury vapor is increased excitability, tremors, and gingivitis.[60]

Inorganic mercury is associated with severe toxic effects, particularly if reduced to elemental mercury, which can pass through the blood-brain barrier. The primary effects are gastrointestinal (nausea, vomiting, hemorrhagic gastroenteritis), renal (tubular necrosis), and oral (gingivitis, ashen mucosa, discoloration of the gums, foul breath, and loosening of the teeth). *Acrodynia* is an idiosyncratic reaction to chronic mercury exposure, especially in children, which is characterized by erythema of the extremities, chest, and face; photophobia; diaphoresis; anorexia; tachycardia; irritability; and a generalized rash.[60]

There have been several major large-scale human poisonings by alkyl mercurials. The first was in Minamata Bay in Japan in 1956, whereby industrial effluent was dumped into Minamata Bay. Consumption of fish in the bay by humans led to thousands of significant long-lasting disease cases and deaths. This led to the term *Minamata disease associated with mercury exposure.*[61,62]

Another incident involved the use of alkyl mercurials as a fungicide in Iraq in 1972. Fungicide-contaminated grain was inadvertently used to make flour. As a result, more than 6500 people were hospitalized and 500 died.[63]

Analysis

Specimen Types and Characteristics

Blood, urine, tissues, and hair have been used to identify recent and/or chronic exposure to mercurials. It has been suggested that creatinine-corrected urine mercury concentrations correlate well with blood concentrations.[56] Alkyl mercurials generally reside in red blood cells, with very little excreted in urine; thus, urine should not be used in suspected exposures.[10]

Modes of Analysis

Analysis for mercury in biological materials is complex and difficult. Some challenges are based on its volatility and the species present. Common analytical techniques today include cold vapor atomic absorption spectroscopy (CVAAS), plasma atomic emission spectrometry (AES), and ICP-MS. Speciation can be performed using such techniques as GC/ICP-MS and capillary electrophoresis with various modes of detection including atomic fluorescence spectrometry and ICP-MS.

Clinical Issues

Unexpected positive or highly elevated results should be confirmed with a newly collected specimen with an appropriate collection method to mitigate the risk of contamination. Besides supportive care, chelation with BAL, N-acetyl-D,L-penicillamine (NAP) succimer (dimercapto succinic acid [DMSA]), D-penicillamine, or DMPS is effective for inorganic mercury intoxication. BAL should not be used for organic mercurials since it has been shown to redistribute mercury to the CNS. Succimer and NAP have been shown to be effective in animals for organic mercurials.[59,64]

Thallium

Origin and Uses

Thallium is an often-overlooked metal in respect to toxicity. It is one of the most toxic of metals, with an estimated lethal dose of 10 mg/kg to 15 mg/kg. While it can be found in the minerals vrbaite, hutchinsonite, lorandite, and crookosite, it is usually present as a byproduct of cadmium production and zinc and lead smelting. Salts of thallium, especially thallium sulfate, were popular rodenticides in the US and Europe but have been supplanted by safer compounds. Thallium was banned as a rodenticide in the US in 1965. However, due to warfarin resistance in some rodents, it is being used again in some countries. Thallium is used for medical imaging, in the electronics industry, and in semiconductors and scintillation counters. Workers are often exposed to thallium via dust inhalation. The general population is exposed to thallium usually via environmental contamination.[65,66] Thallium has been, and continues to be, used as a homicidal and suicidal agent.

Toxicology

Mechanism of Action

It is believed that thallium exerts its actions by mimicking potassium ions, substituting for potassium in the (Na^+/K^+)-ATPase, and interacting with sulfhydryl groups in proteins and biomolecules.[66]

Toxicokinetics

Much of the toxicokinetic information is derived from animal studies. These studies indicate that thallium is well absorbed by oral, inhalation, and dermal means. It is subsequently widely distributed, with the majority of the element found in the kidney. Hair is a good specimen for detecting thallium since it seems to increase in concentration over time. Blood appears to be rapidly cleared of the substance. Thallium is excreted mainly by the kidneys and intestines, with a half-life in humans of approximately 30 days.[11]

Acute Exposure

Acute thallium toxicity is best described as a three-stage process. Initially, there is intravascular distribution over an approximate 4-hour period, which is followed by distribution into the CNS over a 48-hour period. The last stage is elimination mainly by gastrointestinal and renal means. The signs and symptoms associated with these stages include abdominal pain, gastric distress with vomiting, and diarrhea. Hypersensitivity (pain and burning) to touch with severe pain in lower and upper extremities (hands and feet) are a result of axonopathy and demyelination. Psychiatric derangements are common as well.[65,67]

Chronic Exposure

The main features of chronic thallium exposure include nondescript ill health, paresthesias (distal neuropathies, numbness or pain, especially of the feet and hands) progressing to proximal neuropathies, optic neuropathy (atrophy), loss of hair (but not in all cases), and Mees' lines. *The condition is often misdiagnosed as Guillain-Barré syndrome.* Death following significant thallium exposure is not uncommon, especially due to a failure to diagnose speedily.[66-68]

Analysis

Specimen Types and Characteristics

Blood, urine, internal organs (especially kidney), hair, and nails represent satisfactory specimens for identifying exposure to thallium.

Modes of Analysis

Typical analytical techniques include ICP-MS, GFAAS, and anodic stripping voltammetry (ASV).

Clinical Issues

Unexpected positive or highly elevated results should be confirmed with a newly collected specimen with an appropriate collection method to mitigate the risk of contamination. Once absorption has occurred, hemodialysis may promote decontamination. Also, prussian blue forms a complex with thallium and has been shown to be an effective antidote by both decreasing GI absorption and reducing enterohepatic circulation of the metal.[65,67,69]

References

1. Duffus JH. "Heavy metals" – a meaningless term? *Pure Appl Chem.* 2002;74:793-807.
2. Fishbein A, Hu H. Occupational and environmental exposure to lead. In: Rom WN, ed. *Environmental and Occupational Medicine.* Philadelphia, PA: Wolter Kluwers/Lippincott Williams & Wilkins; 2007.
3. Mertz W. The essential trace elements. *Science.* 1981;213:1332-1338.
4. Taylor A. Detection and monitoring of disorders of essential trace elements. *Ann Clin Biochem.* 1996;33:486-510.
5. Sherlock, JC. Cadmium in foods and the diet. *Experientia.* 1984;40:152-156.
6. Lead. Agency for Toxic Substances and Disease Registry. Toxic Substances Portal. https://www.atsdr.cdc.gov/ToxProfiles/tp13.pdf. Accessed June 29, 2018.
7. Aitio A, Bernard A, Fowler BA, Nordberg GF. Biological monitoring and biomarkers. In: Nordberg GF, Fowler BA, Nordberg M, Friberg LT, eds. *Handbook on the Toxicology of Metals.* New York, NY: Academic Press; 2007.
8. Arsenic. Agency for Toxic Substances and Disease Registry. Toxic Substances Portal. https://www.atsdr.cdc.gov/ToxProfiles/tp2.pdf . Accessed June 29, 2018.
9. Cadmium. Agency for Toxic Substances and Disease Registry. Toxic Substances Portal. http://www.atsdr.cdc.gov/substances/toxsubstance.asp?toxid=15. Accessed May 8, 2019.
10. Berlin M, Zalups RK, Fowler BA. Mercury. In: Nordberg GF, Fowler BA, Nordberg M, Friberg LT, eds. *Handbook on the Toxicology of Metals.* New York, NY: Academic Press; 2007.
11. Kazantis G. Thallium. In: Nordberg GF, Fowler BA, Nordberg M, Friberg LT, eds. Handbook on the Toxicology of Metals. New York, NY: Academic Press; 2007.
12. Skerfving S, Bergdahl IA. Lead. In: Nordberg GF, Fowler BA, Nordberg M, Friberg LT, eds. *Handbook on the Toxicology of Metals.* New York, NY: Academic Press; 2007.
13. Fowler BA, Chou C-HSJ, Jones RL, Chen C-J. Arsenic. In: Nordberg GF, Fowler BA, Nordberg M, Friberg LT, eds. *Handbook on the Toxicology of Metals.* New York, NY: Academic Press; 2007.
14. Nordberg GF, Nogawa K, Nordberg M, Friberg LT. Cadmium. In: Nordberg GF, Fowler BA, Nordberg M, Friberg LT, eds. *Handbook on the Toxicology of Metals.* New York, NY: Academic Press; 2007.
15. Rabin R. Warnings unheeded: a history of child lead poisoning. *Am J Public Health.* 1989;79:1668-1674.
16. Landrigan PJ, Todd AC. Lead poisoning. *West J Med.* 1994; 161: 153-159.
17. Gottesfeld P. Time to ban lead in industrial paints and coatings. *Front Pub Health.* 2015;3:Article 144.
18. US Consumer Product Safety Commission. Office of Compliance. Ban of Lead-Containing Paint and Certain Consumer Products Bearing Lead-Containing Paint. 16 CFR 1310. January 2001. https://www.cpsc.gov/s3fs-public/pdfs/blk_pdf_leadpaint.pdf. Accessed June 29, 2018.
19. Kitman, JL. The secret history of lead. *The Nation.* March 20, 2000.
20. Liu J, Goyer RA, Waalkes MP. Toxic effects of metals. In: Klassen CD, ed. *Casarett and Doull's Toxicology.* New York, NY: McGraw-Hill; 2008.
21. Patrick L. Lead toxicity, a review of the literature, part I: exposure, evaluation, and treatment. *Altern Med Rev.* 2006;11:2-20.
22. Wedeen RP. Lead, the kidney, and hypertension. In: Needleman HL, ed. *Human Lead Exposure.* Boca Raton, FL: CRC Press; 1992.
23. Alexander FW, Delves HT. Deaths from acute lead poisoning. *Arch Dis Child.* 1972;47:446-448.
24. Pearce JMS. Burton's line in lead poisoning. *Eur Neurol.* 2007;57:118-119.
25. Case Studies in Environmenetal Medicine: Lead Toxicity. CDC Prevention Guidelines Database (Archive). https://wonder.cdc.gov/wonder/prevguid/p0000017/P0000017.asp. September 1, 1992. Accessed June 29, 2018.
26. Calello DP, Henretig FM. Lead. In: Goldfrank LR, Flomenbaum NE, Lewin NA, et al, eds. *Goldfrank's Toxicologic Emergencies.* New York, NY: McGraw Hill; 2015.
27. Klaasen CD. Heavy metals and heavy-metal antagonists. In: Brunton LL, ed. *Goodman and Gilman's the Pharmacological Basis of Therapeutics.* New York, NY: McGraw Hill, 2006.
28. Needleman H. Lead poisoning. *Annu Rev Med.* 2004;55:209-222.
29. Bellinger DC. Lead. *Pediatrics.* 2004;113:1016-1022.
30. Canfield RL, Henderson CR, Cory-Slechta DA, Cox C, Jusko TA, Lanphear BP. Intellectual impairment in children with blood lead concentrations below 10 ug per deciliter. *New Engl J Med.* 2003;348:1517-1526.
31. Lead. Health Effects. https://www.atsdr.cdc.gov/ToxProfiles/tp13-c2.pdf. Accessed July 1, 2019.
32. Landrigan PJ, Boffetta P, Apostoli P. The reproductive toxicity and carcinogenicity of lead: a critical review. *Am J Indust Med.* 2000;38:231-243.
33. Recommended Actions Based on Blood Lead Level. Centers for Disease Control and Prevention. https://www.cdc.gov/nceh/lead/advisory/acclpp/actions-blls.htm. Accessed October 14, 2019.

34. FDA warns against using Magellan Diagnostics LeadCare testing systems with blood obtained from a vein. FDA Safety Communication. https://www.fda.gov/medicaldevices/safety/alertsandnotices/ucm558733.htm. Accessed July 1, 2018.
35. Calello DP, Henretig FM. Lead. In: Goldfrank LR, Flomenbaum NE, Lewin NA, et al, eds. *Goldfrank's Toxicologic Emergencies.* New York, NY: McGraw Hill; 2019.
36. Mandal BK, Suzuki KT. Arsenic round the world: a review. *Talanta.* 2002;58:201-235.
37. Miller WH Jr, Schipper HM, Lee JS, Singer J, Waxman S. Mechanisms of action of arsenic trioxide. *Cancer Res.* 2002;62(S2):3893-3903.
38. Borak J, Hosgood HD. Seafood arsenic: implications for human risk assessment. *Reg Toxicol Pharmacol.* 2007;47:204-212.
39. Hughes MF. Arsenic toxicity and potential mechanisms of action. *Toxicol Lett.* 2002;133:1-16.
40. Fowler BA, Weissberg JB. Arsine poisoning. *N Engl J Med.* 1974;291:1171-1174.
41. Vahter M and Concha G. Role of metabolism in arsenic toxicity. *Pharmacol Toxicol.* 2001;89:1-5.
42. Gossel TA, Bricker JD. Metals. In: *Principles of Clinical Toxicology.* 2nd ed. New York, NY: Raven Press; 1990.
43. Mees' lines. http://www.pathguy.com/lectures/nejm_transverse_leukonychia.gif. Accessed May 9, 2019.
44. What are the Physiologic Effects of Arsenic Exposure? Agency for Toxic Substances and Disease Registry. Arsenic Toxicity. https://www.atsdr.cdc.gov/csem/csem.asp?csem=1&po=11. Accessed May 9, 2019.
45. Harvard University. Arsenic Project. http://wilsonweb.physics.harvard.edu/arsenic/pictures/Inner%20Mongolia/arsenic_project_pictures2.htm#A. Accessed May 9, 2019.
46. Ford M. Arsenic. In: Goldfrank LR, Flomenbaum NE, Lewin NA, et al, eds. *Goldfrank's Toxicologic Emergencies.* Stamford, CT: Appleton & Lange; 1998.
47. Jarup L. Health effects of cadmium exposure – a review of the literature and a risk estimate. *Scand J Work Environ Health.* 1998;24:1-51.
48. Yoshida F, Hata A, Tonegawa H. Itai-itai disease and the countermeasures against cadmium pollution by the Kamioka mine. *Environ Econ Policy Studies.* 1999;2:215-229.
49. Waalkes MP. Cadmium carcinogenesis in review. *J Inorg Biochem.* 2000;79:241-244.
50. Bernhoft RA. Cadmium toxicity and treatment. *ScientificWorldJournal.* 2013;394652.
51. Schonwald S. Cadimium. In: Dart RC, ed. *Medical Toxicology.* Philadelphia, PA: Lippincott Williams & Wilkins; 2004.
52. Itai-itai. https://people.ucsc.edu/~flegal/migrated/etox80e/Images/itai-itai.jpg. Accessed May 9, 2019.
53. Prozialeck WC, Edwards JR. Early biomarkers of cadmium exposure and nephrotoxicity. *Biometals.* 2010;23:793-809.
54. Traub SJ, Hoffman RS. Cadmium. In: Goldfrank LR, Flomenbaum NE, Lewin NA, et al, eds. *Goldfrank's Toxicologic Emergencies.* New York, NY: McGraw Hill; 2015.
55. Clarkson TW, Magos L. The toxicology of mercury and its chemical compounds. *Crit Rev Toxicol.* 2006;36:609-662.
56. Bernhoft RA. Mercury toxicity and treatment: a review of the literature. *J Environ Public Health.* 2012;460508.
57. Harris HH, Pickering IJ, George GN. The chemical form of mercury in fish. *Science.* 2003;301:1203.
58. Guidelines for Eating Fish that Contain Mercury. US Environmental Protection Agency. https://www.epa.gov/mercury/guidelines-eating-fish-contain-mercury. Accessed May 9, 2019.
59. Sue YJ. Mercury. In: Goldfrank LR, Flomenbaum NE, Lewin NA, et al, eds. *Goldfrank's Toxicologic Emergencies.* New York, NY: McGraw Hill; 2015.
60. Chang LW. Mercury-related neurological syndromes and disorders. In: Yasui M, Strong MJ, Ota K, Verity MA, eds. *Mineral and Metal Neurotoxicology.* Boca Raton, FL: CRC Press; 1997.
61. Ekino S, Susa M, Ninomiya T, Imamura K, Kitamura T. Minamata disease revisited: an update on the acute and chronic manifestations of methyl mercury poisoning. *J Neurol Sci.* 2007; 262:131-144.
62. Eto K. Minamata disease. *Neuropathology.* 2000;20:S14-S19.
63. Bakir F, Damluji SF, Amin-Zaki L, Murtadha M, et al. Methylmercury poisoning in Iraq. *Science.* 1973;181:230-241.
64. Aremu DA, Madejczyk MS, Ballatori N. N-Acetycysteine as a potential antidote and biomonitoring agent of methylmercury exposure. *Environ Health Perspect.* 2008;116:26-31.
65. Riyaz R, Pandalai SL, Schwartz M, Kazzi ZN. A fatal case of thallium toxicity: challenges in management. *J Med Toxicol.* 2013;9:75-78.
66. Galvan-Arzate S, Santamaria A. Thallium toxicity. *Toxicol Lett.* 1998;99:1-13.
67. Al Hammouri F, Darwazeh G, Said A, Ghosh RA. Acute thallium poisoning: series of ten cases. *J Med Toxicol.* 2011;7:306-311.
68. Mercurio-Zappala M, Hoffman RS. Thallium. In: Goldfrank LR, Flomenbaum NE, Lewin NA, et al, eds. *Goldfrank's Toxicologic Emergencies.* New York, NY: McGraw Hill; 2015.
69. Yumoto T, Tsukahara K, Naito H, Iida A, Nakao A. A successfully treated case of criminal thallium poisoning. *J Clin Diag Res.* 2017;11:1-2.

Chapter 29

Common Household and Environmental Toxicants

Christine L.H. Snozek, PhD
Leland B. Baskin, MD

Introduction

There are myriad toxins and toxicants in the environment. This chapter presents select environmental toxic compounds that are frequently encountered and for which some form of laboratory testing is available. While few of these compounds are detected directly in clinical laboratories, all are associated with clinical laboratory correlates and biomarkers, and toxicology laboratories are frequently queried about them.

Carbon Monoxide

Origin

Carbon monoxide (CO) is the most significant acute intoxicant in most fires, cigarette smoke, and automotive exhaust. The most abundant air pollutant worldwide, it is also one of the leading non-pharmaceutical causes of death from poisoning, often due to malfunctioning home heating systems.[1] Cigarette smoke contains 4% CO, while automobile exhaust contains 0.5% to 10% CO. The threshold limit value (TLV)—that concentration below which chronic exposure creates no unreasonable risk of disease or injury—for CO is 25 ppm to 50 ppm (0.0025-0.005 mL/L air).[1-3]

Descriptive Chemistry

CO is a clear, colorless, odorless gas with specific gravity 0.968 (slightly lighter than air). The primary exogenous source of CO is incomplete combustion of organic fuels.[1-4]

Synonyms: None

Formula: CO

Molecular mass = 28.0101 Daltons

CAS-630-08-0

$^{+}C\equiv O^{-}$

Pharmacology

Mechanism of Action

Toxicity related to CO exposure manifests as tissue hypoxia occurring through several mechanisms including displacement of O_2 from hemoglobin (Hb), contributing to reduced availability of O_2 to tissues and a variety of Hb-independent effects in tissues. Due to the high affinity of Hb for CO (~200-250 times greater than that for O_2), CO displaces O_2 from Hb to form COHb. CO binding to Hb also increases the O_2 affinity for the remaining three units of the Hb tetramer, reducing Hb-O_2 dissociation and making less O_2 available to tissues. CO binding to other heme proteins, such as myoglobin, cytochrome P450, and cytochrome oxidase a3, may also limit tissue O_2 utilization. Finally, CO increases production of reactive oxygen species and nitric oxide, increasing oxidative damage throughout the body. The organ systems most susceptible to CO-induced cellular injury are the neurologic, cardiovascular, pulmonary, and renal systems. Acute mortality is attributed to cardiac dysrhythmia due to hypoxia.[1,3]

Toxicokinetics

CO is produced endogenously during Hb metabolism at a rate of 0.4 mL/h, generating a background carboxyhemoglobin (COHb) concentration of up to 2% to 3% (higher in smokers). As a gas, CO is excreted via pulmonary expiration, and less than 1% is metabolized. The half-life of CO in resting adults at sea level is 4 to 6 hours. With administration of pure O_2, half-life is decreased to less than 90 minutes. Under hyperbaric conditions (2-3 atm pressure), half-life is further reduced to about 15 to 25 minutes.[1-5]

Acute physiological effects after exposure roughly correlate with COHb concentration (Table 29-1). Toxicity is increased with length of exposure, metabolic activity, and underlying cardiac or cerebrovascular disease. Metabolic acidosis is common due to accumulation of lactic acid, while respiratory acidosis occurs less commonly but may be severe. Survivors of CO exposure may exhibit residual effects to various degrees. Those suffering mild poisoning have no measurable long-term effects. Those more severely injured can have immediate or delayed-onset neurological deficits, including drowsiness, seizures, headache, subtle personality changes and memory loss, and gross deficits including Parkinsonism and persistent vegetative state. Because various factors affect the degree of chronic toxicity, the COHb concentration is not a reliable indicator of long-term prognosis.[2,3,5]

Analysis

Specimen Types and Characteristics

The optimal sample for measurement of COHb concentration is fresh whole blood, which can be

Table 29-1. Signs and Symptoms Associated With Acute Carbon Monoxide Intoxication

COHb Level	Effects
10%	Frontal headache; decreased ability to perform complex tasks or strenuous labor; aggravation of existing heart disease; confused with gastroenteritis, food poisoning, or a viral syndrome
20%	Throbbing headache, dyspnea on exertion
30%	Dizziness, nausea
40%	Confusion, syncope
50%	Coma, seizures
60%	Hypotension, respiratory failure
70%	Death

COHb, carboxyhemoglobin.

stored at 4°C or frozen if analysis is delayed. Direct measurement of CO from exhaled breath with approximation of COHb from that measurement can also be done.[5,6]

Modes of Analysis

COHb can be measured by spectrophotometry (co-oximetry) and gas chromatography (GC); pulse oximetry and other methods are less reliable, although the introduction of pulse co-oximetry has improved noninvasive measurement somewhat.[7] GC and other chromatographic methods are most accurate and are commonly used for postmortem analysis, after liberation of CO from hemoglobin for quantification. In order to calculate the COHb concentration, the CO binding capacity must be measured on a saturated aliquot of blood. COHb concentration is then calculated using the formula:

$$\%COHb = (CO_{content}/CO_{binding\ capacity}) \times 100$$

Because it is both rapid and convenient, the most commonly used method for quantifying COHb concentration, particularly in the clinical setting, is multiple-wavelength co-oximetry. The COHb concentration is determined along with the concentrations of other forms of hemoglobin including deoxyhemoglobin (deoxy-Hb), oxyhemoglobin (O_2-Hb), and methemoglobin (met-Hb). This method correlates well with GC at COHb levels greater than 3%. Two-wavelength spectrophotometry is less reliable for the quantification of COHb concentration due to the influence of different forms of hemoglobin and other interferences. Pulse co-oximetry has shown some utility as a noninvasive measure, with some limitations.[4-7]

Known Analytical Issues

Bacterial contamination of specimens must be avoided because bacteria can produce CO and denature Hb. Fresh whole blood is preferred because aging erythrocytes produce methemoglobin, which may falsely elevate COHb by some laboratory methods. Other potentially interfering forms of Hb include cyanmethemoglobin and sulfhemoglobin.[4]

Clinical Issues

Interpretation

Fetal hemoglobin (Hb F) has different spectral properties from Hb A that cause COHb concentration to be overestimated by 4% to 7% in neonates. Conventional pulse oximetry falsely measures COHb as O_2-Hb, leading to a falsely high %O_2 saturation. The difference between %O_2 saturation by pulse oximetry and two-wavelength spectrophotometry is called the *saturation gap* and usually represents COHb.[5,7]

Overdose and Toxicity

Although not a reliable predictor of the severity of an exposure, the COHb concentration is usually between 50% to 70% in most CO-related deaths, and values above 50% are typically considered to be incompatible with life. Factors such as old or very young age, pulmonary or cardiovascular disease, physical stress, and exposure to other intoxicating agents may contribute to fatality at lower concentrations. On the other hand, occasionally survivors at rest may have values >70%. The most significant postmortem characteristic is a bright cherry-red color of blood, fingernails, mucous membranes, and skin. This is not specific and may be seen with exposure to cyanide, cold, and with early decomposition.[1-3]

Immediate removal from the environment is the first step in treatment of acute CO intoxication. Depending on the clinical condition, 100% O_2 replacement is instituted to accelerate the elimination of CO for at least 2 hours. Indications for hyperbaric oxygen include syncope, coma, seizure, altered mental status, COHb >25%, abnormal cerebellar examination, older age, and fetal distress in pregnancy. Extent of recovery depends on loss of consciousness and duration of CO exposure.[3,8]

Cyanide

Origin

Cyanide (CN) is a byproduct of numerous manufacturing processes and is also found in cassava roots and the seeds of numerous fruits. CN is a constituent of vitamin B_{12}, cyanocobalamin, and is released during normal metabolism and postmortem putrefaction. It is also a metabolite of the arterial vasodilator, nitroprusside, used to treat heart failure and can be generated in toxic concentrations. There is controversy as to the significance of the contribution of fires to CN poisoning. Probably most poisoning by CN is due to direct exposure, either intentional or unintentional, to hydrogen cyanide (HCN) or a cyanide salt.[2,3,9,10]

Descriptive Chemistry

HCN is a weakly acidic, colorless, volatile liquid that boils at 26.5°C (79.7°F). The colorless gas has a density of air and an odor of bitter almonds, which can only be detected by about 80% of humans at a concentration of 0.2 ppm to 5.0 ppm.[2,4]

Synonyms: Hydrocyanic acid, prussic acid

Formula: HCN

Molecular mass = 27.0253 Daltons

CAS-57-12-5

$HC\equiv N$

Pharmacology

Mechanism of Action

CN is a rapidly acting poison that inhibits cellular utilization of oxygen. This is accomplished by binding to heme iron and the reduced form of cytochrome a3 oxidase. It stops cellular respiration by inhibiting electron transport at cytochrome c oxidase. This stops oxidative phosphorylation, which, in turn, stops the Krebs cycle, leading to accumulation of pyruvate, which is converted anaerobically to lactic acid, causing metabolic acidosis.[11]

Toxicokinetics

CN toxicity depends upon compound, route of exposure, and dose. HCN readily diffuses through biological membranes and is efficiently absorbed via inhalation. Symptoms are immediate and death occurs within minutes. Cyanide salts in solution absorb readily across skin. Oral ingestion of cyanide salts or cyanogenic precursors (eg, nitriles) delays symptom onset due to the need for absorption and, in the case of cyanogens, metabolism.[2]

Symptoms are nonspecific: headache, tachypnea, and dizziness occur within seconds of inhaling HCN gas. Hypoxia causes hyperpnea followed by dyspnea, with Cheyne-Stokes breathing, lactic acidosis, bradycardia, arrhythmia, hypotension, coma, opisthotonus, seizures, and death. Venous oxygen saturation approaches arterial oxygen saturation. The classic findings of CN poisoning are hypoxia, lactic acidosis, and metabolic acidosis; in the setting of house fires, these findings may also be due to an oxygen-deficient atmosphere (10-15% O_2) contaminated with carbon monoxide. CN intoxication is high on the list of differential diagnoses of rapid onset coma, metabolic acidosis, and severe anoxia without cyanosis.[2,3,10]

As a product of normal metabolism, CN is detoxified primarily in the liver by generation of thiocyanate (SCN) via rhodanese (thiosulfate-cyanide sulfotransferase) and beta mercaptopyruvate-cyanide sulfurtransferase and renal excretion. Normal blood CN concentrations are up to 0.25 mg/L in nonsmokers and up to 0.5 mg/L in smokers. The respective half-lives of CN and SCN are 20 to 60 min and 3 to 9 days, depending on renal function.[2,3,10]

Analysis

Specimen Types and Characteristics

Since CN is concentrated in erythrocytes, it is usually measured after extraction from whole blood. SCN may also be measured in serum or plasma.[4,5]

Modes of Analysis

CN can be measured by spectrophotometry, ion-selective electrode and gas chromatography with nitrogen-phosphorous or electron capture detection, or by gas or liquid chromatography coupled to mass spectrometry. SCN is usually measured colorimetrically or by mass spectrometry.[2,4,5,11]

Known Analytical Issues

The need for extraction of whole blood precludes measuring CN within the time frame that is necessary to treat a patient successfully. Measurement of CN is only useful for forensic purposes.[3,10]

Clinical Issues

Interpretation

Due to the time required to measure CN directly, clinical treatment is instituted based upon patient history and supporting laboratory data such as blood gases (pH, O_2, CO_2) and serum lactate. SCN measurements may be used to monitor CN clearance but most often are used to assess smoking status or nitroprusside toxicity.[3,10]

Overdose and Toxicity

The lethal dose of HCN is about 100 mg, while that of CN salts is about twice that. Death can occur at HCN as low as 150 ppm. Toxicity occurs at blood concentrations >0.5 mg/L, with coma and death at 1 mg/L to 3 mg/L.[3,10]

Rapid support for CN exposure includes administration of 100% O_2 and decontamination. Several antidotes have been proposed for CN toxicity. Hydroxocobalamin chelates CN- to form cyanocobalamin (vitamin B_{12}) and can be used for treatment of acute cyanide toxicity as well as prophylaxis against toxicity due to nitroprusside therapy. Hydroxocobalamin does result in red coloration of skin and urine, with uncommon side effects including anaphylaxis. It also interferes with co-oximetry measurements of COHb, met-Hb, and O_2-Hb, which is of particular relevance if co-exposure to CO occurred, eg, in smoke inhalation. The other common antidote is intravenous sodium nitrite, followed by IV sodium thiosulfate. Amyl nitrite is no longer Food and Drug Administration approved as an antidote due to diversion risk and uncertain utility. The nitrites induce met-Hb, which strongly binds CN to form cyanomethemoglobin. Sodium thiosulfate is used as a sulfur donor to generate SCN, which is readily excreted in urine. Less commonly used antidotes include dimethylaminophenol and dicobalt edetate. Like the nitrites, the mechanism of dimethylaminophenol is also to produce met-Hb; dicobalt edetate chelates CN- to form cobalticyanide. Prognosis is a function of quantity, form, route of exposure, and support.[3,11]

Organophosphates

Origin

The term *pesticide* encompasses a wide range of chemicals that are used to control pests of all sorts, both plants and animals. Organophosphates (OPs) are used widely as insecticides; a few highly potent OPs also comprise the class of chemical warfare agents called *nerve agents.* The first OP insecticide was synthesized in 1854; several others were developed in Germany beginning in the 1930s, and recognition of OP toxicity increased at the same time. Worldwide, over 200,000 deaths due to OP pesticide poisoning occur annually, with 95% in underdeveloped nations. In the US, there are some 10,000 reported OP exposures each year, with low mortality.[12-15]

Descriptive Chemistry

OPs are substituted phosphoric acids with two organic side chains that are used primarily as agricultural insecticides. OP nerve agents have no industrial use due to their high potency and toxicity. The general structure of OPs is:

$$R_1, R_2, X\text{-}P{=}O \text{ (or S)}$$

where R1 and R2 are alkyl, alkyl ester, or aryl ester groups; and X is a "leaving group," which may consist of a halogen, CN, SCN, or electron withdrawing moiety. OPs are highly volatile, nonpolar, lipid-soluble liquids that are rapidly absorbed by the central nervous system (CNS). Characteristics of parathion are described as a representative example.[4,12,15]

Parathion

Synonyms: Phosphorothioic acid, *O*,*O*-Diethyl *O*-(4-nitrophenyl) ester

Trade names: Alkron, Aphamite, Folidol, Fosyex E, Niran, Nitrostogmine, Paraphos, Thiophos

Formula: $C_{10}H_{14}NO_5PS$

Molecular weight = 291.3 Daltons

CAS-56-38-2

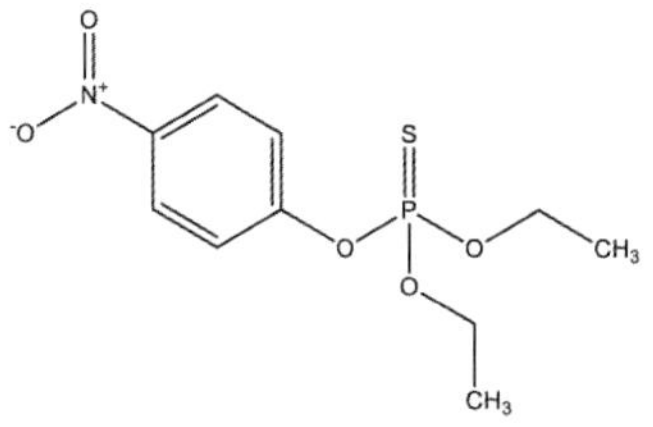

Pharmacology

Mechanism of Action

The mechanism of action is competitive inhibition of acetyl cholinesterase (AChE) by binding at the enzyme active site. Covalent binding occurs when the OP leaving group is replaced by nucleophilic substitution of oxygen from serine in the enzyme active site. Acetyl choline (ACh) is a key neurotransmitter at neuromuscular synapses throughout the central and peripheral nervous systems. AChE inhibition leads to accumulation of ACh within the synapse, with subsequent paralysis of cholinergic neural transmission. Spontaneous dissociation of the stable OP-AChE intermediate requires several hours; loss of one of the alkyl side groups from the bound OP, termed *aging,* results in irreversible AChE inhibition.[12-14]

Toxicokinetics

OPs have highly variable onset and degree of acute toxicity. Acute toxicity of AChE inhibitors during the first 48 hours after exposure, known as the *cholinergic phase,* may manifest in several different patterns. The most common effects are pulmonary and central such as visual disturbances (miosis, ocular pain, blurred vision), lacrimation, and respiratory difficulties (wheezing, chest tightness), whereas muscle twitching, weakness, and secretions are indicative of increasing toxicity. Symptoms are often described by the mnemonics SLUDGE: Salivation, secretion, Lacrimation, Urination, Diarrhea, diaphoresis, Gastrointestinal distress, and Emesis; or DUMBBELSS: Diarrhea, Urination, Miosis/muscle weakness, Bronchorrhea, Bradycardia, Emesis, Lacrimation, Salivation, Sweating. CNS effects include headache, drowsiness, confusion, weakness, lethargy, fatigue, depression, seizure, paralysis, and coma.[5,13-14]

The route of exposure influences the time of onset and type and degree of symptoms. Although all routes are efficient, inhalation causes symptoms to occur earlier than ingestion and percutaneous absorption. Ingestion most often produces gastrointestinal symptoms such as anorexia, cramps, nausea, vomiting, and diarrhea. Dermal exposure manifests as localized symptoms such as diaphoresis, fasciculations, and tremors, although severe exposures or potent agents such as VX can result in systemic effects up to and including death.[15]

Toxicity of the various OPs depends upon several factors, including affinity for the histidine-serine active site, route of exposure, metabolic activity, lipid solubility, blood flow, and concentration. Some OPs are indirect inhibitors that require activation, primarily by the cytochrome P450 system. This may delay onset of intoxication as occurs with the conversion of parathion to the more toxic paraoxon through a reaction mediated by CYP2B1. Oxons, molecules with double-bonded oxygens, tend to be much more toxic than thions, which have double-bonded sulfurs. Also, some OPs preferentially inhibit different forms of cholinesterase. Normal metabolism consists of hydrolysis by enzymes in plasma or endoplasmic reticulum of hepatocytes yielding phosphoric acid derivatives such as phosphates. One common metabolite of all OPs is *p*-nitrophenol. Minor metabolic pathways include dealkylation of side chains.[12,14]

Analysis

Specimen Types and Characteristics

Erythrocyte AChE is identical to the enzyme found in the CNS and peripheral nerves, while butyryl cholinesterase (BuChE, also known as pseudocholinesterase) is the principal cholinesterase enzyme found in plasma. Whole blood cholinesterase (ChE) testing may be used to measure both AChE and BuChE. Tests for plasma or serum BuChE activity are more widely available and tend to show decreased enzyme activity sooner after exposure than erythrocyte ChE tests.[13,14,16]

Modes of Analysis

The classical method for measuring blood ChE activity is the potentiometric method, in which ChE activity is correlated with pH changes caused by the production of acetic acid when acetylcholine is hydrolyzed. Enzyme inhibition results in less acetic acid production and a smaller change in pH. This may also be measured spectrophotometrically with a pH indicator. In the colorimetric method, propionylthiocholine is hydrolyzed to propionic acid and thiocholine. Thiocholine is then oxidized to 5-thio-2 nitrobenzoic acid, which is measured at 420 nm.

Table 29-2. Relationship Between Butyryl Cholinesterase (BuChE) Activity and Degree of Organophosphate Intoxication

BuChE Activity (% of Baseline)	Degree of Intoxication
≥60	None
20 - 60	Mild
10 - 20	Moderate
<10	Severe

Mass spectrometric testing can provide definitive identification through measurement of either OP-adducted BuChE peptides or compound-specific metabolites. A common metabolite of some organophosphates, *p*-nitrophenol, can be measured in urine by GC or mass spectrometry. Also, OP may be identified in urine spectrophotometrically at 820 nm.[4,16-18]

Known Analytical Issues

ChE activity or definitive testing for OP exposure is generally not available quickly enough to guide clinical management. In addition to OP intoxication, erythrocyte AChE is decreased by all conditions that decrease erythrocytes such as anemia and hemoglobinopathies. Among other causes of decreased BuChE are liver disease (hepatitis, carcinoma), chronic nonhepatic diseases, malnutrition, pregnancy and infancy, drugs (opiates), and atypical forms of BuChE. Causes of increased BuChE include recovery from liver damage, nephrotic syndrome, and anxiety.[5,12-13]

Clinical Issues

Interpretation

Diagnosis of OP intoxication is based on history of exposure, physical signs and symptoms of ACh hyperactivity, response to therapy, and supporting laboratory evidence. The most suggestive are the muscarinic symptoms of salivation, lacrimation, weakness, and miosis. The combination of miosis and muscle fasciculation is considered essentially pathognomonic for OP intoxication. Favorable response to an intravenous challenge of 2 mg atropine is a fairly reliable indicator of OP exposure, and decreased BuChE activity is very specific. Finally, elevated urine *p*-nitrophenol concentration is considered diagnostic. A guideline for using BuChE activity as a predictor of degree of OP intoxication is provided in Table 29-2. Since there is wide interindividual variability in BuChE activity, inhibition can only be certain if preexposure values are known. Thus, individuals who are expected to be exposed occupationally to OP compounds should have baseline measurements.[12-15]

Overdose and Toxicity

For OP pesticides, the fatal adult dose ranges from 0.05 g (TEPP) to 60.0 g (malathion). The OP nerve agents have toxicity 100 to 500 times that of the insecticides, with lethal doses as low as 10 mg dermal exposure to VX.[4,15]

Treatment for OP exposure is based on the principles of decontamination, maintaining an airway, and restoring breathing and circulation. Decontamination is accomplished by hydrolysis with alkaline solutions such as bleach and sodium hydroxide. Pharmacologic treatment includes two specific antidotes, atropine and pralidoxime (2-PAM). Atropine is an antagonist of the muscarinic and CNS effects of ACh; it has no effect on nicotinic receptors. Atropine is the first choice for both OP and carbamate exposure. The end point of therapy is adequate respiration with control of respiratory secretions. Pralidoxime has weak anticholinergic activity and is used to detoxify OPs remaining in the system by removing the phosphoryl group to regenerate AChE activity. It does not enter the CNS and is not effective against "aged" AChE so it must be used within 24 hours of exposure. Despite its routine use in treating OP intoxication, the efficacy of pralidoxime as an OP antidote remains uncertain.[19]

Prognosis depends on the degree of toxicity and the timing of therapy. If untreated, severe intoxication leads to death within minutes to 24 hours. The mechanism is asphyxia due to respiratory and cardiac failure, bronchoconstriction, laryngospasm, and bronchorrhea. If treated adequately, full recovery can be expected within days. A small number of patients will experience occasional persistent CNS effects and peripheral neuropathy.[3,12-14,19]

Warfarins

Origin

Hemorrhagic disorder outbreaks in cattle associated with consumption of spoiled yellow clover silage were reported in 1924, and the causative compound was identified in 1939 as bis-hydroxycoumarin (dicoumarol). Subsequently, coumarin was synthesized and marketed as a rodenticide under the name "warfarin." The "superwarfarins" were developed due to the development of resistance by some rodents to the first-generation compounds, warfarin and dicoumarol. In contrast to the first-generation compounds, the second-generation compounds are much more toxic (up to 100 times more than warfarin). Exposure to warfarins may occur as an accidental overdose during therapeutic use of coumadin, accidental ingestion of a rodenticide, or intentional ingestion of either. The most common accidental ingestions of rodenticides occur in young children.[3,12,20]

Descriptive Chemistry

The anticoagulant drug coumadin (crystalline warfarin sodium) is a racemic mixture of 3-(α-acetonylbenzyl)-4-hydroxycoumarin ($C_{19}H_{15}NaO_4$) enantiomers. It is a white, odorless, crystalline powder, discolored by light and soluble in alcohol and water. Rodenticides in this same class of compounds include warfarin and dicoumarol, discussed further as examples below, and the second-generation compounds known as *superwarfarins,* which include brodifacoum, bromadiolone, coumatetralyl, difenacoum, difethialon, and flocoumafen.[4,12,20]

Warfarin

Synonym: 4-Hydroxy-3-(3-oxo-1-phenylbutyl)-sH-1-benzopyran-2-one

Trade names: Biotrol, Dethmor, Sorexa (rodenticides)

Formula: $C_{19}H_{16}O_4$

Molecular mass = 308.3279 Daltons

CAS-81-81-2

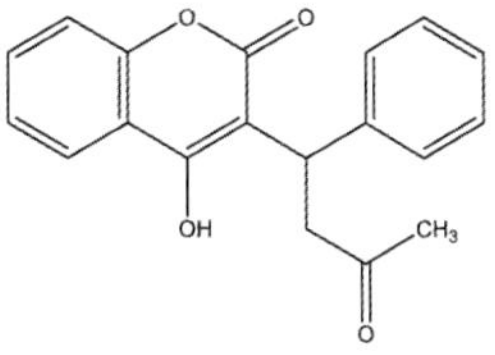

Dicoumarol

Synonyms: Bishydroxycoumarin, dicoumarin, dicumarol, melitoxin; 3,3'-methylenebis-[4-hydroxy-2H-1-benzopyran-2-one

Trade name: Dufalone

Formula: $C_{19}H_{12}O_6$

Molecular mass = 336.2950 Daltons

CAS-66-76-2

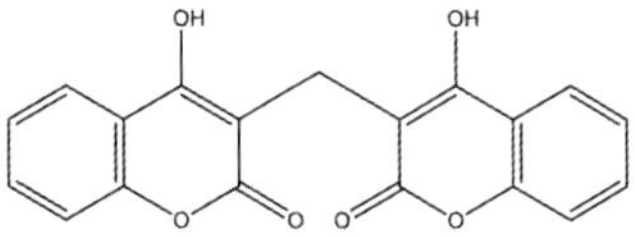

Pharmacology

Intended Use

The potential for human therapeutic anticoagulation by warfarin and related compounds was demonstrated in a patient surviving a suicide attempt with high-dose warfarin in 1951. Today, numerous associated compounds are used both for human anticoagulation medication and as rodenticides.[3,12,20]

Mechanism of Action

The vitamin K-dependent coagulation factors II, VII, IX, and X, and proteins C and S are activated by gamma carboxylation, in which gamma glutamyl carboxylase transfers a carboxyl group from the reduced form of vitamin K to the inactive factor, which activates the coagulation factors by enabling calcium binding. The end-products of this reaction are the oxidized form of vitamin K (vitamin K epoxide) and activated coagulation factors. The reduced form of vitamin K is regenerated by vitamin K epoxide reductase. Derivatives of 4-hydroxycoumarin exert their impact by inhibiting vitamin K epoxide reductase complex subunit 1 (VKORC1) and, to a lesser degree, vitamin K reductase.[3,20]

Toxicokinetics

Coumadin is absorbed almost completely orally, with peak concentration reached in approximately 4 hours. Highly protein bound (>99%), its volume of distribution is small, about 0.14 L/Kg, indicating that most of it remains in the plasma. Due to the half-lives of vitamin K-dependent coagulation factors, anticoagulant effects start 12 to 24 hours after the initial dose and peak after 72 to 96 hours. Gastrointestinal hemorrhage may manifest as abdominal pain, vomiting with or without hematemesis, and heme-positive feces.[12]

The major route of warfarin metabolism is transformation by hepatic microsomal enzymes, primarily the cytochrome P450s (CYPs). Since the *S* enantiomer is two to five times more active than the *R* form, hydroxylation of *S*-warfarin to 7-hydroxywarfarin by CYP2C9 is the major clinically relevant metabolic pathway. *R*-warfarin is largely metabolized by CYP1A2, with minor contributions from CYP2C19 and CYP3A4. All metabolites are cleared through urine and to a lesser extent in bile. In contrast to the onset of anticoagulation, the half-lives of the 4-hydroxycoumarin derivatives will dictate the duration of anticoagulation effect. The half-life of warfarin is approximately 42 hours, while those of the second-generation compounds have been reported to be up to 120 days.

Variants in *VKORC1* and *CYP2C9* can have a significant impact on warfarin action. Alleles with reduced expression or activity of the gene products are associated with lower warfarin requirements to maintain proper anticoagulation; such variants are common for both *VKORC1* and *CYP2C9*. To date, no *CYP2C9* variants with increased activity on warfarin have been described, although variants in *CYP4F2* have been associated with increased dose requirements of warfarin.[21] Numerous drugs, botanical compounds, and medical conditions are also known to affect the apparent potency of warfarin through an effect on serum protein binding, enzyme metabolism, or inherent anticoagulant properties. For the reasons given above, the effect of a given dose of warfarin may be dramatically different for different individuals and for the same individual under different conditions. It is presumed that these principles will also apply to the other 4-hydroxycoumarin derivatives.[22,23]

Analysis

Specimen Types and Characteristics

Warfarins are usually not analyzed directly; although serum/plasma or urine measurement of the individual compounds is possible, concentrations do not correlate well with clinical effects. Serum testing for brodifacoum is available in some reference laboratories and can inform the duration of treatment required. The most common specimen for testing associated with warfarin exposure is plasma anticoagulated with sodium citrate to assess the individual's coagulation status.[3,12,24]

Modes of Analysis

The most useful analyte for following the anticoagulant status of someone exposed to a 4-hydroxycoumarin derivative is the prothrombin time, usually reported as the international normalized ratio (INR). The most common method for measuring 4-hydroxycoumarin derivatives or metabolites of specific warfarins directly is high-performance liquid chromatography alone or coupled to mass spectrometry. Both first- and second-generation compounds may be measured simultaneously, although chiral separation of isomers may be required.[12,20,24]

Clinical Issues

Interpretation

For intentional dosing, anticoagulation targets for INR are usually in the range of 2 to 3.5 depending on the clinical indication for anticoagulation. Therapeutic benefit decreases and the risk of hemorrhage increases at an INR above 4.0. A normal INR is the usual end point of treatment for anticoagulant rodenticide exposure; a normal INR 24 to 48 hours after suspected ingestion of a warfarin or superwarfarin, respectively, essentially rules out significant exposure. The identification and concentration of the ingested compound can aid in determining the expected duration of therapy.[3,12,24]

Overdose and Toxicity

For unintentional ingestion of a small quantity of a first-generation compound, the patient may be asymptomatic, and neither laboratory analysis nor treatment may be necessary. In cases of acute toxicity, the typical clinical signs and symptoms include hemorrhage, prolonged INR, and decreased factor VII. However, since anticoagulation is dependent on the half-lives of coagulation factors, the effects generally appear >12 hours after ingestion. All signs and symptoms may be corrected by administration of vitamin K1 (phytonadione). For large ingestions, gastrointestinal decontamination should be performed as soon as possible. Monitoring for hemorrhage and INR determination should occur within 24 to 48 hours. Treatment could require transfusion with fresh-frozen plasma and/or 4-factor prothrombin complex concentrate to replenish the vitamin K-dependent coagulation factors.[3,20,25]

References

1. Roderique JD, Josef CS, Feldman MJ, Spiess BD. A modern literature review of carbon monoxide poisoning theories, therapies, and potential targets for therapy advancement. *Toxicology.* 2015;334:45-58.
2. Levine B, ed. *Principles of Forensic Toxicology.* 3rd ed. Washington, DC: AACC Press; 2009.
3. Olson KR, Anderson IB, Benowitz NL, et al, eds. *Poisoning and Drug Overdose.* 7th ed. New York, NY: McGraw-Hill; 2018.
4. Baselt RC. *Disposition of Toxic Drugs and Chemicals in Man.* 11th ed. Foster City, CA: Biomedical Publishing; 2017.
5. Rifai N, Horvath AR, Wittwer CT, eds. *Tietz' Textbook of Clinical Chemistry.* 6th ed. St Louis, MO: Elsevier; 2018.
6. Eberhardt M, Powell A, Bonfante G, et al. Noninvasive measurement of carbon monoxide levels in ED patients with headache. *J Med Toxicol.* 2006;2:89-92.
7. Feiner JR, Rollins MD, Sall JW, Eilers H, Au P, Bickler PE. Accuracy of carboxyhemoglobin detection by pulse co-oximetry during hypoxemia. *Anesth Analg.* 2013;117:847-858.
8. Weaver LK, Valentine KJ, Hopkins RO. Carbon monoxide poisoning: risk factors for cognitive sequelae and the role of hyperbaric oxygen. *Am J Respir Crit Care Med.* 2007;176:491-497.
9. Kirk JD. Pharmacologic stabilization and management of acute heart failure in the emergency department. *Heart Fail Clin.* 2009;5(1):43-54.
10. Barillo DJ. Diagnosis and treatment of cyanide toxicity. *J Burn Care Res.* 2009;30:148-152.
11. Lawson-Smith P, Jansen EC, Hyldegaard O. Cyanide intoxication as part of smoke inhalation: a review on diagnosis and treatment from the emergency perspective. *Scand J Trauma Resusc Emerg Med.* 2011;19:14.
12. Brunton LL, Lazo JS, Parker KL, eds. *Goodman and Gilman's The Pharmacological Basis of Therapeutics.* 11th ed. New York, NY: McGraw-Hill; 2006.
13. Eddleston M, Buckley NA, Eyer P, Dawson AH. Management of acute organophosphorus pesticide poisoning. *Lancet.* 2008;371:597-607.
14. Roberts JR, Reigart JR, eds. *Recognition and Management of Pesticide Poisonings.* 6th ed. Washington, DC: US EPA; 2013.
15. Nerve agents. https://www.opcw.org/about-chemical-weapons/types-of-chemical-agent/nerve-agents/. Accessed April 19, 2018.
16. Dass P, Mejia M, Landes M, Jones R, Stuart B, Thyssen J. Cholinesterase: Review of Methods. ASCP Check Sample, Clinical Chemistry, CC94-10. Chicago, IL: American Society of Clinical Pathologists; 1994:135-158.
17. Yan L, Chen J, Xu B, et al. A liquid chromatography tandem mass spectrometric method on in vitro nerve agents poisoning characterization and reactivator efficacy evaluation by determination of specific peptide adducts in acetylcholinesterase. *J Chromatogr A.* 2016;1450:86-93.
18. Hamelin EI, Schulze ND, Shaner RL, et al. Quantitation of five organophosphorus nerve agent metabolites in serum using hydrophilic interaction liquid chromatography and tandem mass spectrometry. *Anal Bioanal Chem.* 2014;406: 5195-5202.
19. Eddleston M, Chowdhury FR. Pharmacological treatment of organophosphorous insecticide poisoning: the old and the (possible) new. *Br J Clin Pharmacol.* 2016;81:462-470.
20. King N, Tran MH. Long-acting anticoagulant rodenticide (superwarfarin) poisoning: a review of its historical development, epidemiology, and clinical management. *Transfus Med Rev.* 2015;29:250-258.
21. Johnson JA, Caudle KE, Gong L, et al. Clinical Pharmacogenetics Implementation Consortium (CPIC) guideline for pharmacogenetics-guided warfarin dosing: 2017 update. *Clin Pharmacol Ther.* 2017;102:397-404.
22. Daly AK, Rettie AE, Fowler DM, Miners JO. Pharmacogenomics of CYP2C9: functional and clinical considerations. *J Pers Med.* 2018;8:1.
23. Shaw K, Amstutz U, Kim RB, et al. Clinical practice recommendations on genetic testing of CYP2C9 and VKORC1 variants in warfarin therapy. *Ther Drug Monit.* 2015;37:428-436.
24. Booth GS, Mody PZ. Brodifacoum inhalation and its clinical manifestations in a 21-year-old Caucasian man. *Lab Med.* 2016;47:63-66.
25. Lankiewicz MW, Hays J, Friedman KD, Tinkoff G, Blatt PM. Urgent reversal of warfarin with prothrombin complex concentrate. *J Thromb Haemost.* 2006;4:967-970.

Section IV

Appendices and Index

Barbarajean Magnani, PhD, MD, Editor

Appendix A. Urine Toxic Screen Template
Nicholas Heger, PhD, and Barbarajean Magnani, PhD, MD

Appendix B. Serum Toxic Screen Template
Nicholas Heger, PhD, and Barbarajean Magnani, PhD, MD

Appendix C. Therapeutic Drug Monitoring Template
Nicholas Heger, PhD, and Barbarajean Magnani, PhD, MD

Appendix D. Frequently Asked Questions on Clinical Urine Drugs-of-Abuse Testing
Tai C. Kwong, PhD

Appendix E. CAP Proficiency Testing Surveys for Toxicology
Annabel Dizon, MT(ASCP)

Index

Preface

Appendix A, *Urine Toxic Screen Template,* and Appendix B, *Serum Toxic Screen Template,* provide a general guide for screening toxicology testing in the clinical laboratory. Each laboratory should customize the appendices based on the current assays offered in house using both the assay package inserts or application sheets and the specific panels or analytes. Cross-reactivity, cutoff concentrations, and interferences may vary depending on the assay used. Appendix C, *Therapeutic Drug Monitoring Template,* provides information on therapeutic drug specimen collection, therapeutic range, laboratory turnaround time, serum half-life, and general comments regarding specific drugs. Each laboratory should modify this guide to fit current protocols (therapeutic ranges, turnaround time, in-house assay versus send-out test, time required for specimen to be in the laboratory), test menu, and other pertinent assay information, as needed.

Appendix A

Urine Toxic Screen Template

Nicholas Heger, PhD
Barbarajean Magnani, PhD, MD

URINE TOXICOLOGY TESTING AT [Your Hospital's Name]

The basic urine immunoassay toxicology screen is appropriate for both the emergency department and all other locations for drugs-of-abuse testing. Nonemergency testing of urine is performed either to determine medication compliance (eg, opioids prescribed for chronic noncancer pain) or to detect the presence of illicit drugs.

The **Urine Toxic Screen at [Your Hospital's Name]** includes **amphetamines, barbiturates, benzodiazepines, buprenorphine, cannabinoids, cocaine metabolite, fentanyl, methadone, opiates, and oxycodone.** Thirty to 40 milliliters (30-40 mL) of urine should be collected in a clean cup for analysis. Immunoassays for **amphetamines, barbiturates, benzodiazepines, and opiates** yield only qualitative class-specific information. Specific agents within a drug class are not identified.* (Note: Each laboratory should determine whether or not to include phencyclidine—PCP—as the use of this drug is specific to certain geographic areas. Also, depending on the clinical practice, tramadol can also be included in the initial screen. Additionally, comments included under the "Comments" column can be modified if used for clinical staff rather than for laboratory staff only.)

Results are reported as presumptive positive ("Detected") or negative ("Not Detected") according to the cutoff values listed below. Presumptive-positive results only indicate the presence of the drug or metabolite in urine and do not indicate or measure intoxication, efficacy of elimination, when the drug was last taken, or how much was taken. Negative screening results reflect concentrations that fall below the cutoff and do not necessarily exclude the presence of the drug or metabolite.

Results obtained from urine immunoassay toxicology screening are to be used for medical purposes only. Definitive testing by a more sensitive and specific method such as mass spectrometry is not automatically performed on substances in this screen but can be requested. Unconfirmed screening results must not be used for nonmedical purposes (eg, employment testing, legal testing).

** Note: The specific drugs detected within each drug class may vary with the vendor-specific assay. Polyclonal antibody-based immunoassays that measure class compounds may exhibit lot-to-lot variation with respect to sensitivity to various compounds within the class. This template should be compared with package inserts from the kit the laboratory is using. Some brand names are included.*

Drug Class or Drug	Cutoff Concentration and Calibrator*	Duration of Positive Result**	Comments***
AMPHETAMINES *d*-AMPHETAMINE Component of Adderall, Mydayis, Benzedrine, Dexedrine, ProCentra, and others *d*-METHAMPHETAMINE MDA (methylenedioxy-amphetamine) MDMA (methylenedioxy-methamphetamine) or Ecstasy	1000 ng/mL of *d*-amphetamine	Urine may test positive within 3 hours after use and for up to 1 or 2 days after last use.	• Prodrugs benzphetamine (Didrex, Recede), lisdexamphetamine (Vyvanse), and L-deprenyl (Selegiline, Emsam) are metabolized into amphetamine and /or methamphetamine. • Possible false positives (manufacturer-specific): Chlorpromazine (Thorazine), promethazine, ranitidine (Zantac), aripiprazole (Abilify), Trazodone metabolite meta-chlorophenylpiperazine (m-CPP), dimethylamylamine (DMMA energy supplement). • Depending on the assay, MDMA/MDA may also be detected.
BARBITURATES BARBITAL BUTABARBITAL (Butisol) BUTALBITAL (Fiorinal, Fioricet) PENTOBARBITAL (Nembutal) PHENOBARBITAL SECOBARBITAL (Seconal) THIOPENTAL (Pentothal)	200 ng/mL of secobarbital	Urine may test positive for 2 to 20 days after use depending on specific agent.	• Prodrug primidone (Mysoline) is metabolized into phenobarbital. • Check vendor-specific cross-reactivities of various barbiturates versus that of the calibrator drug.
BENZODIAZEPINES ALPRAZOLAM (Xanax) CHLORDIAZEPOXIDE (Librium) CLONAZEPAM (Klonopin) DIAZEPAM (Valium) FLURAZEPAM (Dalmane) LORAZEPAM (Ativan) MIDAZOLAM (Versed) NITRAZEPAM (Mogadon) OXAZEPAM (Serax) PRAZEPAM (Centrax) TEMAZEPAM (Restoril) TRIAZOLAM (Halcion)	200 ng/mL of oxazepam	Urine may test positive for 1 to 14 days after use depending on specific agent.	• Many benzodiazepines share common metabolic pathways and may be both byproducts of metabolism or sold as standalone drugs (eg, oxazepam is the active metabolite of temazepam). Cross-reactivities of parent drug and metabolite may differ significantly. Only high concentrations of some benzodiazepines may cross-react, and therefore only toxic concentrations and not therapeutic concentrations may be detected. Check assay package insert section on specificity/cross-reactivity. Clinicians should contact the laboratory if the patient is prescribed a benzodiazepine and the screen is unexpectedly negative. • *Note: Incorporating a hydrolysis step improves detection by assays that target the parent drug, not the glucuronide metabolites.* • Possible false positives (manufacturer-specific): sertraline (Zoloft), oxaprozin (Daypro). • Flunitrazepam (Rohypnol) is NOT available in the USA but may be smuggled across the border. The concentration needed to produce a positive result with this assay is 50 ng/mL.

Drug Class or Drug	Cutoff Concentration and Calibrator*	Duration of Positive Result**	Comments***
BUPRENORPHINE Buprenex Subutex Suboxone (buprenorphine with naloxone)	5 ng/mL of buprenorphine (This cutoff concentration can be set at 10 ng/mL if the laboratory determines increased assay cross-reacts with opiates such as morphine or codeine.)	Urine may test positive for 2 to 4 days after use.	• Possible false positives (manufacturer specific): hydroxychloroquine (Plaquenil), chloroquine (Aralen), tramadol (Ultram), codeine, dihydrocodeine, hydrocodone (Zohydro), naltrexone (Vivitrol), morphine (MS Contin), methadone (Methadose). • Buprenorphine is metabolized into active norbuprenorphine. Most immunoassays will also cross-react with norbuprenorphine.
CANNABINOIDS DELTA-9-THC 11-NOR-DELTA-9-THC-9-CARBOXLIC ACID 11-OH-DELTA-9-THC CANNABINOL	50 ng/mL of 11-Nor-delta-9-THC-9-carboxlic acid	Urine may test positive for 2 to 7 days after use or up to 1 month after chronic use.	• Detects **metabolites** of delta-9-tetra-hydrocannabinol (THC), the primary psychoactive component of marijuana, as most cannabinoids immunoassays have minimal reactivity for THC. Some assays will also detect delta-9-THC. • Possible false positives (manufacturer specific): efavirenz (Sustiva). • Peak plasma concentrations reached within 10 minutes of inhalation. • Passive inhalation is unlikely to be detected by this assay (however this may be cutoff dependent). • Dronabinol (Marinol) is also picked up by this assay. • Hemp seed ingestion may produce a positive result. • Cannabidiol (CBD), a nonregulated nonpsychoactive component of marijuana sold as a supplement, is not detected by this assay.
COCAINE METABOLITE BENZOYLECGONINE COCAINE ECGONINE	300 ng/mL of benzoylecgonine	Urine may test positive up to 48 to 72 hours after use. May be positive longer after use in chronic high-dose abusers.	• Immunoassays are designed to detect benzoylecgonine, a major cocaine metabolite. • Highly specific assay. • Cocaine has a half-life of 30 to 60 minutes. Blood cocaine levels do not guide management. • In the presence of ethanol, cocaine will undergo transesterification to form cocaethylene.
FENTANYL Duragesic Actiq Fentora Ionsys Matrifen	1 ng/mL of fentanyl	Urine may test positive up to 48 to 72 hours after use.	• Possible false positives (manufacturer specific): labetalol (Normodyne), risperidone (Risperdal), trazodone, haloperidol (Haldol). • Immunoassays may also cross-react with some known fentanyl analogs (eg, acetyl fentanyl, butyryl fentanyl, sufentanil, despropionyl fentanyl) as well as newly emerging fentanyl analogs. • Most immunoassays will also cross-react with the metabolite norfentanyl.

Drug Class or Drug	Cutoff Concentration and Calibrator*	Duration of Positive Result**	Comments***
METHADONE METHADONE (Methadose) METHADOL	300 ng/mL of methadone	Urine may test positive for 5 to 10 days after use.	• Possible false positives (manufacturer specific): quetiapine (Seroquel), tramadol (Ultram), verapamil (Verelan), tapentadol (Nucynta). • Single-analyte methadone immunoassays will not detect the metabolites EDDP (2-ethylidene-1,5-dimethyl-3,3-diphenyl pyrrolidine) or EDMP (2-ethyl-5-methyl-3,3-diphenyl-1-pyrroline). However, combined immunoassays for methadone/EDDP are available.
Or			
EDDP (methadone metabolite)	100 ng/mL (300 ng/mL)		• Specific for EDDP (2-ethylidene-1,5-dimethyl-3,3-diphenyl pyrrolidine); does not detect methadone. • May be used as a supplementary test for methadone use as the metabolite remains in the urine for longer than the parent compound.
OPIATES (Opioids) CODEINE (Robitussin AC: codeine + guaifenesin) MORPHINE (MS Contin) MORPHINE-3-GLUCURONIDE DIHYDROCODEINE (Drocode) HEROIN HYDROCODONE (Vicoprofen: hydrocodone + ibuprofen) (Vicodin: hydrocodone + acetaminophen) HYDROMORPHONE (Dilaudid)	300 ng/mL of morphine	Urine may test positive for 2 to 3 days after use.	• Nonopiate opioids (methadone, naloxone, tramadol, etc) do not cross-react with this assay. • Possible false positives (manufacturer specific): naloxone (Narcan), ofloxacin (Floxin), levofloxacin (Levaquin), rifampicin/rifampin (Rifadin). • Oxycodone (in OxyContin/Percocet/Percodan) is variably and not reliably detected with this assay even in cases of suspected overdose. Order specific oxycodone immunoassay if detection of this analyte is required. • Poppy seed ingestion may cause a positive result. The urine concentration of morphine and codeine from poppy seeds peaks within 2 to 4 hours and may be positive up to 72 hours. • Many opiates/opioids share common metabolic pathways. Check with the laboratory if confirmation testing is needed to determine the specific opiate/opioid triggering the positive result or if an unexpected negative result is obtained. • The heroin metabolite 6-acetylmorphine (6-AM) may be detected with this assay (vendor specific). 6-AM is rapidly metabolized into morphine, which is also detected. Only definitive testing to identify 6-AM can confirm heroin use.

Drug Class or Drug	Cutoff Concentration and Calibrator*	Duration of Positive Result**	Comments***
OXYCODONE OxyContin (Oxycodone HCL) Oxyfast Oxyir Roxicodone Percodan (oxycodone + aspirin) Percocet (oxycodone + acetaminophen) Combunox (oxycodone + ibuprofen)	100 ng/mL of oxycodone	Urine may test positive for 1 to 4 days after use.	• Oxycodone is variably and not reliably detected by the opiates class immunoassay screen even in cases of suspected overdose. • Oxycodone is metabolized into active oxymorphone, which is also detected by this immunoassay. (Noroxycodone and noroxymorphone are inactive metabolites and are not detected by the immunoassay.) • Oxymorphone is sold under the trade names Opana, Numorphan, Numorphone, and others.
PHENCYCLIDINE (PCP) and metabolites Sernylan (discontinued veterinary anesthetic)	25 ng/mL of PCP	Urine may test positive for 10 to 20 days after use.	• Possible false positives (manufacturer specific): venlafaxine (Effexor), dextromethorphan (antitussive agent in many cough syrups/tablets), dextrorphan (DXO; illicit psychoactive hallucinogen), tramadol (Ultram), MDPV (3,4-methylenedioxypyrovalerone; component of illicit bath salts), chlorpromazine (Thorazine), meperidine (Demerol). • Usually does not cross-react with ketamine.
TRAMADOL Ultram	200 ng/mL of tramadol	Urine may test positive for 2 to 3 days or longer after use.	• Tramadol is not reliably detected with opiates/opioids immunoassays. • Tramadol is metabolized into *N*-desmethyltramadol and *O*-desmethyltramadol, which may also cross-react with tramadol immunoassays.

* The cutoff concentration reflects the assay threshold for a positive result relative to the calibrator concentration. Each assay may be more or less sensitive to additional compounds within the same assay class. **Refer to the package insert for specific information on sensitivity and specificity**.

Note: Where multiple cutoff concentrations are available, each lab should assess which cutoff would be most appropriate for the given clinical practice.

** The duration of positive results fields are estimates and will vary with individual user's dose, metabolism, and elimination. Adulteration of the urine sample may also cause erroneous results. In general, if the sample pH is outside the range of 4.5 to 8.0, adulteration should be suspected and another specimen should be obtained.

*** *Note: The specific information listed under the **"Comments"** heading should be vendor specific. Each laboratory should check the package insert for each assay and modify the comment as appropriate.*

Bibliography

Baron JM, Griggs DA, Nixon AL, Long WH, Flood JG. The trazodone metabolite meta-chlorophenylpiperazine can cause false-positive urine amphetamine immunoassay results. *J Anal Toxicol.* 2011;35:364-368.

Birch MA, Couchman L, Pietromartire S, et al. False-positive buprenorphine by CEDIA in patients prescribed amisulpride or sulpiride. *J Anal Toxicol.* 2013;37(4):233-236.

Brahm NC, Yeager LL, Fox MD, Farmer KC, Palmer TA. Commonly prescribed medications and potential false-positive urine drug screens. *Am J Health Syst Pharm.* 2010;67(16):1344-1350.

D'Nicuola J, Jones R, Levine B, Smith ML. Evaluation of six commercial amphetamine and methamphetamine immunoassays for cross-reactivity to phenylpropanolamine and ephedrine in urine. *J Anal Toxicol.* 1992;16(4):211-213.

Gilbert RB, Peng PI, Wong D. A labetalol metabolite with analytical characteristics resembling amphetamines. *J Anal Toxicol.* 1995;19(2):84-86.

Lippi G, Romero A, Cervellin G, Mercadanti M. Unusual false-positive case of urinary screening for buprenorphine. *J Clin Lab Anal.* 2011;25(4):244-245.

Melanson SEF, Snyder ML, Jarolim P, Flood JG. A new highly specific buprenorphine immunoassay for monitoring buprenorphine compliance and abuse. *J Anal Toxicol.* 2012;36:201-206.

Nasky KM, Cowan GL, Knittel DR. False-positive urine screening for benzodiazepines: an association with sertraline? A two-year retrospective chart analysis. *Psychiatry.* 2009;6(7):36-39.

Reidy L, Walls HC, Steele BW. Crossreactivity of bupropion metabolite with enzyme-linked immunosorbent assays designed to detect amphetamine in urine. *Ther Drug Monit.* 2011;33(3):366-368.

Straseski JA, Stolbach A, Clarke W. Opiate-positive immunoassay screen in a pediatric patient. *Clin Chem.* 2010;56(8):1220-1225.

Yee LM, Wu D. False-positive amphetamine toxicology screen results in three pregnant women using labetalol. *Obstet Gynecol.* 2011;117(2.2):503-506.

Appendix B

Serum Toxic Screen Template

Nicholas Heger, PhD
Barbarajean Magnani, PhD, MD

SERUM TOXICOLOGY TESTING AT [Your Hospital's Name]

The basic serum (immunoassay) drug screen (SDS) is appropriate for the Emergency Department (including acute psychiatric services). **Patient floors or doctor's offices rarely need serum drug screens and should instead be ordering serum/plasma concentrations of therapeutic drugs as appropriate (individual drugs are listed on the requisition form or computerized provider order entry [CPOE]).**

The SDS **at** [**your hospital's name**] includes **acetaminophen, salicylates, barbiturates, benzodiazepines, ethanol, and tricyclic antidepressants.** *Note: Barbiturates and benzodiazepines screening assays are also included in routine urine toxicology testing.*

Enzyme immunoassays (EIAs) for barbiturates, benzodiazepines, and tricyclic antidepressants yield only qualitative class-specific information. Specific agents within a drug class are not identified.* Results are reported as positive ("Detected") or negative ("Not Detected") according to the cutoff values listed below. Specific drugs such as acetaminophen, salicylates, and ethanol are quantitated.

Blood for serum drug screens should be collected in a plain red top tube. However, serum separator tubes (SST; barrier, gel, marble top, camouflage, tiger top, or gold top) may be allowed for specimens that are processed immediately. (Some laboratories may choose to use plasma and should determine equivalency with serum as appropriate.)

For suspected toxicity of a therapeutic drug (see appendix C, *Therapeutic Drug Monitoring*), order a quantitative concentration of the specific drug in question or consult the Clinical Laboratory or Laboratory Medicine Resident on call (beeper XXXX) if the drug is not assayed in house.

For suspected heavy metal toxicity, consult the Clinical Laboratory or Laboratory Medicine Resident on call. Depending on the heavy metal involved, either urine or serum/plasma may be the preferred specimen. Urine heavy metal testing requires special acid-washed containers and may necessitate avoidance of certain foods (eg, seafood) prior to collection. Heavy metal testing in blood requires specific collection tubes (ie, tan for lead testing, royal blue for other metals) to reduce inadvertent contamination.

* *Note: The specific drugs detected within each drug class may vary with the specific assay. This template should be compared with package inserts from the kit the laboratory is using. Some brand names are included.*

Drug Class or Drug	Drugs Detected*	Reported Therapeutic Range**	Assay Threshold for Positive Result	Serum Half-Life	Comments
ACETAMINOPHEN	TYLENOL, DATRIL, PARACETAMOL Consider other drugs containing acetaminophen, eg, Percocet (acetaminophen/oxycodone), Talacen (acetaminophen/Pentazocine), OTC cold/pain/headache preparations.	μg/mL 10-30	3.0 μg/mL	1-3 h In toxicity, serum half-life will be extended.	Toxicity greater than 200 μg/mL at 4 hours or 50 μg/mL at 12 hours post ingestion. Follow Rumack nomogram (appended) to determine treatment protocol. (For extended-release medications, additional levels may be required to assure peak concentration.)

Acetaminophen toxicity: In acute overdose, initial symptoms include anorexia, nausea, or vomiting. Obtain baseline levels of electrolytes, glucose, BUN, creatinine, liver transaminases (AST, ALT), and prothrombin time (PT, INR). Obtain a 4-hour postingestion acetaminophen concentration or a level at the time of presentation if the ingestion time is unknown. Use the Rumack-Matthew nomogram (see end of appendix) for the prediction of acetaminophen hepatotoxicity in **acute** overdose. Treatment for acetaminophen toxicity is *N*-acetylcysteine (NAC). After 24 to 48 hours, transaminase levels usually rise, and, in untreated cases, fulminant hepatic failure may occur with encephalopathy, metabolic acidosis, and increased PT. Note: Serum specimens collected immediately after administration of NAC may show significantly reduced concentrations of acetaminophen depending upon the assay. A serum sample assayed prior to the administration of NAC is preferred. Other possible sources of interference include hemolysis, icterus, lipemia, and elevated concentrations of NAPQI (*N*-acetyl-4-benzoquinone imine) or metamizole. Consult the assay package insert for assay-specific information.

Drug Class or Drug	Drugs Detected*	Reported Therapeutic Range**	Assay Threshold for Positive Result	Serum Half-Life	Comments
BARBITURATES CLASS SCREEN		μg/mL	1.0 μg/mL of secobarbital		Phenobarbital can be quantitated in house; order a phenobarbital level.
	BARBITAL	5-30		2 d	
	BUTALBITAL (Fiorinal, Fioricet)	1-10		35-88 h	
	PENTOBARBITAL (Nembutal)	1-5		15-48 h	
	PHENOBARBITAL	15-40		2-6 d	
	SECOBARBITAL (Seconal)	1-5		22-29 h	

Barbiturates are sedative hypnotic agents used as anticonvulsant therapy, as inductive agents for anesthesia, or to reduce intracranial pressure and reduce cerebral oxygen demand in severe head trauma. Toxicity depends on the specific drug and route of administration. Mild to moderate intoxication produces lethargy, slurred speech, ataxia, and nystagmus, while higher doses produce hypotension, coma, and respiratory arrest. Additional laboratory studies include electrolytes, glucose, BUN, creatinine, and arterial blood gases.

Drug Class or Drug	Drugs Detected*	Reported Therapeutic Range**	Assay Threshold for Positive Result	Serum Half-Life	Comments
BENZODIAZEPINES CLASS SCREEN		ng/mL	50 ng/mL diazepam		Many benzodiazepines share common metabolic pathways and may be both byproducts of metabolism or sold as standalone drugs (eg, oxazepam is the active metabolite of temazepam).
	ALPRAZOLAM (Xanax)	25-55		6-27 h	
	CHLORDIAZEPOXIDE (Librium)	100-3000†		6-27 h	
	CLONAZEPAM (Klonopin)	20-60		19-60 h	
	DIAZEPAM (Valium)	100-1500		21-37 h	

Drug Class or Drug	Drugs Detected*	Reported Therapeutic Range**	Assay Threshold for Positive Result	Serum Half-Life	Comments
BENZODIAZEPINES CLASS SCREEN *(continued)*	FLUNITRAZEPAM (Rohypnol)	N/A		9-25 h	Cross-reactivities of parent drug and metabolite may differ significantly. Only high concentrations of some benzodiazepines may cross-react, and therefore only toxic concentrations and not therapeutic concentrations may be detected. Check assay package insert section on specificity/cross-reactivity. Clinicians should contact the laboratory if the patient is prescribed a benzodiazepine and the screen is unexpectedly negative. † *Therapeutic range includes parent compound and metabolite.*
	FLURAZEPAM (Dalmane)	0-30		1-3 h	
	LORAZEPAM (Ativan)	50-240		9-16 h	
	NITRAZEPAM (Mogadon)	30-100		17-48 h	
	OXAZEPAM (Serax)	200-500		4-11 h	
	PRAZEPAM (Centrax)	100-2200		1.3 h	
	TEMAZEPAM (Restoril)	50-1000		3-13 h	
	TRIAZOLAM (Halcion)	5-20		1.8-3.9 h	

Benzodiazepines are central nervous system depressants used clinically as sedatives, hypnotics, anxiolytics, muscle relaxants, antiepileptics, and in the treatment of alcohol withdrawal. Generally the toxic-to-therapeutic ratio for benzodiazepines is high, and death from a benzodiazepine-alone overdose is rare. However, the short-acting triazolobenzodiazepines (triazolam, alprazolam, and midazolam) have been associated with respiratory arrest. Benzodiazepines combined with other CNS-acting drugs such as ethanol, opiates/opioids, or barbiturates may also increase toxicity. Specific serum concentrations of a benzodiazepine are not helpful in the treatment of a suspected benzodiazepine overdose. A glucose level and arterial blood gases may be helpful in overdose. Flumazenil is a benzodiazepine receptor antagonist used to reverse coma.

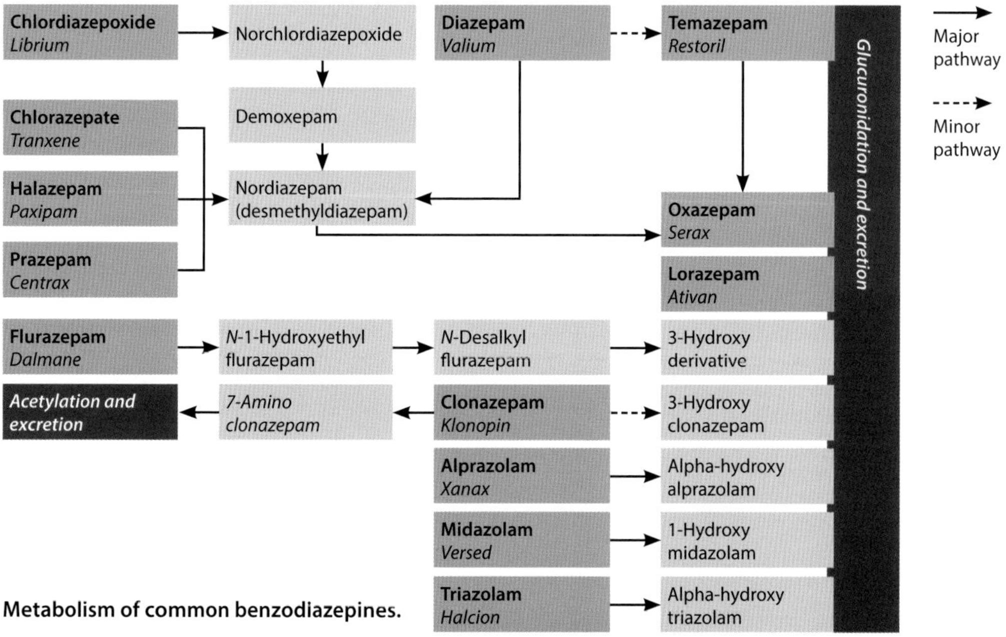

Metabolism of common benzodiazepines.

Drug Class or Drug	Drugs Detected*	Reported Therapeutic Range**	Assay Threshold for Positive Result	Serum Half-Life	Comments
ETHANOL	ETHYL ALCOHOL Consider OTC preparations containing ethanol, eg, perfumes, aftershaves, food flavorings (vanilla, almond, lemon extracts).	mg/dL 0.0	10.0 mg/dL	2-14 h Zero-order kinetics are independent of the dose. However, at lower doses, elimination may be first-order kinetics.	This assay is specific for ethanol and does not detect isopropanol and methanol. The serum ethanol concentration is approximately 12% higher than whole blood ethanol concentrations, which are reported in g/dL or grams percent. Assay uses enzymatic methodology. **A false-positive ethanol may occur in patients with a high lactic dehydrogenase or lactic acid (lactate) concentration. Positive results with a high concentration of either analyte should be confirmed by a gas chromatographic assay.**

Ethanol is metabolized approximately 12 to 25 mg/dL/h depending on the individual's sex, ethnicity, and history of ethanol use. Approximately 3 to 4 drinks or 0.7g/kg of ethanol will generate a blood ethanol concentration of 100 mg/dL. Mild intoxication produces euphoria, mild incoordination, ataxia, nystagmus, and impaired judgment, while deep intoxication may result in respiratory depression and coma. Hypoglycemia may occur in children or individuals with depleted hepatic glycogen. Additional laboratory studies include electrolytes, glucose, BUN, creatinine, arterial blood gases, LFTs, and a serum osmolality. A calculated olmolarity and measured serum osmolality should be obtained from the same blood sample. Calculated Serum Osmolarity = $2[Na^+] + [glucose]/18 + [BUN]/2.8$ (reference interval for measured serum osmolality = ~290 mOsm/L). An osmolal gap greater than 10 (measured – calculated) indicates additional osmotically active substances in the blood. If the measured osmolality is greater than that of the contribution of measured ethanol alone, consider co-ingestants such as isopropanol, methanol, or ethylene glycol, among others.

Specimen collection: Prepare skin with a nonalcohol disinfectant or ensure the skin is dry prior to needle insertion if an isopropanol pad is used. Due to the volatility of ethanol, the collection tube must be tightly sealed immediately after collection.

Drug Class or Drug	Drugs Detected*	Reported Therapeutic Range**	Assay Threshold for Positive Result	Serum Half-Life	Comments
SALICYLATES	ASPIRIN (salicylic acid) Consider other drugs containing aspirin, eg, combination drugs such as Percodan (aspirin/oxycodone), OTC cold preparations, Pepto-Bismol, Bengay topical.	mg/dL Analgesic: <10 Anti-inflammatory: 15-20 Critical alert value: >30 at peak	1.5 mg/dL salicylic acid	13-20 min for acetylsalicylic acid; 3-20 h for salicylic acid (dose dependent)	Toxicity greater than 30 mg/dL 2 hours post ingestion. If large concentrations have been ingested, then the peak may be delayed. Repeat level every 2 hours. Elevated concentrations of sulfapyridine or sulfasalazine may produce erroneous results.

Drug Class or Drug	Drugs Detected*	Reported Therapeutic Range**	Assay Threshold for Positive Result	Serum Half-Life	Comments
Salicylate toxicity: Acute ingestion results in vomiting and hyperventilation. An initial respiratory alkalosis is usually followed by a compensatory metabolic acidosis. Severe intoxication may produce coma, seizures, hypoglycemia, and pulmonary edema. Chronic intoxication is nonspecific, and patients (especially elderly) may present with confusion, dehydration, and metabolic acidosis. Additional laboratory studies include electrolytes, glucose, BUN, creatinine, arterial blood gases, and a PT. To calculate the anion gap: $[Na^+] - [Cl^-] - [HCO_3] = 8\text{-}12$ mEq/L.					
TRICYCLIC ANTIDEPRESSANTS CLASS SCREEN	*Primarily detects:*	ng/mL	300 ng/mL nortriptyline		A positive result in this assay indicates the presence of tricyclic antidepressants (TCAs) either in the high therapeutic range or greater, depending on the specific TCA. Other compounds that have been reported to cross-react with TCA assays in general include therapeutic concentrations of chlorpromazine, thioridazine, and cyproheptadine, and high concentrations of cyclobenzaprine, diphenhydramine, and orphenadrine. *If there is suspicion of a cross-reacting substance, the specimen can be sent out for confirmation testing by a different methodology. Contact the laboratory for further information.* A negative result in this assay indicates either the absence of TCAs or concentrations of TCA that fall into the therapeutic or subtherapeutic range. TCA concentrations do not correlate well with toxicity. Monitor ECG and clinical presentation for toxicity.
	AMITRIPTYLINE (Elavil, Emitrip, Endep)	75-250†		8-51 h	
	DESIPRAMINE (Norpramin)	50-150 (150-300)		12-54 h	
	IMIPRAMINE (Tofranil)	100-300†		6-20 h	
	NORTRIPTYLINE (Aventyl, Pamelor)	50-150		15-90 h	
	Should be detectable at higher concentrations:				
	CLOMIPRAMINE (Anafranil)	70-200		12-36 h	
	DOXEPIN (Adapin, Sinequan)	90-250		8-25 h	
	PROTRIPTYLINE (Vivactil)	50-170		54-92 h	
	TRIMIPRAMINE (Surmontil)	50-300		16-39 h	

Continued on next page

Drug Class or Drug	Drugs Detected*	Reported Therapeutic Range**	Assay Threshold for Positive Result	Serum Half-Life	Comments
TRICYCLIC ANTIDEPRESSANTS CLASS SCREEN *(continued)*					Combined parent and metabolite concentrations >500 ng/mL increase the risk of cardiac toxicity, and levels >1000 ng/mL are associated with severe, sometimes fatal, cardiac and CNS side effects. † *Therapeutic range includes parent compound and metabolite.*

Tricyclic antidepressant toxicity results from the anticholinergic effects and the inhibition of reuptake of catecholamines. Patients may exhibit dilated pupils, altered mental status, tachycardia, dry skin and mucous membranes, hypothermia secondary to impaired sweating, decreased bowel sounds, and urinary retention. Cardiovascular manifestations include abnormal cardiac conduction (quinidine-like effect), arrhythmias, and hypotension. Prolongation of the QRS interval >0.12 s in the limb leads is associated with severe toxicity. Seizures may result from the inhibition of norepinephrine or serotonin in the brain. Additional laboratory studies include electrolytes, glucose, BUN, creatinine, arterial blood gases, and a total CK. *Note: This assay does not detect selective serotonin reuptake inhibitors such as fluoxetine, paroxetine, sertraline, and others. However, these drugs are less cardiotoxic and do not require serum concentrations in overdose.*

* Some brand names included; others may exist.

** Reported ranges may vary according to laboratory, method, and clinical indication. These are only suggested guidelines.

Rumack-Matthew nomogram for determining hepatotoxicity in acute acetaminophen overdose.

Adapted from Rumack B, Matthew M. Acetaminophen poisoning and toxicity. *Pediatrics.* 1975;55(6):871.

Bibliography

Baselt RC. *Disposition of Toxic Drugs and Chemicals in Man.* 10th ed. Seal Beach, CA: Biomedical Publications; 2014.

Olsen K, ed. *Poisoning and Drug Overdose.* 7th ed. Norwalk, CT: Appleton and Lange; 2007.

Dade Behring (Syva) package insert (acetaminophen).

Microgenics Corp package insert (tricyclic antidepressants, benzodiazepines, salicylates, barbiturates, ethanol).

Sekisui Sekure package insert (acetaminophen).

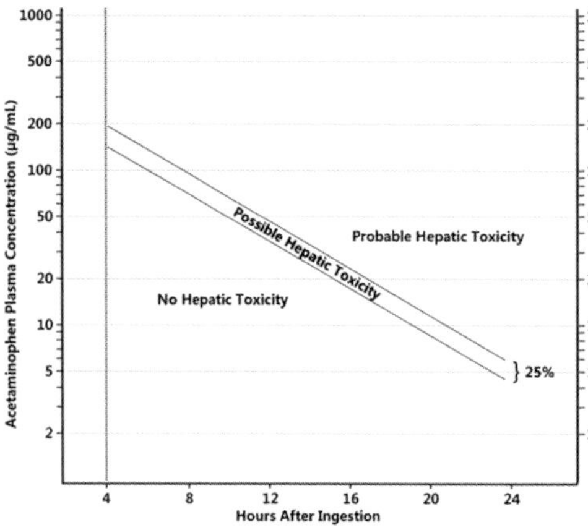

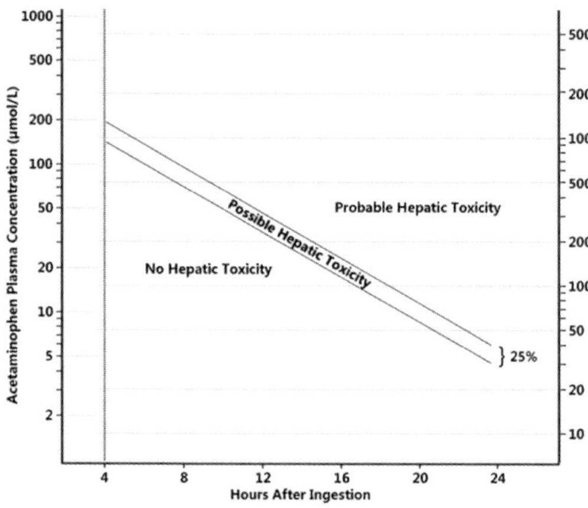

Appendix C

Therapeutic Drug Monitoring Template

Nicholas Heger, PhD
Barbarajean Magnani, PhD, MD

THERAPEUTIC DRUG MONITORING AT [Your Hospital's Name]

It is important to record the time of blood collection on the requisition form (or computerized provider order entry [CPOE]) to ensure accurate interpretation of drug concentrations. For inpatients, specimen collection should be accurately timed according to the table below. For outpatients, every effort should be made to obtain the specimen at the appropriate time to avoid misinterpretation of drug concentrations. For suspected toxicity, blood may be drawn immediately, but note that certain drugs (eg, acetaminophen) should be assayed at the peak absorption for best assessment.

Questions regarding Therapeutic Drug Monitoring (TDM) may be directed to the Clinical Chemistry Laboratory (XXXX), the Laboratory Medicine (Clinical Pathology) Resident on-call (beeper XXXX), or, for specific interpretation or questions regarding aminoglycosides, call the Pharmacy Department (XXXX). *These tables are suggested examples for presenting information on TDM. Modify according to your own laboratory's protocol.*

Toxicity: Therapeutic drugs may be potentially toxic at concentrations lower than the Critical Alert Value (CAV). However, only CAVs will prompt a call to the ordering provider. It is recommended that results be reviewed in a timely manner and be evaluated in conjunction with the patient's history, physical exam, or other pertinent clinical findings. To aid in your assessment, information on toxic concentrations is listed for some drugs.

Specimen collection: See specific drug for collection tube guidelines.

Availability: *These are suggested examples of test availability on TDM. Modify according to your own laboratory's protocol. Some tests listed here may be assayed in house in your institution, and others listed as in-house may be sent out.*

Unless noted in the table, most therapeutic drugs **assayed in house** are available 24 hours a day, 7 days a week. Specimens sent out to a reference laboratory (send-out test) might only be available 5 to 6 days a week. **Turnaround time (TAT)** for routine monitoring of in-house drugs is approximately 2 hours. Most in-house assays are available stat. For drugs not listed below, call the Clinical Laboratory (XXXX) for information. Some send-out tests may require the Pathologist's approval. The Laboratory Medicine (Clinical Pathology) Resident is available for consultation by paging beeper number XXXX.

Methods:

CLCI: Chemiluminescent competitive immunoassay
EMIT: Enzyme multiplied immunoassay technology
GC-MS: Gas chromatography-mass spectrometry
LC-MS/MS: Liquid chromatography-tandem mass spectrometry
PETINIA: Particle enhanced turbidimetric inhibition immunoassay

Drug*	Specimen Collection	Therapeutic Range	TAT	Serum Half-Life	Comments
ACETAMINOPHEN (Tylenol, Datril, paracetamol)	Serum/Plain red top tube; gold top tube 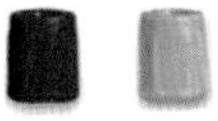 Plasma/ Lithium or sodium heparin green top tube 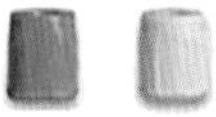 Therapeutic monitoring: TROUGH: Collect just prior to next dose.	µg/mL 10-30 Critical alert value: See Comment	Routine 2 h Available stat	1-3 h	Toxicity greater than 200 µg/mL at 4 hours (or 50 µg/mL at 12 hours) post ingestion. Follow Rumack-Matthew nomogram to determine treatment protocol. (For extended-release medications additional specimens may be required to assure peak concentration.) A negligible acetaminophen concentration 2 to 4 hours after ingestion rules out toxicity. See Serum Toxic Screen guideline for additional information. Note: Serum specimens collected immediately after administration of NAC (*N*-acetylcysteine) may show significantly reduced concentrations of acetaminophen depending upon the assay. A serum specimen assayed prior to the administration of NAC is preferred. Other possible sources of interference include hemolysis, icterus, lipemia, and elevated concentrations of NAPQI (*N*-acetyl-4-benzoquinoneimine) or metamizole. Consult the assay package insert for assay-specific information. Method: Enzymatic
AMIKACIN** (Amikin)	Serum/Plain red top tube; gold top tube 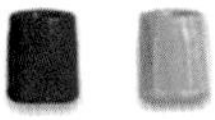 Plasma/ Lithium or sodium heparin green top tube 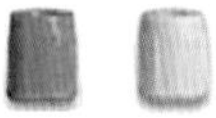 Therapeutic monitoring: TROUGH: Collect within 1 h of next dose or just before next dose. PEAK: Collect 60 min after IM injection, or 30 min after end of 30-min IV infusion or at end of 60-min IV infusion.	mg/L Traditional dosing Trough: 4-8 Toxic: >10 Peak: 20-35 Toxic: >40	Available Mon-Sun 24-48 h	1.9-2.8 h	Draw specimen at steady state around third dose if given by traditional dosing. Potentially nephrotoxic and ototoxic. Method: PETINIA

Drug*	Specimen Collection	Therapeutic Range	TAT	Serum Half-Life	Comments
AMITRIPTYLINE** (Elavil)	Serum/Plain red top tube; no gel tubes  Therapeutic monitoring: Collect 10-14 hours post oral dose.	µg/L Amitriptyline + nortriptyline 80-250 Toxic: >500 µg/L (consider parent compound and metabolite)	Available Mon-Fri 48 h	15 h (range: 8-51 h)	Includes metabolite nortriptyline. Monitor serum TCA to evaluate compliance, to verify therapeutic concentrations, to evaluate potential toxicity, to establish the effects of drug-drug interaction on steady state TCA concentrations. For semiquantitative TCA compliance or suspected toxicity screen; see Serum Toxic Screen guideline for additional information. Method: LC-MS/MS
CARBAMAZEPINE (Tegretol)	Serum/Plain red top tube; gold top tube 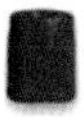  Plasma/ Lithium or sodium heparin green top tube 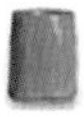 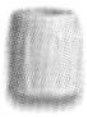 Therapeutic monitoring: TROUGH: Collect within an hour of next dose.	µg/mL 4-12 Critical alert value: >15	Routine 2 h Available stat	18-65 h (single dose)	Draw specimen at steady state reached at approximately 2 weeks. Some patients may reach steady state after 3 to 4 weeks. Half-life decreases to 12 to 17 hours after multiple doses over several weeks due to autoinduction of its own metabolism by its active metabolite. Cross-reactivity with 10,11-epoxide metabolite is ~7.3%. Method: PETINIA
CYCLOSPORINE (Sandimmune, Neoral)	Whole blood/ Lavender top tube (EDTA) 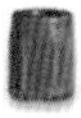 Therapeutic monitoring: TROUGH: Collect within an hour of next dose.	ng/mL 50-350 Therapeutic range is organ specific and dependent on time interval post transplant. For other clinical conditions, therapeutic goals may be lower.	Available Mon-Fri/ Sat-Sun Specimens must be in the lab by 10:30 AM for same day results and 9:30 AM for week-ends	19 h (6-27 h)	Levels can also be collected 12 to 18 hours post oral dose or 12 hours post intravenous dose. Cyclosporine adheres to plastic IV lines, so blood should be drawn from a site other than where the drug is being infused. Immunoassay methods for cyclosporine may variably detect metabolites, which may accumulate if elimination is impaired. Results are not interchangeable between methodologies. Method: LC-MS/MS

TCA, Tricyclic antidepressant.

Drug*	Specimen Collection	Therapeutic Range	TAT	Serum Half-Life	Comments
DESIPRAMINE** (Norpramin, Pertofrane)	Serum/Plain red top tube; no gel tube  Therapeutic monitoring: Collect 10-14 h post oral dose (single daily dose regimen) or 4-6 h post divided daily dose regimen.	µg/L 100-300 Toxic: >400	Available Mon-Fri 48 h	17 h (12-54 h)	Monitor TCA: To evaluate compliance, to verify therapeutic concentrations, to evaluate potential toxicity, to establish the effects of drug-drug interactions on steady state (reached after 3 to 5 days) TCA concentrations. For semiquantitative TCA, compliance, or suspected toxicity screen, see Serum Toxic Screen guidelines for more information. Method: LC-MS/MS
DIGOXIN (Lanoxin)	Serum/Plain red top tube; gold top tube 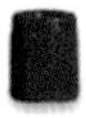 Plasma/ Lithium or sodium heparin green top tube 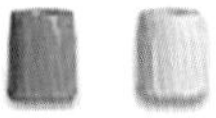 Therapeutic monitoring: TROUGH: Collect just prior to next dose. May also be collected within 6-8 h after IV or oral dose.	µg/L 0.8-2 Critical alert value: >3	Routine 2 h Available stat	30-45 h	Draw specimen at steady state reached at approximately 5 to 7 days. Digibind (digoxin immune Fab) drug therapy affects immunoassay results. Some assays will variably cross-react with Digoxin-like immunoreactive factors (DLIF) or substances (DLIS). % cross–reactivity with this assay: Digoxigenin bis-digitoxoside, 112% Digoxigenin mono-digitoxoside, 78.2% Digoxigenin, 4.0% Digitoxin, 3.0% Digitoxigenin, 0.5% Method: PETINIA
ETHOSUXIMIDE** (Zarontin)	Serum/Plain red top tube; gold top tube 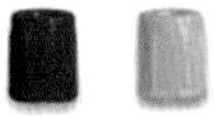 Therapeutic monitoring: Collect specimen just prior to next dose.	mg/L Adults: 40-100 Toxic: >120	Available Mon-Sun 24-48 h	48-60 h (dose dependent)	An anticonvulsant that requires 5 to 8 days to achieve a steady-state plasma level. Method: EMIT

TCA, Tricyclic antidepressant.

Drug*	Specimen Collection	Therapeutic Range	TAT	Serum Half-Life	Comments
GENTAMICIN (Garamycin)	Serum/Plain red top tube; gold top tube 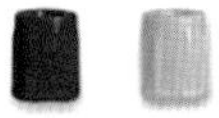 Plasma/ Lithium or sodium heparin green top tube 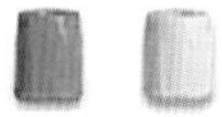 Therapeutic monitoring: TROUGH: Collect just prior to next dose. PEAK: 60 min after IM injection, or 30 min after end of 30-min IV infusion, or at end of 60-min IV infusion.	µg/mL Traditional dosing Trough: 1- 2 Critical alert value: >2 Peak: 5-10 Critical alert value: >12	Routine 2 h Available stat	1-3 h	Draw specimen at steady state around third dose if given as traditional dosing. Specimens containing cephalexin, netilmicin, sisomicin, sagamicin, kanamycin B, neomycin, or tobramycin may cause falsely elevated results with some assays. Specimens containing β-lactam antibiotics may yield falsely low results in some assays when analysis is delayed more than 8 hours. Potentially nephrotoxic and neurotoxic. Method: CLCI
LIDOCAINE** (Xylocaine)	Serum/Plain red top tube; gold top tube 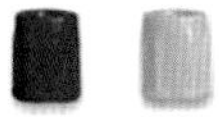 Collect at a trough just prior to the next dose.	mg/L 1.5-5.0 Toxic: >6.0	Available Mon-Fri 48 h	0.7-1.8 h	Method: EMIT
LITHIUM (Eskalith, Lithobid)	Serum/ Plain red top tube; gold top tube; NO lithium heparin tubes 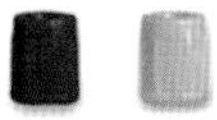 Draw specimen at least 12 hours after last dose. Use consistent sampling time.	mEq/L Acute mania: 0.5-1.2 Maintenance: 0.6-1.0 Critical alert value: >1.5	Routine 2 h Available stat	17-58 h	Increased toxicity with thiazide diuretics, nonsteroidal anti-inflammatory drugs (NSAIDs), haloperidol, phenothiazines, neuromuscular blockers, carbamazepine, fluoxetine, and ACE inhibitors. Method: Spectrophotometric

Drug*	Specimen Collection	Therapeutic Range	TAT	Serum Half-Life	Comments
METHOTREXATE (Rheumatrx, Trexall)	Serum/Plain red top tube; gold top tube 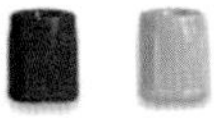 Plasma/ Lithium or sodium heparin green top tube 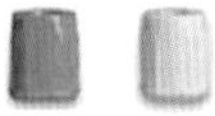	µmol/L Dependent on indication. High-dose regimes produce concentrations between 0.1 and 1.0.	Routine available with same day results Available stat	Low dose: 3-10 h High dose: 8-15 h	Draw specimen at steady state reached 24 to 48 hours. Some assays may cross-react with triamterene or trimethoprim to produce falsely elevated result. Patients given glucarpidase (Voraxaze) as a high-dose rescue therapy will have high concentrations of 2,4-diamino-N(10)-methylpteroic acid (DAMPA), which may cross-react with some assays to produce a falsely elevated result. DAMPA may continue to circulate for up to 7 days. Assay instead by LC-MS/MS. Method: EMIT
NORTRIPTYLINE** (Allegron, Aventyl, Pamelor)	Serum/Plain red top tube; no gel tubes 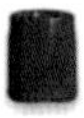 Therapeutic monitoring: Collect just prior to next dose (divided daily dose regimen) or 10-14 h post oral dose (once daily regimen).	µg/L 50-150 Toxic: >300	Available Mon-Fri 48 h	15-90 h	Monitor TCA: to evaluate compliance, to verify therapeutic concentrations, to evaluate potential toxicity, to establish the effects of drug-drug interaction on steady state TCA concentrations. For semiquantitative TCA, compliance, or suspected toxicity screen, see Serum Toxic Screen guideline. Method: LC-MS/MS
PENTOBARBITAL** (Nembutal)	Serum/Plain red top tube  Plasma/ Lithium heparin green top tube 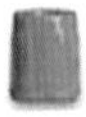 No gel tubes Collect specimen just prior to next dose.	mg/L 1-5 Toxic: >10	Available Mon-Sun 72 h	15-48 h	In conjunction with supportive therapy, pentobarbital is given IV to reduce intracranial pressure and lower cerebral oxygen demand in patients with severe head trauma. Adult intracranial pressure reduction therapy range 25 to 35 mg/L; child: 20 to 30 mg/L. Method: GC-MS

TCA, Tricyclic antidepressant.

Drug*	Specimen Collection	Therapeutic Range	TAT	Serum Half-Life	Comments
PHENOBARBITAL	Serum/Plain red top tube; gold top tube 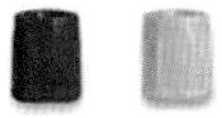 Plasma/ Lithium or sodium heparin green top tube 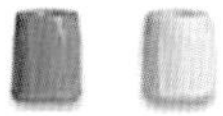 Chronic monitoring: Any consistent sampling time.	µg/mL 15-40 Critical alert value: >50	Routine 2 h Available stat	2-6 d	IV: Collect 2 to 4 hours post loading dose. Check level 2 to 3 weeks after a change in dose. Method: PETINIA
PHENYTOIN (Dilantin)	Serum/Plain red top tube; gold top tube 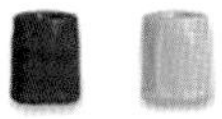 Plasma/ Lithium or sodium heparin green top 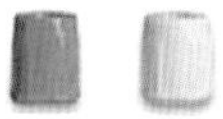 IV infusion: At least 2-4 h post loading dose. Chronic monitoring: Any consistent sampling time.	µg/mL 10-20 Critical alert value: >30	Routine 2 h Available stat	14 h 8-60 h (dose dependent)	Check concentration at least 3 to 4 days after a change in dose. Specimens from patients taking fosphenytoin should be drawn at least 2 hours after IV administration or 4 hours after IM administration. Method: CLCI
PROCAINAMIDE AND NAPA** (Procan, Pronestyl)	Serum/Plain red top tube; gold top tube 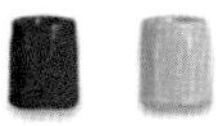 Therapeutic monitoring: TROUGH: Collect prior to next dose.	mg/L PA: 4-10 NAPA: 10-30 Or combined PA + NAPA: 5-30 Toxic: PA: >12 Or combined PA+NAPA: >30	Available Mon-Sun 24 h	PA: 2-5 h NAPA: 5-7 h	Both procainamide (PA) and its active metabolite N-acetylprocainamide (NAPA) should be measured, especially when establishing acetylator status. Fast acetylator status is defined as a measurement 3 hours after the last dose that shows NAPA concentrations higher or equal to that of Procainamide. Method: EMIT

Drug*	Specimen Collection	Therapeutic Range	TAT	Serum Half-Life	Comments
QUINIDINE** (Duraquin, Quinaglute, Quinora)	Serum/Plain red top tube; gold top tube 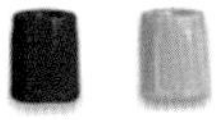 Plasma/ Lithium or sodium heparin green top tube 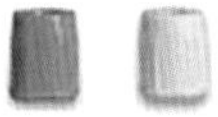 Therapeutic monitoring: TROUGH: Collect just prior to next dose.	mg/L 2-5 Toxic: >6	Available Mon-Sun 48 h	5-12 h	Draw specimen at steady state reached approximately at 1 to 2 days. Check level 1 to 2 days after a change in dose. Some immunoassays may cross-react with closely related compounds including quinine, quinidine-n-oxide, dihydroquinidine, and others. Method: PETINIA
SALICYLATES (Aspirin; component of Percodan, Pepto Bismol, and others)	Serum/Plain red top tube; gold top tube 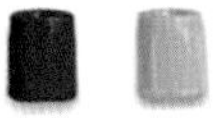 Plasma/ Lithium or sodium heparin green top tube 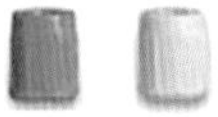 Therapeutic monitoring: TROUGH: Collect within an hour of next dose.	mg/dL Analgesic: <10 Anti-inflammatory: 15-30 Critical alert value: >30 at peak	Routine 2 h Available stat	Acetylsalicylic acid 13-20 min; 3-20 h for salicylic acid (dose dependent)	Toxicity greater than 30 mg/dL 2 hours post ingestion. If large concentrations have been ingested, the peak may be delayed. Repeat concentration every 2 hours. See Serum Toxic Screen guideline for additional information. Method: Enzymatic
SIROLIMUS (Rapamycin, Rapamune)	Whole blood/ Lavender top tube (EDTA) 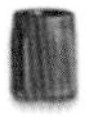	ng/mL 3-20	Available Mon-Fri/ Sat-Sun Specimens must be in the lab by 10:30 AM for same day results, 9:30 AM for weekends	46-86 h	Time to steady state is 5 to 7 days. Immunoassay methods for sirolimus may variably detect metabolites. Results are not interchangeable between methodologies. Method: LC-MS/MS

Drug*	Specimen Collection	Therapeutic Range	TAT	Serum Half-Life	Comments
TACROLIMUS (Prograf, FK506)	Whole blood/ Lavender top tube (EDTA) 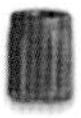 Therapeutic monitoring: TROUGH: Collect within an hour of next dose.	ng/mL 3-20	Available Mon-Fri/ Sat-Sun Specimens must be in the lab by 10:30 AM for same day results, 9:30 AM for weekends	12-30 h	Optimal whole blood concentrations of tacrolimus will vary with each patient's clinical state and sensitivity to the immunosuppressive effects of the drug. Before treatment adjustments are made, each patient should have a thorough clinical evaluation. Individual whole blood tacrolimus values cannot be used as the single indicator for making changes in the treatment protocol. Immunoassay methods for tacrolimus may variably detect metabolites. Results are not interchangeable between methodologies. Method: LC-MS/MS
THEOPHYLLINE (Theo-24, Elixophylline, Theochron)	Serum/Plain red top tube; gold top tube 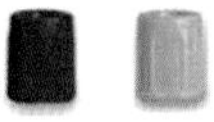 Plasma/ Lithium or sodium heparin green top tube 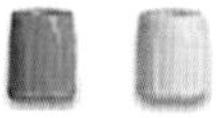 Oral: Liquid or immediate release: TROUGH: Collect just prior to next dose. Sustained release: As above or any consistent time within the dosing interval. Continuous infusion: 4-6 h after starting infusion; the infusion should be stopped for 15 min before the sample is taken. Post load level, if necessary, ≥1 h after bolus.	µg/mL 10-20 Neonatal apnea: 6-11 Critical alert value: >25	Routine 2 h Available stat	8.7 h 3-11 h, higher in neonates	Draw specimen at steady state reached approximately at 2 to 3 days in adults and at approximately 5 days in newborns. If toxicity suspected, draw anytime during continuous IV or 2 hours after oral dose. Method: EMIT

Drug*	Specimen Collection	Therapeutic Range	TAT	Serum Half-Life	Comments
THIOCYANATE**	Serum/Plain red top tube 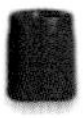 Plasma/ Lithium heparin green top tube 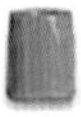 No gel tubes	mg/L Nonsmokers: <4 Smokers: <8	Available Mon, Wed, Fri 72 h	3 d	For monitoring nitroprusside therapy in patients receiving therapy >48 hours. Not for **acute** cyanide overdose. Hemolyzed specimens are unacceptable. Lab must centrifuge and separate immediately; submit specimen in a plastic vial. Method: Spectrophotometric
TOBRAMYCIN (Nebcin, Tobrex)	Serum/Plain red top tube; gold top tube 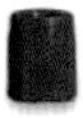  Plasma/ Lithium or sodium heparin green top tube 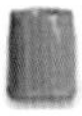 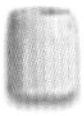 Therapeutic monitoring: TROUGH: Collect just prior to next dose. PEAK: 60 min after IM injection, or 30 min after end of 30-min IV infusion, or at end of 60-min IV infusion.	mg/L Traditional dosing Trough: 1-2 (ideal goal ≤1) Critical alert value: >2 Peak: 5-10 Critical alert value: >12	Routine 2 h Available stat	2-4 h	Draw specimen at steady state around third dose if traditional dosing used. Indicated therapeutic or toxic ranges should not be used for patients on pulse dosing schedules, when other methods such as AUC or nomograms may be more reliable. Method: PETINIA

Drug*	Specimen Collection	Therapeutic Range	TAT	Serum Half-Life	Comments
VALPROIC ACID (Depakene, Depakote)	Serum/Plain red top tube; gold top tube 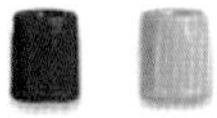 Plasma/ Lithium or sodium heparin green top tube 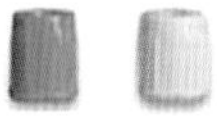 Therapeutic monitoring: TROUGH: Collect within an hour of next dose. Sample preferably before the AM dose.	µg/mL 50-100 Critical alert value: >150	Routine 2 h Available stat	8-12 h	Draw specimen at steady state reached at approximately 2 to 4 days. Check concentration if dosing changed or if additional anticonvulsants are given. Amikacin, kanamycin A, kanamycin B, or 3',4'-dideoxykanamycin B may cross-react with some immunoassays to produce an elevated result. Method: PETINIA
VANCOMYCIN (Vancocin, Vancoled)	Serum/Plain red top tube; gold top tube 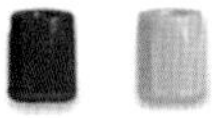 Plasma/ Lithium or sodium heparin green top tube 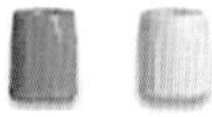 Therapeutic monitoring: TROUGH: Collect within an hour of next dose.	µg/mL Trough: 10-15† Critical alert value: >30 Peak: 30-40 Critical alert value: >60 *† 15-20 µg/mL appropriate for deep or invasive infections.*	Routine 2 h Available stat	2.6-7.8 h	Draw specimen at steady state around third dose. PEAK concentrations should **not** be measured unless approved by pharmacy. Method: PETINIA

* Some brand names included; others may exist.
** Send-out test.

Bibliography

Baselt RC. *Disposition of Toxic Drugs and Chemicals in Man*. 10th ed. Seal Beach, CA: Biomedical Publications; 2014.

Hammett-Stabler C, Dasgupta A, eds. *Therapeutic Drug Monitoring Data: A Concise Guide*. 3rd ed. Washington DC: AACC Press; 2007.

Hiemke C, Bergemann N, Clement C, et al. Consensus guidelines for therapeutic drug monitoring in neuropsychopharmacology: update 2017. *Pharmacopsychiatry*. 2018;51(01/02):9-62.

IBM Watson Health. Micromedex Clinical Knowledge. http://www.micromedex.com. Accessed May 16, 2019.

Jacobs DS, et al. *Laboratory Test Handbook*. 5th ed. Hudson, OH: Lexi-Comp; 2001.

Li D, Nichols J. *Specimen Collection and Stability for Therapeutic Drug Monitoring: Therapeutic Drug Monitoring and Toxicology*. Vol 18, No 1. Washington, DC: American Association for Clinical Chemistry; 1997.

Rybak MJ, Lomaestro BM, Rotschafer JC, et al. Vancomycin therapeutic guidelines: a summary of consensus recommendations from the Infectious Diseases Society of America, the American Society of Health-System Pharmacists, and the Society of Infectious Diseases Pharmacists. *Clin Infect Dis*. 2009;49(3):325-327. Erratum in: *Clin Infect Dis*. 2009;49(9):1465.

Winter ME, ed. *Basic Clinical Pharmacokinetics*. 3rd ed. Vancouver, WA: Applied Therapeutics Inc; 1994.

Zandvliet ML, Jacobs B, den Boer E, et al. Monitoring of methotrexate levels following glucarpidase rescue treatment requires detection by mass spectrometry since immunoassay is not applicable. *Eur J Hosp Pharm*. 2012;19:198.

Appendix D

Frequently Asked Questions on Clinical Urine Drugs-of-Abuse Tests

Tai C. Kwong, PhD

Introduction

Directors of clinical laboratories receive many requests to consult on urine drugs-of-abuse test results. These requests come from physicians, nurses, and counselors of drug treatment programs and pain management services. Many of these questions are repetitive, dealing mostly with the basics of immunoassay-based drug tests. Included in this collection are a sampling of some of the most frequently asked questions from actual practice, each illustrating an important feature of urine drug tests as they are typically performed in hospital-based clinical laboratories. The questions are organized into four main categories: analytical false positives, clinical false positives, window of detection, and false negatives. Additional information on these parameters can also be found in appendix A, *Urine Toxic Screen Template*. The answers provided are as simple and straightforward as they should be when given over the telephone or within an email. When appropriate, the reader is referred to the relevant chapters in this book for additional information or more detailed discussion.

1. What is clinical urine drugs-of-abuse testing?

It is drug testing for medical purposes, not forensic testing for the workplace or criminal justice system.

It is usually not a broad-spectrum drug screen (eg, for suspected drug overdose) but typically is a targeted panel of drugs of abuse by immunoassays (except ethanol):

Amphetamines
Barbiturates
Benzodiazepines
Buprenorphine
Cannabinoids
Cocaine metabolite (benzoylecgonine)
Ethanol
Fentanyl
Hydrocodone/hydromorphone
MDMA/MDA
Methadone
Opiates
Oxycodone/oxymorphone
Phencyclidine (PCP)

2. How is testing performed?

It can be a one- or two-step testing process.

One Step

1. Initial test ("screen") by immunoassays.

Use a cutoff to define a result as negative or positive:

result ≥ cutoff = positive
result < cutoff = negative
eg, THC metabolite assay cutoff = 50 ng/mL
50 ng/mL = positive
49 ng/mL = negative

Negative does not mean devoid of drug.

Positive result by immunoassay is a presumptive positive only. Definitive test will determine if it is a true or false positive.

Two Steps

1. Initial test as described above.

2. Definitive test. Initial test positive result confirmed by second test (not mandatory in clinical testing; see questions 11 through 13).

3. What are the SAMHSA Guidelines for drug testing?

These refer to the Mandatory Guidelines for Federal Workplace Drug Testing Programs first promulgated by the National Institute on Drug Abuse (NIDA) and later by the Substance Abuse and Mental Health Services Administration (SAMHSA). These guidelines, and also those issued by the Department of Transportation (DOT), are mandatory for workplace drug testing programs for federal agency employees only, or industries regulated by the DOT, and do not apply to nonregulated workplace drug testing programs or clinical drug testing. The initial immunoassay test and definitive test cutoffs, however, have been adopted in many clinical testing programs.

Guidelines available at https://www.samhsa.gov/sites/default/files/workplace/frn_vol_82_7920_.pdf. (See also chapter 6, *Workplace Drug Testing*.)

4. What should one look for in a clinical urine drug test laboratory report?

Drugs/metabolites tested.

Drugs/metabolites test results (negative or positive).

Assay cutoffs. Assays with different cutoffs give different results on the same urine sample, eg, a urine containing 35 ng/mL of THC-metabolite will test positive by a 20-ng/mL cutoff assay but test negative by a 50-ng/mL cutoff assay.

Positive result (unconfirmed positive or confirmed positive by definitive testing).

5. What are some of the frequently asked questions about clinical urine drug test results?

Questions are grouped into four categories:

I. Analytical false positives
II. Clinical false positives
III. Negatives
IV. Window of detection

I. Questions Relating to Analytical False Positives

6. What is an analytical false positive?

It is when a test detects substance(s) other than the target drug or the metabolite due to nonspecificity of the initial immunoassay, eg, a positive phencyclidine (PCP) assay result given by dextromethorphan.

An immunoassay is not specific for one analyte; it will detect all substances that have immunoreactivity with the assay antibody. Thus, a positive result can be a true positive or false positive and is therefore a presumptive positive only, to be confirmed by a definitive test. Check the assay kit package insert for cross-reacting substances.

Definitive testing eliminates analytical false positives.

(See chapter 11, *Laboratory-Based Screening Assays in Support of Pain Management;* and chapter 12, *Approaches to Broad-Spectrum Drug Testing in the Clinical Laboratory.*)

7. My patient has a positive amphetamines immunoassay result. She is on bupropion. Can bupropion explain the positive amphetamines result?

Bupropion is detected by some amphetamines immunoassays and can give a false-positive result. (See also appendix A, *Urine Toxic Screen Template.*)

Answer 1

Definitive testing was performed and reported the presence of amphetamine and methamphetamine: The patient was taking more than just bupropion.

Answer 2

Definitive testing was not performed: Bupropion may or may not be the only drug taken. Check the assay kit package insert for cross-reacting substances.

(See chapter 12, *Approaches to Broad-Spectrum Drug Testing in the Clinical Laboratory.*)

8. My patient tested positive for cocaine metabolite but swears he is not a cocaine user. What else can give a positive cocaine (metabolite) result?

Answer 1

Definitive testing was performed and the cocaine metabolite (benzoylecgonine) was confirmed: The patient was exposed to cocaine.

Answer 2

Definitive testing was not performed: Although the cocaine metabolite immunoassay is "quite specific" for benzoylecgonine, a false-positive result cannot be ruled out definitively. Check assay kit package insert for cross-reacting substances.

See also question 9.

(See chapter 11, *Laboratory Based Screening Assays in Support of Pain Management.*)

9. My patient claimed her use of Anbesol for her sore gum caused her positive "cocaine" result. Is it a valid claim?

The "cocaine" assay is actually an assay for the metabolite benzoylecgonine, not cocaine. Anbesol contains benzocaine, which is not detected by the cocaine metabolite assay (neither are lidocaine, mepivacaine, bupivacaine, procaine, or chloroprocaine). Use of extemporaneous formulation containing cocaine, eg, TAC (tetracaine, adrenaline, cocaine) or 1% cocaine solution (for ophthalmic procedures) can give a true-positive result.

See also question 8.

10. Definitive tests eliminate analytical false-positive results. What is an acceptable definitive test?

Repeat analysis by the same assay is not definitive testing. A definitive assay should be:

- Based on an analytical principle different from that of initial test (eg, do not use a different amphetamines immunoassay to confirm the initial amphetamines positive result)
- More specific and equally or more sensitive than initial test (eg, do not use an amphetamines immunoassay to confirm a positive result given by liquid chromatography-tandem mass spectrometry [LC-MS/MS])
- Performed on a fresh aliquot obtained from the original container

11. When should one order a definitive test?

In clinical drug testing, definitive tests are not always done automatically for confirmation of initial immunoassay positive results. They are ordered at the discretion of the physician or in consultation with the laboratory scientist/pathologist, eg, when the initial test result is *clinically unexpected* or probably performed prior to taking an administrative action (eg, expelling a patient from a drug treatment program).

12. What does a confirmed positive result mean?

It is an *analytical true-positive* result that suggests the patient was *exposed* to the drug prior to urine collection. Do not overinterpret a positive result in terms of:

- When (was exposure)
- How (active or passive exposure)
- How much (dose)
- Impairment (at time of collection)

13. Is a confirmed positive result a true-positive result?

A confirmed positive result is an *analytical true* positive.

But

An *analytical true* positive can be a *clinical false* positive.

Therefore, there has to be a clinical interpretation of an analytical true-positive result (see next question).

II. Questions Relating to Clinical False Positives

14. What is a clinical *true*-positive result? What is a clinical *false*-positive result?

Interpret an analytical true-positive as being a clinical true-positive or a clinical false-positive result in the context of identifying illicit drug use.

Clinical true positive (for illicit drug use): The patient does not have a legitimate reason for testing positive, eg, hydrocodone use without prescription.

Clinical false positive (for illicit drug use): The patient has a legitimate reason for testing positive, eg, a positive opiates result due to prescription opiate use, poppy seed ingestion.

15. What are examples of clinical false-positive results?

Clinical false-positive result (for illicit drug use):

- The medication contains the target drug: acetaminophen with codeine, medical marijuana, thus giving analytical true positive for the target drug, but patient has a valid prescription for the medication.
- The substance metabolizes to the target drug: selegiline is metabolized to methamphetamine (and amphetamine), thus giving an analytical true positive for the amphetamines test; hydrocodone is metabolized to hydromorphone, thus giving an analytical true positive for hydromorphone.
- A food item may contain the target drug: poppy seeds contain morphine, hemp seed oil contains THC, thus giving analytical true positives for the opiates and cannabinoids tests, respectively.
- Passive exposure: passive inhalation of marijuana smoke can give an analytical true positive for the cannabinoids test.

For additional listing of prescription and nonprescription drugs that could affect a drug test, consult the *Medical Reviewer Officer Manual for the Federal Workplace Drug Testing Program,* available at https://www.samhsa.gov/sites/default/files/workplace/mro_guidance_manual_508_final_march_2018.pdf.

(Kwong TC. Clinical false positives. In: Dasgupta A, ed. *Handbook of Drug Monitoring Methods: Therapeutics and Drugs of Abuse.* Totowa, NJ: Humana Press; 2008:395-406.)

16. Can I assume a confirmed positive morphine is indicative of heroin use? What are the possible sources of morphine found in urine?

Morphine is a metabolite of heroin (diacetylmorphine). There are other sources of the morphine in urine:

- Morphine use
- Codeine use
- Heroin use
- Poppy seed ingestion (some are contaminated with morphine)

The confirmed presence of morphine in urine is therefore not absolute evidence of heroin use.

(See chapter 24, *Opioids 1: Opiates and Semisynthetic Opioids.*)

17. How important is ingestion of poppy seeds to a positive morphine test?

Some batches of poppy seeds are contaminated with morphine and codeine, and the detection of morphine (and codeine) is not a laboratory error (it is an analytical true-positive result).

Using a higher opiates immunoassay cutoff at 2000 ng/mL (instead of 300 ng/mL) eliminates most but not all opiates-positive results due to ingestion of poppy seeds. However, in the clinical context of a hospital setting, 300 ng/mL is the preferred cutoff to ensure that the semisynthetic opiates will be detected.

(Lachenmeier DW, Sproll C, Musshoff F. Poppy seed foods and opiate drug testing: where are we today? *Ther Drug Monit.* 2010;32:11-18. Also see chapter 24, *Opioids 1: Opiates and Semisynthetic Opioids.*)

18. Is there a test to differentiate poppy seed ingestion from heroin use?

Diacetylmorphine (heroin)
↓
Monoacetylmorphine (6-AM)
↑
Codeine → Morphine ← Poppy seeds

6-AM is an intermediary metabolite of heroin metabolism, and its presence indicates heroin use. The short half-life of 6-AM limits its detection window to 10 to 12 hours or less since exposure. 6-AM is usually associated with high morphine concentrations (>2000 ng/mL), but detection of 6-AM in urines that have very low morphine concentrations has been reported.

(See chapter 24, *Opioids 1: Opiates and Semisynthetic Opioids.*)

19. My patient is on Tylenol with codeine, and her drug test is positive for codeine and morphine. Is the patient using morphine too?

Morphine is a metabolite of codeine. The ratio of morphine to codeine in the urine of <2 indicates use of codeine, not consumption of contaminated poppy seeds.

(ElSohly MA, Jones AB. Morphine and codeine in biological fluids: approaches to source differentiation. *Forensic Sci Rev.* 1989;1:13-22. See also chapter 24, *Opioids 1: Opiates and Semisynthetic Opioids.*)

20. A pain clinic patient on MS Contin (morphine; 200 mg/day) tested positive for morphine and hydromorphone. Was the patient using nonprescribed hydromorphone?

Hydromorphone is a minor metabolite of morphine. It can be detected after high doses of morphine, but its concentration is usually <6% that of morphine. Similarly, hydrocodone is detectable after high doses of codeine. Understanding the minor pathways of opiates metabolism is important in making the correct interpretation without wrongly accusing a patient of illicit drug use.

(See chapter 3, *Laboratory Support of Chronic Opioid Therapy;* and chapter 24, *Opioids 1: Opiates and Semisynthetic Opioids.*)

21. A pain clinic patient on OxyContin (oxycodone; 80 mg/day) tested positive for oxycodone (50,000 ng/mL) and hydrocodone (300 ng/mL). Would this be nonprescription use of hydrocodone?

Hydrocodone is not a (minor) metabolite of oxycodone. Presence of hydrocodone can be attributed to illicit use of hydrocodone or as an impurity in the pharmaceutical material used for oxycodone manufacturing. Low concentrations of hydrocodone have been found in urine specimens with very high concentrations of oxycodone (33% of specimens with oxycodone at 50,000 to 100,000 ng/mL were positive for hydrocodone).

(West R, West C, Crews B, et al. Anomalous observations of hydrocodone in patients on oxycodone. *Clin Chim Acta.* 2011;412:29-32. See also chapter 3, *Laboratory Support of Chronic Opioid Therapy;* and chapter 24, *Opioids 1: Opiates and Semisynthetic Opioids.*)

III. Questions Relating to Negative Results

22. I witnessed my patient taking his methadone. Why did he test negative for methadone?

Some patients (~10%) metabolize methadone rapidly; they have low urine methadone and high metabolite concentrations. Therefore, a test that detects only methadone, and not the metabolites, may be negative for the fast metabolizers, but the test for the metabolite EDDP will be positive. The metabolite assay, but not the methadone assay, will be negative if the urine has been spiked with methadone.

(Preston KL, Epstein DH, Davoudzadeh D, Huestis MA. Methadone and metabolite urine concentrations in patients maintained on methadone. *J Anal Toxicol.* 2003;27(6):332-341.)

23. My patient on OxyContin had a negative opiates drug test. Was she noncompliant? (I suspect she might be diverting her OxyContin.)

One possible explanation is that the opiates assay immunoreactivity for oxycodone (check the opiates assay package insert for cross-reactivities) is not sufficient to detect oxycodone after therapeutic doses. "Opiates" assays target morphine and codeine and have lower reactivities for the semisynthetics. For example:

Opiates	*Cross-Reactivity*
Morphine, codeine	+++
Hydromorphone	++
Hydrocodone	++
Oxycodone	+

OxyContin (oxycodone), particularly on low pain-management doses, is not well detected by standard the opiates assays even at the low (300 ng/mL) cutoff. Separate assays specific for oxycodone detection are available.

(See chapter 4, *Clinical Pathology Consultation for Pain Management Services;* and chapter 11 *Laboratory-Based Screening Assays in Support of Pain Management.*)

24. My patient is on 2 Vicodin (hydrocodone-acetaminophen) a day, but her opiates test is negative. She is adamant that she has been compliant. Is there a reason why the test is negative?

The opiates immunoassay targets morphine and codeine and has lesser reactivities with semisynthetic opiates. For example, with one opiates immunoassay, hydrocodone has 50% the reactivity of morphine. Thus, the urine concentration of hydrocodone (or hydromorphone) of a patient on low-dose hydrocodone (or hydromorphone) may not be high enough to give a positive opiates result. This negative result is a clinical false-negative. Immunoassays designed for hydrocodone and hydromorphone detection are now commercially available. Alternatively, the laboratory can bypass initial immunoassay testing and offer direct definitive testing using mass spectrometry-based methodologies, which have lower detection limits for hydrocodone and hydromorphone.

(See chapter 3, *Laboratory Support of Chronic Opioid Therapy;* chapter 4, *Clinical Pathology Consultation for Pain Management Services;* and chapter 11, *Laboratory-Based Screening Assays in Support of Pain Management.*)

25. My patient is on methadone, but her opiates test came back negative. Was she noncompliant? (I suspect she might be diverting her methadone.)

One possible explanation is the opiates assay immunospecificity (check the opiates assay package insert for cross-reactivities) is not sufficient to detect methadone. "Opiates" assays target opiates, not all opioids. These nonopiate opioids are not detected by opiates immunoassays:

- Buprenorphine*
- Fentanyl*
- Meperidine
- Methadone*
- Pentazocine
- Propoxyphene*
- Tramadol*

*Specific immunoassays are available.

(See chapter 11, *Laboratory-Based Screening Assays in Support of Pain Management.* See also question 24.)

26. My patient said there are many easily purchased products for "beating" the drug tests. What are these adulteration products?

False-negative result by adulteration products:

- Dilution products
- Cleansing products
- Adulteration additives
- Substitute urine (reservoir, catheter)

(See also chapter 6, *Workplace Drug Testing,* for additional information on adulteration and specimen validity testing.)

27. Can you give me a list of the most popular adulteration products? Do they work?

This is a moving target. It is a very dynamic marketplace with new products and frequent reformulation of existing products. Not all products are effective. See next the question for common adulteration tests.

28. How can a laboratory detect adulteration?

- Temperature, at time of collection
- Visual inspection
- Urine pH
- Urine specific gravity and creatinine
- Tests for oxidants (nitrite, Chromium VI, halogens, pyridine)
- Others: glutaraldehyde, surfactant, others
- Immunoassay, chromatography, mass spectrometry assay response

(See chapter 6, *Workplace Drug Testing.*)

IV. Questions Relating to Window of Detection

29. How long will a person test positive after drug use?

There is no simple and definitive answer. It will depend on:

- Dose (difficult to estimate)
- History of use (tissue store)
- Pharmacokinetics (absorption, distribution, metabolism, excretion)
- Urine pH
- Degree of hydration
- Assay specificity and cutoff

(See appendix A, *Urine Toxic Screen Template.*)

30. A patient's THC-metabolite assay was positive on Monday, but the patient denied use; claimed passive exposure at Saturday night party. Is it possible?

Detectable amount of THC-carboxylic acid (THCA) is present in urine after passive exposure (secondary smoke). However, after exposure under normal social settings, the urine THCA concentration is usually below the popular assay cutoff of 50 ng/mL. The urine specimen with the highest THCA concentration is the one collected in the first several hours post exposure. It is more difficult to discount the claim of passive exposure if exposure is recent or under extreme conditions.

(See chapter 18, *Cannabis.*)

31. A patient tested positive for "marijuana" today but tested negative last week. Is this indicative of new use or residual drug excretion?

Urine Δ^9-THC-carboxylic acid (THCA) concentrations depend partly on the urine volume (hydration status). The same amount of THCA in a larger urine volume gives a lower concentration, one that might be below assay cutoff, thus giving a negative result. To answer the question of new use versus residual excretion may require serial sampling to construct an "excretion curve," which requires:

- Quantitative measurement of THCA in serially collected urine specimens
- Normalization of THCA concentration to urine creatinine concentration
- Following the trend of THCA-to-creatinine ratios with time

32. A patient's "THC" by an immunoassay went from 35 ng/mL to 42 ng/mL in 1 week. Is the increase indicative of new use?

This is not a real change if assay imprecision is taken into consideration. Urine volume varies with hydration status; concentration can change with time. Immunoassay measures Δ^9-THC-carboxylic acid (THCA) and many other THC metabolites of different immunoreactivities and varying concentrations. The real THCA concentration is not known. The "concentration" result given by a semiquantitative immunoassay is actually the calibrator-equivalent concentration.

33. My patient's latest test shows the urine oxycodone concentration is lower than that of his previous test. I suspect he has taken less than his prescribed dose or has skipped one or more doses.

Urine drug concentrations cannot be extrapolated to serum concentrations or to the amount of drug taken. The urine drug concentration is highly variable, being affected by dose, absorption, distribution, metabolism, excretion, and hydration status.

Appendix E

CAP Proficiency Testing Surveys for Toxicology

Annabel Dizon, MT(ASCP)

For a complete list of Toxicology Surveys and program details, please review the Toxicology Survey program section of the College of American Pathologists (CAP) Surveys and Anatomic Pathology Education Programs catalog (www.cap.org).

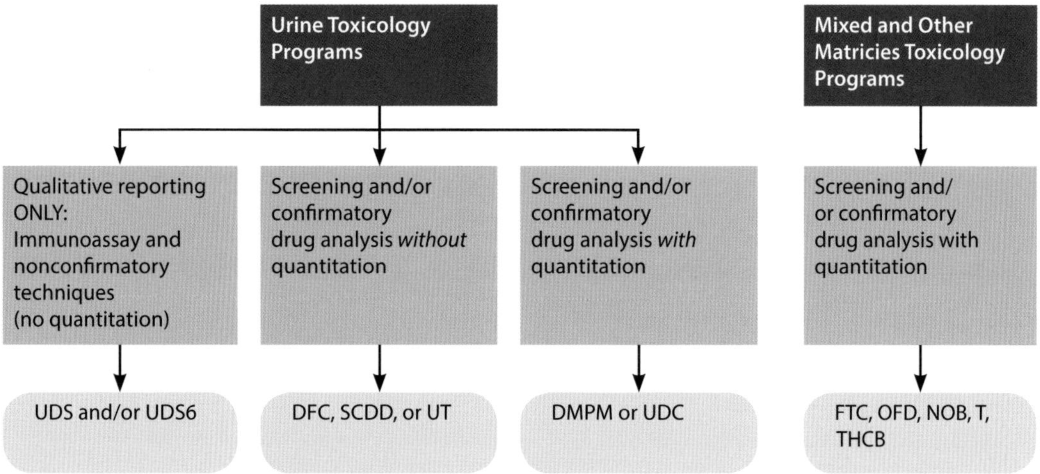

Program Acronym	Program Name	Program Acronym	Program Name
DFC	Drug-Facilitated Crime	DMPM	Drug Monitoring for Pain Management
FTC	Forensic Toxicology, Criminalistics	NOB	Novel Opioids and Benzodiazepines
OFD	Oral Fluid for Drugs of Abuse	SCDD	Synthetic Cannabinoid/ Designer Drugs
T	Toxicology	THCB	Blood Cannabinoids
UDC	Forensic Urine Drug Testing, Confirmatory*	UDS	Urine Drug Testing, Screening*
UDS6	Urine Drug Testing, Screening (Limited)*	UT	Urine Toxicology

* Co-sponsored programs with the AACC (American Association for Clinical Chemistry).

Index

AABB, 77, 78, 84
abacavir, 112, 115, 118
AB-CHMINACA
descriptive chemistry, 283
origin, 282
overdose and toxicity, 284
pharmacokinetics, 284
potency compared to delta-9-THC, 283
absorption, 51-52, 101-102
absorption, distribution, metabolism, and excretion (ADME), 101, 107, 108
accreditation
agencies with deemed status from CMS, 78
condition level requirements for, 78-84
forensic testing, 77-78, 86
acetaminophen, 10, 17, 102
abuse potential and characteristics, 304-305
analytical issues, 306
clinical issues, 306-307
descriptive chemistry, 304
intended use, 304
mechanism of action, 304
metabolism, 305
modes of analysis, 305-306
origin, 304
overdose and toxicity, 306-307
pharmacokinetics, 304
pharmacology, 304-305
results interpretation, 306
Rumack-Matthew nomogram for determining hepatotoxicity, 305-306, 342
specimen types and characteristics, 305
toxic dose and concentration, 302
acetone
analysis, 201-202
analytical issues and problems, 202
analytical parameters, 202
anion gap (AG), 202
clearance, 199
clinical issues, 202-203
context of human use, 198
descriptive chemistry, 197
exposure, 198-199
half-life, 199
hazmat considerations, 198, 199
metabolism and excretion, 199-200
mortality and morbidity, 199
osmolal gap (OG), 202
toxicity, 200
treatment and management, 203
volume of distribution, 199
acetylfentanyl
analgesic activity and potency relative to morphine, 288
descriptive chemistry, 287
dose and duration of action, 289
overdose and toxicity, 289-290
pharmacology, 288-289
6-acetylmorphine (6-AM), 262, 266, 267. *See also* 6-monoacetylmorphine
cutoff for federal workplace drug testing program, 68
FDA-cleared oral fluid immunoassay cutoffs, 161
oral fluid, reported detection time in, 161
adulterant testing, urine, 5
adulterated specimen, 68-69
alcohol, 79, 162-163. *See also* ethanol
blood alcohol concentration (BAC), 189-190, 193
alfentanil, 274
alprazolam, 17. *See also* benzodiazepines
abuse potential and characteristics, 257
analysis, 257-258
analytical issues, 258
descriptive chemistry, 253
detection window in urine, 253
half-life, 255
intended uses, 255
metabolites, active, 256
origin, 253
pharmacokinetics, 256
pharmacology, 255-257
toxic dose and concentrations, 259
volume of distribution, 253
alternative matrices for testing, 8-9
hair, 170-176
meconium, umbilical cord tissue, and breast milk, 179-181
oral fluid, 157-166
sweat, 176-179
American Association for Clinical Chemistry (AACC), 18, 258
proficiency testing with CAP, 81, 84, 85, 86
American Association of Poison Control Centers (AAPCC), 300
American Board of Forensic Toxicology (ABFT) Laboratory Accreditation Program, 77
American College of Physicians Medical Laboratory Evaluation (MLE) program, 81, 84, 85
American Osteopathic Association (AOA), 77, 78
American Proficiency Institute (API), 81, 84-85

American Society for Histocompatibility and Immunogenetics (ASHI), 77, 78, 84
American Society of Addiction Medicine, 18
American Society of Crime Laboratory Directors Laboratory Accreditation Board (ASCLD/LAB), 77
amitriptyline, 17, 102, 103, 109, 115
amobarbital. *See also* barbiturates
- abuse potential and characteristics, 250
- analytical issues, 250
- clearance, 248
- clinical use, 249
- descriptive chemistry, 246
- detection window in urine, 249
- duration of action, 249
- half-life, 248, 249
- origin, 246
- pharmacokinetics, 248, 249
- toxic dose and concentrations, 251
- volume of distribution, 248

amphetamine. *See also* amphetamines
- cutoff for federal workplace drug testing program, 68
- detection time in oral fluid, 165
- FDA-cleared oral fluid immunoassay cutoffs, 161
- proposed initial screening and confirmatory cutoffs for hair testing, 171, 172
- proposed initial screening and confirmatory cutoffs for sweat patch testing, 178

amphetamines, 10. *See also* methamphetamine
- abuse potential and characteristics, 240-241
- analysis, 241
- analytical issues, 243
- clinical issues, 243-244
- cross-reactivity, 242
- descriptive chemistry, 239
- EWDTS recommended initial screening and confirmatory cutoffs for hair testing, 172
- FDA-cleared oral fluid immunoassay cutoffs, 161
- half-life, 240
- intended uses, 239-240
- mechanism of action, 240
- modes of analysis, 241-243
- oral fluid, reported detection time in, 161
- oral fluid testing for, 163
- origin, 239
- overdose and toxicity, 244
- pharmacokinetics, 240
- pharmacology, 239-241
- results interpretation, 243-244
- SAMHSA proposed initial screening and confirmatory cutoffs for hair testing, 171
- SAMHSA proposed initial screening and confirmatory cutoffs for sweat patch testing, 178
- specimen types and characteristics, 241
- volume of distribution, 240

anion gap (AG), 202
ANSI-ASQ National Accreditation Board (ANAB), 77
arsenic, 312-314
- physico-chemical properties, 310

autopsy, hospital, and toxicology testing, 90-98
- external examination, 91-92
- indications for, 90
- medical examiner/coroner (ME/C) involvement in, 96-97
- medical records review, 91
- medicolegal issues, 96-97
- microscopic examination, 92
- National Association of Medical Examiners (NAME) standards, 90
- postmortem redistribution, 95
- specimen collection, 93-94
- specimen selection, 94
- toxicology results, interpretation of, 95-96
- toxicology testing, ordering of, 94-95

barbiturates, 10
- abuse potential and characteristics, 249-250
- analysis, 250
- analytical issues, 250
- clearance, 248
- clinical issues, 251
- clinical uses, 249
- descriptive chemistry, 246-247
- detection window in urine, 249
- duration of action, properties based on, 249
- half-lives, 248
- intended uses, 247-248
- intermediate-acting, 249
- long-acting, 248-249
- mechanism of action, 248
- oral fluid, reported detection time in, 161
- origin, 246
- overdose and toxicity, 251
- pharmacokinetics, 248-249
- pharmacology, 247-250
- results interpretation, 251
- saliva/plasma (S/P) ratio, average, 158
- short-acting, 249
- specimen types and characteristics, 250
- toxic dose and concentration, 251
- ultra-short-acting, 247, 249
- volumes of distribution, 248

benzodiazepines, 10
- abuse potential and characteristics, 257
- analysis, 257-258
- analytical issues, 257-258
- clinical issues, 258-259
- descriptive chemistry, 253-255
- designer, 292-294
- detection window in urine, 256
- duration of action, 256
- EWDTS recommended initial screening and confirmatory cutoffs for hair testing, 172
- half-lives, 256

intended uses, 255
mechanism of action, 256
metabolism of common, 29
metabolites, active, 256
oral fluid, reported detection time in, 161
oral fluid testing for, 163
origin, 253
overdose and toxicity, 259
pharmacokinetics, 256-257
pharmacology, 255-257
results interpretation, 258-259
SAMHSA proposed initial screening and confirmatory cutoffs for sweat patch testing, 178
specimen types and characteristics, 257
toxic dose and concentrations, 259
volumes of distribution, 256-257
benzoylecgonine, 229-231, 234-235
concentrations detected in a population of drivers suspected of impaired driving and in postmortem cases, 234
cutoff for federal workplace drug testing program, 68, 161
FDA-cleared oral immunoassay cutoffs, 161
hair testing for, 232
oral fluid testing for, 161, 163
bioavailability, 101-102
biotransformation, 52-54
blood alcohol concentration (BAC), 189-190, 193
blood testing, comparison with oral fluid, 164-166
breastfeeding, risk of exposure to substances in children, 59-60
breast milk, drugs in, 181
broad-spectrum drug testing, 129-139
analytical approaches, 130-134
gas chromatography-mass spectrometry (GC-MS), 130-130
high-resolution mass spectrometry (HRMS), 133, 135-137
liquid chromatography-mass spectrometry (LC-MS), 131-132
poisoning and overdose trends, 130
quadrupole time-of-flight (QTOF), 133-134
tandem mass spectrometry (MS/MS), 132-133
targeted versus untargeted mass spectral data acquisition, 134-135
time-of-flight (TOF) mass analyzers, 133
buprenorphine, 10, 17. *See also* opioids, synthetic
abuse potential and characteristics, 275-276
analytical issues, 276
descriptive chemistry, 270
EWDTS recommended initial screening and confirmatory cutoffs for hair testing, 172
half-life, 274
intended use, 272
mechanism of action, 273
oral fluid, reported detection time in, 161
origin, 270
overdose and toxicity, 278
pharmacokinetics, 273-274
saliva/plasma (S/P) ratio, average, 158
toxic dose, 277
volume of distribution, 273
bupropion, 17, 177, 243
buspirone, 17, 246
butabarbital. *See also* barbiturates
clearance, 248
clinical use, 249
descriptive chemistry, 246, 247
detection window in urine, 249
duration of action, 249
half-life, 248, 249
origin, 246
pharmacokinetics, 248, 249
toxic dose and concentration, 251
volume of distribution, 248
butalbital. *See also* barbiturates
abuse potential and characteristics, 250
analytical issues, 250
clearance, 248
clinical use, 249
descriptive chemistry, 246
detection window in urine, 249
duration of action, 249
half-life, 248, 249
intended uses, 248
origin, 246
pharmacokinetics, 248, 249
toxic dose and concentrations, 251
volume of distribution, 248
1,4-butanediol (1,4BD)
abuse potential and characteristics, 215-216
analysis, 216
clinical issues, 216-217
descriptive chemistry, 214-215
intended use, 215
interpretation of results, 216
mechanism of action, 215
modes of analysis, 216
origin, 214
overdose and toxicity, 216
pharmacokinetics, 215
pharmacology, 215-216
specimen types and characteristics, 216

cadmium, 315-316
physico-chemical properties, 310
cannabidiol, 206
cannabinoids. *See also* cannabis
EWDTS recommended initial screening and confirmatory cutoffs for hair testing, 172
oral fluid testing for, 164
SAMHSA proposed initial screening and confirmatory cutoffs for hair testing, 171

SAMHSA proposed initial screening and confirmatory cutoffs for sweat patch testing, 178
synthetic, 282-284
cannabinol, 206
cannabis. *See also* cannabinoids; delta-9-tetrahydrocannabinol (THC)
abuse potential and characteristics, 209
adverse effects and complications, 211-212
analysis, 209-210
analytical parameters, 209
cardiovascular effects, 211
clinical issues, 210-211
CNS effects, 211
descriptive chemistry, 205-206
excretion, 209
intended use/medical use, 206-207
mechanism of action, 207
medical, formulations of, 207
metabolism, 208-209
metabolites, principle, 208
modes of analysis, 210
origin, 205
overdose and toxicity, 211
pharmacokinetics, 207-208
reproductive effects, 212
respiratory effects, 211
specimen types, requirements, and characteristics, 209-210
toxic dose, 212
treatment and rehabilitation for overdose and toxicity, 212
volume of distribution, 209
carbamazepine, 9, 17, 79, 102, 109, 110, 115, 177
carbon monoxide (CO), 321-322
signs and symptoms associated with acute intoxication, 322
carboxyhemoglobin (COHb), 9, 58
Centers for Disease Control and Prevention (CDC), 7, 179, 189
estimates of fentanyl potency, 35, 44, 47
guideline for prescribing opioids, 18, 122
reported drug-induced deaths, 90, 275
Centers for Medicare and Medicaid Services (CMS), 76, 142
accreditation, 78-84
exemption from CLIA, 77
chlordiazepoxide, 17. *See also* benzodiazepines
descriptive chemistry, 253
detection window in urine, 256
half-life, 256
intended uses, 255
metabolites, active, 256
origin, 253
pharmacokinetics, 256
toxic dose and concentrations, 259
volume of distribution, 256
clearance (Cl), 103-105
Clinical Laboratory Improvement Amendments of 1988 (CLIA), 76-84
CLIA certification, 76-77
CLIA-exempt laboratories, 76-77, 142
definition of a laboratory under, 76
laboratory director responsibilities, 81, 83
personnel requirements, 81, 83-84
clinical pathology consultation
case examples, 32-48
CPT codes for, 28
clonazepam, 17. *See also* benzodiazepines
abuse potential and characteristics, 257
analytical issues, 258
descriptive chemistry, 253
detection window in urine, 256
half-life, 256
intended uses, 255
metabolite, active, 256
origin, 253
pharmacology, 255-257
toxic dose and concentrations, 259
volume of distribution, 256
clopidogrel, 113, 115, 117
clorazepate, 17
club drugs, 214-227
cocaethylene, 229
concentrations detected in a population of drivers suspected of impaired driving and in postmortem cases, 234
cocaine, 10
absorption, 229
abuse potential and characteristics, 231-232
analysis, 232-234
analytical issues, 233-234
concentrations detected in a population of drivers suspected of impaired driving and in postmortem cases, 234
clinical issues, 234-235
descriptive chemistry, 228
EWDTS recommended initial screening and confirmatory cutoffs for hair testing, 172
excretion, 231
FDA-cleared oral fluid immunoassay cutoffs, 161
hair testing for, 232
half-life, 230
intended use, 228-229
mechanism of action, 229
metabolism, pathways, 230
modes of analysis, 232-233
oral fluid, reported detection time in, 161
oral fluid testing for, 163
origin, 228
overdose and toxicity, 235-236
pharmacokinetics, 229-231
pharmacology, 228-232
SAMHSA proposed initial screening and confirmatory cutoffs for hair testing, 171

SAMHSA proposed initial screening and confirmatory cutoffs for sweat patch testing, 178
saliva/plasma (S/P) ratio, average, 158
specimen types and characteristics, 232
treatment of overdose, 236
codeine, 17, 115, 118-119. *See also* opiates/opioids
cutoff for federal workplace drug testing program, 68, 161
descriptive chemistry, 262
estimated morphine equivalent, 265
half-life, 265
metabolic relationships, 262
modes of analysis, 266
oral fluid, reported detection time in, 161
origin, 261
results interpretation, 267
saliva/plasma (S/P) ratio, average, 158
volume of distribution, 265
College of American Pathologists (CAP), 66, 77, 93
CAP 15189, 84
FDT Accreditation Program, 77
Laboratory Accreditation Program, 141
proficiency testing, 6, 28, 84, 85, 86, 361
Commission on Laboratory Accreditation (COLA), 77, 78, 84
condition level requirements for accreditation
facility administration, 79-80
inspection, 84
personnel, 81, 83-84
proficiency testing, 78-79
quality systems, 80-81
confirmation testing, 4-5, 140
Controlled Substances Act (CSA), 73
CPT codes 80500 or 80502, appropriate use of, 28
cyanide, 322-324
cyclooxygenase-2 inhibitors, 17

DAWN Report, 14
definitive testing, 4-5, 22-24
Department of Health and Human Services (HHS), 66-70, 77. *See also* Substance Abuse and Mental Health Services Administration (SAMHSA)
Department of Transportation (DOT), 66, 69, 73, 162-163
detoxification, 52
dextromethorphan (DXM)
abuse potential and characteristics, 218
analysis, 218
analytical issues, 218
clinical issues, 218
descriptive chemistry, 217
half-life, 215
intended uses, 217
mechanism of action, 217
modes of analysis, 218
origin, 217
overdose and toxicity, 218
pharmacokinetics, 217
pharmacology, 217-218
specimen types and characteristics, 218
volume of distribution, 215
diazepam, 17. *See also* benzodiazepines
abuse potential and characteristics, 257
analytical issues, 258
descriptive chemistry, 254
detection window in urine, 256
half-life, 53, 256
intended uses, 255
modes of analysis, 257
origin, 253
pharmacokinetics, 256-257
pharmacology, 255-257
results interpretation, 259
saliva/plasma (S/P) ratio, average, 158
toxic dose and concentrations, 259
volume of distribution, 256
dicoumarol, 326
digoxin, 9, 79, 95, 102, 107, 109
dilute specimen, 68
distribution, drug, 52, 102-103
Drug Enforcement Administration (DEA), 73, 215, 239, 273, 282
drug screens, 3
duloxetine, 17

ecstasy. *See also* methylenedioxymethamphenamine (MDMA)
assays for, 20, 70
cross-reactivity, 242
elimination rate constant (K_e), 104
emergency department, 3, 4
challenges associated with testing, 10-13
laboratory-specific testing menu, 7-8
point-of-care testing (POCT), 8
stat quantitative serum toxicology assays required to support, 9
supporting, 7-16
Tier 1 tests, 7-9
Tier 2 tests, 10
toxic agents, commonly encountered, 14
toxidromes, commonly encountered, 13-15
turnaround time (TAT), acceptable, 8
l-ephedrine, cross-reactivity, 242
ethanol, 9, 79
abuse potential and characteristics, 189
adverse effects, 189
analysis, 1190-192
analytical issues and problems, 192
back-extrapolation of BAC, 193
biomarkers, 194
clinical issues, 192-193
descriptive chemistry, 189
diseases, common, attributable to, 189

effects on children, 57-58
estimate of dose, 193
EWDTS recommended initial screening and confirmatory cutoffs for hair testing, 172
metabolism and excretion, 190
modes of analysis, 191-192
oral fluid testing for, 162-163
overdose and toxicity, 189
pharmacokinetics, 190
pharmacology, 189-190
plasma/serum versus blood testing, 190
postmortem considerations, 191
saliva/plasma (S/P) ratio, average, 158
sources, other, 193
tolerance, 192-193
toxic dose, 190
treatment and rehabilitation for overdose and toxicity, 193-194
type of agent, 189
urine testing, 190-191
vitreous fluid testing, 191

ethosuximide, 79, 102

ethylene glycol, 9
analysis, 201-202
analytical issues and problems, 202
analytical parameters, 202
anion gap (AG), 202
clearance, 199
clinical issues, 202, 203
context of human use, 198
descriptive chemistry, 197
exposure, 198-199
half-life, 199
hazmat considerations, 198, 199
metabolism and excretion, 201
mortality and morbidity, 199
osmolal gap (OG), 204
toxicity, 201
treatment and management, 204
volume of distribution, 199

etizolam. *See also* benzodiazepines; novel psychoactive substances
abuse potential and characteristics, 257, 293
cross-reactivity, 294, 295
descriptive chemistry, 254
detection window in urine, 256
half-life, 256
intended use, 255, 293
metabolites, active, 256
modes of analysis, 257
origin, 292
overdose and toxicity, 293-294
pharmacokinetics, 256-257, 293
pharmacology, 255-257
toxic dose and concentration, 259
volume of distribution, 256-257

European Monitoring Centre for Drugs and Drug Addiction (EMCDDA), 282

European Workplace Drug Testing Society (EWDTS), 170
recommended initial screening and confirmatory cutoffs for hair testing, 172

excretion, 54, 103

fentanyl, 10, 17, 20. *See also* opioids, synthetic
abuse potential and characteristics, 275-276
analgesic activity and potency relative to morphine, 288
analytical issues, 276
descriptive chemistry, 271
half-life, 275
illicit, 287-290
intended use, 272
mechanism of action, 273
origin, 270
overdose and toxicity, 278
pharmacokinetics, 274
toxic dose, 277
volume of distribution, 275

first-pass metabolism, 102

flunitrazepam. *See also* benzodiazepines
analytical issues, 258
descriptive chemistry, 253, 254
detection window in urine, 256
half-life, 256
intended uses, 255
metabolite, active, 256
modes of analysis, 257
pharmacokinetics, 256
pharmacology, 255-257
toxic dose and concentrations, 259
volume of distribution, 256

flurazepam. *See also* benzodiazepines
descriptive chemistry, 254
detection window in urine, 256
half-life, 256
intended uses, 255
metabolite, active, 256
pharmacokinetics, 256
pharmacology, 255-257
toxic dose and concentrations, 259
volume of distribution, 256

Food and Drug Administration (FDA), 8, 82, 142-143, 272, 277, 278
approved test, 143
and broad-spectrum drug testing, 136
cleared assay cutoffs, 125, 161
cleared immunoassays, 8, 19, 21, 22, 78, 122, 123
cleared oral fluid immunoassay cutoffs, 161
cleared test, 143
510(k) process, 141
general controls, 141
in vitro diagnostic (IVD) products, 81, 141
and laboratory-developed tests, 81, 143
medical cannabis, approved formulations, 207

and *N*-acetylcystine, 14
nonwaived tests, 142
and OTC analgesics, 300, 305
pharmacogenomic testing, drug labeling comments, 115
premarket approval, 141
and propoxyphene, 8
special controls, 141
terminology and approval processes, 141
test categorization, 142
test validation, 140, 143, 144
verification of test performance, 143
waived tests, 4, 19, 76, 78, 142-143
forensic toxicology testing, 77-78
furanylfentanyl, 276
analgesic activity and potency relative to morphine, 288
descriptive chemistry, 288
dose and duration of action, 289
origin, 287
pharmacokinetics, 288

gabapentin, 17, 102
gamma-butyrolactone (GBL)
abuse potential and characteristics, 215-216
analysis, 216
clinical issues, 216-217
descriptive chemistry, 214
intended use, 215
interpretation of results, 216
mechanism of action, 215
modes of analysis, 216
origin, 214
overdose and toxicity, 216
pharmacokinetics, 215
pharmacology, 215-216
specimen types and characteristics, 216
gamma-hydroxybutyric acid (GHB)
abuse potential and characteristics, 215-216
analysis, 216
analytical issues, 216
clinical issues, 216-217
descriptive chemistry, 214
half-life, 215
intended use, 215
interpretation of results, 216
mechanism of action, 215
modes of analysis, 216
origin, 214
overdose and toxicity, 216
pharmacokinetics, 215
pharmacology, 215-216
specimen types and characteristics, 216
volume of distribution, 215
gas chromatography-mass spectrometry (GC-MS), 130-131
gentamicin, 79

hair, drug detection in, 172-174
hair testing, 170-176
adulteration issues, 176
collection and analysis, 170-171
environmental or external contamination, effects of, 174-175
EWDTS recommended initial screening and confirmatory cutoffs, 172
hair color, effects of, 175-176
SAMHSA proposed initial screening and confirmatory cutoffs, 171
half-life ($t_{1/2}$), 106-107
Health Insurance Portability and Accountability Act of 1996 (HIPAA), 6, 10, 97
heavy metals, 91, 95, 309. *See also* metals
in hair samples, 93, 170
in red blood cells, 103
in tissue samples, 94
heroin. *See also* opiates/opioids
abuse potential and characteristics, 265-266
descriptive chemistry, 262-263
half-life, 265
metabolic relationships, 262
origin, 261
results interpretation, 267
volume of distribution, 265
high-resolution mass spectrometry (HRMS), 133
advantages of, 136-137
data analysis, 135-136
hydrocodone, 17. *See also* opiates/opioids
cutoff for federal workplace drug testing program, 68, 161
descriptive chemistry, 263
estimated morphine equivalent, 265
half-life, 265
metabolic relationships, 262
modes of analysis, 266
oral fluid, reported detection time in, 161
origin, 261
volume of distribution, 265
hydromorphone. *See also* opiates/opioids
cutoff for federal workplace drug testing program, 68, 161
descriptive chemistry, 263
estimated morphine equivalent, 265
half-life, 265
metabolic relationships, 262
modes of analysis, 266
volume of distribution, 265

ibuprofen, 17, 300
immunoassay, initial testing by, 19-22
sensitivity, 21-22
immunoassays, use in pain management
microarray-based, 126-127
in oral fluid drug testing, 125-126
in urine drug testing, 122-125

inspection, 84
invalid result, 68
irinotecan, 115, 117
iron, 9
ISO 15189, 84
isopropanol
analysis, 201-202
analytical issues and problems, 202
analytical parameters, 202
anion gap (AG), 202
clearance, 199
clinical issues, 202-203
context of human use, 198
descriptive chemistry, 197
exposure, 198-199
half-life, 199
hazmat considerations, 198, 199
metabolism and excretion, 200
mortality and morbidity, 199
osmolal gap (OG), 202
toxicity, 201
treatment and management, 203
volume of distribution, 199
ivacaftor, 115

Joint Commission, The, 77, 78, 84, 142
JWH-018
descriptive chemistry, 282
overdose and toxicity, 284
pharmacokinetics, 283-284
potency compared to delta-9-THC, 283

ketamine
abuse potential and characteristics, 221
analysis, 221
analytical issues, 221
clinical issues, 221
descriptive chemistry, 220
EWDTS recommended initial screening and confirmatory cutoffs for hair testing, 172
half-life, 215
intended uses, 220
mechanism of action, 220
modes of analysis, 221
origin, 220
overdose and toxicity, 221
pharmacokinetics, 220-221
pharmacology, 220-221
results interpretation, 221
specimen types and characteristics, 221
volume of distribution, 215

laboratory-developed test (LDT), 22, 122, 162
clinical validation, 136
cutoffs, 125
definition, 143
example checklist for validation and institution of new, 82
method validation, 81, 140, 143
results reporting, 154
for testing alternative matrices, 181
laboratory director, responsibilities under CLIA, 81, 83
lead, 79
acute exposure, 311
blood concentrations and indicated treatment in children, 313
chronic exposure, 311-312
clinical issues, 312
effects of, in children and adults, 312
mechanism of action, 311
modes of analysis, 312
origin and uses, 310-311
physico-chemical properties, 310
specimen types and characteristics, 312
toxicokinetics, 311
legal implications, clinical testing with, 5, 78
legal testing, 5-6
liquid chromatography-mass spectrometry (LC-MS), 131-132, 151-153
lithium, 9, 79, 95, 102, 107
lorazepam, 17. *See also* benzodiazepines
analytical issues, 258
descriptive chemistry, 254
detection window in urine, 256
half-life, 256
intended uses, 255
modes of analysis, 257
origin, 253
pharmacokinetics, 256
pharmacology, 255-257
results interpretation, 259
toxic dose and concentrations, 259
volume of distribution, 256

Mandatory Guidelines for Federal Workplace Drug Testing Programs, 66-70, 77
using oral fluid (OFMG), 67, 157, 158, 159, 160, 161
mass spectrometry
definitive testing by, 22-24
sample preparation for, 152
meconium testing, 179-181
medical-legal testing, 5-6
Medical Review Officer (MRO), 67-69, 70-73
actions for primary specimen reports, 72-73
3-MeO-PCP, 291-292
meperidine, 17. *See also* opioids, synthetic
descriptive chemistry, 271
half-life, 53, 275
intended use, 272
mechanism of action, 273
origin, 270
overdose and toxicity, 277-278

pharmacokinetics, 274
toxic dose, 277
volume of distribution, 275
mephobarbital. *See also* barbiturates
clearance, 248
clinical use, 249
descriptive chemistry, 246, 247
detection window in urine, 249
duration of action, 249
half-life, 248, 249
origin, 246
pharmacokinetics, 248, 249
volume of distribution, 248
mercaptopurine, 115, 117
mercury, 316-318
physico-chemical properties, 310
metabolism, 52, 102
metals, 309-320. *See also* heavy metals
arsenic, 310, 312-315
cadmium, 310, 315-316
lead, 310-312
mercury, 310, 316-318
physico-chemical properties, 310
thallium, 310, 318-319
methadone, 17. *See also* opioids, synthetic
analytical issues, 276-277
descriptive chemistry, 271
EWDTS recommended initial screening and confirmatory cutoffs for hair testing, 172
half-life, 275
intended use, 272
mechanism of action, 273
oral fluid, reported detection time in, 161
origin, 270
overdose and toxicity, 278
pharmacokinetics, 274-275
saliva/plasma (S/P) ratio, average, 158
toxic dose, 277
volume of distribution, 275
methamphetamine. *See also* amphetamines
abuse potential and characteristics, 240
cross-reactivity, 242
cutoff for federal workplace drug testing program, 68
descriptive chemistry, 239
pharmacokinetics, 240
saliva/plasma (S/P) ratio, 158
methanol, 9
analysis, 201-202
analytical issues and problems, 202
analytical parameters, 202
anion gap (AG), 202
clearance, 199
clinical issues, 202, 203
context of human use, 198
descriptive chemistry, 197
exposure, 198-199
half-life, 199
hazmat considerations, 198, 199
metabolism and excretion, 200
mortality and morbidity, 199
osmolal gap (OG), 203
toxicity, 200-201
treatment and management, 203-204
volume of distribution, 199
methemoglobin (MetHb), 9, 58
method validation, 140-156
accuracy, 144-145
analyte stability, 150
analytical specificity, 149
calibration, linearity/analytical measurement range (AMR), and reportable range, 144, 145-146
calibration curves, regression models, 146
carryover, 146, 147
clinical claims validation, 151
clinical/diagnostic sensitivity and specificity, 151
cross-reactivity, 150
cutoffs, 148-149
exceptions to CLIA regulations, 142
FDA terminology and approval processes for commercially available new tests, 141-142
interference, 149-150
internal standard (IS), 152
laboratory-developed test (LDT), 81, 140, 143
limit of detection (LOD), 149
limit of quantitation (LOQ), 149
liquid chromatography-mass spectrometry (LC-MS) validation, 151-153
matrix effects, evaluation of, 153-154
measurement range, 152-153
qualitative versus quantitative testing, 140-141
reagent stability, 150
receiver operator characteristics (ROC) curve, 151
reference intervals, 146-147, 148
regression equations, 148
results reporting, 154
role of the FDA, CMS, and CLIA, 142-143
screening versus confirmatory testing, 140
test validation, 143-145
therapeutic ranges, 148
verification/validation parameters, minimum, 144
verification versus validation of test performance, 143
waived versus nonwaived tests, 142
methylenedioxyamphetamine (MDA), 20, 219
cross-reactivity, 241-242
cutoff concentration, 68, 171, 172, 178
oral fluid testing for, 161, 163
methylenedioxyethylamphetamine (MDEA), 20
cross-reactivity, 241-242
cutoff concentration, 171, 172, 178

oral fluid testing for, 163
methylenedioxymethamphetamine (MDMA), 20
abuse potential and characteristics, 219
analysis, 219
analytical issues, 219
clinical issues, 219-220
cross-reactivity, 241-242
cutoff concentration, 68, 171, 172, 178
descriptive chemistry, 218
FDA-cleared oral fluid immunoassay cutoffs, 161
half-life, 215
intended uses, 218-219
mechanism of action, 219
modes of analysis, 219
oral fluid, reported detection time in, 161
oral fluid testing for, 163
origin, 218
overdose and toxicity, 220
pharmacokinetics, 219
pharmacology, 218-219
results interpretation, 219-220
saliva/plasma (S/P) ratio, average, 158
volume of distribution, 215
methylone
descriptive chemistry, 285
intended use and mechanism of action, 285
overdose and toxicity, 287
pharmacokinetics, 286
microarray-based immunoassay testing, 126-127
6-monoacetylmorphine (6-MAM), 23, 31, 94, 263, 265. *See also* 6-acetylmorphine
cutoffs, 171, 172, 178
morphine, 17. *See also* opiates/opioids
analgesic activity and potency, 288
cutoff for federal workplace drug testing program, 68
descriptive chemistry, 262
estimated equivalents of opiates and semisynthetic opioids, 265
half-life, 265
metabolic pathways of, 29, 262
modes of analysis, 266
oral fluid, reported detection time in, 161
origin, 261
saliva/plasma (S/P) ratio, average, 158
volume of distribution, 265

N-acetylcysteine (NAC), 7, 14, 306
naproxen, 17, 300
National Academy of Clinical Biochemistry (NACB), 7, 8, 9
National Highway Traffic Safety Administration (NHTSA), 189
National Institute of Drug Abuse (NIDA), 66
National Laboratory Certification Program (NLCP), 77, 86, 162
25I-NBOMe, 290-291
neonatal abstinence syndrome (NAS), 179
neonate specimens, 179-181
N-ethylpentylone
descriptive chemistry, 285
intended use and mechanism of action, 285
overdose and toxicity, 287
newborn
biological testing relevant to, 179
breast milk, drugs in, 181
characteristics of meconium, umbilical cord tissue, and breast milk for detection and management of a drug exposed, 180
New York Clinical Laboratory Evaluation Program, 77
nonwaived tests, 76, 80, 87, 141-142, 154
minimum test verification requirements, 144
nordiazepam. *See also* benzodiazepines
descriptive chemistry, 255
detection window in urine, 256
half-life, 256
metabolite, active, 256
pharmacokinetics, 256
results interpretation, 259
toxic dose and concentration, 259
volume of distribution, 256
novel psychoactive substances (NPS), 282-299
analysis, 294-295
designer benzodiazepines, 292-294
designer dissociative, 291-292
designer hallucinogen, 290-291
novel illicit opioids, 287-290
synthetic cannabinoids, 282-284
synthetic stimulants, 284-287

Occupational Safety and Health Administration (OSHA), 79-80, 315
on-site testing, 4, 160, 161. *See also* point-of-care/collection testing
opiates/opioids, 10. *See also* opioids, synthetic; opioid therapy, chronic
abuse potential and characteristics, 265-266
analysis, 266-267
analytical issues, 267
clinical issues, 267
descriptive chemistry, 261-264
effects on children, 56-57
estimated morphine equivalents, 265
FDA-cleared oral fluid immunoassay cutoffs, 161
half-life, 265
illicit, 287-290
intended uses, 264
maternal use while breastfeeding, 59-60
mechanism of action, 264
metabolism of, 30, 262
metabolites, 23, 31
modes of analysis, 266-267
novel illicit, 287-290
oral fluid testing for, 163-164

origin, 261
overdose and toxicity, 267
pharmacokinetics, 264-266
pharmacology, 264-266
results interpretation, 267
SAMHSA proposed initial screening and confirmatory cutoffs for hair testing, 171
SAMHSA proposed initial screening and confirmatory cutoffs for sweat patch testing, 178
specimen types and characteristics, 266
volume of distribution, 265
opioids, semisynthetic. *See* opiates/opioids
opioids, synthetic
abuse potential and characteristics, 275-276
analysis, 276-277
analytical issues, 276-277
clinical issues, 277
descriptive chemistry, 270-272
intended use, 272
mechanism of action, 273
modes of analysis, 276
origin, 270
overdose and toxicity, 277-278
pharmacokinetics, 273-275
pharmacology, 272-276
results interpretation, 277
specimen types, requirements, and characteristics, 276
opioid therapy, chronic. *See also* pain management
clinical laboratory, role in pain management, 18
drugs used in treatment of pain, 17
drug test results, interpretation of, 24, 27-31
guidelines for treating patients, 18, 122
immunoassay-based urine drug test (screening), 122-125
laboratory support of, 17-26
oral fluid, 157-169
alcohol in, 162-163
amphetamines in, 163
as analytical specimen, 157-158
benzodiazepines in, 163
blood testing, comparison with, 164-166
cannabinoids in, 164
chromatographic tests, 162
cocaine in, 163
in compliance testing, 159
in criminal justice system testing, 158
detection times of drugs in, 165
in driving under the influence of drugs testing, 158-159
FDA-cleared immunoassay cutoffs, 161
immunoassays for, 125-126, 161-162
laboratory-based testing, 161-162
Mandatory Guidelines for Federal Workplace Drug Testing Programs—Oral Fluid (OFMG), 67, 157, 158, 159, 160, 161
opiates and opioids in, 163-164
pain management drug testing, 125-126, 163-164
point-of-collection testing, use in, 158, 161
proficiency testing, 87, 162
results interpretation, 164-166
saliva/plasma (S/P) ratio, 157-158
specimen collection, 159-160
specimen validity testing, 160-161
split specimen collection, 160
urine testing, comparison with, 164-166
workplace testing, 158
organophosphates, 324-326
parathion chemistry, 324
relationship between BuChE activity and degree of intoxication, 325
osmolal gap (OG), 9, 202, 203, 204, 340
over-the-counter (OTC) analgesics, 300-308. *See also* acetaminophen; salicylates
oxazepam, 17. *See also* benzodiazepines
analytical issues, 258
descriptive chemistry, 255
detection window in urine, 256
half-life, 256
intended uses, 255
modes of analysis, 257
pharmacokinetics, 256
pharmacology, 255-257
toxic dose and concentrations, 259
volume of distribution, 256-257
oxycodone, 10, 17. *See also* opiates/opioids
cutoff for federal workplace drug testing program, 68, 161
descriptive chemistry, 263-264
estimated morphine equivalent, 265
half-life, 265
metabolic relationships, 262
modes of analysis, 266
oral fluid, reported detection time in, 161
urinary excretion kinetics of, 29
volume of distribution, 265
oxygen saturation, carboxyhemoglobin, and methemoglobin, co-oximetry for, 9
oxymorphone, 17. *See also* opiates/opioids
cutoff for federal workplace drug testing program, 68, 161
descriptive chemistry, 264
estimated morphine equivalent, 265
half-life, 265
metabolic relationships, 262
modes of analysis, 266
origin, 261
volume of distribution, 265

pain management, 4. *See also* opioid therapy, chronic
clinical pathology consultation for, 27-48
definitive tests, 125
drugs used in, 17

drug test program, design of, 18-19
drug test results, interpretation of, 24, 27-31
microarray-based immunoassays, 126-127
oral fluid drug testing in, 125-126, 163-164
point-of-collection testing, 122-123
proficiency testing for drug monitoring, 86
role of clinical laboratory in, 18-24
testing menu for, 20-21
urine drug test immunoassays, 122-125
parathion, 324-325. *See also* organophosphates
pediatric toxicology, 49-65
absorption, 51-52
biotransformation (metabolism), 52-54
blood volume, changes in with age, 51
and breastfeeding, 59-60
CYPs, selected, and activity in the developing child, 53
deaths in children, analyses to consider, 60
distribution, 52
esoteric substances of concern unique to children, 56
excretion, 54
fatal substances in small doses in children, 56
general toxicologic principles, 50
half-lives, differences in, of selected compounds at various ages, 53
lead, blood concentration, 312, 313
meconium, cord tissue, and breast milk testing, 179-181
poisonings, 50
size, changes in, 50-51
statistics, 49-50
total body water, differences in, 51
toxic exposures, top categories involved, 49
toxicodynamics, 54-58
toxicokinetics, 51-54
toxicological analyses, 60-61
pentazocine, 17
pentobarbital, 9. *See also* barbiturates
abuse potential and characteristics, 250
clearance, 248
clinical uses, 249
descriptive chemistry, 246, 247
detection window in urine, 249
duration of action, 249
half-life, 248, 249
intended uses, 248
origin, 246
pharmacokinetics, 248, 249
toxic dose and concentration, 251
volume of distribution, 248
personnel, CLIA requirements, 81, 83-84
pharmacogenetics, 113
pharmacogenomics (PGx), 112-113
pharmacogenomic testing, 112-121
abacavir, 118
Chronic Kidney Disease Epidemiology Collaboration (CKD-EPI) equation, 104
clopidogrel, 117
codeine, 118-119
definitions and terminology, 113
drug listing for, 113
examples with the highest levels of evidence, 115
irinotecan, 117
phenotypes, nomenclature for common, 114
tamoxifen, 116-117
thiopurine drugs, 117-118
warfarin, 114-116
pharmacokinetic concepts, 101-111
absorption, 101-102
area under the curve (AUC), 107-108
bioavailability, 101-102
clearance (Cl), 103-105
Cockcroft-Gault equation, 104
drug concentrations, interpretation of, 110
drug distribution, 102-103
elimination rate constant (K_e), 104
first-order kinetics, 105
first-pass metabolism, 102
half-life ($t_{½}$), 106-107
nonlinear, 108-109
one-compartment model, 105
and pharmacodynamics, 101
steady state, 107
therapeutic drug monitoring, 101-102, 109-110
two-compartment model, 106
volume of distribution (V_d), 103
zero-order kinetics, 105, 108
phencyclidine (PCP), 10
abuse potential and characteristics, 222
analysis, 222
analytical issues, 222-223
clinical issues, 223
cutoff for federal workplace drug testing program, 68
descriptive chemistry, 222
FDA-cleared oral fluid immunoassay cutoffs, 161
half-life, 215
intended uses, 222
mechanism of action, 222
modes of analysis, 222
origin, 221
overdose and toxicity, 223
pharmacokinetics, 222
pharmacology, 222
results interpretation, 223
SAMHSA proposed initial screening and confirmatory cutoffs for hair testing, 171
SAMHSA proposed initial screening and confirmatory cutoffs for sweat patch testing, 178
volume of distribution, 215
phenobarbital, 79, 102. *See also* barbiturates
analytical issues, 250
clearance, 248

clinical use, 249
descriptive chemistry, 246, 247
detection window in urine, 249
duration of action, 249
half-life, 248, 249
intended uses, 248
origin, 246
overdose, 251
pharmacokinetics, 248, 249
toxic dose and concentrations, 251
volume of distribution, 248
phentermine, cross-reactivity, 242
phenylpropanolamine (PPA), cross-reactivity, 242
phenytoin, 17, 79, 102, 105, 108-109
point-of-collection/care testing (POCT), 4, 19. *See also* on-site testing
emergency department, 8
in pain management, 122-123
in workplace drug testing, 70
poisoning and overdose trends, 130
polypharmacy, 13-14, 96, 112
pregabalin, 17, 87, 102
primidone, 79, 102
procainamide, 79, 102
proficiency testing, 78-79, 84-87, 361
alcohol and volatiles, 84
and alternative performance assessment, 80-81
American Proficiency Institute (API) program, 85
broad-spectrum urine drug screen, 86
CMS regulated drugs for, 102
College of American Pathologists (CAP), 6, 28, 84, 85, 86, 361
common therapeutically monitored drugs for which proficiency testing is available from CAP, 102
condition level requirement for, 78-79
drug monitoring for pain management, 28, 86
forensic drug testing, 77
forensic toxicology (criminalistics), 87
forensic urine drug testing (confirmatory), 66, 86
immunoassay urine drug screen, 86
Medical Laboratory Evaluation (MLE) program, 85
oral fluid, 87, 162
regulated analytes in toxicology and scoring on, 79
serum drug screening, 86
toxicology, 87
urine drug adulterant integrity, 87
urine drug testing (screening), 85
urine toxicology, 86
vitreous fluid, postmortem, 87
whole blood, serum, and plasma drug screening, 86-87
Wisconsin State Laboratory of Hygiene (WSLH) program, 85-86
propoxyphene, 10, 17, 31, 70, 163. *See also* opioids, synthetic
abuse potential and characteristics, 275
descriptive chemistry, 271
half-life, 275
intended use, 272-273
mechanism of action, 273
origin, 270
overdose and toxicity, 278
pharmacokinetics, 275
toxic dose, 277
volume of distribution, 275
pseudoephedrine, 239, 242, 243
alpha-PVP
descriptive chemistry, 285
intended use and mechanism of action, 285-286
overdose and toxicity, 287
pharmacokinetics, 286

quadrupole time-of-flight (QTOF), 133-134
quality systems, 80-81
quinidine, 79, 102

rasburicase, 115
regulatory issues, 76-89
accreditation, agencies with deemed status from CMS, 78
CLIA certification, 76-77
CLIA-exempt laboratories, 76-77
condition level requirements for accreditation, 78-84
ISO 15189, 84
legal implications, medical testing with, 5, 78
proficiency testing, 78-79, 84-87
regulated analytes, 79
waived tests, 78
release of specimens, 10
example form for, 12
sample policy for, 11

salicylates, 9, 17, 102
abuse potential and characteristics, 301-302
analysis, 302-303
clinical issues, 303-304
descriptive chemistry, 300
effects on children, 56-57
enzymatic assay for, 303
intended use, 300
mechanism of action, 300
metabolism, 301
modes of analysis, 302-303
origin, 300
overdose and toxicity, 303-304
pharmacokinetics, 301-302
pharmacology, 300-302
results interpretation, 303
specimen types and characteristics, 302

symptoms associated with acute and chronic exposure, 302
toxic dose and concentration, 302
saliva/plasma (S/P) ratio, 157-158
Scientific Working Group for Forensic Toxicology (SWGTOX), 140, 153
screening tests, 140
secobarbital. *See also* barbiturates
abuse potential and characteristics, 250
analytical issues, 250
clearance, 248
clinical use, 249
descriptive chemistry, 246, 247
detection window in urine, 249
duration of action, 249
half-life, 248, 249
origin, 246
pharmacokinetics, 248, 249
toxic dose and concentrations, 251
volume of distribution, 248
selective serotonin reuptake inhibitors, 17
serum drug screens, 4
proficiency testing, 86-87
serum drug tests, quantitative, 9
serum toxic screen template, 337
simvastatin, 115
specimen validity testing (SVT), 67-69
steady state, 107
Substance Abuse and Mental Health Services Administration (SAMHSA), 66, 70, 73, 77. *See also* workplace drug testing
approved MRO certification entities, 71
certified laboratories, employment-related drug testing by, 142
Federal Workplace Drug Testing Program, 66
guidelines for oral fluid testing, 157, 159, 160
immunoassay cutoffs, 161
Mandatory Guidelines for Federal Workplace Drug Testing Programs, 66-70, 77
Mandatory Guidelines for Federal Workplace Drug Testing Programs—Oral Fluid (OFMG), 67, 157, 158, 159, 160, 161
National Survey on Drug Use and Health, 66
NCCP accreditation, 77, 86
proposed guidelines for hair testing, 170-171, 174, 272
proposed initial screening and confirmatory cutoffs for sweat patch testing, 177, 178
substituted specimen, 68
sufentanil, 17, 274, 276
superwarfarin, 326, 327
sweat, drug detection in, 177-178
sweat testing, 176-179
adulteration and contamination issues, 178-179
collection and analysis, 177
SAMHSA proposed initial screening and confirmatory cutoffs for sweat patch testing, 178
tacrolimus, 102, 115, 152
tamoxifen, 112, 115, 116
tandem mass spectrometry (MS/MS), 132-133
tapentadol. *See also* opioids, synthetic
analytical issues, 277
descriptive chemistry, 271-272
half-life, 275
intended use, 273
mechanism of action, 273
pharmacokinetics, 275
toxic dose, 277
volume of distribution, 275
targeted versus untargeted mass spectral data acquisition, 134-135
temazepam. *See also* benzodiazepines
descriptive chemistry, 255
detection window in urine, 256
half-life, 256
intended uses, 255
metabolite, active, 256
modes of analysis, 257
pharmacokinetics, 256
pharmacology, 255-257
toxic dose and concentrations, 259
volume of distribution, 256
delta-8-tetrahydrocannabinol, 205
delta-9-tetrahydrocannabinol-9-carboxylic acid (THCA), cutoff concentrations, 68
delta-9-tetrahydrocannabinol (THC), 164. *See also* cannabis
in breast milk, 181
descriptive chemistry
FDA-cleared oral fluid immunoassay cutoffs, 161
hair testing for, 171, 173-175
metabolite, cutoff for federal workplace drug testing program, 68
oral fluid testing for, 165-166
origin, 205
saliva/plasma (S/P) ratio, average, 158
sweat testing for, 178
delta-9-tetrahydrocannabinolic acid, 206
thallium, 318-319
physico-chemical properties, 310
theophylline, 9, 56, 79, 102
therapeutic drug monitoring (TDM), 3
indications for, 101
common drugs for which proficiency testing is available, 102
considerations in interpretation of results, 109-110
therapeutic drug monitoring template, 343
thiopental. *See also* barbiturates
clearance, 248
clinical use, 249
descriptive chemistry, 246, 247
detection window in urine, 249
duration of action, 249

half-life, 248, 249
origin, 246
pharmacokinetics, 248, 249
toxic dose and concentration, 251
volume of distribution, 248
thiopurine drugs, 117-118
Tier 1 tests, 7-9
Tier 2 tests, 10
time-of-flight (TOF) mass analyzers, 133
tobramycin, 79, 102
toxic agents, commonly encountered, 14
toxicants, household and environmental, 321-328
carbon monoxide (CO), 321-322
cyanide, 322-324
organophosphates, 324-326
warfarins, 326-328
toxicodynamics (TD), in pediatric population, 54-58
toxicokinetics (TK), in pediatric population, 51-54
toxidromes, 13-15
symptoms, agents, and antidotes, 13
tramadol, 17. *See also* opioids, synthetic
abuse potential and characteristics, 276
analytical issues, 277
descriptive chemistry, 272
half-life, 275
intended use, 273
mechanism of action, 273
origin, 270
overdose and toxicity, 278
pharmacokinetics, 275
saliva/plasma (S/P) ratio, average, 158
toxic dose, 277
volume of distribution, 275
transferrin, 9, 209
triazolam. *See also* benzodiazepines
descriptive chemistry, 255
detection window in urine, 256
half-life, 256
intended uses, 255
metabolite, active, 256
pharmacokinetics, 256
pharmacology, 255-257
toxic dose and concentrations, 259
volume of distribution, 256
tricyclic antidepressants (TCIs), 10, 13, 17, 56, 102, 209, 241
in tissue specimens, 94
tyramine, cross-reactivity, 242

U-47700
analgesic activity and potency relative to morphine, 288
descriptive chemistry, 288
dose and duration of action, 289
origin, 287
pharmacokinetics, 289
umbilical cord testing, 180
urine adulterant testing, 5
urine drug screens, 3-4
broad-spectrum, 86
immunoassays for, 70, 85
oral fluid, comparison with, 164-166
in pain management, 122-125
urine drug tests, qualitative, 9-10
urine toxic screen template, 331

valproic acid, 9, 79, 102, 110
venlafaxine, 17, 223
volume of distribution (V_d), 103

waived tests, 4, 19, 76, 78, 142-143
method validation, 142
warfarin, 114-116
descriptive chemistry, 326
warfarins, 326-328
Washington State Office of Laboratory Quality Assurance, Washington Medical Test Site Licensure Program, 77
Wisconsin State Laboratory of Hygiene (WSLH), 81, 84, 85-86
workplace drug testing, 66-75
cutoff concentrations, 68, 161
Mandatory Guidelines for Federal Workplace Drug Testing Programs, 66-70, 77
Mandatory Guidelines for Federal Workplace Drug Testing Programs—Oral Fluid (OFMG), 67, 157, 158, 159, 160, 161
and Medical Review Officer, 67, 71-73
nonregulated, 69-71
point-of-collection/care (POC) testing, 70
regulated, 67-69
specimen validity testing (SVT), 67-69

XLR-11
descriptive chemistry, 283
overdose and toxicity, 284
pharmacokinetics, 284
potency compared to delta-9-THC, 283